Lecture Notes in Networks and Systems 956

The series "Lecture Notes in Networks and Systems" publishes the latest developments in Networks and Systems—quickly, informally and with high quality. Original research reported in proceedings and post-proceedings represents the core of LNNS.

Volumes published in LNNS embrace all aspects and subfields of, as well as new challenges in, Networks and Systems.

The series contains proceedings and edited volumes in systems and networks, spanning the areas of Cyber-Physical Systems, Autonomous Systems, Sensor Networks, Control Systems, Energy Systems, Automotive Systems, Biological Systems, Vehicular Networking and Connected Vehicles, Aerospace Systems, Automation, Manufacturing, Smart Grids, Nonlinear Systems, Power Systems, Robotics, Social Systems, Economic Systems and other. Of particular value to both the contributors and the readership are the short publication timeframe and the world-wide distribution and exposure which enable both a wide and rapid dissemination of research output.

The series covers the theory, applications, and perspectives on the state of the art and future developments relevant to systems and networks, decision making, control, complex processes and related areas, as embedded in the fields of interdisciplinary and applied sciences, engineering, computer science, physics, economics, social, and life sciences, as well as the paradigms and methodologies behind them.

Indexed by SCOPUS, INSPEC, WTI Frankfurt eG, zbMATH, SCImago.

All books published in the series are submitted for consideration in Web of Science.

For proposals from Asia please contact Aninda Bose (aninda.bose@springer.com).

Kevin Daimi · Abeer Al Sadoon
Editors

Proceedings of the Second International Conference on Advances in Computing Research (ACR'24)

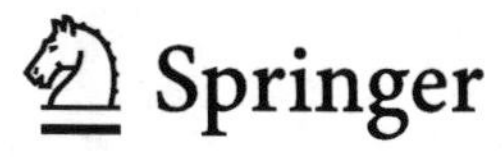

Editors
Kevin Daimi
University of Detroit Mercy
Farmington Hills, MI, USA

Abeer Al Sadoon
Asia Pacific International College (APIC)
Sydney, NSW, Australia

ISSN 2367-3370 ISSN 2367-3389 (electronic)
Lecture Notes in Networks and Systems
ISBN 978-3-031-56949-4 ISBN 978-3-031-56950-0 (eBook)
https://doi.org/10.1007/978-3-031-56950-0

This Springer imprint is published by the registered company Springer Nature Switzerland AG
The registered company address is: Gewerbestrasse 11, 6330 Cham, Switzerland

Paper in this product is recyclable.

Preface

ACR'2024, the Second International Conference on Advances in Computing Research, was held in Madrid, Spain, from June 3 to 5, 2024, at the IE University. ACR'24 was sponsored by the Spanish National Research Council (CSIC), Spain, Australian Computer Society (ACS), Australia, Polytechnic Institute of Porto, Portugal, University of Detroit Mercy, USA, Features Analytics, Belgium, and Flexens Ltd. Finland.

The 2024 International Conference on Advances in Computing Research (ACR'24) is organized by the Institute for Innovations in Computer Science and Engineering Research (IICSER). The goal of this conference is to bring together researchers from academia, business, industry, and government to exchange significant and innovative contributions and research ideas and to act as a platform for international research collaboration. To this extent, ACR'24 sought submissions that furnish innovative ideas, techniques, methodologies, and applications.

We would like to thank the leadership of the IE University for hosting our ACR'24 Conference. Special thanks are due to Dr. Robert Polding, Dr. Federico Castanedo, and Ms. Maria Paula Salinas for their kind help.

The conference received 178 submissions. Only 43 papers were selected by the Program Committee for presentation at the conference. The Program Committee also accepted five posters, two of which were from undergraduate students to encourage undergraduate research. There were two presentation modes: remote (virtual) and in-person at IE University. 24 papers were presented online, and 19 papers were presented on-site. These proceedings contain the revised versions of the papers that took the comments of the reviewers into consideration. Only the Program Committee members were used as reviewers and no secondary reviewers were allowed. The revisions were not re-reviewed. The authors assume full responsibility for the contents of their final papers. All papers were checked for plagiarism using the Turnitin App.

It gave us great pleasure to appreciate the great dedication of the Conference Chair, Advisory Committee, Organization Committee, and the Program Committee. This dedication greatly contributed to the success of ACR'24. Without the excellent papers that were accepted by the Program Committee, this conference would have not existed. Therefore, we are delighted to thank all the authors for their hard work to come up with excellent original papers and for their productive cooperation with us to incorporate the comments of the reviewers and editors who participated in improving their papers and submitting their camera-ready papers on time.

The Proceedings are published by the Springer book series: Lecture Notes in Networks and Systems (LNNS). LNNS is currently indexed by SCOPUS, DBLP, INSPEC, Norwegian Register for Scientific Journals and Series, SCImago, WTI Frankfurt eG, and zbMATH.

It gives us great pleasure to thank Dr. Thomas Ditzinger, the Editorial Director in charge of the Springer book series: Lecture Notes in Networks and Systems (LNNS). We very much appreciate his valuable help and support. We would also like to thank

Varsha Prabakaran, the project coordinator of ACR'24 proceedings book project for her cooperation.

June 2024

Kevin Daimi
Abeer Al Sadoon

ACR'2024

The Second International Conference on Advances in Computing Research (ACR'24), IE University, Madrid, Spain, June 3–5, 2024

Advisory Committee

Luis Hernandez Encinas	Spanish National Research Council (CSIC), Spain
Guilermo Francia III	University of West Florida, USA
Solange Ghernaouti	Swiss Cybersecurity Advisory & Research Group, Switzerland
Åsa Hedman	Flexens Ltd., Finland
Hiroaki Kikuchi	Meiji University, Japan
Slobodan Petrovic	Norwegian University of Science and Technology (NTNU), Norway
Professor Stefan Pickl	University of the Federal Armed Forces Munich, Germany
Cristina Soviany	Features Analytics SA, Belgium

Organization Committee

Honorary Conference Chair

Federico Castanedo	IE University, Spain

Conference Chair

Solange Ghernaouti	University of Lausanne, Switzerland

Program Chairs

Abeer Alsadoon	Charles Sturt University, Australia
Kevin Daimi	University of Detroit Mercy, USA

Posters Chairs

Oli Buckley	University of East Anglia, UK
Eleftheria Katsiri	Democritus University of Thrace, Greece
Sandi Ljubic	University of Rijeka, Croatia

Sessions/Workshops Chairs

Ioanna Dionysiou	University of Nicosia, Cyprus
Robert Polding	IE University, Spain
Alessandro Ruggiero	University of Salerno, Italy

Publicity Chairs

Anna Allen	IICSER, Australia
Carl Wilson	ZRD Technology, USA

Web Chairs

Deshao Liu	Western Sydney University, Australia
Teresa Martinez	Kent Institute Australia, Australia

Program Committee

Computational Intelligence

Khaled R. Ahmed	Southern Illinois University, USA
Dariusz Barbucha	Gdynia Maritime University, Poland
Luís Coelho	Polytechnic Institute of Porto, Portugal
Ireneusz Czarnowksi	Gdynia Maritime University, Poland
Farhad Ahamed	Western Sydney University, Australia
Thair Al-Dala'in	Western Sydney University, Australia
Hasan AlMarzouqi	Khalifa University, UAE
Abdussalam Mohamad Ali	Melbourne Institute of Technology (MIT), Australia
Maryna Averkyna	The National University of Ostroh Academy, Ukraine
Mahmoud Bekhit	Australian Catholic University, Australia
Nadire Cavus	Near East University, Cyprus

Cybersecurity Engineering

Violeta Bulbenkiene	Klaipeda University, Lithuania
Sarra Cherbal	University Ferhat Abbas Setif 1, Algeria
Feng Cheng	University of Potsdam, Germany
Ahmed Dawoud	University of South Australia, Australia
George Dimitoglou	Hood College, USA
Ioanna Dionysiou	University of Nicosia, Cyprus
Muhammad Iqbal Hossain	Brac University, Bangladesh
Charan Gudla	Mississippi State University, USA
Ezhil Kalaimannan	University of West Florida, USA
Irene Kopaliani	Princeton University, USA
Arash Habibi Lashkari	York University, Canada
Luis Hernández Encinas	Spanish National Research Council, Spain
Jide Edu	King's College London
Hanady Hussien Issa	Arab Academy for Science, Technology and Maritime Transport, Egypt
Funminiyi Olajide	University of Westminster, UK
Junfeng Qu	Clayton State University, USA
Narasimha Shashidhar	Sam Houston State University, USA
Sorin Soviany	National Institute for Research and Development in Informatics ICI-Bucharest, Romania
Elochukwu Ukwandu	Cardiff Metropolitan University, UK
Kevin Kam Fung Yuen	Hong Kong SAR, China
David Zeichick	California State University, Chico, USA

Data Analytics Engineering

Thair Al-Dala'in	Western Sydney University, Australia
Ghazi Al-Naymat	Ajman University, UAE
Nawzat Sadiq Ahmed	Duhok Polytechnic University, Iraq
Farhad Ahamed	Western Sydney University, Australia
Ali A. Alwan Al-juboori	Ramapo College of New Jersey, USA
Rawhi Alrae	UAE University-Al Ain, United Arab Emirates
Suhair Amer	Southeast Missouri State University, USA
Karim Baïna	Mohammed V University in Rabat, Morocco
Wolfgang Bein	University of Nevada, USA
Abdussalam Mohamad Ali	Catholic University, Australia
Mahmoud Bekhit	Australian Catholic University, Australia
Violeta Bulbenkiene	Klaipeda University, Lithuania
Birgitta Dresp-Langley	UMR7357 CNRS and Strasbourg University, France

Iman M. A. Helal	Cairo University, Egypt
Muhammad Iqbal Hossain	Brac University, Bangladesh
Waleed Ibrahim	Central Queensland University, Australia
Fathe Jeribi	Jazan University, Saudi Arabia
Rajeev Kanth	Savonia University of Applied Sciences, Finland
William Klement	University of Ottawa, Canada
Asma Musabah Alklabani	University of Technology and Applied Sciences, Oman
Marie Khair	Notre Dame University, Lebanon
Majdi Maabreh	The Hashemite University, Jordan
Nevine Makram	The Institute of National Planning, Egypt
Deepa Mary Mathews	Federal Institute of Science And Technology (FISAT), India
Dmitry Namiot	Lomonosov Moscow State University, Russia
Panicos Masouras	Cyprus University of Technology, Cyprus
Edwin Montoya	Universidad EAFIT, Colombia
Marian Sorin Nistor	Universität der Bundeswehr München, Germany
Mohammad Zavid Parvez	Australian Catholic University, Australia
Robert Polding	IE University, Spain
Aleksandra Popovska-Mitrovikj	Cyril and Methodius University in Skopje, Macedonia
Junfeng Qu	Clayton State University, USA
Khem Poudel	Middle Tennessee State University, USA
Roozbeh Sadeghian	Harrisburg University of Science and Technology, USA
Ahmed Salah	Zagazig University, Egypt
Biswaranjan Senapati	University of Arkansas, USA
Sergiy Shevchenko	National Technical University, Ukraine
Hang Su	Politecnico di Milano, Italy
Haitao Zhao	The University of North Carolina at Pembroke, USA
Suhad A. Yousif	Al-Nahrain University, Iraq
Mohamed Chrayah	University Abdelmalek Essaadi Morocco, Morocco
Wafaa M. Salih Abedi	City University Ajman, UAE
Karwan Jacksi	University of Zakho, Iraq
Martin Qiang Zhao	Mercer University, USA

Mobile and Cloud Computing

Ali A. Alwan Al-juboori	Ramapo College of New Jersey, USA
Ke-Lin Du	Concordia University, Canada

Jonathan Kavalan	University of Florida, USA
Irene Kopaliani	Princeton University, USA
Panicos Masouras	Cyprus University of Technology, Cyprus
Michele Melchiori	University of Brescia, Italy
Hung Ba Ngo	Can Tho University, Vietnam
Małgorzata Pańkowska	University of Economics in Katowice, Poland
Javad Rezazadeh	Victoria University (VU), Australia
Razwan Mohmed Salah	University of Duhok, KRI, Iraq
Rao Naveed Bin Rais	Ajman University, UAE
Celia Ghedini Ralha	University of Brasilia (UnB), Brazil
N. Deniz Sarier	University of Lleida, Spain
Santosh Subedi	Pixii AS, Norway
Marwa Thabet	University of Sousse, Tunisia
Amjad Gawanmeh	University of Dubai, UAE
Jeong Yang	Texas A&M University-San Antonio, USA

Networking and Communication

Fawaz Alazemi	Kuwait University, Kuwait
Marco Javier Suarez Baron	Universidad Pedagógica y Tecnológica de Colombia, Colombia
Grigorios N. Beligiannis	University of Patras, Greece
Marek Bolanowski	Rzeszow University of Technology, Poland
Liquan Chen	Southeast University, China
Cheng Siong Chin	Newcastle University, UK
Rodrigo Pérez Fernández	Universidad Politécnica de Madrid, Spain
Przemyslaw Falkowski-Gilski	Gdansk University of Technology, Poland
Smain Femmam	UHA University, France
Chadi El Kari	University of the Pacific, USA
Natasha Ilievska	Ss. Cyril and Methodius University, Republic of North Macedonia
Attila Kertesz	University of Szeged, Hungary
Pascal Lorenz	University of Haute Alsace, France
Lemia Louail	Université de Lorraine, France
Sabina Rossi	Università Ca' Foscari Venezia, Italy
Addisson Salazar	Universitat Politècnica de València, Spain
Grzegorz Sierpiński	Silesian University of Technology, Poland
Pokkuluri Kiran Sree	Shri Vishnu Engineering College for Women, India
Radwa A. Roshdy	Higher Technological Institute, Egypt
Mario Versaci	DICEAM–University Mediterranea, Italy
Anita Yadav	Harcourt Butler Technical University, India

Contents

Computational Intelligence

Networking and Communication

Cloud and Mobile Computing

Robotics and Automation

Posters

Posters Abstracts

Data Analytics Engineering

Evaluating Study Between Vision Transformers and Pre-trained CNN Learning Algorithms to Classify Breast Cancer Histopathological Images

Maali Altulayhi and Ashwaq Alhrgan(✉)

College of Computing and Informatics, Saudi Electronic University, Riyadh, Saudi Arabia
a.alhrgan@seu.edu.sa

Abstract. Breast cancer exhibits a higher incidence rate among women compared to other forms of cancer. In the Kingdom of Saudi Arabia, there exists a higher propensity for the development of breast cancer in women aged 40 and above, as compared to their younger counterparts. Convolutional neural networks (CNNs) are the well-known approach for classifying breast cancer mammographic images. The utilization of convolutional neural networks has proven to be effective in the interpretation of mammograms and the study of medical imaging recent times, a new revelation called Vision Transformers (ViT) has been able to attend to global information in earlier layers, facilitating a more adaptable methodology for the exploration and identification of features. This study conducted a comparative analysis between the vision transformer ViT_16 and the ResNet18 convolutional neural network, which is considered the current leading model in the field. The models were trained using datasets obtained from the King Abdulaziz University Breast Cancer Mammography Dataset (KAU-BCMD) version 1. The results have been identified by evaluating the accuracy metrics. ResNet18 outperformed ViT_16 by 8% in overall accuracy. However, ViT_16 exhibit superior performance in detecting suspicious abnormality. This emphasizes the potential benefit of ViT_16 model in classifying breast cancer images. Overall, ViT_16 model performance could be improved when trained with sufficient data.

Keywords: Breast Cancer · Medical Imaging · Vision Transformer · Convolutional Neural Networks · ResNet18

1 Introduction

1.1 Breast Cancer Statistics in KSA

Breast cancer is a heterogeneous illness that typically begins as a small lesion in the breast and then slowly progresses to other portions of the body, where it targets the lymph nodes in the armpits and other organs. Numerous factors influence the type, duration of treatment, and success and serve as a warning [1].

K. Daimi and A. Al Sadoon (Eds.): ACR 2024, LNNS 956, pp. 3–14, 2024.
https://doi.org/10.1007/978-3-031-56950-0_1

In the KSA, breast cancer affects women more frequently than any other type of cancer. Women over the age of 40 in Saudi Arabia are more likely to develop breast cancer than younger women. In the Kingdom, more than 50% of breast cancer cases are discovered late, compared to 20% in developed nations. Because of this, there is a higher mortality rate from breast cancer, a worse chance of recovery, and a higher cost of care. Through mammography and radiography, early detection of breast cancer considerably improves the prognosis and chances of survival [1]. In the year 2016, the number of breast cancer cases in Saudi Arabia amounted to about 31,000, as depicted in the subsequent Table 1.

Table 1. Breast Cancer Statistics in KSA 2016 [1].

Saudis			Non-Saudis			Total
Males	Females	Total	Males	Females	Total	16,698
5,803	7,358	13,161	1,872	1,826	3,698	

Mammography plays a critical role in breast cancer diagnosis because early detection is one of the most effective strategies for preventing breast cancer. Early diagnosis of breast cancer is important for treatment. It increases the chance of being cured by more than 95% and cuts the chance of dying by up to 30% [2].

Breast cancer diagnosis involves multiple tests and procedures, including mammograms, ultrasounds, and MRIs. Mammograms are X-rays of the breast, while ultrasounds use sound waves to create images of the body's deepest structures. MRI uses a magnet and radio waves to provide images of the breast's interior, without radiation [2].

1.2 Computer-Aided Methods are Needed to Diagnose Cancer

As mentioned earlier, diagnosis of breast cancer is a crucial step in increasing a patient's chances of being treated and surviving. To do so pathologists interpreted the tests and procedures images to analyze tissue appearance and spot aberrant diseases. The characteristics of these medical images include their typically high resolution, numerous magnification scales, multiple acquisition processes, and diverse staining techniques. The findings of the interpretation of these medical images differ from one pathologist to another and sometimes from different analyses done by the same pathologist. Leading to inter-observer and intra-observer variability and uncertainty in the decision-making process. Therefore, there is a motivation to develop efficient computer-aided methods for analyzing and interpreting medical imaging [3].

Computer-aided methods are a collection of artificial intelligence, pattern recognition, and image-processing technologies that can help professionals diagnose cancer. In this context, they can diagnose and detect malignant tumors in several organs, including the skin, blood, uterus, and breast. These methods also can considerably improve image quality and spot worrisome spots and present them to radiologists for further inspection [2].

1.3 Comparing Vision Transformers and CNN

Deep Learning (DL), which achieves high success in the detection of breast cancer through digital mammography image classification and object recognition with unprecedented levels of accuracy, is one of the most promising computer-aided methods. Especially Convolutional Neural Network (CNN) which showed excellent performance in solving various problems such as segmentation, interpretation, and registration in analyzing medical images. The reason for this achievement is that CNN can extract the features that accurately describe the data for the underlying issue [3]. Although long-range dependencies are crucial for effectively recognizing or mapping corresponding breast lesion features derived from unregistered numerous mammograms, CNNs typically are unable to model them well because of the intrinsic locality of the convolution operation. This encourages us to make use of the sequence-view Vision Transformers (ViT) architecture to record the long-range associations between numerous mammograms taken from the same patient during a single examination [4].

This study proposes the utilization of pre-trained convolutional neural networks, specifically the ResNet algorithm and ViT method, for the classification of breast cancer images. The objective is to detect and differentiate between benign and malignant tumors in breast mammography images based on the BI-RADS classifications. Subsequently, a comparative analysis is conducted on the performers of both algorithms, followed by an assessment of the effectiveness of these networks. Finally, a comprehensive assessment of the networks is conducted, with a focus on analyzing the distinctive characteristics of each method.

2 Literature Review

2.1 The Transformers

Transformers architecture was originally introduced to solve some of the RNN lack, RNN or Recurrent neural networks are deep-learning models that use dynamic recurrent connections to carry information across consecutive time steps, The model generates a sequence of hidden states ht, based on the function of the input for position t and the previously hidden state ht-1 respecting the temporal order of the data [5]. Due to memory limitations, batching across examples cannot be parallelized within training examples due to the inherent sequential character of the data, which is crucial for longer sequence durations [6].

In 2017, Google issued a paper titled "Attention is All You Need" that introduced transformers [6]. Transformers is a model architecture that completely depends on an attention mechanism (hint at the title) to draw global dependencies between input and output avoiding recurrence. This enables significantly greater parallelization and, after only twelve hours of training on eight P100 GPUs, may achieve a new state-of-the-art level of translation quality. to compute a representation of the sequence an attention mechanism known as "self-attention" is introduced to relate different positions of a single sequence. Also, the transformer uses Multi-Head Attention to learn dependencies between distant positions by averaging attention-weighted positions [6]. From that transformer models were the model of choice in Natural Language Processing (NLP)

[7]. For instance, the well-known ChatGPT AI chatbot uses transformers as a language model. It uses the GPT (Generative Pre-trained Transformer) architecture, which uses self-attention techniques to model the dependencies between words in a text [8].

2.2 The Vision Transformer (ViT)

The Transformers architecture has gained substantial acceptance and usage in Computer Vision after their enormous success in Natural Language Processing. Since its release in October 2020 [7], Recently, ViT have been used for numerous computer vision applications, including image classification, object recognition, and semantic picture segmentation, in a very competitive manner [8]. A research article titled "An Image is Worth 16*16 Words: Transformers for Image Recognition at Scale" that was published by Google [7] as a conference paper at ICLR 2021 revealed the Vision Transformer model architecture as seen in Fig. 1. The ImageNet and ImageNet-21k datasets served as the pre-training data for the ViT models [7].

To understand vision transformer architecture let us assume an input square image of size $X \times X \times C$ spatially patched into $M \times M$ patches of a fixed size $P \times P$ then flatten each patch, which is a small crop from the image with dimensions $P \times P \times C$ into a single vector of size $P \cdot P \cdot C$ Then using trainable linear layer, the model will map every single vector to an embedding of dimension D. The resulting vectors are called patch embeddings, and they are taken to be the input tokens that represent the data that is included in each small patch of the square image. Finally, the flattened $M \times M$ patch embeddings provide the Transformer with a sequence of tokens of length $N = M \cdot M$ which is fed into the Transformer [9]. Then this sequence of tokens is passed to the Transformer encoder made up of many multi-headed self-attentions and MLP layers, shown on the right in Fig. 1 [9].

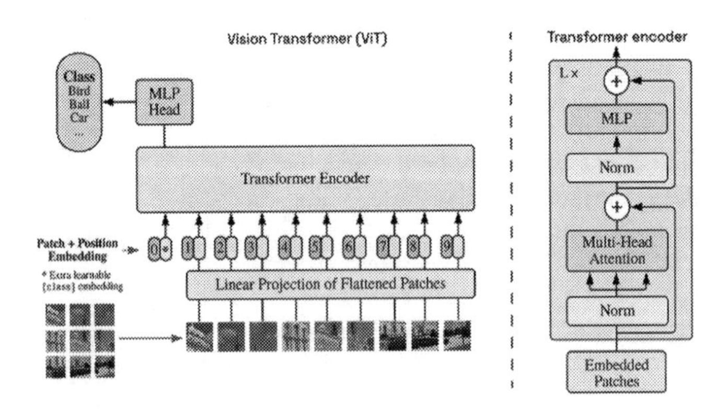

Fig. 1. The Vision Transformer architecture [7].

2.3 The Residual Network

The Residual Network, known as ResNet, is a type of neural network architecture that was first proposed in 2015 by [10]. The ResNet models have demonstrated remarkable success. That can facilitate the training process of neural networks with significantly greater depth compared to earlier approaches. The layers are reformulated in a manner that involves explicitly learning residual functions by referencing the layer inputs, rather than learning functions that lack reference. In this study, residual networks obtained an error rate of 3.57% on the ImageNet test dataset [10].

2.4 Related Work

As previously indicated, ViT architecture was introduced in 2021 which uses a variants model to train the datasets as detailed in Table 2 below.

Table 2. Details of Vision Transformer model variants [7].

Model	Layer	Hidden size D	MLP size	Heads	Params
ViT-Base	12	768	3072	12	86 M
ViT_Large	24	1024	4096	16	308 M
ViT-Huge	32	1280	5120	16	632 M

Using ResNet as a CNN baseline, the current study finds that Vision Transformer models pre-trained on the JFT-300M dataset outperform ResNet-based baselines on all datasets. This experiment demonstrates an improvement in image classification when employing transformations and this work has provided numerous researchers with the opportunity to scale up ViT further, which could improve performance [7].

For the care and treatment of patients with breast cancer, histopathology images are essential. With the aid of an innovative method based on image processing, pathologists can produce more precise diagnoses.

This method is an ensemble model of the Vision Transformer and Data-Efficient Image Transformer (DeiT) models of pre-trained vision transformers. The suggested ViT-DeiT model divides the histopathological images of breast cancer into eight classes, four of which are classified as benign and the others as malignant. The proposed model was assessed using the BreakHis open dataset. The testing findings indicated a 98.12% F1 score, 98.17% accuracy, 98.18% precision, and 98.08% recall [11].

Another Vision Transformer approach was proposed by [12]. That demonstrates that breast cancer histopathological image recognition is a difficult process. The staining characteristics of histological pictures are not fully utilized by many deep learning models, even though these models have produced positive classification results for histopathological image classification tasks. Introducing a unique Deconv-Transformer (DecT) network model in this paper that includes color deconvolution as convolution layers. To mirror the independent characteristics of the HED channel information discovered through color deconvolution, this model employs a self-attention mechanism. Additionally, it employs a technique comparable to the residual connection to combine the data from RGB and HED color space images, which can make up for the information lost during the conversion of RGB images to HED images. To better tailor the settings of the deconvolution layer to various kinds of histopathology pictures, the DecT model's training procedure is split into two parts. To lessen overfitting during the model training procedure, we apply the color jitter in the image data augmentation step. On the BreakHis dataset, the DecT model achieves an average accuracy of 93.02% and an F1-score of 0.9389; on the BACH and UC datasets, the average accuracy is 79.06% and 81.36%, respectively [12].

3 The Dataset

King Abdulaziz University Breast Cancer Mammography Dataset (KAU-BCMD) version 1 is a public mammography dataset that is presented in this study. KAU-BCMD is the first dataset in Saudi Arabia that we are aware of that deals with a significant number of mammography scans. The Sheikh Mohammed Hussein Al-Amoudi Center of Excellence in Breast Cancer at King Abdulaziz University provided the data for this study. Provided the dataset from April 2019 to March 2020. Between April and June 2020, the dataset was annotated. The collection includes images from 1416 instances, totaling 5662 mammography images. Each case includes images with two different views (CC and MLO) for both breasts (right and left). According to BI-RADS categories, the dataset was divided into 1 to 5 groups [13], as follows:

- Category 0: To provide a category, more imagery is required. Inconclusive findings were obtained.
- Category 1: The test came back negative. Your mammography shows no noteworthy or obvious abnormalities. At regular intervals, screening should continue.
- Category 2: It was determined that the growth was benign. A benign calcification or fibroadenoma exists, however, it is unimportant. Maintain your routine mammograms. Category 2 is missing from the dataset.
- Category 3: There was discovered growth that is probably benign. To check for changes, you should have mammograms more frequently (every six months).
- Category 4: A suspicious abnormality that could be malignant is present. The outcome calls for a biopsy.
- Category 5: The growth is almost certainly cancerous and highly likely to be malignant. The outcome calls for a biopsy [14]. The distribution of (BI-RADS) classes is shown in Fig. 2, correspondingly.

In this study, the mammography method used for breast imaging has proven to be a reliable tool for breast cancer screening, exceedingly even ultrasound (US) as a tool for breast cancer detection, since breast US misses early cancer signs such as microcalcifications (small calcium deposits), it is rarely employed as a diagnostic tool for the disease. Each mammography screening case includes the recording of two views for each breast: the mediolateral oblique (MLO), which is a side view, and the craniocaudal (CC), which is a top-to-bottom view. To categorize breast anomalies, a (BI-RADS) classification system was used to provide mammography reports that include categories for the description of breast cancer stages, enabling uniform breast imaging reporting [13].

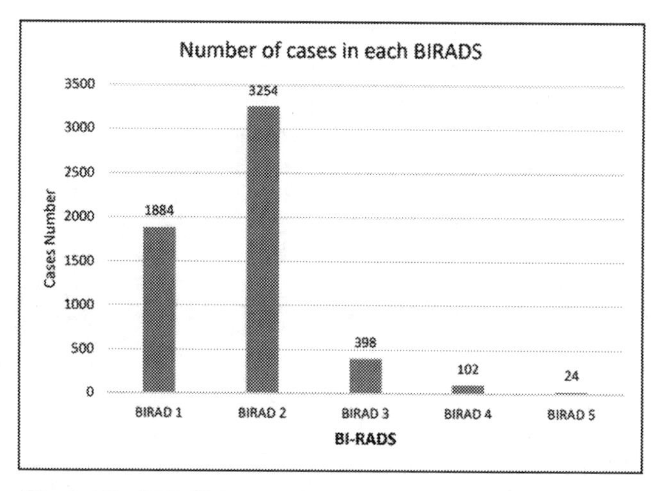

Fig. 2. The BI-RADS categories in the KAU-BCMD dataset [14].

4 The Synthesis and Analysis Phases

Starting by loading the data and then image processing since the dataset has some unbalanced data as shown in Fig. 3. Generally, in biomedical datasets patients with malignant tumors are less than patients with benign tumors. Data augmentation is a technique used for expanding the size of the input data by creating additional data from the original input data, as result. Then splitting the data into train, test, and validation sets, then assembled, fine-tuned, and evaluated the model.

There are several methods for enhancing data; the one utilized in this publication is rotation. Rotations of 0, 60, 120, 180, and 240 degrees are applied to each original image. As a result, each image is increased to five images [2]. Then splitting the data into train, test, and validation sets, then assembled, fine-tuned, and evaluated the models.

5 Research Results and Discussions

This section contains the findings of the comparison between the ResNet18 and ViT_16 models. Using the confusion matrix to evaluate the model's performance alongside its accuracy and loss curves. Every model was trained using 10 epochs. Additionally, as previously indicated, the data has significant imbalance issues, so a comparison of balanced and imbalanced data using ViT_16 will be conducted to determine how the model can manage imbalance data.

5.1 ResNet18 vs ViT_16

A confusion matrix was presented to compare the performance and accuracy of the two models before beginning the comparison between ResNet18 and ViT_16 model predictions, as shown in Fig. 4 and Table 3. Both models RestNet18 and ViT_16 did very well in identifying the first class which is BI-RADS 1 with 99% and 98% accuracy,

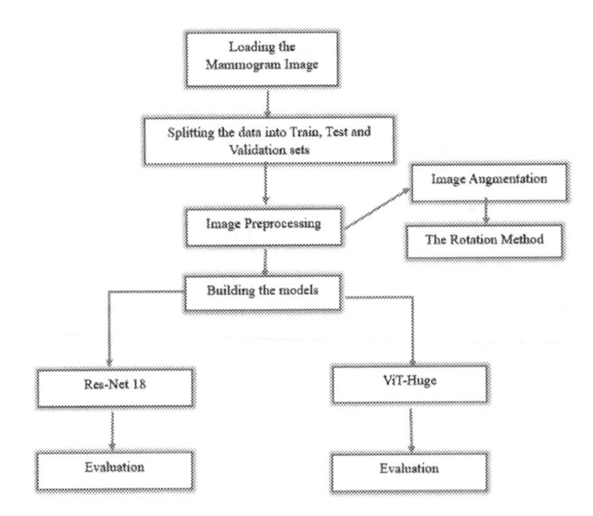

Fig. 3. The proposed system.

respectively. BI-RADS 1 class has 1884 images and no augmented images added to it and has distinguished features from the other classes since it is the negative test mammography that shows no noteworthy or obvious abnormalities [14].

Moving to the following classes, both models face difficulties in discerning BI-RADS 3 from the BI-RADS 4 category. However, according to the data presented in Table 3, the accuracy of ResNet18 was 78%, while ViT_16 achieved an accuracy of 28%. Nonetheless, the ResNet18 model performs better than ViT_16. BI-RADS 3 has 390 images and had over 900 augmented images added to it this may affect the classification performance. Since the diagnosis for BI-RADS 3 is that the discovered growth is probably benign and the diagnosis for BI-RADS 4 is a suspicious abnormality that could be malignant present, both classes have a shared feature which is the peasant of suspicious growth that differentiates one from another hard.

The BI-RADS 4 class comprises a total of 92 images, which have been further enhanced by the addition of almost 1000 augmented images. The potential impact on classification performance is shown in Table 3. The accuracy of the ResNet18 model was found to be 29%, while the ViT_16 model achieved an accuracy of 66%. Due to the similarity of the classes and the large, augmented images that was added to the class as previously mentioned. For BI-RADS 4 and BI-RADS 3, both models struggled to distinguished from one another. Nonetheless, the ViT_16 model performs better than ResNet18.

Of all the classes BI-RADS 4 is the most dangerous class where the diagnosis is a suspicious abnormality that would be highly cancerous if present. Additionally, the patient requires a biopsy. Misclassifying this class could lead to dire consequences. ViT_16 classifies 16 out of 24 images correctly but classifies 3 of the misclassified images as BI-RADS 1 which is very dangerous to send a patient that highly has cancer out of the hospital without a further diagnosis and misclassified 5 out of 24 images as

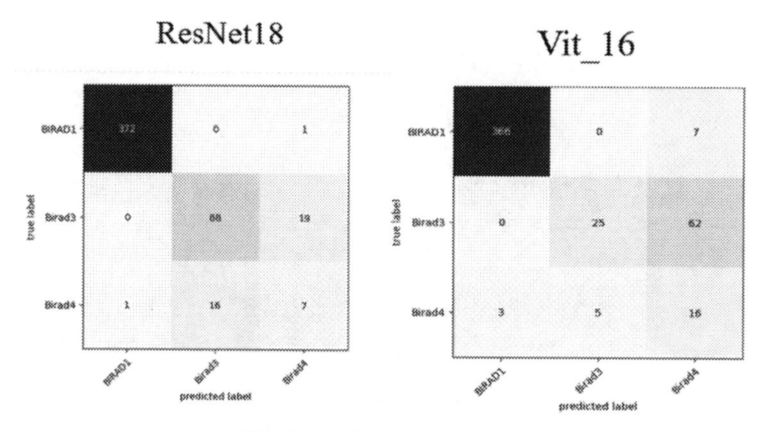

Fig. 4. ResNet18 *vs* ViT_16.

Table 3. Classification Accuracy.

Accuracy	BI-RADS 1	BI-RADS 3	BI-RADS 4	Overall Accuracy
ResNet_18	99%	78%	29%	92%
ViT_16	98%	28%	66%	84%

BI-RADS 3. On the other hand, ResNet18 misclassified 16 out of 24 images and only classify 7 out of 24 images correctly.

The overall outcomes indicate that the ResNet18 model exhibited better results compared to the ViT_16 model, with a difference of 8% in accuracy. Specifically, Table 3 illustrates that the accuracy of the ResNet18 model was 92%, whereas the ViT_16 model achieved an accuracy of 84%. However, for BI-RADS 4 ViT_16 showed superior performance, by 37% accuracy. Suggesting that breast cancer diagnoses can be improved using ViT-based model compared to CNN-based model.

Before diving into the loss curves and the accuracy curves for each epoch, it should be noted that the augmentation was applied only to the training dataset, the test dataset does not have any augmented images.

It clearly appears that both the loss curves for the train and the test are going down for the ViT_16 model as shown in Fig. 5. Additionally, it is harder to fit the model to the train set than the test set as the loss curves interpret. For the accuracy curves for each epoch, the model did well on the test set but struggled with the training set this could be due to the augmentation images that were added to the training dataset as a result, the model has a harder time extracting more features.

For the loss curves and accuracy curves for the ResNet18, the model performed well on the training dataset for both curves the model struggled only on the test set this could be due to few images in the test set as the ResNet18 model have a different structure then ViT_16 and can generalize over augmented images but needed more data to do so as shown in Fig. 6.

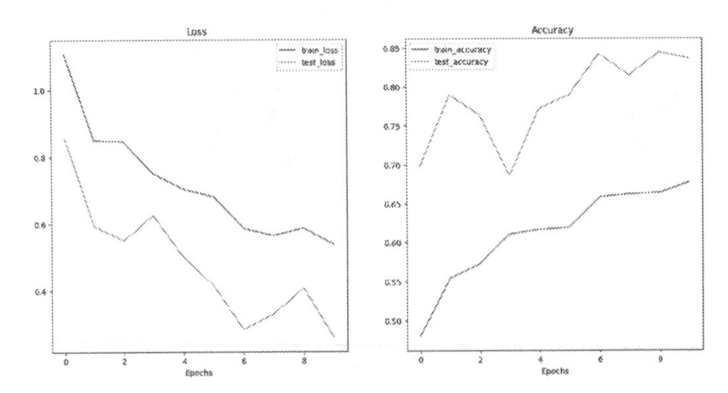

Fig. 5. The loss curves and the accuracy curves for ViT_16.

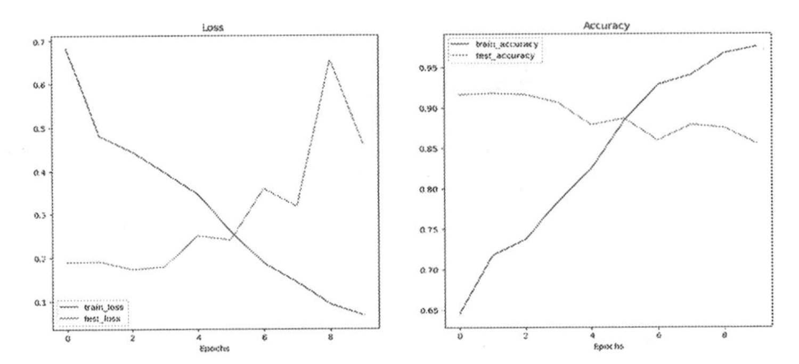

Fig. 6. The loss curves and the accuracy curves for ResNet18.

5.2 ViT_16 With Augmentation vs ViT _16 Without Augmentation

This section investigates the impact of data augmentation on ViT_16 model performance. The class distribution for the ViT_16 without augmentation is as follows: 1884 for BI-RADS 1, 398 for BI-RADS 3, and 126 for BI-RADS 4. The confusion matrix given in Fig. 7, illustrates that the model handled the imbalanced data quite well, misclassifying all samples of the BI-RADS 4 only, which has few points. After applying data augmentation classification accuracy for BI-RADS 4 was improved, with 16 images correctly classified. Suggesting that training with augmented data would lead to better results. Additionally, it is worth investigating other techniques for handling data imbalance. For instance, Xu et al. [15] showed that ViT can enhance classification accuracy for highly imbalanced data by using Masked Generative Pretraining (MGP) without the need to apply data augmentation.

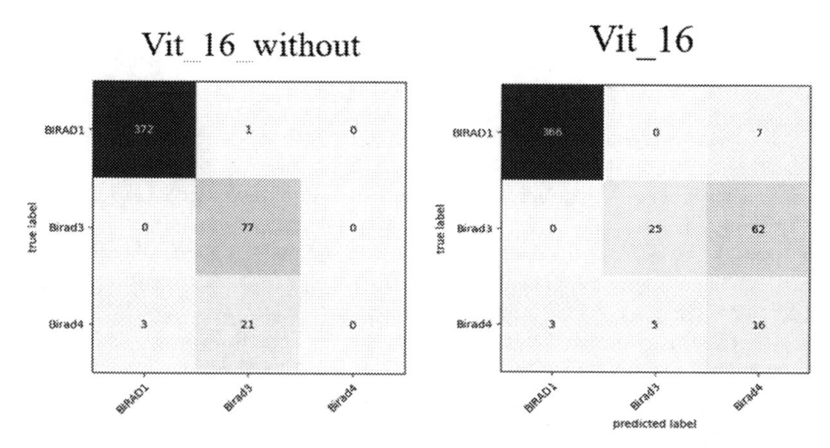

Fig. 7. ViT _16 with augmentation vs ViT _16 without augmentation.

6 Conclusions

In this paper, a comparative analysis of two models was proposed to classify breast cancer learning using unbalanced data.The models were ViT_16 and ResNet18. The performance and accuracy of the ResNet18 and ViT_16 models were compared by using a confusion matrix. Both models performed well in identifying the first class, BI-RADS 1, which consisted of a total of 1884 images and did not include any augmented images. Nevertheless, the BI-RADS 3 class consisted of a total of 398 images, with an additional inclusion of more than 900 augmented images. On the other hand, the BI-RADS 4 class consisted of 92 original images, and an additional 1000 augmented images were included. This augmentation process has the potential to impact the overall performance of the classification task for both classes. The ResNet18 model outperformed the ViT_16 model by 8% in accuracy, with a 92% overall accuracy rate, compared to the 84% achieved by the ViT_16 model. Conversely, ViT_16 detected suspicious abnormality (BI-RADS 4 category) more precisely compared to RestNet18, by 37% accuracy. These findings recommend that breast cancer diagnoses can be improved using ViT-based models over CNN-based models.

7 Future Work

The imbalance data set is the most crucial component of this study. Therefore, other models can be investigated to handle imbalanced dataset in breast cancer diagnosis, such as Few-Shot Learning models that use meta-learning rather than supervised learning. Additionally, different data augmentation methods such as GAN will be investigated in the future to mitigate class imbalance and understand the impact on classification accuracy.

References

1. Arabia, M.O.H.S.: Ministry of health Saudi Arabia (2020). https://moh.gov.sa/en/HealthAwareness/EducationalContent/wh/Breast-Cancer/Pages/default.aspx
2. Ragab, D.A., Sharkas, M., Marshall, S., Ren, J.: Breast cancer detection using deep convolutional neural networks and support vector machines. PeerJ **1**, 2019 (2019). https://doi.org/10.7717/peerj.6201
3. Karuppasamy, A.D., Abdesselam, A., Hedjam, R., Zidoum, H., Al-Bahri, M.: Recent CNN-based techniques for breast cancer histology image classification. J. Eng. Res. **19**(1), 41–53 (2022). https://doi.org/10.53540/tjer.vol19iss1pp41-53
4. Chen, X., et al.: Transformers improve breast cancer diagnosis from unregistered multi-view mammograms. Diagnostics **12**(7) (2022). https://doi.org/10.3390/diagnostics12071549
5. Zhang, A., Lipton, Z.C., Li, M., Smola, A.J.: Dive into Deep Learning. Cambridge University Press (2023)
6. Vaswani, A., et al.: Attention is all you need (2017)
7. Dosovitskiy, A., et al.: An image is worth 16X16 words: transformers for image recognition at scale (2020). https://github.com/
8. Boesch, G.: Vision transformers (ViT) in image recognition – 2023 Guide, viso.ai (2023). https://viso.ai/deep-learning/vision-transformer-vit/
9. Momentum, M.: A brief history of vision transformers: revisiting two years of vision research (2022). https://medium.com/merantix-labs-insights/a-brief-history-of-vision-transformers-revisiting-two-years-of-vision-research-26a6bd3251f3
10. He, K., Zhang, X., Ren, S., Sun, J.: Deep residual learning for image recognition (2015). http://image-net.org/challenges/LSVRC/2015/
11. Alotaibi, A., et al.: ViT-DeiT: an ensemble model for breast cancer histopathological images classification (2022). http://arxiv.org/abs/2211.00749
12. He, Z., et al.: Deconv-transformer (DecT): a histopathological image classification model for breast cancer based on color deconvolution and transformer architecture. Inf. Sci. (N Y) **608**, 1093–1112 (2022). https://doi.org/10.1016/j.ins.2022.06.091
13. Alsolami, A.S., Shalash, W., Alsaggaf, W., Ashoor, S., Refaat, H., Elmogy, M.: King Abdulaziz university breast cancer mammogram dataset (KAU-BCMD). Data (Basel) **6**(11) (2021). https://doi.org/10.3390/data6110111
14. What to know about your BI-RADS score (2021). https://www.webmd.com/breast-cancer/what-to-know-about-bi-rads-score
15. Xu, Z., Liu, R., Yang, S., Chai, Z., Yuan, C.: Learning imbalanced data with vision transformers. (2022). http://arxiv.org/abs/2212.02015

TNEST: Training Sparse Neural Network for FPGA Based Edge Application

Rammi Das[1], Rupesh Raj Karn[2(✉)], Jukka Heikkonen[3], and Rajeev Kanth[4]

[1] Nepal College of Information Technology, Pokhara University, Kathmandu, Nepal
[2] Center for Cyber Security, New York University, Abu Dhabi, United Arab Emirates
rupesh.k@nyu.edu
[3] Department of Computing, University of Turku, Turku, Finland
jukhei@utu.fi
[4] Department of Information Technology, Savonia University of Applied Sciences, Kuopio, Finland
rajeev.kanth@savonia.fi

Abstract. Machine learning (ML) hardware inference has developed ultra-low-power edge devices that accelerate inferential applications performance. An FPGA (Field Programmable Gate Array) is a popular option for such systems. The FPGA has power budget, memory, compute resource, area, etc. constraints but possesses several key advantages, including bandwidth saving, speed, real-time inference, offline activity, etc. Neural networks have been extensively used in Edge systems due to their significant popularity in AI. Requirements of complex neural networks have only been recently realized for edge applications, so the research community has yet to develop a standard model for such applications. The sparse neural architecture reduces the active neurons and connections, making the entire system computationally more efficient and utilizing less memory. Such essential facts are more and more evident in edge-based IoT applications. In this work, we have customized neural network training algorithms to fit precisely for the Edge systems. Rather than a traditional top-down approach where MLs are fully trained and then pruned to fit within edge device resources, we adopted a generative approach where MLs are prepared with the least number of parameters, and further components are added as the need arises to improve inference accuracy. Our generative model shows significant savings in FPGA resource consumption compared to the top-down approach for the same precision.

Keywords: Sparse Model · Neural Network · FPGA · High-level Synthesis · Edge Application

1 Introduction

Using machine learning in edge hardware enhances applications such as machine vision, automotive vehicles, and robotics to make them intelligent and improve operational performance. Over the decades, embedded microcontrollers and

K. Daimi and A. Al Sadoon (Eds.): ACR 2024, LNNS 956, pp. 15–28, 2024.
https://doi.org/10.1007/978-3-031-56950-0_2

lightweight processors have been used to simplify repeated operations. However, deploying machine-learning algorithms on edge devices is still in the early stages. The advancement in ultra-low-power machine learning called TinyML hardware has shown promising outcomes, however, the continued progress is due to the lack of standard ML models specific to the edge inference applications [1]. Artificial neural network (ANN) has been the most commonly adopted machine learning technology across various edge inference domains. As expected, ANN models have a higher capacity for learning than other traditional machine learning models. Such capability is mainly due to the large number of ANN parameters and hyper-parameters variables [2], which can be tuned extensively to build accurate models. The exponential growth of the network dimension and the associated increases in computational complexity and memory consumption are a clear trend in ANNs [3]. However, because of the limited space and power budget, the performance and energy performance of the edge inference system is constrained and restricted by technical size [4]. An FPGA (Field Programmable Gate Array) is the prime example of such a constrained edge device.

Sparse neural architectures can be distinctly well-suited for edge-based applications for several reasons. Edge devices often have limited computational resources, including processing power, memory, and energy. By reducing the number of active neurons and connections, Sparse neural architectures can significantly reduce the computational demands of neural networks. This makes them more feasible to deploy on resource-constrained edge devices. Memory is often a precious resource on edge devices. Sparse neural architectures can considerably reduce the memory footprint of the model, making it easier to deploy on devices with limited memory capacity. The research community is still searching for the standard training procedures of the machine learning model for edge inference. By "standard training procedure," we imply that no well-known training approach includes a mechanism for selecting between the platform or use cases where the inference might execute, such as on a software server or an edge device. In this paper, we attempt to solve such requirements through the following strategies:

1. Select a fully connected or convolution neural network architecture as an ML model.
2. Prescribe a set of rules to map edge resources and ML's size using their hyper-parameters.
3. Measure the edge resource footprint versus ML's accuracy trade-offs.

For such an ML model, we present a methodology to generate constrained neural architecture for an FPGA to simulate an edge device. Specifically, the constraints of edge hardware are used to design the neural architecture. The size of computing and memory resources of hardware are applied as constraints during the architecture search process to select the hyper-parameters of the neural network model. In summary, our contributions are as follows:

1. We provide a training mechanism to develop the sparse neural network work for the edge application.

2. We use FPGA as the edge device to accelerate the sparse model and show the trade-off between accuracy vs. resource utilization.

2 Literature Review

In [5], an FPGA-based edge device for IoT is suggested to offload significant communication stack functions to specialized hardware to increase system performance. It focuses on edge-device communication and interoperability by building an IoT protocol stack on a low-cost SoC FPGA architecture with an embedded hardcore CPU. A TCP/IP application is made in RTOS in [6] with the motive that RTOS, like FPGA, in hardware does not lose application flexibility while maintaining energy efficiency equivalent to application-specialized hardware. The benefits of FPGA and edge computing are merged in [7] to create a new network-assisted computing model, FPGA-based edge computing. Three computer vision (CV)-based mobile interactive apps are chosen as edge applications, with their back-end computation engines implemented on FPGA. Experiments show that this strategy effectively reduces application response time and overall system energy usage when compared to typical CPU-based edge/cloud offloading approaches. The survey paper [8] reveals that FPGAs are ideal candidates for speeding neural network inference due to their programmability. FPGA has a quicker design and verification cycle compared to ASIC design and does not require as much fabrication [9]. Because of the reconfigurability and speed of design verification, developers may create ASIC accelerator prototypes on FPGA to test both the logic and the algorithm for the intended applications. For computer vision applications, an FPGA accelerator is shown in [10] while [11] shows the same for the cyber-security applications. Using Neural Architecture Search (NAS) and AutoML allows for the automated generation of efficient neural network models. A recent work [12] shows a prior-arts assessment of neural network models designed particularly for resource-constrained devices. Other examples of NAS on resource-constrained devices are [13,14]. The present state of research on computing sparse neural networks is shown in [15], emphasizing sparse algorithms, software frameworks, and hardware accelerations.

3 Motivation for Edge Computing

Consider the instance A, $\mathbf{H_A}$ that does nothing more than shuffle data between sensors and the cloud. Let $\mathbf{P_A}$ be the power required to send a frame of those signals denoted by $\mathbf{X_A}$ to the cloud. Let $\mathbf{t_A}$ be the time to receive the inference result at $\mathbf{H_A}$ after sending the signals. Again, consider another instance, B, $\mathbf{H_B}$, that contains an ML model, computes inference or decision-making from those signals, and occasionally sends signals $\mathbf{X_B}$ to the cloud. Let $\mathbf{P_B}$ be its power consumption which is divided into $\mathbf{P'_B}$ and $\mathbf{P''_B}$, $\mathbf{P'_B}$ = power used for signal transmission between cloud and sensors, $\mathbf{P''_B}$ = power used for computation in ML inference. Let $\mathbf{t_B}$ be the time to receive the inference result at $\mathbf{H_B}$ after feeding the signals to the ML model. It has been successfully inspected the following aspects for edge application in a selected time-period $\mathbf{T}$ for $\mathbf{N}$ inference data samples:

1. Bandwidth saving $= \frac{dim(\mathbf{X_A}) - dim(\mathbf{X_B})}{\mathbf{T}}$.
2. Power Utility, whether $\mathbf{P_B^{''}} > \mathbf{P_A} - \mathbf{P_B^{'}}$ and excessive power requirement $= \mathbf{P_B} - \mathbf{P_A}$. It is noted that $\mathbf{P_B} = \mathbf{P_B^{'}} + \mathbf{P_B^{''}}$.
3. Latency improvement factor $= \frac{1}{\mathbf{T}} \sum_{\mathbf{i=1}}^{\mathbf{N}} [\mathbf{t_{A_i}} - \mathbf{t_{B_i}}]$

As a result, edge computing decreases latency, allows real-time analytics, improves data security, and provides a cost-effective solution. Edge computing avoids forwarding all data signals between edge devices and the server. Consequently, the computations at the edge could be performed in an encrypted domain using the homomorphic encryption (HE) approach. Some of the HE neural network and its FPGA implementation are given in [16–18]. This will use less power and cause less delay than transferring all encrypted data signals between the edge device and the server.

4 Constrained Neural Architecture Generator

Traditionally, the ML model is trained offline on a cloud server in software, and it is further compressed and optimized to fit into a target hardware platform at the expense of inference accuracy. Some compression techniques include quantizing floating-point weights into smaller bit sizes, reducing the fan-in and fan-out of neurons in ANN, and dropping the least significant connections based on their importance on loss function, etc. Typically, this strategy does not consider the best solutions overall. This article discusses the design automation methods of architecture search based on hardware constraints. Our architecture search method is based on the following assumptions:

1. Size of memory $\mathbf{M}$ of edge device imposes constraints on the number of compute parameters $\mathbf{p}$ of an ML model since these parameters are saved into the device's memory.
2. The compute resource $\mathbf{C}$ of edge device is measured as the number of multiplier and adder.
3. The floating-point weights are quantized into the bit size of the data bus of the edge device.
4. The search process is run for a fully connected neural network model.
5. The number of input nodes of ML is equal to the number of data features $\mathbf{X}.size$ and output nodes is equal to the number of classes $\mathbf{K}$ of the dataset.

Architecture design of the ML model, including the number of layers, nodes, connections, and the number of filters per layer, has emerged as an increasingly expensive method called art rather than science by many researchers [19]. Furthermore, suppose the hardware limitations and design considerations imposed by underlying hardware are considered. In that case, the capacity of a human expert to identify the best-performing ML model can be significantly compromised. Works that optimize both the hardware efficiency and the precision of the ML model have become increasingly important. The architectural attributes, like feature maps, the number of branches, and so forth, are selected to minimize inference costs subject to maximum error constraints.

For any ML, an architecture space $\mathbf{\Lambda}$ is defined where a point $\lambda_i = [\lambda_{i,1}, \lambda_{i,2}, ...] \in \mathbf{\Lambda}$ is a vector of hyper-parameters of ML. One of the members of λ_i for the ANN model can be the number of nodes in different hidden layers denoted by $\eta_1, \eta_2, ..., \eta_{\mathbf{L}}$.

Consider a case for simple feed-forward vanilla ANN. Let $\mathbf{X} \in \mathbb{R}^{n \times N}$ be the input data record of the feature space and $\mathbf{y} \in \mathbb{R}^{1 \times N}$ the output record. Let $\boldsymbol{\theta} \in \mathbb{R}^n$ be the weight vector based on $\mathbf{X}$ and $\mathbf{y}$ and ϕ be the activation function. The predicted output is given by

$$\hat{\mathbf{y}} = \phi(\boldsymbol{\theta}^T \mathbf{X}) \tag{1}$$

The output of the next hidden layer is:

$$\mathbf{y}_l = \phi(\boldsymbol{\theta}_l^T \mathbf{y}_{l-1}), 1 \leq l \leq \mathbf{L} \tag{2}$$

$$\mathbf{y}_{L+1} = \hat{\mathbf{y}} = \phi(\boldsymbol{\theta}_{L+1}^T \mathbf{y}_L) \;\; and \;\; \mathbf{y}_1 = \phi(\boldsymbol{\theta}_0^T \mathbf{X}) \tag{3}$$

where, $\boldsymbol{\theta}_0$ is a vector of weights of input layer and $\boldsymbol{\theta}_{L+1}$ is that of output layer. The cost function equation is:

$$\begin{aligned} \mathbf{J}(\mathbf{y}, \hat{\mathbf{y}}) = -\frac{1}{\mathbf{N}} \sum_{i=1}^{\mathbf{N}} [\mathbf{y}^i \log \phi(\boldsymbol{\theta}_{L+1}^T \mathbf{y}_L^i) \\ + (1 - \mathbf{y}^i) \log(1 - \phi(\boldsymbol{\theta}_{L+1}^T \mathbf{y}_L^i))] \end{aligned} \tag{4}$$

Total number of weights or parameters in ANN architecture is:

$$\mathbf{p} = \sum_{l=0}^{\mathbf{L+1}} n(\boldsymbol{\theta}_l) \;\; and \;\; \mathbf{p}_{min} = n(\boldsymbol{\theta}_0) + n(\boldsymbol{\theta}_{\mathbf{L+1}}) \tag{5}$$

The number of weights $n(\boldsymbol{\theta}_l)$ depends on the number of nodes η_l in any hidden layer l.

$$n(\boldsymbol{\theta}_l) = \eta_l \times \eta_{l-1} \tag{6}$$

Hardware constrained training function is given by:

$$Min \; \mathbf{J}(\mathbf{y}, \hat{\mathbf{y}}) \; s.t. \; \mathbf{p} \leq M \tag{7}$$

Different value of L and $\eta_l, l \in \mathbf{L}$ results in different ANN characteristics in terms of $\mathbf{J}(\mathbf{y}, \hat{\mathbf{y}})$ and computational capacity $\mathbf{C}$. A model can be loaded on the edge device only if $\mathbf{M} \geq \mathbf{p}_{min}$. The performance constraint for validation dataset $[\mathbf{X}_{val}, \mathbf{y}_{val}]$ is

$$\mathbf{J}[\mathbf{y}(\mathbf{X}_{\mathbf{val}}), \hat{\mathbf{y}}] \leq Obj_{accuracy} \; s.t. \; \mathbf{p} \leq M \tag{8}$$

To train the model with hardware constraints, there are two possible approaches to fulfill $\mathbf{p} \leq M$.

1. A densely connected ANN with less $\mathbf{L}$ and minimal nodes $\eta_l, 1 \leq l \leq \mathbf{L}$.
2. A sparsely connected ANN with comparatively large $\mathbf{L}$ and $\eta_l, 1 \leq l \leq \mathbf{L}$ but many $n(\boldsymbol{\theta}_l)$ weights equal to zero.

This work adopts the second approach, where the model is made highly sparse. After every training epoch, a set of parameters in each hidden layer is set to zero. During gradient descent back-propagation, the weight update is discounted for those parameters. This is different from the traditional sparse network generation method where the ANN model is trained with all parameters in the architecture, and later, the pruning or fine-tuning is performed to remove the unimportant parameters to meet the constraints of Eq. (8). Please note that we have set the value to $\mathbf{L}$ before training the sparse neural network. It is recommended to start training with a smaller value $\mathbf{L}$ and increase its value gradually only if the last training cannot produce the desired accuracy score. The tuning of $\mathbf{L}$ is covered in Sect. 5 and 6, where we have shown the hyper-parameter tuning approach to achieve a highly sparse model with smaller parameter sizes. We adopt the training setup described in Algorithm 1.

Algorithm 1: Sparse neural network training.

Input : $\mathbf{X}$, $\mathbf{y}$, $Obj_{accuracy}$, $\mathbf{M}$
Output: ANN model

```
1  l = 1
2  η = y.size
3  sparsity= 0.99
4  model = sequential() // incremental model
5  model.add(Dense(input=X.size, output=K, L = 0, η = NULL ))
6  model.fit(X,y)
7  p ← from equ (5) while p ≤ M do
8      if model.eval(X_val,y_val) ≥ Obj_accuracy then
9          return model
10     end
11     else
12         η = η + 1
13         sparsity = sparsity-0.1
14         model.add(Sparse(L = l, num_of_params = η, sparse= sparsity))
15     end
16 end
```

The zeroed weights don't consume memory and don't contribute in $\hat{\mathbf{y}}$ prediction in Eqs. (1) and (3). In this algorithm, at line 14, the added hidden layer is sparse such that the fan-in of any neuron is limited, i.e., only a few non-zero weights or connections directed to each neuron. Let's call this a case I. Several ANN sparse connectivity are built and trained to locate the minima of the cost function that verifies the constraints in line 7. If the objective accuracy $Obj_{accuracy}$ is unable to be achieved, then the neuron's fan-in is increased gradually. The algorithm stops whichever criteria $\mathbf{p} \geq M$ or model.eval($\mathbf{X}_{val}$, $\mathbf{y}_{val}$) $\geq$ $Obj_{accuracy}$ arrives first. Although we have shown the sparsity of the first hidden layer, the same applies to other hidden layers. If the layer $l = 1$ reaches non-sparse without meeting the objective accuracy, then the Algorithm 1 is called further by adding a more hidden layer, and this cycle repeats.

5 Methodology

5.1 Sparsity Mechanism

To create the neural network model, we have used the Keras library. Keras does not provide an API to build a sparse layer. Furthermore, the training function employs vector-matrix algebra. There is no mathematical equation in such a training function for freezing a portion of elements in a weight matrix/vector during the gradient-descent phase of training. As a result, we employ Keras callbacks to build a sparse layer. We zero the value of a random set of parameters $\boldsymbol{\theta}^s$ in an array called *zero_weight*. The connections in $\boldsymbol{\theta}^s$ are selected randomly across different neurons in the hidden layer to match the sparsity quantity of Algorithm 1. It is then fed into the training function through a callback. The Keras training proceeds as usual where all the parameters $\boldsymbol{\theta}$ are updated in gradient-descent. But after every epoch, the value of $\boldsymbol{\theta}^s$ is reverted back to the *zero_weight*. We make use of two functions, 'on_train_begin' and 'on_batch_end,' as shown in the pseudocode:

```
class LossHistory(keras.callbacks.Callback):
    def on_train_begin(self, θ^s, logs={}):
        for layer in model.layers:
            self.model.layer.set_weights([θ^s, zero_weights])
    def on_batch_end(self, theta_tau_minus_1, logs={}):
        for layer in model.layers:
            self.model.layer.set_weights([θ^s, zero_weights])
model.fit(D_τ, batch_size, epochs, callbacks=[LossHistory()])
```

5.2 Connections Re-wiring

One of the primary criteria of whether a neural network can be efficiently implemented in hardware or simulated in software is a network connection. Memory references, for example, require more than two orders of magnitude more energy than ALU operations in an implementation of a long short-term memory network (LSTM) [20]. This implementation barrier will become much more severe in future deep learning applications as the number of neurons in layers increases, resulting in a quadratic increase in the number of connections between them. Thus it needs an additional step after sparsity that makes it possible to evaluate different connectivity.

The rewiring strategy randomly rewires the network during supervised training with the expectation that numerous random samplings will create the connections where they are most needed to improve the classification accuracy, but their total number is always rigidly constrained by the sparsity percentage [21]. Several random samplings result in diverse weight distributions, with the value scattered on both sides of the zero axis. The register to hold the weights will be smaller when the dispersion spread is narrow. Alternatively, the small distribution will aid in representing the floating point weights with limited bits. It additionally boosts the optimal utilization of FPGA resources.

5.3 Layer Size Tuning

As explained in Algorithm 1, the mechanism to build training is to dynamically grow the neural architecture by adding more neurons to the hidden layers. The neural architecture is expanded whenever the model fails to achieve the desired inference accuracy. Over-expansion with too many nodes increases training time, compute resource usage, and the likelihood of overfitting. On the other hand, under-expansion would not be adequate to achieve reasonable inference and generalization accuracy in the generated model.

There is no mathematical equation for calculating "Which way to increase the layer size and construct the model to fulfill expectations?" As a result, the general process is to evaluate several options and automatically select the best model design from the evaluated choices. In other words, the state-of-the-art often relies on an investigation to discover what works best from the available configurations to develop the optimal model design. That is also the basis for our work.

6 Experiments Evaluation

6.1 Experiment Testbench

To showcase our generative model building, Algorithm 1, we use two applications: image recognition for the MNIST dataset and intrusion detection for the

Table 1. Dataset description.

Attributes	UNSW	MNIST
Description	Both normal and contemporary synthesized attack activities of LAN network traffic [23,24]	Primitive image dataset [25]; collection of gray-scale images of handwritten digits from 0 to 9
Number of features	43	784
Number of labels	10	10
Training size	175, 341	60, 000
Validation size	82, 332	10, 000
Feature data types	Binary, float, nominal and integer	Integer
Some feature names	port numbers, service names, protocols, IP addresses, packet transmission statistics, etc	Pixel grayscale values

UNSW dataset. They are compared in Table 1. All of them perform multi-label classification. We use Xilinx *Artix-7 35T cpg236-1* FPGA board [22] board as the edge device. In this work, we apply such an application on the *Artix-7* FPGA.

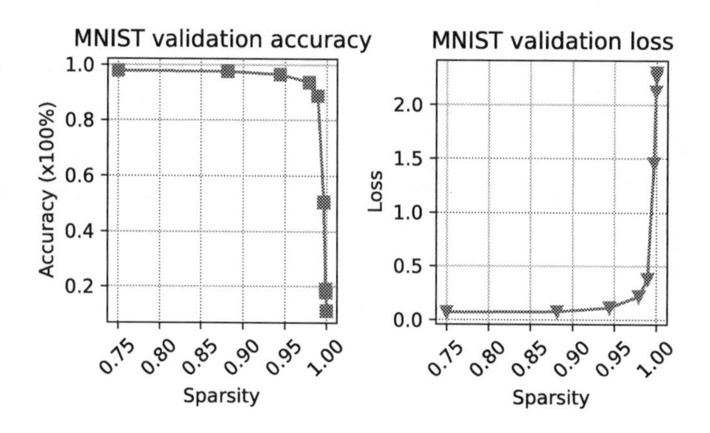

Fig. 1. MNIST model evaluation across various sparsity.

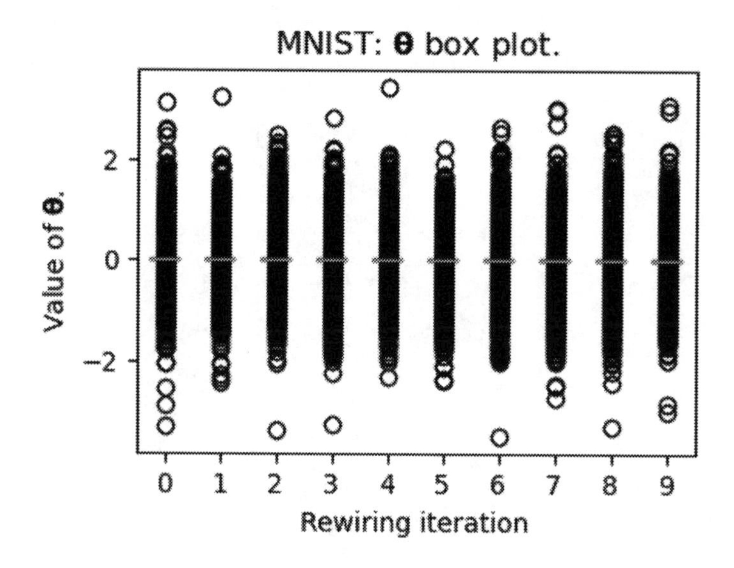

Fig. 2. MNIST model evaluation across various sparsity.

6.2 Software Implementation

The experimental outcome of pseudocode for Listing 5.1 for several sparsity percentages is displayed in Fig. 1. With such a heuristic approach, the value of

$\boldsymbol{\theta}^s$ are frozen to zero and the distribution of $\boldsymbol{\theta}$ values lies on either side of the zero axis.

The experimental outcome of rewiring, with respect to Sect. 5.2, for ten random samples is shown in Fig. 2. For all the rewiring cases, the sparsity is the same. The experimental outcome in Fig. 2 shows that iterations $\{4, 5, 6\}$ has a narrower spread than other iterations. The small spread aids quantization, allowing a lightweight neural network model to be run on an FPGA without sacrificing inference accuracy. The narrow spread reduces the number of bits necessary to hold the weights, reducing the width of the FPGA's register or RAM. For iteration $\{4, 5, 6\}$, except for a few outliers, most weights are between -2 and 2. As a result, two bits would suffice to indicate the integer component of the weights, one of which is the sign bit. When the spread is more comprehensive, quantization causes a significant loss in weight value, resulting in a considerable deterioration in inference accuracy.

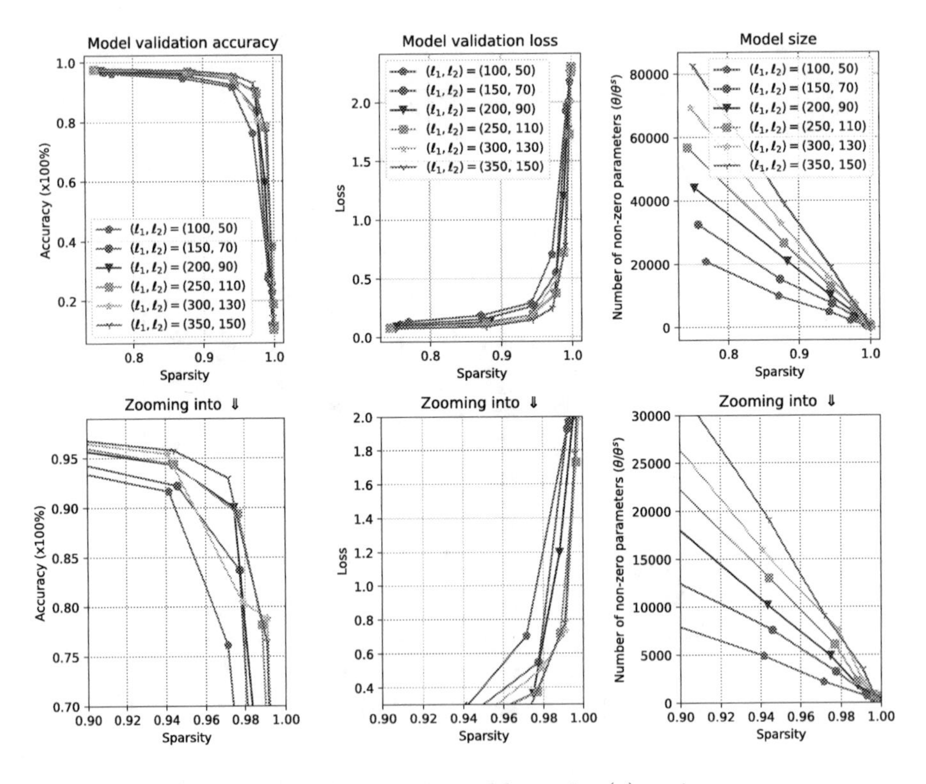

Fig. 3. MNIST sparsity and layer size (η) tuning.

It is to be noted that unlike [21], ([21] described in Sect. 5.2) we obtain the same value of the model's inference accuracy for each rewiring iteration.

To showcase the layer size tuning given in Sect. 5.3, we have tuned the two hidden layers for different sparsity percentages. The outcome is shown in Fig. 3.

The plots below each of the subplots show the *zoom-in* area to show the comparison between different experiment cases. We developed a pandas data frame out of all the experimental evaluation metrics and neural architectures and sorted it based on accuracy and layer size. It is shown in Table 2. From this data frame, it could be observed that the minimum size of the layer to achieve more than 90% accuracy is 200 and 90 for the first and second layers, respectively at a sparsity of 0.941605.

The source code to perform the training and generate the plots for Figs. 1, 2, 3, and pandas frame, Table 2, is available. We have extensively shown the experimental results for the MNIST dataset only. Nonetheless, we conducted similar research for the UNSW datasets. The outcome of for UNSW dataset is available at our source code link [26] (https://github.com/rkarn/Constrained-Neural-Network).

Table 2. MNIST training summary in a Pandas dataframe short by $\boldsymbol{\theta}/\boldsymbol{\theta}^s$ and validation accuracy.

	ℓ_1	ℓ_2	Sparsity	Validation Acc	Validation Loss	Nonzero $\|\theta\|$	$\|\theta\|$	Centroid of θ
2	200	90	0.941605	0.9162	0.288913	4873	84060	0.003255
12	300	90	0.945974	0.9219	0.264279	7570	129030	0.001381
53	350	110	0.971807	0.9296	0.244130	9127	328910	0.001370
1	150	70	0.871192	0.9457	0.183184	10011	84060	0.002555
22	400	90	0.943422	0.9433	0.186692	10194	176000	0.001412
63	450	110	0.974962	0.9336	0.228893	10511	383880	0.001272
73	150	110	0.975001	0.9348	0.215994	11919	440850	0.000967
32	100	90	0.944229	0.9435	0.188803	13021	224970	0.001554
11	250	70	0.873349	0.9545	0.150629	15239	129030	0.003352
42	200	90	0.940895	0.9541	0.156316	15959	275940	0.000976
52	300	90	0.944251	0.9575	0.146827	19134	328910	0.000996
0	100	50	0.769394	0.9616	0.131913	20882	84060	0.005350
21	350	70	0.883847	0.9611	0.127569	20929	176000	0.002024
62	400	90	0.945332	0.9581	0.146918	22182	383880	0.001188
72	100	90	0.941187	0.9624	0.125418	25384	440850	0.001285
31	450	70	0.878756	0.9672	0.116704	26636	224970	0.001562
10	200	50	0.758687	0.9680	0.107122	32454	129030	0.002516
41	150	70	0.874892	0.9703	0.100194	32840	275940	0.001651
51	250	70	0.879268	0.9718	0.088362	39173	328910	0.001723

6.3 FPGA Implementation

We make use of the HLS4ML tool to perform the FPGA synthesis. HLS4ML is an open-source software-hardware co-design methodology for interpreting and

Table 3. Xilinx's *Artix-7* FPGA resource consumption for MNIST dataset. LUT: Look-up Table, FF: Flip-flops, BRAM_18K: Block RAM with 18 kilobytes, DSP48E: Digital signal processor.

Attributes	Sparsity = 75%	Sparsity = 0%
LUT	21024	71763
FF	71103	228552
BRAM_18K	2	2
DSP48E	562	2067

Table 4. Xilinx's *Artix-7* FPGA resource consumption for UNSW dataset. LUT: Look-up Table, FF: Flip-flops, BRAM_18K: Block RAM with 18 kilobytes, DSP48E: Digital signal processor.

Attributes	Sparsity = 75%	Sparsity = 0%
LUT	32890	114368
FF	113863	412489
BRAM_18K	2	2
DSP48E	1060	4139

translating machine learning algorithms for FPGA and ASIC implementation. It is a framework that enables digital hardware implementations of machine learning algorithms to be more accessible, interpretable, and (re)usable to developers. While hardware implementations eventually necessitate fully built solutions, HLS4ML enables developers to co-design algorithms depending on their system and application constraints. This tool is tremendously helpful in decreasing engineering time and promoting faster design iterations.

This work uses such a tool to convert the *Keras*-based trained sparse neural network model, Sect. 4, into the Verilog-based hardware representation. Finally, such hardware representation is synthesized with Vivado. The synthesis report showing FPGA resource utilization for sparse and non-sparse models is demonstrated in Table 3 and 4 for MNIST and UNSW datasets respectively. As expected, the DSPs, LUTs, and FFs used for the non-sparse network are much higher than those of the sparse model. The extra DSPs are used in the multiplication operation between extensive weights in the non-sparse architecture. The same is the case for additional LUTs. Further, extra weights $\boldsymbol{\theta}'s$ must be stored, so the non-sparse model shows high flip-flops utilization.

The last step of the verification is the bit-stream generation and finally loading onto FPGA. The FPGA board is connected to the host machine (containing the Vivado design suite) through a serial port. We have used the UART protocol to transfer the data between the host machine and the FPGA board to test the inference. We set the baud rate to 119200 bits per second. The inference data

$\mathbf{X}_{test}$ is sent through the serial port. The inference is made at the FPGA, and the inference outcome ($\mathbf{y}$) is sent from the FPGA to the host machine.

7 Conclusion

This research demonstrates how to tailor neural network training techniques to fit Edge systems. In particular, a generative approach is used, in which MLs are sparsely trained with the fewest components, then additional components are added as needed to increase inference accuracy while meeting the resource limits of the edge device. The generative model is demonstrated on the Artix-7 FPGA for two edge applications: image recognition and intrusion detection. Compared to the non-sparse model, the generative model shows considerable reductions in FPGA resource use with negligible accuracy drop. Our generative model-building approach could effectively be applied for image classification on convolution neural networks and language modeling on recurrent neural networks. In a forthcoming article, we will discuss and demonstrate those potential use cases on an ASIC accelerator board.

References

1. Banbury, C.R., et al.: Benchmarking tinyml systems: challenges and direction. arXiv preprint arXiv:2003.04821 (2020)
2. Schmidhuber, J.: Deep learning in neural networks: an overview. Neural Netw. **61**, 85–117 (2015)
3. Xu, X., et al.: Scaling for edge inference of deep neural networks. Nat. Electron. **1**(4), 216–222 (2018)
4. Yang, K., Shi, Y., Yu, W., Ding, Z.: Energy-efficient processing and robust wireless cooperative transmission for edge inference. IEEE Internet Things J. (2020)
5. Gomes, T., Pinto, S., Tavares, A., Cabral, J.: Towards an FPGA-based edge device for the internet of things. In: 2015 IEEE 20th Conference on Emerging Technologies and Factory Automation (ETFA). IEEE, pp. 1–4 (2015)
6. Maruyama, N., Ishihara, T., Yasuura, H.: An RTOS in hardware for energy efficient software-based TCP, IP processing. In: IEEE 8th Symposium on Application Specific Processors (SASP). IEEE 2010, pp. 58–63 (2010)
7. Xu, C., et al.: The case for FPGA-based edge computing. IEEE Trans. Mob. Comput. **21**(7), 2610–2619 (2020)
8. Wu, R., Guo, X., Du, J., Li, J.: Accelerating neural network inference on FPGA-based platforms - a survey. Electronics **10**(9), 1025 (2021)
9. Yi, Q., Sun, H., Fujita, M.: FPGA based accelerator for neural networks computation with flexible pipelining. arXiv preprint arXiv:2112.15443 (2021)
10. Liu, X., et al.: Collaborative edge computing with FPGA-based CNN accelerators for energy-efficient and time-aware face tracking system. IEEE Trans. Comput. Soc. Syst. **9**(1), 252–266 (2021)
11. Rodríguez, A., Valverde, J., Portilla, J., Otero, A., Riesgo, T., De la Torre, E.: FPGA-based high-performance embedded systems for adaptive edge computing in cyber-physical systems: the ARTICo^3 framework. Sensors **18**(6), 1877 (2018)

12. Yang, Y., Zhan, J., Jiang, W., Jiang, Y., Yu, A.: Neural architecture search for resource constrained hardware devices: a survey. IET Cyber-Phys. Syst. Theory Appl. (2023)
13. Lyu, B., Yuan, H., Lu, L., Zhang, Y.: Resource-constrained neural architecture search on edge devices. IEEE Trans. Netw. Sci. Eng. **9**(1), 134–142 (2021)
14. Loni, M., Mousavi, H., Riazati, M., Daneshtalab, M., Sjödin, M.: TAS: ternarized neural architecture search for resource-constrained edge devices. In: Design, Automation and Test in Europe Conference and Exhibition (DATE). IEEE 2022, pp. 1115–1118 (2022)
15. Sun, F., Qin, M., Zhang, T., Liu, L., Chen, Y.-K., Xie, Y.: Computation on sparse neural networks: an inspiration for future hardware. arXiv preprint arXiv:2004.11946 (2020)
16. Yang, Y., Kuppannagari, S.R., Kannan, R., Prasanna, V.K.: FPGA accelerator for homomorphic encrypted sparse convolutional neural network inference. In: IEEE 30th Annual International Symposium on Field-Programmable Custom Computing Machines (FCCM). IEEE 2022, pp. 1–9 (2022)
17. Ye, T., Kuppannagari, S.R., Kannan, R., Prasanna, V.K.: Performance modeling and FPGA acceleration of homomorphic encrypted convolution. In: 2021 31st International Conference on Field-Programmable Logic and Applications (FPL). IEEE, pp. 115–121 (2021)
18. Turan, F., Roy, S.S., Verbauwhede, I.: Heaws: an accelerator for homomorphic encryption on the amazon AWS FPGA. IEEE Trans. Comput. **69**(8), 1185–1196 (2020)
19. Marculescu, D., Stamoulis, D., Cai, E.: Hardware-aware machine learning: modeling and optimization. In: Proceedings of the International Conference on Computer-Aided Design, pp. 1–8 (2018)
20. Han, S., et al.: ESE: Efficient speech recognition engine with sparse LSTM on FPGA. In: Proceedings of the 2017 ACM/SIGDA International Symposium on Field-Programmable Gate Arrays, pp. 75–84 (2017)
21. Bellec, G., Kappel, D., Maass, W., Legenstein, R.: Deep rewiring: training very sparse deep networks. arXiv preprint arXiv:1711.05136 (2017)
22. Przybus, B.: Xilinx redefines power, performance, and design productivity with three new 28 nm FPGA families: Virtex-7, kintex-7, and artix-7 devices. In: Xilinx White Paper (2010)
23. UNSW-NB15 Dataset Features and Size Description. https://www.unsw.adfa.edu.au/australian-centre-for-cyber-security/cybersecurity/ADFA-NB15-Datasets/. Accessed 16 Aug 2017
24. Moustafa, N., Slay, J.: UNSW-NB15: a comprehensive dataset for network intrusion detection systems (UNSW-NB15 network dataset). In: Military Communications and Information Systems Conference (MilCIS), pp. 1–6. IEEE (2015)
25. LeCun, Y., Bottou, L., Bengio, Y., Haffner, P.: Gradient-based learning applied to document recognition. Proc. IEEE **86**(11), 2278–2324 (1998)
26. Sparse neural network training mechanims. https://github.com/rkarn/Constrained-Neural-Network

Public Policy Decision Making: Confirmatory Factor Analysis

Maryna Averkyna[1,2](✉) and Oleksandr Skarbarchuk[2]

[1] Estonian Business School, A. Lauteri, 3, Tallinn, Estonia
Maryna.Averkyna@ebs.ee
[2] The National University of Ostroh Academy, Seminarska, 2, Ostroh, Ukraine

Abstract. The paper deals with creation a model influence of interest of groups on public policy decision making. The results of the study showed that the use of Likert data is a very important element in research. In this case, it allowed us to understand who influences decision-making. It is worth noting that we obtained quite interesting results based on using the method of principal components and confirmatory factor analyses. The application of existing modeling tools helped us to determine the factor loads and assess the significance of the obtained models for choosing the best appropriate. Confirmatory Factory Analysis is very important approach in determining the influence of stakeholders on public policy decision-making. However, this approach has some limitations, forming data, it is necessary to form groups with an equal number of participants. There is some limitation usage descriptive statistics for discrete data. The authors point out that there is the strong covariance between latent factors Policy and Administrative. This investigation shown that Authorities, Political parties and Domestic business strong legislative influence on formation of state policy and approving of management decisions. On the other hand, Government analytical centers, non-governmental analytical centers, foreign donor organizations, Ukrainian donor organizations, ordinary citizens, participants of street actions executively influence on formation of state policy and approving of management decisions.

Keywords: Public Policy · Decision Making · Interest of Groups · Confirmatory Factor Analysis

1 Introduction

Public authorities and local governments often face the problem of decisions making under uncertainties. These decisions must be optimal, relevant and to be made quickly [1, 2]. Every government and other institution through the world try to make decisions as rationally as it is possible. More officials, and more of the citizens they represent, are asking which of the options available to them does the best job of trading off relevant values against each other [4]. The decisions in organizations usually are made by humans. Michael Mintrom pointed out that the human limits are both cognitive and informational. 'All relevant information about future consequences of actions cannot be

K. Daimi and A. Al Sadoon (Eds.): ACR 2024, LNNS 956, pp. 29–37, 2024.
https://doi.org/10.1007/978-3-031-56950-0_3

readily accessed. Even if it could be, cognitive limits would inhibit effective analysis in service of good decision-making. The number of alternatives to be assessed stretch brain power' [9]. The public always makes a fundamental decision about the implementation of any program or project. That decision is whether or not to become involved in supporting or opposing the public agency's decision to implement the project or program. Experience and research have convinced the author that, in general, when the public agency's decision is announced, most citizens decide not to become involved in. If citizens decide on involvement, it is nearly always to oppose the public agency's decision; therefore, subsequent discussion will refer only to the public's decision for involvement in opposition [5]. Unlike corporate or governmental decisions, there are not so widely discussed models such as rationality or bounded rationality theory to explain public decisions. Perhaps that is because the public (groups and individuals with special interest) is suspected of making decisions either emotionally or irrationally but the decisions are no less valid because of it! Psychologists, anthropologists and sociologists generally agree that individual and group decisions are based in large measure on values. In the case of the decision to become involved, deeply held convictions are perceived as threatened, which motivates individuals and groups who hold those convictions to defend them against the threat (Firth, 1998) [5].

As noted by Papadakis and Barwise [10], the influence of context on decision making is largely unexplored. Contextual influences arise from an organization's role in a society, such as being an instrument of public policy or a means for creating wealth for shareholders. This role dictates the governance arrangements that are needed to exercise control for different types of owners, such as elected officials or shareholders [10].

The research problem is formulated as follow who influence on Public Policy Decision Making?

The purpose of the study is to obtain some generalized data under the condition of a limited sample (about 240 respondents). The study was to reveal the personal perception of the target groups of the products of the analytical centers and to obtain from them an assessment of various aspects of their work.

In this paper we will consider on meaning of public policy decision making and create a model which will show who influence on public decision making.

2 Public Policy Decision Making

Public policy decision making refers to actions taken within governmental settings to formulate, adopt, implement, evaluate, or change environmental policies. These decisions may occur at any level of government (Center for American Politics and Public Policy) [7].

Public policy is a combination of basic decisions, commitments, and actions made by those who hold authority or affect government decisions. The policy-making process weighs and balances public values. Often there is no 'right' choice or correct technical answer to the issue at hand [7]. Kenneth Arrow as the researcher of social choice theory tried to solve the problem of group decision-making [3]. He pointed out that 'If we exclude the possibility of interpersonal comparisons of utility, then the only methods of passing from individual tastes to social preferences which will be satisfactory and which will be defined for a wide range of sets of individual orderings are either imposed or dictatorial' (Forman, 2001) [6]. In general impossibility theorem, often named after him, Arrow theorized that it was impossible to formulate a social preference ordering that satisfies all of the following conditions: nondictatorship, individual sovereignty, unanimity, freedom from irrelevant alternatives, uniqueness of group rank [1]. One of the basic implicit assumptions of economic theory is that decisions matter: wrong decisions have a negative impact (a loss of possible utility gains) on the decision-maker [6]. G. Kirchgässner pointed out that this assumption is non-controversial for nearly all 'economic decisions', be it production decisions or consumption decisions. In such situations, there are strong incentives for individuals to behave rationally and self-interestedly. However, once the economic model of behaviour is applied to other areas, this assumption is no longer non-controversial. In the political and judicial sphere, we find beside others the following two types of decisions:

i) decisions where the individual decision is irrelevant for the individual himself/herself and for all other individuals, but the collective decision is relevant for all individuals (Low-Cost Decision Type I), and
ii) decisions where the individual decision is irrelevant for the individual himself/herself, but it is highly relevant for other individuals (Low-Cost Decisions Type II) [6, 305–306].

We suppose that public policy decision making is related with maintenance sustainable development in order to achieve balance between economy, ecology and social spheres. We should take under the consideration that different stockholders can influence on public policy decision making. The key element of the public policy decision-making is interest of groups. There is little evidence of the concrete benefits that could be brought by interest groups' influence on decision making. In general, interest groups may improve policy-making by providing valuable knowledge and insight data on specific issues. They also represent interests which may be negatively and involuntarily impacted by a poorly deliberated public policy [8]. Moreover, as such groups keep track of legislative and regulatory processes, they also have an important role in holding government accountable [8]. For our theoretical framework we use the model based on Maira Martini "Influence interest of groups on policy making" which is presented on the Fig. 1.

Kiev International Institute of Sociology presented the Technical report about Expert survey of representatives of 6 target groups on their assessment of the use of products of key providers of policy research (think tanks) in Ukraine.

An expert survey of representatives of six target groups on their assessment of the use of products of key policy research providers (think tanks) in Ukraine.

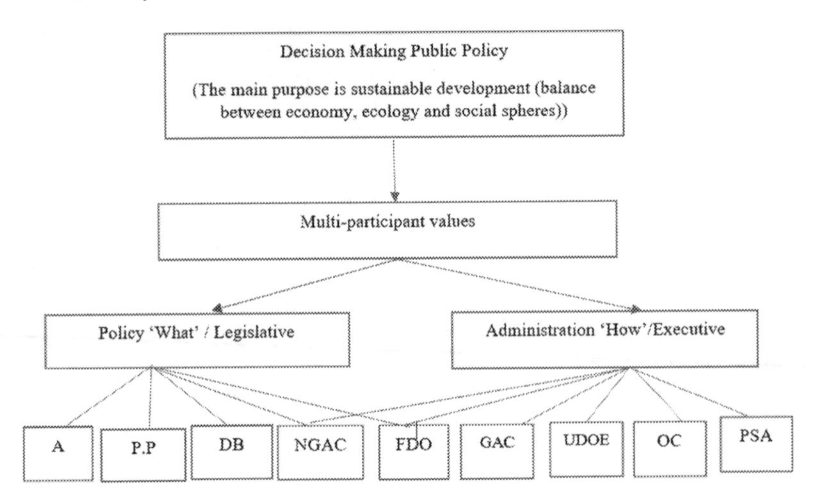

Fig. 1. Theoretical model

Where:

A	Authorities influence on formation of state policy and approving of management decisions
P.P	Political parties influence on formation of state policy and approving of management decisions
DB	Domestic business influence on formation of state policy and approving of management decisions
GAC	Government analytical center influence on formation of state policy and approving of management decisions
NGAC	Non-governmental analytical centers influence on formation of state policy and approving of management decisions
FDO	Foreign donor organizations / international technical assistance projects influence on formation of state policy and approving of management decisions
UDOE	Ukrainian donor organizations and foundations influence on formation of state policy and approving of management decisions
OC	Ordinary citizens influence on formation of state policy and approving of management decisions
PSA	Participants of street actions influence on formation of state policy and approving of management decisions.

2.1 Sample and Descriptive Statistics

Sample size: 240 scheduled interviews were conducted with respondents of 6 categories (groups), namely (Table 1):

1) decision makers (deputies) - 40 respondents;
2) representatives of executive bodies - 40 respondents;
3) scientists - 20 respondents;
4) representatives of non-governmental organizations - 60 respondents;

5) media representatives - 45 respondents;
6) representatives of business associations - 35 respondents

There is an important question: In what way according to you the mentioned above parties in interest would influence on formation of state policy and approving of management decisions?

Table 1. Measurement of the impact

Do not affect at all	Rather not affected	It is difficult to say for sure whether they affect or not	Rather affect	Very influential	It's hard to say / I don't know
1	2	3	4	5	6

We can indicate the following demographics of our study, shown in Table 2. In general, the average age of respondents was 39 years, ranging from 23 to 61. The average age of male and female is 39.

Table 2. Descriptive Statistics

Statistics	N	Mean	St. Dev.	Min	Pctl (25)	Pctl (75)	Max
ID.	240	120.500	69.426	1	60.8	180.2	240
Age	240	39.388	8.147	23	34	45	61
Gender	240	0.506	0.501	0.000	0.000	1.000	1.000
A	240	4.362	1.202	1	4	5	6
P.P	240	3.767	1.126	1	3	5	6
DB	240	3.746	1.112	1	3	5	6
GAC	240	3.096	1.041	1	2	4	6
NGAC	240	2.679	1.125	1	2	3	6
FDO	240	3.004	1.163	1	2	4	6
UDOE	240	2.658	1.075	1	2	3	6
OC	240	1.842	1.082	1	1	2	6
PSA	240	2.392	1.184	1	2	3	6

The average age of the next groups is followed:

- business associators are 37
- deputies are 42
- executive powers are 42
- journalists are 36

- representatives of business associations are 37
- scientists are 43.

As stated, we have 9 attitudinal items in our survey.

3 Reliability of the Scales

First, we calculate the reliability of the scales measure by applying Cronbach's alpha. The threshold for reliability is conventional, meaning that Cronbach's alpha should be bigger or equal to 0.7. According to the obtained results Cronbach's raw alpha is 0.97 and the standardized measure is 0.97. This is high value. See more in Table 3, where it is clearly visible that dropping A and PSA will increase Cronbach's alpha and will meet the threshold. Variables are nicely distributed (see Fig. 2).

Table 3. Reliability if an item is dropped

	raw alpha	std. Alpha	G6 (smc)	average r
A	0.97	0.97	0.97	0.80
P.P	0.96	0.97	0.97	0.78
DB	0.96	0.96	0.97	0.76
GAC	0.96	0.96	0.97	0.75
NGAC	0.96	0.96	0.97	0.76
FDO	0.96	0.96	0.97	0.76
UDOE	0.96	0.96	0.97	0.76
OC	0.97	0.97	0.97	0.79
PSA	0.96	0.96	0.97	0.77

3.1 Confirmatory Factor Analysis

At the next stage we decide to conduct confirmatory factor analysis and further to exploration of "good model fit" based optimal factor structure using modification indexes. We initiate our model estimation from M0 (Fig. 1). The fit statistics in Table 4 for model M0 suggest to revise and modify the final model. We report the following model fit characteristics: Chi-square (cut-off value $p < 0.05$); the Comparative Fit Index (CFI), which compares the fit of a target model to the fit of the null model (the target cut-off value CFI > 0.90); and the Root Mean Square Error of Approximation (RMSEA), where values close to 0 represent a good fit.

According to the theoretical model we assume that Factor Administration includes such items as GAC, NGAC, FDO, OC, PSA and UDOE. Factor Policy includes such items as A, P.P, NGAC, FDO and DB. Based on results fit statistics we can see that coefficient Chi-square (cut-off value $p < 0.05$); the Comparative Fit Index (CFI), which

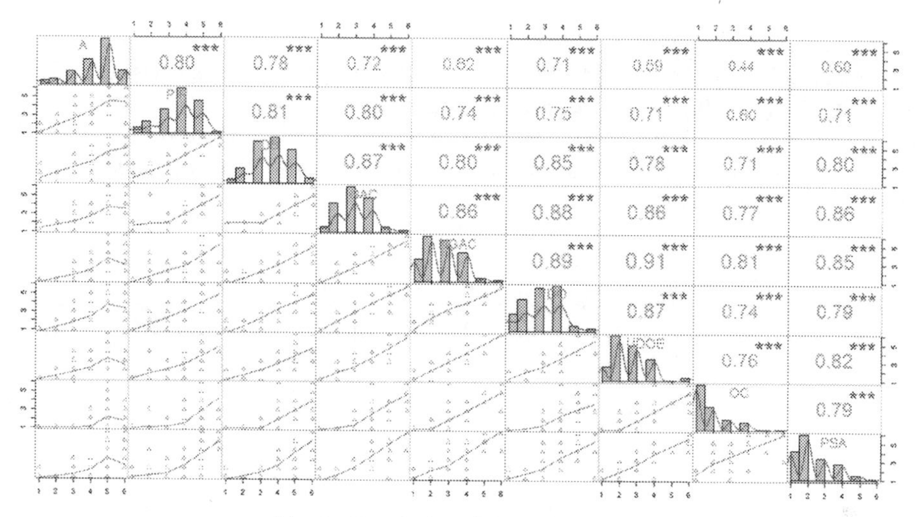

Fig. 2. Correlation of observable items

Table 4. Model fit statistics: comparison of CFA (M0) and CFA (M1-M4)

Model	Chi2 (df, p)	CFI	TLI	RMESA (CI90)	Chi2(df)
M0: theoretical final	205,329 (24, .000)	0.937	0.905	0.177 (0.155–0.20)	
M1	330.304 (26, .000)	0.894	0.853	0.221 (0.200–0.242)	
M2	253.460 (26, .000)	0.921	0.890	0.191 (0,170–0,213)	
M3	330.304 (26, .000)	0.894	0,853	0.221 (0.200–0.0.242)	
M4 (the best results from iteration) – EFA model	181.43 (19, .000)	0.940	0.910	0.165 (0.150–0.20)	23.902***(5)

compares the fit of a target model to the fit of the null model (the target cut-off value CFI > 0.90); and the Root Mean Square Error of Approximation (RMSEA), where values close to 0 shown that model represents good fit. Then we saw on the modification indexes and built the next model M1. According to this model Factor Administration includes such items as GAC, NGAC, FDO, OC, PSA and UDOE. Factor Policy includes such items as A, P.P, NDEO and DB. Based on results fit statistics we can see that all coefficients are less than in Theoretical model (M0). At the next stage we created the third model (M2). According to Model 2 Factor Administration includes such items as GAC, NGAC, FDO, OC, PSA, NDEO and UDOE. Factor Policy includes such items as A, P.P, and DB. The results of fit statistics also less than in theoretical model. Then we propose to form model based on principal components (M4). Due to Factor Administration includes such items as GAC, NGAC, FDO, OC, PSA, NDEO and UDOE. Factor Policy includes A, P.P and DB. So, we can see that this model performs the best fit statics (see Table 4). We make a decision that Model 4 is the final model, all with positive factor loadings (see Fig. 3). The highest loading has A (Authorities influence on formation of state policy and approving of management decisions).

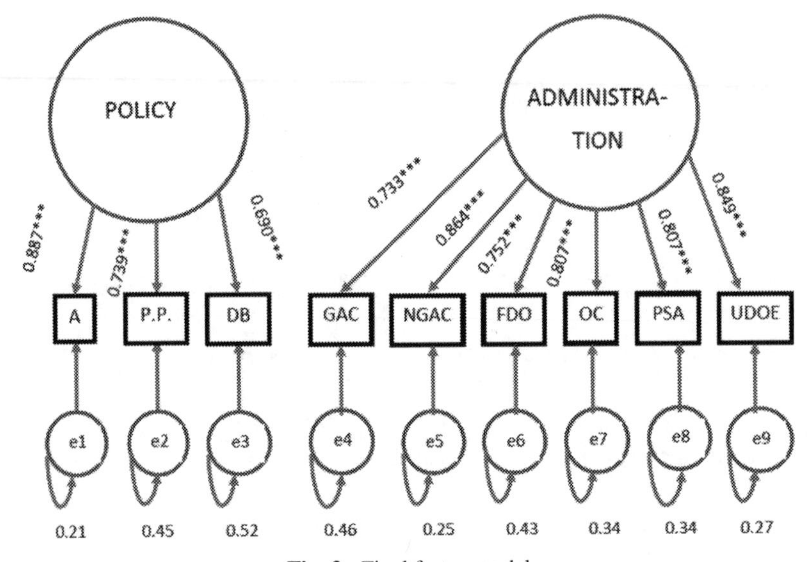

Fig. 3. Final factor model

Discussion. Based on the study, we can saw that the use of confirmatory factor analyses is very important in determining the influence of stakeholders on public policy decision-making such as helps us to determine whether the theoretical model "Public policy decision making" proposed by authors to clarify connections between variables. However, this approach has some limitations (i.e. data formation requires to form groups with an equal number of participants).

4 Conclusion

The results of the study showed that the use of Likert data is a very important element in research. In this case, it allowed us to understand who influences decision-making. It is worth noting that we obtained quite interesting results based on using the method of principal components and confirmatory factor analyses. The application of existing modeling tools helped us to determine the factor loads and assess the significance of the obtained models for choosing the best appropriate model. We saw that there is the strong covariance between latent factors Policy and Administrative. This investigation shown that Authorities, Political parties and Domestic business strong legislative influence on formation of state policy and approving of management decisions. On the other hand, Government analytical centers, non-governmental analytical centers, foreign donor organizations, Ukrainian donor organizations, ordinary citizens, participants of street actions executively influence on formation of state policy and approving of management decisions.

References

1. Averkyna, M.: Situation similarity calculus based modeling of decision-making processes in Urban transportation management. Doctoral Thesis in Management, Estonian Business School, Tallinn (2023)
2. Averkyna, M.: Theoretical Aspects of the Local Government's Decision-Making Process. In: Ahram, T.Z., Karwowski, W., Kalra, J. (eds.) AHFE 2021. LNNS, vol. 271, pp. 107–115. Springer, Cham (2021). https://doi.org/10.1007/978-3-030-80624-8_14
3. Arrow, K.A.: Difficulty in the Concept of Social Welfare. J. Polit. Econ. **58**(4), 328–346 (1950)
4. Baron, J.: Biases in the quantitative measurement of values for public decisions. Psychol. Bull. **122**, 72–88 (1997)
5. Firth, L.J.: Role of values in public decision-making: where is the fit? Impact Assess. Proj. Appraisal **16**(4), 325–329 (1998)
6. Kirchgässner, G.: Towards a theory of low-cost decisions. Eur. J. Polit. Econ. **8**(2), 305–320 (1992)
7. Local government policy-making processal: Municipal research & services center of Washington (1999)
8. Martini, M.: Influence of interest groups on policy-making, u4.no (2012)
9. Mintrom, M., Herbert Simon, A.: Oxford Handbooks (2016)
10. Papadakis, V., Barwise, P.: Strategic decisions. Kluwer, Boston (1998)

An Analytical Study of Traffic Accidents in Connecticut, USA Using Python

Prudhvinath Reddy Sureddy, Saifuddin Mohammed, Venkata Sai Veerendranath Magathala, Yamuna Koppala, and Samah Senbel(✉)

Sacred Heart University, Fairfield, CT, USA
{sureddyp2,mohammeds21,magathalav, koppalaY}@mail.sacredheart.edu, senbels@sacredheart.edu

Abstract. Amidst the growing traffic networks, the need for nuanced perspectives on traffic safety becomes increasingly apparent. Traffic patterns are affected by different factors in different parts of the world. This study focuses on the state of Connecticut, conducting a careful analysis of road accidents to discern patterns and trends affecting traffic accidents. Using a comprehensive dataset from the Connecticut Department of Transportation, we use Python and its data analytics libraries to unveil the dynamics shaping road safety in the state. We concentrated on five different aspects of a car accident: frequency of accidents, spatial distribution of accidents in the different towns, the time of day of the accident, the distribution of vehicle colors, and age demographics among vehicle proprietors. Our findings show that some of these factors in our analysis are unique to the state of Connecticut while other show a following of general trends in the USA and the world. By showing the specific dynamics of the state, we lay the groundwork for state-targeted methods and strategies to minimize traffic accidents. This would potentially lead to a safer traffic landscape in the future.

Keywords: Road Accidents · Data Analytics · Python · Traffic paterns · Road safety

1 Introduction

The contemporary landscape of urban living is defined by relentless urbanization and continuous advancements in transportation technologies. In this dynamic era, understanding the intricacies of vehicular dynamics takes center stage, with a heightened emphasis on unraveling the key determinants of traffic accidents. As the symbiotic relationship between technology, societal behaviors, and vehicular trends evolves, there is an escalating demand for data-driven insights that can decode the underlying patterns shaping road safety [8]. This paper embarks on a meticulous exploration of traffic accidents in the state of Connecticut. The goal is to discover the layers of complexity inherent in traffic incidents, with a particular focus on vehicle characteristics, weather effect, time of day, driver age, insurance dynamics, and the broader contextual landscape of vehicular mishaps. We aim to discover the unique pattern of traffic accidents in the state of Connecticut, and compare it to USA and global trends.

K. Daimi and A. Al Sadoon (Eds.): ACR 2024, LNNS 956, pp. 38–46, 2024.
https://doi.org/10.1007/978-3-031-56950-0_4

By scrutinizing the dataset with rigor, conducting sophisticated analyses, and employing strategic visualizations, our endeavor is to distill meaningful insights that not only illuminate current trends but also provide a solid foundation for informed policymaking [12]. Beyond this, we aim to contribute to intervention strategies and drive scholarly advancements within the realm of transportation and public safety. Through this research, we seek to enrich the discourse surrounding traffic safety by offering a comprehensive understanding of the multifaceted factors influencing vehicular incidents.

For temporal analysis, our work utilizes Python code to conduct an extensive analysis of road traffic accidents in Connecticut, focusing on the months of January and June for the years 2019 and 2022. The initial component of the analysis involves a temporal examination of road traffic accidents, specifically in the months of January and June. By leveraging the Pandas library, the code loads and preprocesses accident data from data files for these specific months and years.

The multi-faceted analysis, presented through interactive visualizations and numerical summaries, provides a nuanced understanding of how the frequency of accidents has evolved over time. To further enhance the temporal analysis, the code explores daily accident trends by hour. Through line plots, we illustrate how the number of accidents varies throughout the day, offering insights into peak hours of accident occurrence [6]. This temporal granularity aids in identifying patterns that may be influenced by factors such as commuting patterns, weather conditions, or enforcement measures.

This work also introduces a town-wise analysis, presenting the distribution of accidents across different towns. By combining data from both January and June, the code creates insightful visualizations, highlighting towns with the highest and lowest accident frequencies. This town-wise breakdown provides a localized perspective, assisting policymakers and local authorities in prioritizing interventions based on geographical accident hotspots. The Python code presented here offers a holistic exploration of road traffic accidents in Connecticut, unraveling temporal, spatial, and intersection-related patterns. The integration of data visualization libraries such as Matplotlib, Seaborn, and Geopandas enhances the interpretability of the findings. This comprehensive analysis provides a valuable foundation for evidence-based policymaking, allowing stakeholders to formulate targeted interventions aimed at improving road safety. Moreover, the code serves as a versatile framework that can be adapted for similar analyses in different regions, contributing to a broader understanding of the complex dynamics of road traffic accidents.

The paper is organized as follows: Sect. 2 summarizes relevant research in traffic pattern analysis, Sect. 3 describes our methodology for obtaining, organizing, cleaning, and processing our dataset. Section 4 shows our results of the analysis of seven different aspects of traffic accidents factors, and Sect. 5 concludes the paper.

2 Background

The study of traffic accidents has long been a focal point in transportation research, with scholars extensively examining the multifaceted factors that contribute to road safety challenges. Notably, seasonal variations have emerged as a recurrent theme in this literature. Research by Ashraf et al. [1] and Bao et al. [2] has underscored the influence of weather conditions, particularly during winter months, on both the frequency and severity of accidents. This emphasis aligns with the scope of our research, which homes in on the month of January, marked by adverse weather in Connecticut. Fritz et al. [6] also studied the time-of-day factor in accident analysis and the effect of daylight-saving time on accidents. By investigating the interplay between climatic factors and accident patterns, we aim to contribute nuanced insights to the broader discussion on mitigating the impact of seasonal variations on road safety.

As car accidents depend on different environmental and road design factor, Mohamed [8] and Buehler [4] both did a comparative analysis of accidents in the USA versus other countries in urban accidents with an emphasis on type of injuries and number of fatalities. Our research concentrates on one state in the northeast USA, the state of Connecticut.

Other factors affecting car accidents were studied as well: Sheykhfard [11] compared accident rates and type in urban versus rural roads, by concentrating on the pedestrian involved in those accidents. Östling [10] and Brühwiler [3] worked on predicting the occurrence of accidents based on different geospatial factors and driving trajectory. Ospina-Mateus [9] did a similar study but the concentration was on motorcycles and not regular cars.

3 Method

3.1 Data Collection

The data for this research was collected from the Connecticut Department of Transportation's records of traffic accidents that occurred during the January 2017 to June 2023 time period [5]. These records are comprehensive and include detailed information about each accident, making them a valuable source for understanding the dynamics of traffic incidents. The dataset encompasses a wide array of variables, providing insights into temporal, spatial, and contextual aspects of each accident.

3.2 Data Inspection

The initial phase of this study involves a meticulous inspection of the dataset, a comprehensive repository derived from real-world traffic observations. The dataset comprises key variables, including vehicle make, model year, colors, owner details, insurance expiration dates, and demographic information. Notably, during the inspection, we observed mixed data types in certain columns, prompting a conscientious approach to handle these variations effectively. The dataset's magnitude, boasting over a million entries, necessitates careful consideration of potential biases, missing values, and outliers that could impact the robustness of subsequent analyses. This scrutiny is particularly crucial given the diverse nature of the data, ranging from categorical information such as vehicle colors to numerical data like vehicle model years.

Upon closer examination, the dataset revealed some intriguing patterns. Noteworthy is the presence of mixed data types in certain columns, signifying potential challenges that need to be addressed during the preprocessing stage. Additionally, discrepancies in data completeness across columns, evident in variables like insurance expiration dates and owner details, underscore the need for a nuanced approach to data cleaning. This initial phase sets the foundation for subsequent analyses, ensuring that the insights derived are not only statistically sound but also reflective of the dataset's true nuances. As we navigate this trove of information, our commitment to data integrity and precision remains paramount to unveil accurate and meaningful insights into the dynamics of traffic incidents.

3.3 Data Cleaning and Preprocessing

In the wake of a comprehensive data inspection, the next critical step in our analysis involves data cleaning and processing to ensure the integrity and reliability of our findings. We used the Python coding language, the pandas and seaborn libraries in our work. One prominent issue identified during inspection pertains to the mixed data types present in certain columns, most notably in the 'Vehicle Model Year' and 'Month' columns. To address this, a careful conversion process is initiated, transforming these columns into appropriate data types. For 'Vehicle Model Year,' the conversion involves mapping the values to the nearest whole number, aligning with the nature of model years. Simultaneously, for the 'Month' column, we ensure a consistent format and datatype to facilitate subsequent temporal analyses.

Addressing missing values is another pivotal facet of our data cleaning endeavor. Given the substantial dataset size, our strategy involves meticulous handling of missing entries across columns, prioritizing preservation of data integrity. This includes leveraging appropriate imputation techniques tailored to the nature of each variable. For instance, in columns such as 'Insurance Expiration Date' and 'Owner City,' where missing values are prevalent, we employ strategies like forward-fill or backward-fill based on the context of the dataset to infer accurate information.

Furthermore, to enhance the interpretability of the dataset and facilitate downstream analyses, we introduce additional features. The 'Vehicle Color' column, originally denoting color abbreviations, is enriched by creating a new column, 'Vehicle Color Name,' where color abbreviations are mapped to their corresponding full names. This not only aids in clarity but also contributes to the visualizations that will follow. Overall, this meticulous data cleaning and processing phase aims not only to rectify inconsistencies and mitigate missing values but also to enrich the dataset for more robust exploratory analyses.

To facilitate a comparative temporal analysis between the winter and summer seasons, the dataset has been filtered to segregate accidents based on their occurrence in the month of January for winter and June for summer. This partitioning enables an in-depth examination of any discernible variations in accident patterns during these contrasting temporal contexts.

4 Results

4.1 Temporal Analysis

Table 1 shows the number of traffic accidents in a sample winter month (January) and a sample summer month (June). Two years were chosen from the dataset 2019 and 2022 to avoid the disruption of traffic during the pandemic period (2020–2021). Therefore, we have about 18,000 accidents in each sample month.

Table 1. Dataset Samples

Year	January Accidents	June Accidents
2019	9,166	9,417
2022	9,083	8,603
Total	18,249	18,020

The temporal analysis reveals interesting trends. In January, the number of crashes remained relatively stable, with a slight decrease from 9,166 in 2019 to 9,083 in 2022. However, June exhibited a more pronounced shift, with crashes dropping from 9,417 in 2019 to 8,603 in 2022. These findings suggest a potential variability in road safety dynamics, with January showing consistency over the years, while June experiences a notable reduction in crash incidents, perhaps due to decreased traffic in general after the pandemic.

4.2 Town-Wise Analysis

For this analysis we chose the five biggest cities in Connecticut and plotted their number of accidents in both January and June. Figure 1 shows the number of accidents for each town in January or June.

We observe from the chart that for big towns in general, there were more accidents in June than in January, except for the town of Waterbury, an industrial hub in the center of the state, where the June accidents far exceeds that of January.

4.3 Hourly Analysis

Figure 2 shows the distribution of accidents throughout the day for January (blue) and June (orange). We note that there is a slightly different traffic pattern for winter vs summer.

During the early hours there are more accidents in June, with a sharp rise during the morning rush hour. The trend is reversed after that with more January accidents during mid-day and the evening rush hour. This could be due to the difficult weather conditions and earlier sunset during the winter.

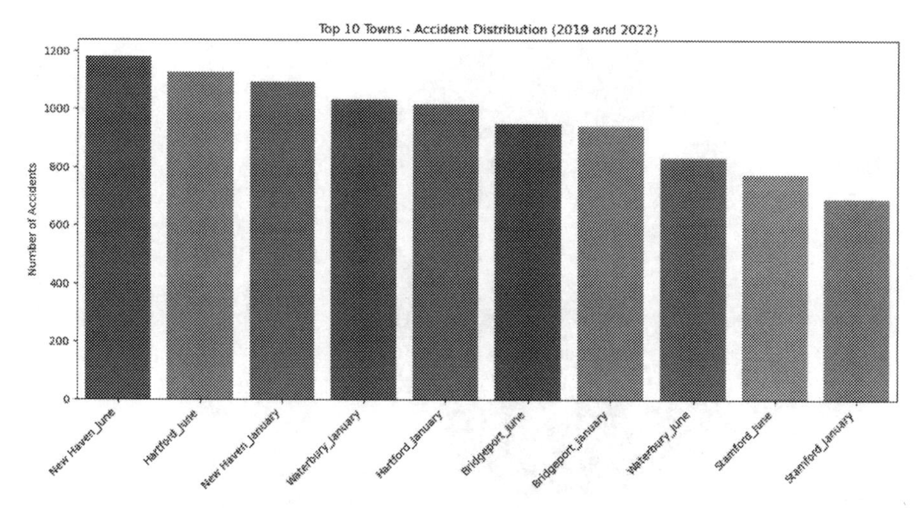

Fig. 1. Winter and summer accidents in major towns

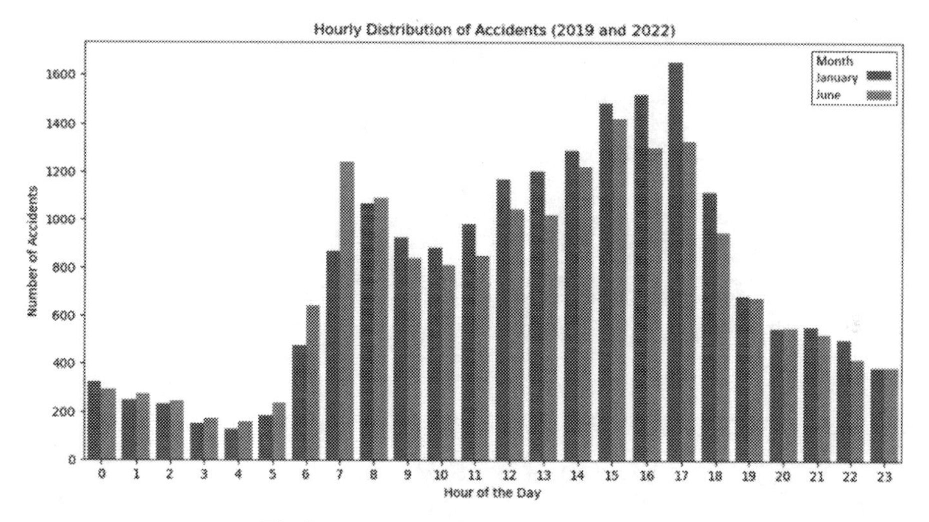

Fig. 2. Hourly distribution of car accidents

4.4 Vehicle Color Analysis

Figure 3 shows the colors of the vehicles involved in crashes in our dataset for all 6 years, as well as the overall percentage of each color in the dataset. The high percentage of red and blue colored vehicles is particularly interesting when compared with the popular car colors in the USA [13], shown in Table 2. Red and Blue cars account for about 50% of Connecticut car crashes colors, but only compose about 23% of colors used in cars in the USA.

While there is some alignment in the popularity of certain colors (White Black, and Gray), there are notable differences in rankings and the inclusion/exclusion of specific

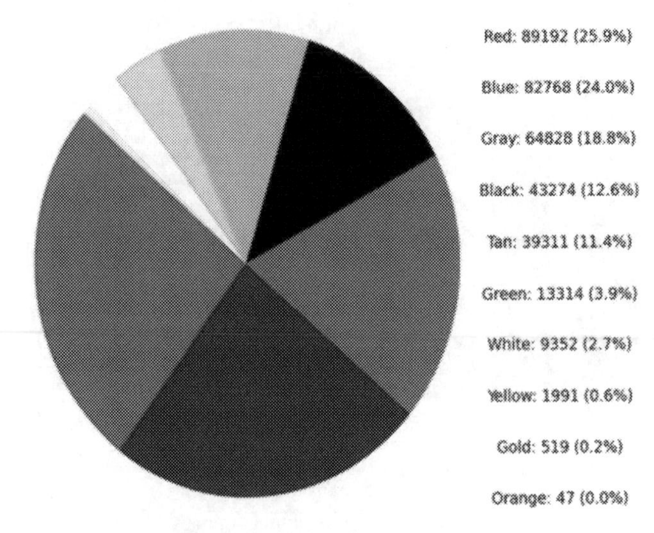

Fig. 3. Vehicle color percentages.

Table 2. Popular vehicle colors in the USA

Rank	Color	Percentage share
1	White	24.9%
2	Black	20%
3	Gray	19.2%
4	Silver	12.6%
5	Blue	10%
6	Red	9%
7	Brown	1.8%
8	Green	1.4%
9	Orange	0.6%
10	Gold	0.3%

colors between the Connecticut accident dataset and popular USA colors. These variations could be influenced by factors such as regional preferences or changes in consumer tastes over time.

4.5 Driver Age Analysis

Figure 4 shows the histogram of the age of the driver in the CT accident dataset. The largest group was the 15–30 age range with about 300,000 accidents. This is typical results for car crash driver ages [7]. It is important to note that this age group has the lowest percentage of car ownership, as shown in Table 3. Therefore, we can conclude that a significant percentage of the car crashes are made by someone who is young and may not be the owner of the vehicle.

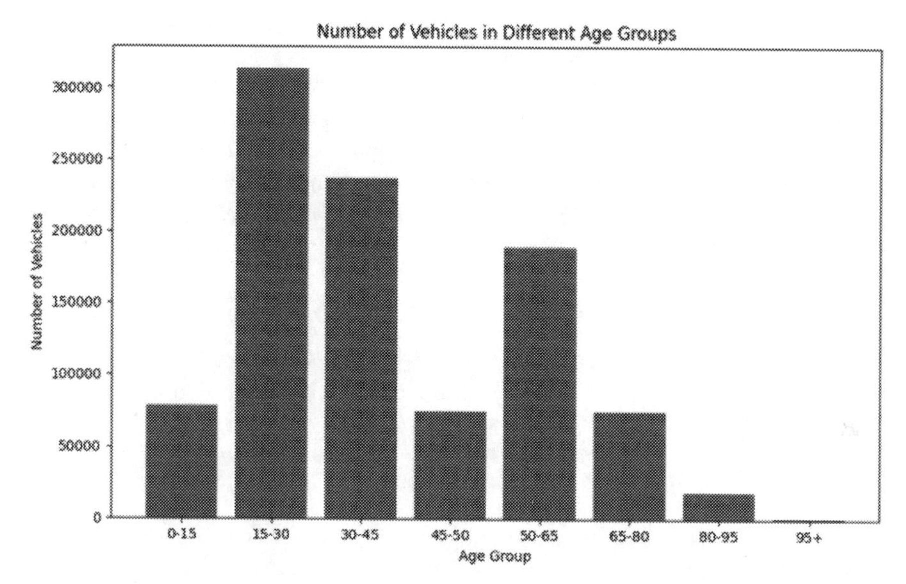

Fig. 4. Crash driver age in the Connecticut dataset

Table 3. Car ownership percentage in the USA in 2017

Age group	Percentage of cars owned
15–34	14%
34–44	14%
45–54	20%
55–64	25%
65 and older	27%

5 Conclusion

In this paper, we presented a comprehensive analysis of traffic accidents in the state of Connecticut in the period 2017–2023. The dataset was obtained from the official state of Connecticut accident registry, and it encompasses all aspects about an accident, from information about the location and type of accident to information about the driver and passengers, to vehicle model, maker, color, and model. Insurance information, weather information, and injury type is also recorded. Our analysis shows some interesting observations: There is little change in the number of accidents over the different seasons in the state overall, but inside bigger towns, there is a trend for more accidents in summer than in winter. Also, in the summer the peak accident time of day is between 5 and 6 pm, but earlier in the winter when it peaks at around 3 pm and another morning peak around 7 am. Also, it seems that cars with a color of blue or red have a higher rate of accidents proportional to their overall population percentage. While white cars, who are generally the most common color have a much lower accident number. An analysis of car crash accident driver age shows a peak in the age range 15–30, while the ownership percentage is typically low for that age range, which fits the general country trend. By understanding the specific dynamics at play in Connecticut, we lay the groundwork for targeted strategies that can navigate the intersection of crises and road safety effectively, fostering a safer and more resilient transportation landscape for the future.

References

1. Ashraf, I., Hur, S., Shafiq, M., Park, Y.: Catastrophic factors involved in road accidents: underlying causes and descriptive analysis. PLoS ONE **14**(10), e0223473 (2019)
2. Bao, W., Yu, Q., Kong, Y.: Uncertainty-based traffic accident anticipation with spatio-temporal relational learning. In: Proceedings of the 28th ACM International Conference on Multimedia, pp. 2682–2690 (2020)
3. Brühwiler, L., Fu, C., Huang, H., Longhi, L., Weibel, R.: Predicting individuals' car accident risk by trajectory, driving events, and geographical context. Comput. Environ. Urban Syst.. Environ. Urban Syst. **93**, 101760 (2022)
4. Buehler, R., Pucher, J.: The growing gap in pedestrian and cyclist fatality rates between the United States and the United Kingdom, Germany, Denmark, and the Netherlands, 1990–2018. Transp. Rev. **41**(1), 48–72 (2021)
5. Connecticut car crash repository. https://www.ctcrash.uconn.edu/. Accessed 27 Dec 2023
6. Fritz, J., VoPham, T., Wright, K.P., Vetter, C.: A chronobiological evaluation of the acute effects of daylight saving time on traffic accident risk. Curr. Biol.. Biol. **30**(4), 729–735 (2020)
7. Hamed, M.M., Al-Eideh, B.M.: An exploratory analysis of traffic accidents and vehicle ownership decisions using a random parameters logit model with heterogeneity in means. Anal. Methods Acid. Res. **25**, 100116 (2020)
8. Mohammed, A.A., Ambak, K., Mosa, A.M., Syamsunur, D.: A review of traffic accidents and related practices worldwide. Open Transp. J. **13**(1), 65–83 (2019)
9. Ospina-Mateus, H., Quintana Jiménez, L.A., Lopez-Valdes, F.J., Salas-Navarro, K.: Bibliometric analysis in motorcycle accident research: a global overview. Scientometrics **121**, 793–815 (2019)
10. Östling, M., Lubbe, N., Jeppsson, H., Puthan, P.. Passenger car safety beyond ADAS: defining remaining accident configurations as future priorities. In: Proceedings of 26th international technical conference on the enhanced safety of vehicles (ESV) (2019). https://bit.ly/2IHtHWV
11. Sheykhfard, A., Haghighi, F., Nordfjærn, T., Soltaninejad, M.: Structural equation modelling of potential risk factors for pedestrian accidents in rural and urban roads. Int. J. Inj. Contr. Saf. Promot.Saf. Promot. **28**(1), 46–57 (2020)
12. Zhang, J., et al.: Immediate effects of the COVID-19 pandemic on road safety in China: a nationwide cross-sectional study. Transp. Res. Part A: Gen. **136**, 334–342 (2020)
13. Zou, X., Vu, H.L., Huang, H.: Fifty years of accident analysis & prevention: a bibliometric and scientometric overview. Accid. Anal. Prev.. Anal. Prev. **144**, 105568 (2020)

Improving the Efficiency of Multimodal Approach for Chest X-Ray

Jiblal Upadhya[1(✉)], Jorge Vargas[2], Khem Poudel[3], and Jaishree Ranganathan[3]

[1] Computational and Data Science, Middle Tennessee State University, Murfreesboro, TN 37132, USA
ju2i@mtmail.mtsu.edu

[2] Department of Engineering Technology, Middle Tennessee State University, Murfreesboro, TN 37132, USA
jorge.vargas@mtsu.edu

[3] Department of Computer Science, Middle Tennessee State University, Murfreesboro, TN 37132, USA
{khem.poudel,jaishree.ranganathan}@mtsu.edu

Abstract. Medical data analysis with limited data has been a challenging problem in machine learning. Privacy regulations limit the sharing and use of patient data, making it challenging to access and aggregate large datasets for research purposes. To address this challenge, we propose a deep learning-based Multimodal network that incorporates data from multiple data sources: images, and text in the learning process. When faced with limited data of one type, incorporating data from multiple sources can enhance the model's performance and generalization. Our approach integrates the text sub-model and image sub-model with deep network of Dense 512 using the transfer learning process. Specifically, the goal is to explore the impact of hyperparameter adjustments on the performance of the model with different learning rates. Evaluation of our proposed approach on the Indiana University Chest X-ray dataset that consists of textual (radiological reports) and visual (X-ray images) show that our approach significantly outperforms several baseline methods in classification accuracy.

Keywords: Transfer Learning · Deep learning · Multimodal · Fusion · clinical data

1 Introduction

With the proliferation of machine learning in healthcare, we face numerous challenges due to the inherent characteristics of medical data, including its complexity, high dimensionality, and privacy concerns. One of these challenges involves medical data analysis in situations where data availability is limited. Privacy regulations often restrict the sharing and utilization of patient data, posing a formidable obstacle in the gathering and aggregating of substantial datasets for research objectives. This constraint critically impairs the training of robust

K. Daimi and A. Al Sadoon (Eds.): ACR 2024, LNNS 956, pp. 47–59, 2024.
https://doi.org/10.1007/978-3-031-56950-0_5

machine learning models, thereby undermining their performance and generalizability.

To mitigate the problem of data scarcity, this study presents a deep learning-based Multimodal network for medical data analysis. This innovative approach makes use of multiple data sources, including images and textual data, such as radiological reports, to improve the model's performance and adaptability in cases of data limitation.

The significance of our study lies in the incorporation of a Multimodal approach that provides a solution to the aforementioned data constraint issue in healthcare. We fuse an image sub-model, and a text sub-model via a deep network of Dense 512, leveraging transfer learning to enhance the model's efficiency and accuracy. This fusion of different modalities, such as text and image data, creates a more robust model capable of delivering superior results compared to the conventional, single modality approaches.

Our evaluation on the Indiana University Chest X-ray dataset [3], encompassing both textual and visual data, shows that our proposed method outperforms several baseline techniques in terms of classification accuracy. This research underscores the potential of Multimodal learning in addressing the shortage of data in the medical field, offering profound implications for future machine learning applications in healthcare.

Moreover, the societal impact of this research is worth noting. By improving the accuracy of disease classification, we can enhance the diagnostic process, thus potentially leading to better patient outcomes and an overall improvement in healthcare delivery.

While our findings are promising, the scarcity of data in medical analysis still remains a key challenge. This paper will further discuss these challenges, elaborate on our Multimodal deep learning approach, and provide a comprehensive evaluation of its performance in comparison to traditional approaches.

Our objective is to enhance the model's accuracy and effectiveness by implementing several modifications and optimizations. We explain the specific changes made to the Baseline model, highlighting the rationale behind each modification. Additionally, we conduct a comparative analysis by benchmarking the proposed model against the Baseline model [1]. Through our analysis, we aim to provide insights into the effectiveness of our enhancements and contribute to the ongoing research in the field of Multimodal learning and optimization.

2 Literature Review

Various researchers have worked on Multimodality healthcare data, like combining different image modalities, CT-scan and X-ray, CT-scan with MRI, or combining textual data like lab reports with medical imaging, etc., for disease identification [4,9,10,16]. The researchers mainly use two different medical imaging modalities to develop efficient disease identification approaches [13].

Mukhi et al. [15] suggested a deep learning classification strategy for COVID-19 detection in chest X-ray and CT scan modalities. Data was used from the

Kaggle repository to evaluate the models' efficacy. Following data preprocessing, CNN models based on deep learning are optimized and compared using measures of accuracy. Models under consideration include Xception, Inception v3, VGG-19, and ResNet-50. This study suggests that chest X-rays are more effective than CT scans at detecting lung cancer. High levels of accuracy in detecting COVID-19 were achieved using the fine-tuned VGG-19 model, as high as 94.17 for chest X-rays and 93 for CT scans. This study suggests that VGG-19 is the most effective model for detecting COVID-19 and that chest X-rays are more accurate for the model than CT scans.

Likewise, Moon et al. [14] proposed a Medical Vision Language Learner (MedViLL) with better generalizations across a range of vision-language tasks like detection, healthcare image-report extraction, and healthcare visual question answering using a BERT-based framework and a unique multimodal attention masked method.

Yu et al. [17] also suggested a Multimodal Multitask Deep Learning (MMDL) strategy for a content-based image retrieval system. Training on a multimodal database, the proposed method then learns semantic feature representations for each modality before mapping them into a common subspace. During testing, the query and database's similarities are scored using representations from the common subspace. The dataset used is the data from 227,835 investigations contained in the MIMIC Chest X-ray (MIMIC-CXR) dataset [7]. The findings show significant efficiency gains compared to a conventional single-mode approach, achieving an mAP of 0.541.

Otherwise, Jain et al. [6] presented RadGraph, a collection of relationships and entities in the entire text chest X-ray imaging reports that are extracted using an innovative information extraction schema. The MIMIC-CXR dataset's radiology reports have been annotated with 14,579 entities and 10,889 relations and released as a development dataset; the CheXpert dataset's 100 radiology reports have also been annotated and provided as a test dataset. In training and testing with these datasets, the deep learning model known as RadGraph Benchmark achieves F1 scores of 0.82 and 0.73, respectively, on relation extraction when applied to the MIMIC-CXR and CheXpert test sets.

On the other hand, Manocha & Bhatia [12] proposed a Deep Learning-based Multi-modal Data Analysis (DMDA) approach, which is developed to determine COVID-19 symptoms through the use of acoustic data like cough, breathing, and speech signals and image-based data, which is necessary for dealing with the complicated symptoms of COVID-19. In addition, the proposed Dynamic Fusion Strategy (DFS) receives the classified events in order to verify the patient's health state. It is highly reliable, with an accuracy of 95.64, even when testing without any of the data modalities.

Most of the research studies are divided into two categories, one that uses only images and the other using images, text, or sound. In the case of the first category, two different modalities like, CT-scan, X-ray are used to develop the healthcare model. In this case, mostly the problem solved is a diagnosis of covid19 or the classification of images to identify covid 19. However, in the second case, along with identifying of covid-19 patients, the other problems resolved are text-based image retrieval, automated report creation or generation from the medical images, and many more. Even a few researchers are using sound due to the limitation of open-source datasets. Most of the models developed using deep learning approaches, specifically transfer learning, i.e., pre-trained models due to the storage of the data available in the case of text and sounds (Fig. 1).

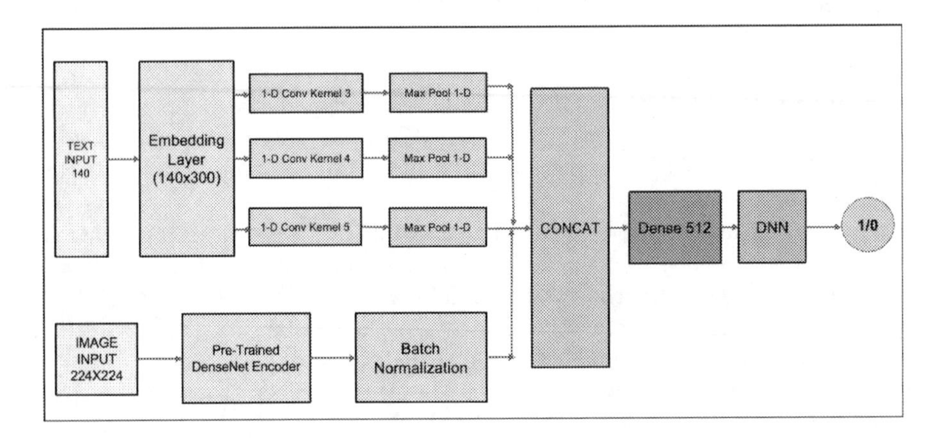

Fig. 1. Multi-Modal Architecture

3 Data

The Indiana University Chest X-ray collection, often referred to as IU-CXR [3], includes a comprehensive assortment of 7470 chest X-rays and 3955 corresponding radiological reports. Each report is linked to a set of two images that provide both a frontal and lateral view. The report itself is divided into various sections including Comparison, Indication, Findings, and Impression. The Comparison section evaluates the current study in relation to any past imaging studies of the same patient. The Indication section, on the other hand, provides crucial patient information such as age, gender, and any pertinent clinical details, encompassing existing ailments and symptoms. The Findings section gives an assessment of each part of the image, determining whether it's normal, abnormal, or possibly abnormal. Arguably the most significant part of the report is the Impression section. It summarizes the results, the patient's clinical history, and the study's rationale, which is crucial for medical decision-making.

4 Methods

Multimodal healthcare machine learning refers to the process of integrating and evaluating various forms of data, such as medical images and clinical text, using advanced machine learning algorithms [2]. By combining multiple modalities, this technique offers a more comprehensive sight of patient health and permits a wider understanding of complex medical situations. The synergy between image and text data allows for a more accurate and holistic analysis of disease diagnosis, prognosis, medicine recommendations, and patient supervision [11].

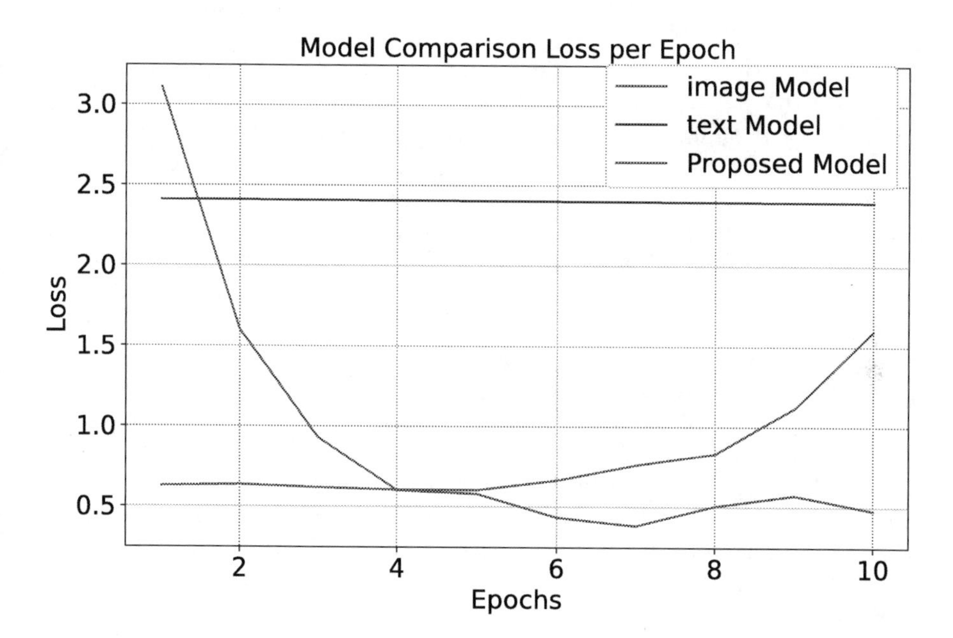

Fig. 2. Validation loss comparing each text, image and proposed model

The implication of multi-modal healthcare machine learning rests in its capability to modify the healthcare prospect. By efficiently integrating image and text records, healthcare experts can make more informed choices, individualize treatment plans, and ameliorate patient care. This extensive approach has the potential to boost disease identification, empower early interruption, optimize resource allocation, and eventually contribute to better healthcare results.
In this present work, we are adopting the Text and Image submodel architecture from [1], with considerable changes in the hyperparameter optimization strategy. Also, we are experimenting with only 3000 samples of data, which helps to understand how with less data, model performance can be improved or not. We acknowledge that the Class Imbalance is an important factor for medical data analysis. But due to the resource limitations and the computational constraints that we encountered during our study, this is not considered.

4.1 Image Submodel

The concept of transfer learning serves as the driving force for the Image submodal. We pretrained a variety of encoders (VGG, DenseNet, ResNet, etc.)

using ImageNet and ChestX-ray14 dataset from the National Health Institutes. Because of better classification performance, we selected the DenseNet121 model [5] to serve as the encoder. This encoder is then fed into a simple batch normalization which is then fed into a decoder for binary classification.

4.2 Text Submodel

Indiana University Chest X-ray dataset [3] was used for this experiment which consists of the radiological reports in the form of text data corresponding to the frontal and lateral views of the chest X-ray images of a patient. In this text submodel, we opted for a text classifier based on Convolutional Neural Network (CNN) as described by [8] due to elegance in classifying the sentences of the reports. Both static and non-static versions of the CNN model were tested which was built on top of `word2vec`. In the static version, word vectors are kept static and are not fine-tuned, while in the non-static version, they are fine-tuned during training. Our text classifier able to classify the abstract labels like findings, impressions, or conditions that can be identified in a chest X-ray which are derived from the textual contents of the radiological reports.

The final design of the text classifier employs pre-existing embedding layers that are specifically tailored to the text dataset being categorized. These embeddings are fed separately to Kernels used in the 1-D CNN, which are of length 3, 4, and 5. A kernel is a set of weights that the network learns to apply to input data. These weights help the model extract relevant features from the input. In a 1-D CNN used for text, the kernel length of 3 would look at three-word sequences (trigrams), a kernel of length four would look at four-word sequences (4-grams), and so on. Using different kernel lengths can help the model pick up on different language patterns. The outputs of the 1-D Conv layers are then passed to separate Max Pooling 1-D layers before concatenating. Finally, the output is fed into a decoder containing the Dense 512 layer and Deep Neural Network for the downstream classification task.

4.3 Multimodal Fusion Techniques

Multimodal fusion techniques play a crucial role in integrating image and text data for multimodal healthcare machine learning. These techniques aim to combine the complementary information from different modalities to enhance the overall performance and understanding of the data. Early fusion techniques combine the data from different modalities at the input level. These methods aim to merge the modalities' information into a single representation, allowing for joint processing and analysis. Concatenation-based fusion involves concatenating the features from different modalities into a single vector. This approach creates a unified representation that incorporates both the image and text data. By concatenating the features, the resulting fused representation preserves the information from all modalities.

The focal point of multimodal architecture, which incorporates a Text submodal and an Image submodal, both heavily leverage transfer learning. The

Text submodal is crafted by harnessing the network layers - from input layers to feature vectors - of a pre-existing text classifier. In a similar fashion, the Image submodal is constructed using the network layers of a trained image classifier, ranging from the input layers to the feature vectors.

Following this, the text and image feature vectors that have been encoded are merged into a singular, flattened feature vector. This integrated feature vector is then forwarded to a densely interconnected decoder for binary classification. The application of transfer learning to these two encoders enables the multimodal architecture to function effectively even with limited datasets, such as those below 3K. The transposed text and image encoders comprise the pre-trained embedding and residual layers. These pretrained encoders are then subtly refined using low learning rates.

4.4 Modification for Enhanced Comparison

In this work, significant changes were made to the code format to enable training the model with various learning rates. This modification allows for a more comprehensive comparison and a greater overview of the model's performance under different settings.

By introducing different learning rates during the training process, we can systematically explore the model's behavior and evaluate its robustness and adaptability. This approach helps in identifying the optimal learning rate that yields the best results in terms of convergence speed, accuracy, and generalization.

4.5 Model Improvement

In our proposed model, significant enhancements have been made to the Text submodal and training parameters aimed at improving the model's performance and generalization capabilities. The following sections outline the specific improvements and their rationale:

A notable improvement in the text sub-model involves adjusting the L2 regularization parameter in the create channel function for the (CNN) layer. Specifically, the regularization parameter has been increased from 0.03 to 0.1 indicated by the modification `regularizers.l2(0.1)`. The increase in the regularization strength aims to prevent overfitting and enhance the model's ability to generalize to unseen data. By imposing a higher penalty on the model's weights, larger weight values are discouraged, leading to simpler and more robust models. This adjustment helps in reducing the risk of over-relying on specific features in the text sub-model, promoting a more balanced representation.

4.6 Training Parameters

Another crucial modification lies in the training parameters, specifically the dropout rate after the first Dense layer. The dropout rate has been increased from 0.3 to 0.5, represented by `x = Dropout(.5)(x)`. Increasing the dropout rate introduces a stronger regularization effect during training. By randomly dropping a larger fraction of the learned features, the model becomes less reliant on any particular set of features and learns more robust representations. This adjustment aids in mitigating overfitting and improves the model's ability to generalize to unseen data, resulting in enhanced performance.

4.7 Output Activation Function

In our proposed model, a notable change has been made to the activation function of the final output layer. Instead of using softmax, the activation function has been switched to sigmoid, as indicated by `out = Dense(1, activation='sigmoid')(x)`. Since the task at hand appears to be a binary classification, with a single output dimension representing the probability of the positive class, the sigmoid activation function is more suitable. The sigmoid function maps the output to a range between 0 and 1, allowing for intuitive interpretation as a probability. This adjustment ensures the model's output is aligned with the desired classification task, enhancing its suitability and performance.

5 Model Evaluation Metrics

To assess the performance of the improved model, various evaluation metrics, including loss, accuracy, F1 score, and recall, have been calculated for each learning rate separately. These metrics are then stored in a metrics dictionary for

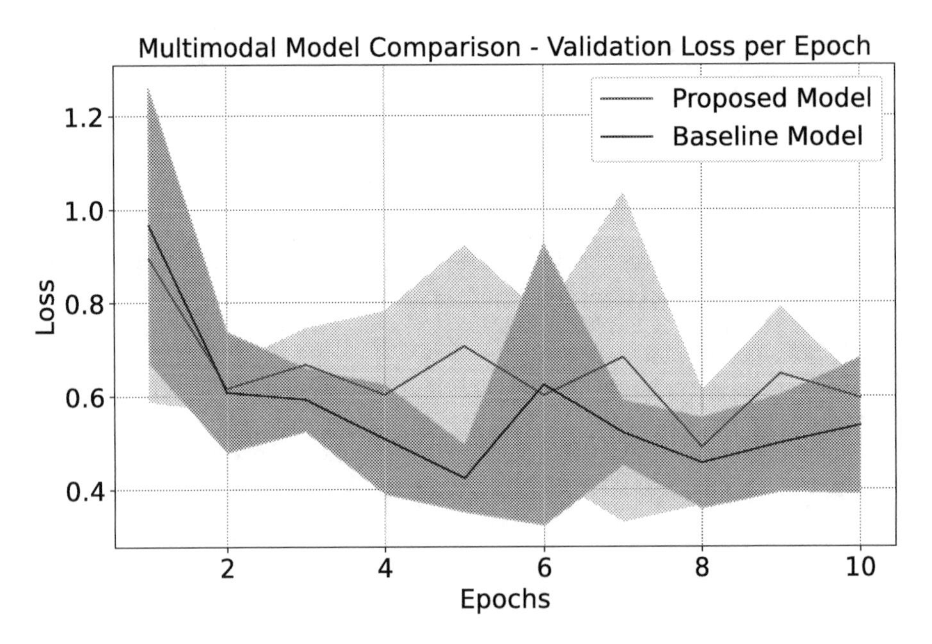

Fig. 3. Comparison of Validation loss per epoch for Baseline and Proposed Model

further analysis and comparison. By tracking and comparing the metrics for different learning rates, a comprehensive analysis of the model's performance can be obtained. This enables informed decision-making and facilitates the selection of the optimal learning rate that yields the best results. The evaluation metrics serve as valuable indicators to measure the model's effectiveness and guide further improvements (Fig. 3).

6 Results and Discussion: Proposed Model vs Baseline Model

The proposed model exhibits significant enhancements compared to the Baseline model. In terms of accuracy, the proposed model demonstrates a notable improvement, showcasing its ability to make more accurate predictions. Ablation studies has been performed to know the individual contributions of the text and image models with increase in the overall classification accuracy ranging from 4% to 12% on average of 20 epochs. As shown in Fig. 2, the superior performance of our proposed Multimodal compared to two baseline models which are individual text model and image model on Indiana University dataset tuned with low learning rate ranging from 0.001, 0.0005 to 0.0001. Similarly, the model's F1 score showcases a substantial increase, indicating a better balance between precision and recall. Moreover, the improved model achieves a commendable recall rate, indicating its effectiveness in capturing positive instances. Overall, the enhancements made to the model have resulted in substantial improvements across multiple evaluation metrics, surpassing the performance of the Baseline model (Figs. 4, 5 and 6).

The changes made to the text sub-model included adjusting the L2 regularization parameter, while the image sub-model remained unchanged. Training parameters were also modified, such as increasing the dropout rate. The evaluation of the proposed model revealed significant enhancements across multiple metrics compared to the original model. The applied modifications successfully improved the model's performance, showcasing the benefits of strategic changes in building Multimodal learning models. These findings contribute to the advancement of image and text classification tasks. The comparison with the Baseline models further demonstrated the superiority of the improved model. The improvements resulted in higher F1 score, accuracy, and recall values, indicating better performance (Fig. 7).

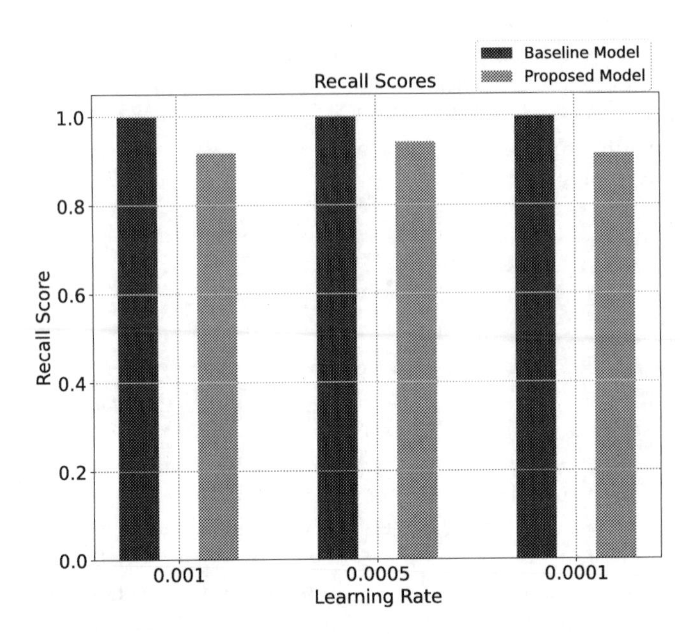

Fig. 4. Recall Score for the comparisons of the models for three learning rates: 0.001, 0.0005, 0.0001

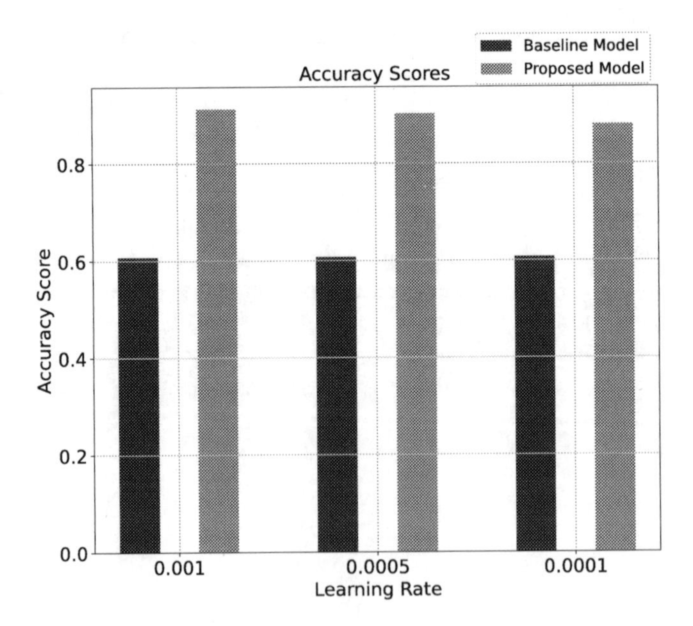

Fig. 5. Accuracy Score for the comparisons of the models for three learning rates: 0.001, 0.0005, 0.0001

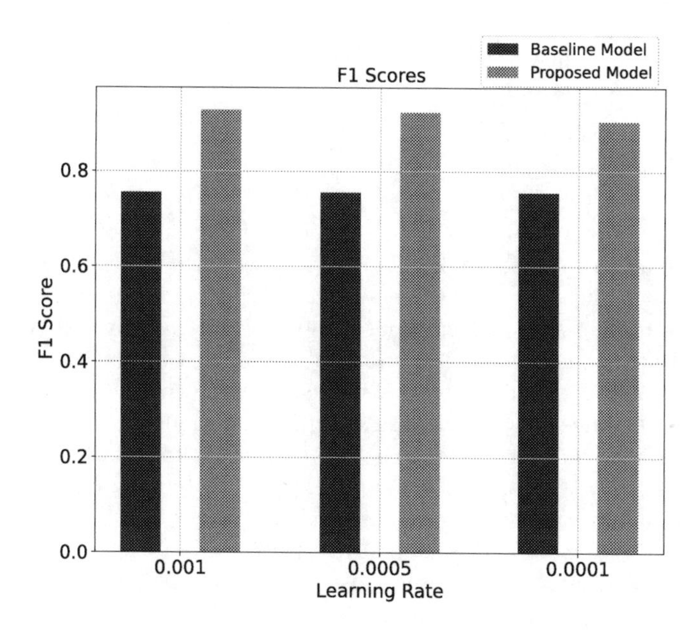

Fig. 6. F1 Score for the comparisons of the models for three learning rates: 0.001, 0.0005, 0.0001

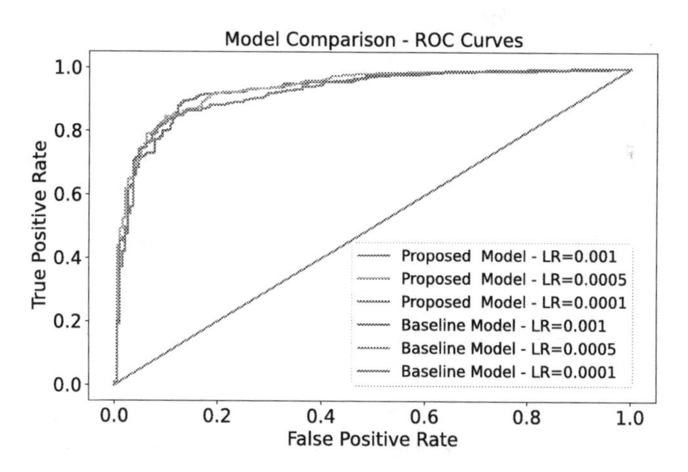

Fig. 7. ROC Curve for Proposed model

The ROC curve analysis further illustrates the superiority of the Proposed model over the Baseline model. The proposed model exhibits a higher area under the ROC curve, indicating its superior ability to discriminate between positive and negative instances. On the other hand, the baseline model shows consistent ROC curves across the three learning rates, suggesting that its predictive performance remains unchanged regardless of the learning rate. This comparison clearly demonstrates that the improvements made to the model have substantially enhanced its ability to classify instances accurately and distinguish between positive and negative cases.

7 Conclusion

We present an improved framework for Multimodal learning with the hyperparameters tuning strategy through different learning rates. The experiments show promising results in improving the classification performance in the validation data. Also, the evaluation of the proposed model on the test data shows that the proposed Multimodal framework performed better in comparison to the baseline model. In our experiments, we achieved an accuracy of 88% compared to the baseline model, which was around 63%. Multimodal models offer the promise of enhanced explainability by leveraging complementary information from different modalities, but they also pose unique challenges. In the present context, it is evident that different conditions obtained from the Chest X-ray data using our image and text sub-models helped to identify those abstract labels in the classification of images. Our evaluations on the test data give us the binary classification result as normal or abnormal images of a patient.

We plan to explore multi label classification problem with different data fusion techniques, such as early fusion, late fusion, and sketching, to enhance the model's performance further.

References

1. Aydin, F., Zhang, M., Ananda-Rajah, M., Haffari, G.: Medical multimodal classifiers under scarce data condition. arXiv preprint arXiv:1902.08888 (2019)
2. Baltrušaitis, T., Ahuja, C., Morency, L.P.: Multimodal machine learning: a survey and taxonomy. IEEE Trans. Pattern Anal. Mach. Intell. **41**(2), 423–443 (2018)
3. Demner-Fushman, D., et al.: Preparing a collection of radiology examinations for distribution and retrieval. J. Am. Med. Inform. Assoc. **23**(2), 304–310 (2016)
4. Hadjiyski, N., Vosoughi, A., Wismueller, A.: Cross modal global local representation learning from radiology reports and x-ray chest images. arXiv preprint arXiv:2301.10951 (2023)
5. He, K., Zhang, X., Ren, S., Sun, J.: Deep residual learning for image recognition. In: Proceedings of the IEEE Conference on Computer Vision and Pattern Recognition, pp. 770–778 (2016)
6. Jain, S., et al.: Radgraph: extracting clinical entities and relations from radiology reports. arXiv preprint arXiv:2106.14463 (2021)
7. Johnson, A.E., et al.: Mimic-CXR, a de-identified publicly available database of chest radiographs with free-text reports. Sci. Data **6**(1), 317 (2019)
8. Kim, Y.: Convolutional neural networks for sentence classification. arXiv preprint arXiv:1408.5882 (2014)
9. Kline, A., et al.: Multimodal machine learning in precision health: a scoping review. NPJ Digit. Med. **5**(1), 171 (2022)
10. Kohankhaki, M., Ayad, A., Barhoush, M., Leibe, B., Schmeink, A.: Radiopaths: deep multimodal analysis on chest radiographs. In: 2022 IEEE International Conference on Big Data (Big Data), pp. 3613–3621. IEEE (2022)

11. Lopez, K., Fodeh, S.J., Allam, A., Brandt, C.A., Krauthammer, M.: Reducing annotation burden through multimodal learning. Front. Big Data **3**, 19 (2020)
12. Manocha, A., Bhatia, M.: A novel deep fusion strategy for COVID-19 prediction using multimodality approach. Comput. Electr. Eng. **103**, 108, 274 (2022)
13. Meedeniya, D., Kumarasinghe, H., Kolonne, S., Fernando, C., De la Torre Díez, I., Marques, G.: chest x-ray analysis empowered with deep learning: a systematic review. Appl. Soft Comput. 109319 (2022)
14. Moon, J.H., Lee, H., Shin, W., Kim, Y.H., Choi, E.: Multi-modal understanding and generation for medical images and text via vision-language pre-training. IEEE J. Biomed. Health Inform. **26**(12), 6070–6080 (2022)
15. Mukhi, S.E., Varshini, R.T., Sherley, S.E.F.: Diagnosis of COVID-19 from multimodal imaging data using optimized deep learning techniques. SN Comput. Sc. **4**(3), 212 (2023)
16. Singh, S., Karimi, S., Ho-Shon, K., Hamey, L.: From chest x-rays to radiology reports: a multimodal machine learning approach. In: 2019 Digital Image Computing: Techniques and Applications (DICTA), pp. 1–8. IEEE (2019)
17. Yu, Y., Hu, P., Lin, J., Krishnaswamy, P.: Multimodal multitask deep learning for x-ray image retrieval. In: de Bruijne, M., et al. (eds.) MICCAI 2021, Part V. LNCS, vol. 12905, pp. 603–613. Springer, Cham (2021). https://doi.org/10.1007/978-3-030-87240-3_58

Wrist Crack Classification Using Deep Learning and X-Ray Imaging

Biswaranjan Senapati[1](✉), Awad Bin Naeem[2], Muhammad Imran Ghafoor[3], Vivek Gulaxi[4], Friban Almeida[5], Manish Raj Anand[6], Saroopya Gollapudi[7], and Chandra Jaiswal[8]

[1] Parker Hannifin Corp, Chicago, USA
BSENAPATI@ualr.edu
[2] National College of Business Administration and Economics, Multan, Pakistan
[3] Pakistan Television Corporation, Lahore, Pakistan
[4] Publix Corporation, Lakeland, USA
[5] Computer Science Department Inc., Wilmington, USA
[6] Medline Pharmaceuticals, Waukegan, USA
[7] Deloitte Consulting LLP, New York, USA
[8] Hanes Brands Inc., Winston-Salem, USA

Abstract. Wrist cracks are the most prevalent kind of crack and have a high incidence rate. Although wrist cracks are often identified with X-ray medical imaging, the portrayal of cracks may sometimes provide issues. Wrist cracks are common in humans' wrist bones as a result of unintentional traumas like sliding. Many hospitals lack qualified specialists to identify wrist cracks. As a result, an automated method is necessary to lessen the strain on physicians while also identifying cracks. A CNN model for detecting wrist cracks obtained 0.98 accuracy, surpassing competitors, minimizing erroneous diagnoses and saving time in clinician assistance.

Keywords: Wrist Cracks · VGG16 · VGG19 · Image processing · CNN

1 Introduction

A bone fracture occurs when a strong force is applied to a bone. Trauma, osteoporosis, and overuse may all lead to bone fractures [1]. According to recent (WHO) research, a fracture affects a large number of individuals, and the repercussions of an untreated fracture may result in serious harm or even death [2]. Wrist fractures are a rather frequent ailment, with positive instances growing daily. Accidents, such as sliding over with an extended hand, may result in wrist fractures [3]. Weak bone looks to shatter more quickly in osteoporosis. Numerous cases need the examination of fractures by healthcare personnel. Inexperienced clinicians, physical weariness, diversions, poor observation settings, and time restrictions all contribute to radiography analysis mistakes [4].

The development of radiography technology has greatly enhanced the early detection of fractures. X-rays, on the other hand, are most often used in bone fracture diagnosis

K. Daimi and A. Al Sadoon (Eds.): ACR 2024, LNNS 956, pp. 60–69, 2024.
https://doi.org/10.1007/978-3-031-56950-0_6

due to their cheap cost and accessibility [5]. However, in contrast to the high number of fractural patients, there is a severe shortage of qualified radiologists. As a consequence of the large volume of medical imaging, many radiologists feel exhausted [6]. X-rays are essential for assessing suspected fractures in people, but manual inspection takes time and requires skilled radiologists or orthopedic surgeons. Insufficient radiologists and inadequate clinical resources lead to delays in diagnosis and treatment [7]. As existing bone fracture detection techniques evolve with computerized frameworks and health informatics consoles [8], the project seeks to employ deep learning to diagnose fractures on wrist X-ray images, assisting physicians in emergency services [9].

The study outlines five stages: data preparation and data collection, comparison of bone fracture diagnostic models, investigation of therapies for bone fracture observations using classical and deep learning methodologies [10, 18], and comparison of contemporary DL-based bone fracture diagnosis models [11, 20]. The feature extraction data is fed into 12 different machine learning classifiers, and the research is evaluated for 10-fold cross-validation [6, 22]. In the EL2 model, a CNN-based deep learning algorithm achieved good test accuracy and Cohen's kappa values [12, 22], intending to construct an image processing system for effectively recognizing bone fractures utilizing X-ray and CT images [13, 17]. The contribution of this study is as follows: 1) A unique RN-21 CNN model is suggested to properly categorize crack locations in an X-ray picture, easing the load on doctors. 2) Our suggested model can extract the characteristics required for bone fracture recognition. 3) Our proposed model attained the greatest classification accuracy of 98.0.

2 Literature Review

In emergency services, bone fractures are prevalent in many regions of the body, such as the wrists, shoulders, and arms. These fractures might be partial or full, and they can be open or closed. Falls, trauma, direct blows, repeated activities, osteoporosis, and cancer are all potential causes. Sudden discomfort, bruising, swelling, visible deformity, warmth, or redness are all possible symptoms [14, 22]. Despite the requirement for physical inspection and erroneous bone data extraction owing to inadequate clinical resources and medical support systems, the research used a two-stage R-CNN approach to properly identify fractures on around 4,000 arm fracture X-ray photographs [7, 20]. The stages covered in this paper include data preparation, data collection, comparative analysis of bone fracture diagnostic models, treatment versus conventional and deep learning approaches, relative diagnosis solutions, treatment advantages, and comparison with new DL-based models [15, 19, 23]. Undiagnosed or misdiagnosed bone fractures are a major issue in orthopedics, resulting in inaccurate diagnoses or treatments, extended treatment times, and wrong diagnosis or therapy [4, 21]. This work uses machine learning approaches to identify and categorize fractures in a dataset that includes both normal and damaged bones. Following that, the data is exposed to 12 different algorithms, with LDA attaining the greatest accuracy rate of 0.88% and 0.89 AUC [16, 17, 23].

3 Materials and Methods

This section includes the study's methodology.

3.1 Dataset Descriptions

The dataset was utilized to test and train the suggested model. The dataset was developed using X-Ray Medical Imaging on patients ranging in age from 16 to 40 years. The collection has 200 X-ray pictures in total, including 120 crack images and the remaining are normal. Figure 1 depicts a graphical depiction of X-ray pictures of (a) Crack, (b) Normal Wrist.

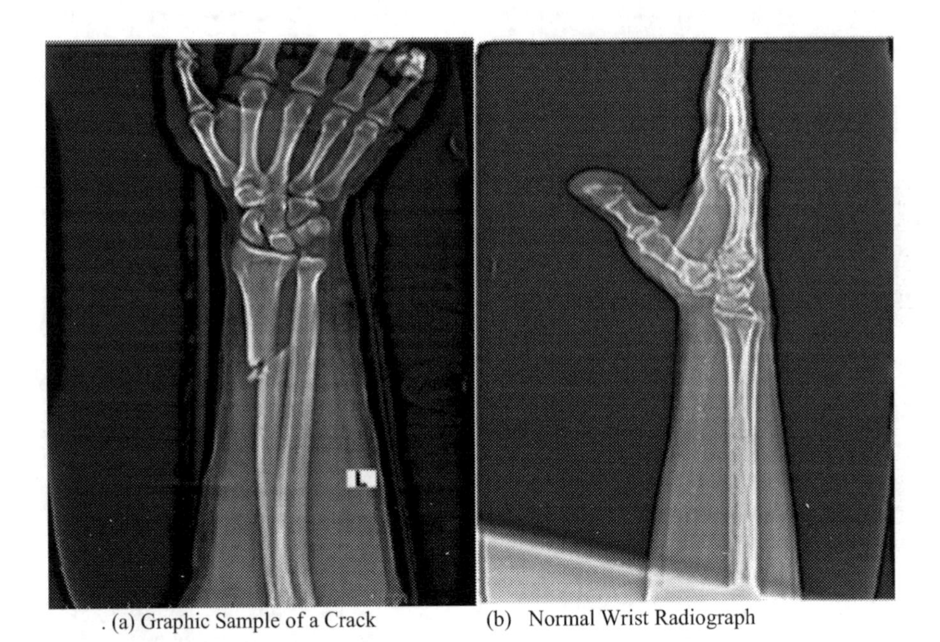

Fig. 1. (a) Graphic Sample of a Crack (b) Normal Wrist Radiograph

3.2 Data Preprocessing

Images obtained as samples are available in a range of sizes. To improve the training process, the dataset was shrunk to 150*150 pixels and data normalization was conducted. During training, data augmentation methods were used to prevent overfitting and increase dataset size.

3.3 Proposed CNN

A model that takes form, texture, spatial relationship, and target color into account is necessary for the wrist crack categorization medical imaging task. Researchers often employ local features to interpret images because textural characteristics are the main variation in wrist crack types. There aren't many accessible explanations of textures, however. Figure 2 depicts the architecture of the model we presented. To bridge the gap between anticipated and actual values, the proposed model employs a residual network-based CNN. It overcomes poor fitting effects by increasing the number of neural network layers. The model trains neurons and stores texture data using a ReLU function and a convolution section while keeping the original network's goal in mind.

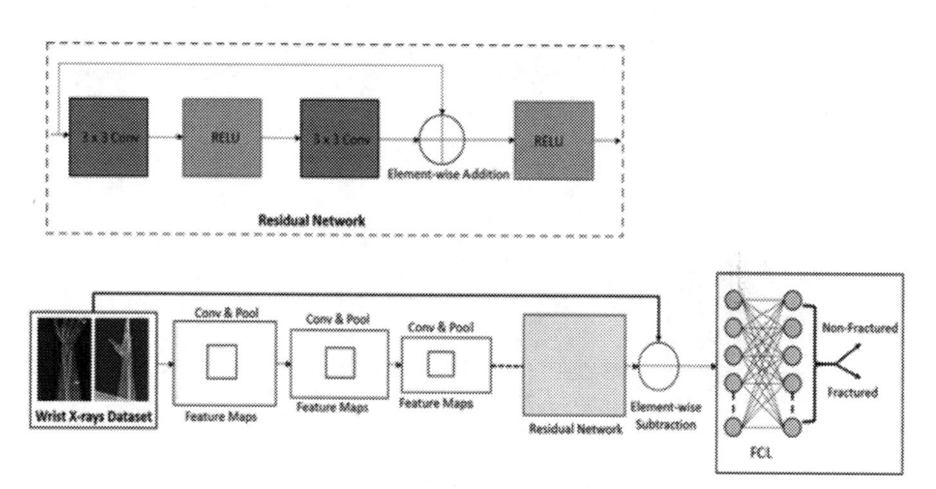

Fig. 2. Proposed CNN Architecture

3.4 Training Process of Proposed Method

The Adam Optimizer was employed in the research to decrease cross-entropy loss in neural networks. The Adam Optimizer is a stochastic gradient descent extension that adjusts neural network weights depending on training data. Calculating the gradient's first and second sequence moment estimates provides a customizable learning rate for numerous components. When assessed in the early phases of patient wrist crack classification, the model reduced the learning rate tenfold on the verification set and decreased after 10 epochs.

3.5 Methodology

This research is divided into three stages: preprocessing, feature engineering, and a transfer learning model. The dataset was split into three groups for training, validation, and testing, and the authors employed data augmentation techniques to avoid overfitting. Preprocessing techniques were also applied to determine the ROI. Pre-trained transfer learning classifiers used 1.3 M naturally occurring images from the ILSVR collection to determine their weights. Each pre-trained CNN model's final classification layer was swapped out for a single sigmoid function neuron. The resolution of wrist radiographs was changed to 150. The output of the preceding layer was utilized as data in the layers of the suggested models that feature classifiers employed, and the output layer was linked as a contribution to the next layers. The convolution layer and maximum pooling outputs were merged to create feature maps, which are 2-D planes. The final output layer from the convolution approach was flattened to provide the final dense layer with a single extended vector to use for its final classification using sigmoid processes. To address classification issues, a soft-max classifier was implemented between the dense layers and the activation stage. The loss function was calculated using binary cross-entropy loss, and the optimal hyperparameters, including learning rate and batch size, were found using grid search. Using a stochastic gradient descent optimizer with a momentum of 0.9 depending on the initial learning rate, the pre-trained model was adjusted. Epochs were terminated early with a maximum of 30 epochs executed to avoid overfitting. Figure 3 displays the suggested framework for classifying wrist cracks.

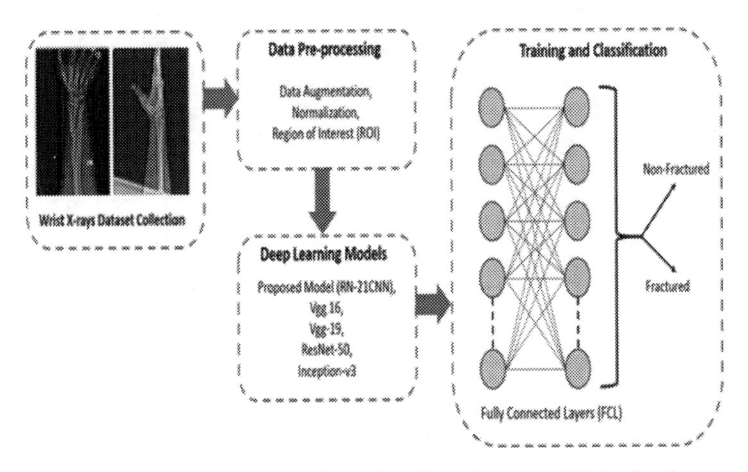

Fig. 3. Proposed Framework for The Classification of Wrist Cracks

4 Results and Discussions

This research focuses on the implementation, evaluation strategy, and experimental results of CNN models on the wrist crack database. The model was trained on the dataset's training set, validation set, and test set to assess diagnostic performance and classification accuracy. The confusion matrix approach was used to determine metrics like sensitivity, specificity, accuracy, and f1-score. The AUC was strategized to compare the model with four well-known architectures for illness detection in clinical imaging.

4.1 Results Analysis

Validation is applied to the suggested model in order to enhance performance. The first convolutional layer's partial filter result feature maps are shown in (Fig. 4), showcasing its edge detection skills. The output of the network's max pooling layer is also included in the visualization. The main and ultimate bottleneck designs' partial result feature maps are also shown by the model. Figure 5 depicts the proposed model's training loss and accuracy validation concerning epochs. The CNN model was run over 30 epochs. The highest acquired accuracy for training was 0.99, while the maximum obtained accuracy for validation was 0.96.

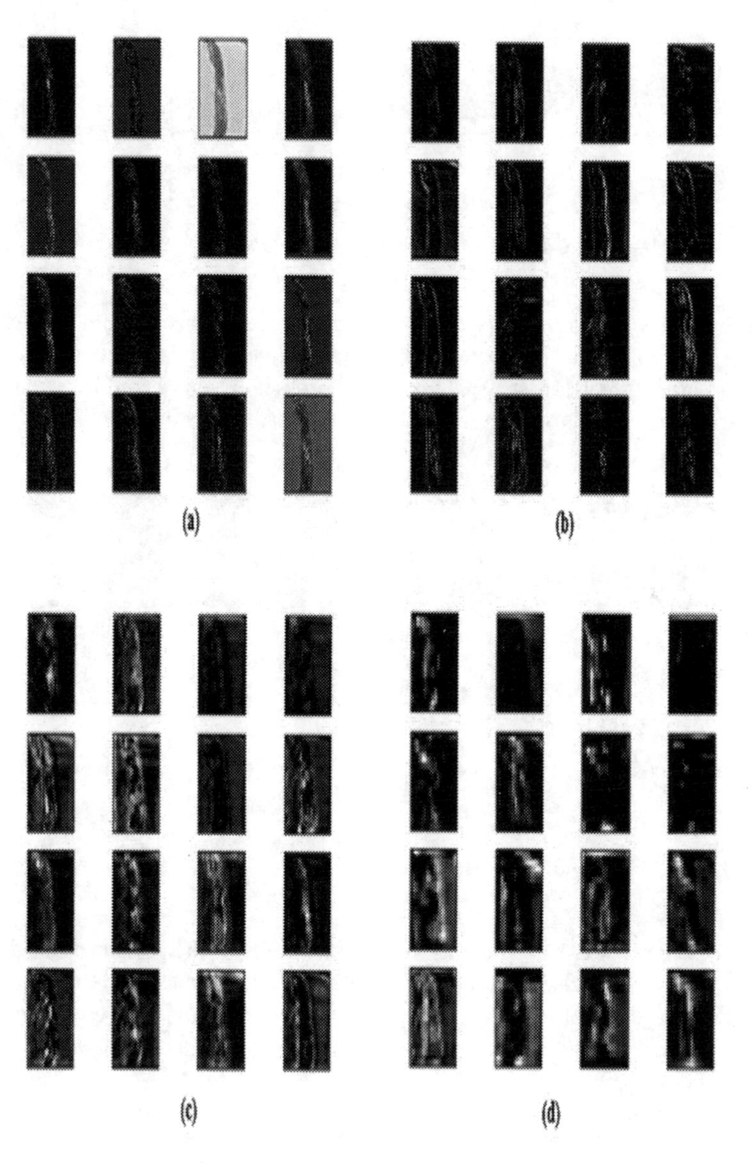

Fig. 4. Partial validation process outcomes of proposed method.

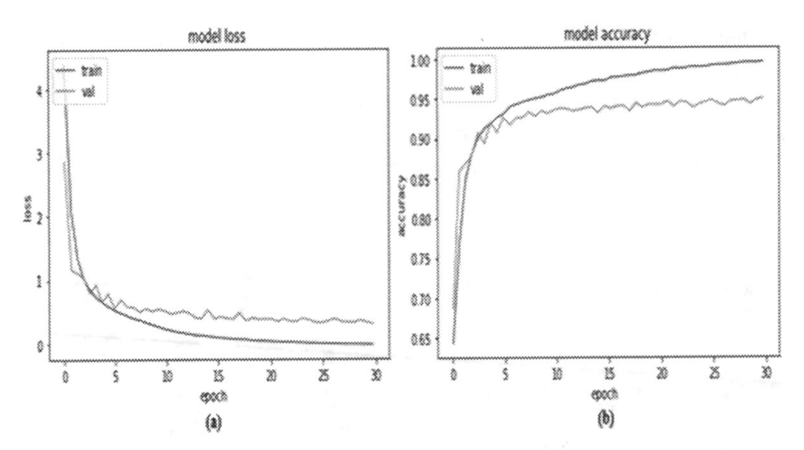

Fig. 5. Training loss and accuracy validation of proposed 21 layers of CNN.

Our CNN classifier accurately classifies wrist cracks against normal wrists, with a validation and training loss of 0.026 and 0.021, respectively. Figure 6 shows the accuracy of CNN this model's performance parameters were assessed, and a confusion matrix was created, arranging actual examples in rows and expected cases in columns.

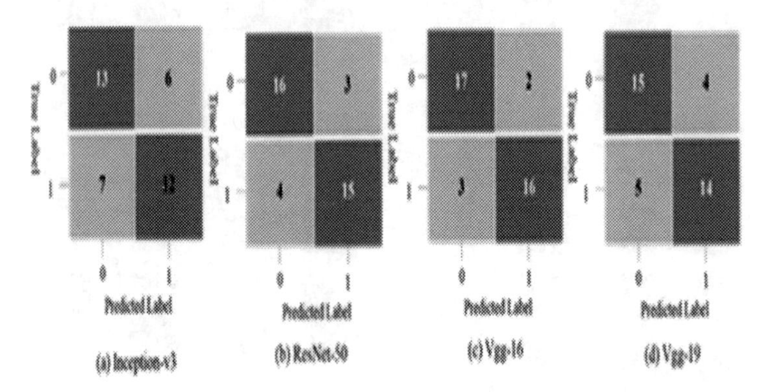

Fig. 6. Training loss and accuracy validation of proposed 21 layers of CNN

The model detects 17 cases out of 19 wrist crack cases, with 2 instances misclassified as normal. ResNet's precise class label predicts all normal instances, while Inception V3 predicts 13 instances and 6 cases as normal. Our suggested approach recognizes all 19 instances and misclassifies 0 cases as normal. Table 1 displays a comparison of different classifier models.

The performance of several models, including ResNet 50, Inception V3, and ResNet 50, is shown in (Fig. 7). The F1 score for the Vgg-16 model was 84.1%, while the F1 score for the Vgg-19 model was 78%. ResNet 50 had an F1 rating of 83%, whereas Inception V3 received a rating of 66%. The suggested model attained a 98% accuracy, precision, sensitivity, and F1-Score.

Table 1. Comparison of Proposed Method with Four Pre-Trained Classifiers

Model	Accuracy	Specificity	Sensitivity	F1-Score	AUC
VGG 16	84%	85.6%	88.7%	84.1%	89%
VGG 19	78%	75%	79%	76%	85%
Inception V3	69%	65%	70%	66%	61%
ResNet 50	84%	79%	86%	83%	90%
Proposed Method	98%	96%	99%	96%	98%

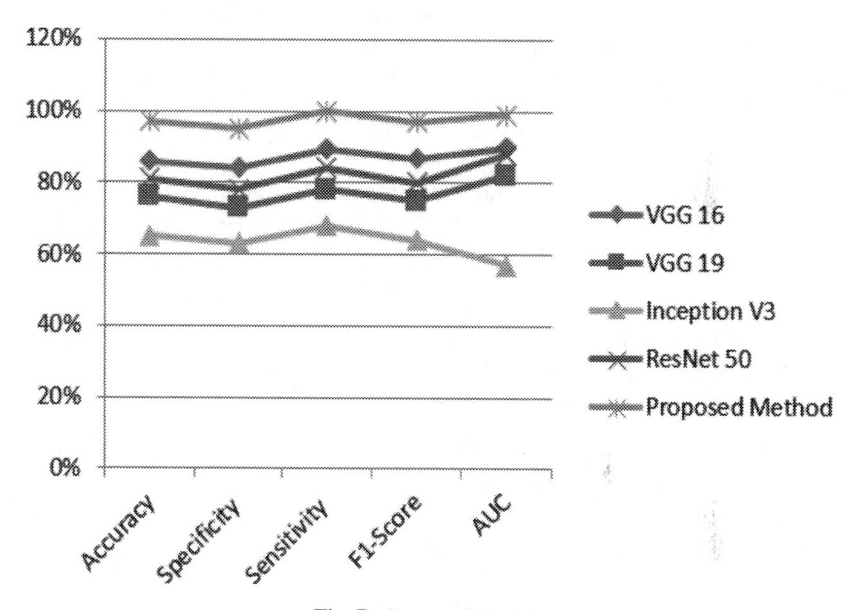

Fig. 7. Proposed Model.

5 Conclusions and Future Work

The paper provides an automated diagnostic approach for determining whether wrist radiographs are normal or broken. To comprehend the textural features of wrist tissues, it employs a novel network design with residual structures. The algorithm employs 21 Convolutional layers, two thick layers, and ReLU activation. Cross-entropy loss is minimized using the Adam optimizer and dilated convolutions. Transfer learning overcomes the issue of missing information and speeds up neural network training. The approach enhances classification presentation and has the potential to be spread to economically depressed areas for telemedicine training and local medical imaging diagnostics. Future work will improve the approach for MRI and CT medical imaging analysis, perhaps extending to economically undeveloped places for telemedicine training and local medical imaging diagnostic improvement.

References

1. Bin, N.A., et al.: Early gender identification of date palm using machine learning. J. Comput. Biomed. Inform. **4**(02), 128–141 (2023). https://www.jcbi.org/index.php/Main/article/view/147
2. Ghoti, K., Baid, U., Talbar, S.: MURA: bone fracture segmentation using a U-net deep learning in X-ray images. In: Pawar, P.M., Balasubramaniam, R., Ronge, B.P., Salunkhe, S.B., Vibhute, A.S., Melinamath, B. (eds.) Techno-Societal 2020: Proceedings of the 3rd International Conference on Advanced Technologies for Societal Applications—Volume 1, pp. 519–531. Springer, Cham (2021). https://doi.org/10.1007/978-3-030-69921-5_52
3. Ha, Y.J., et al.: Spatio-temporal split learning for privacy-preserving medical platforms: case studies with COVID-19 CT, X-Ray, and cholesterol data. IEEE Access **9**, 121046–121059 (2021). https://doi.org/10.1109/ACCESS.2021.3108455
4. Hardalaç, F., et al.: Fracture detection in wrist X-ray images using deep learning-based object detection models. Sensors **22**(3), 1285 (2022). https://doi.org/10.3390/s22031285
5. Joshi, D., Singh, T.P.: A survey of fracture detection techniques in bone X-ray images. Artif. Intell. Rev. **53**(6), 4475–4517 (2020). https://doi.org/10.1007/s10462-019-09799-0
6. Naeem, A.B., et al.: Hypothyroidism disease diagnosis by using machine learning algorithms. Int. J. Intell. Syst. Appl. Eng. **11**(3), 368–373 (2023). https://www.ijisae.org/index.php/IJISAE/article/view/3178
7. Naeem, A.B., Soomro, A.M., Saim, H.M., Malik, H.: Smart road management system for prioritized autonomous vehicles under vehicle-to-everything (V2X) communication. Multimedia Tools Appl. (2023). https://doi.org/10.1007/s11042-023-16950-1
8. Ma, Y., Luo, Y.: Bone fracture detection through the two-stage system of crack-sensitive convolutional neural network. Inform. Med. Unlocked **22**, 100452 (2021). https://doi.org/10.1016/j.imu.2020.100452
9. Naeem, A.B., Senapati, B., Chauhan, A.S., Kumar, S., Orosco Gavilan, J.C., Abdel-Rehim, W.M.F.: Deep learning models for cotton leaf disease detection with VGG-16. Int. J. Intell. Syst. Appl. Eng. **11**(2), 550–556 (2023). https://www.ijisae.org/index.php/IJISAE/article/view/2710
10. Naeem, A.B., et al.: Intelligent four-way crossroad safety management for autonomous, non-autonomous and VIP vehicles. In: 2023 IEEE International Conference on Emerging Trends in Engineering, Sciences and Technology (ICES&T), 9–11 January 2023, pp. 1–6, (2023). https://doi.org/10.1109/ICEST56843.2023.10138829
11. Sathish Kumar, L., Prabu, A.V., Pandimurugan, V., Rajasoundaran, S., Malla, P.P., Routray, S.: A comparative experimental analysis and deep evaluation practices on human bone fracture detection using x-ray images. Concurrency Comput. Pract. Exper. **34**(26), e7307 (2022). https://doi.org/10.1002/cpe.7307
12. Rashid, T., Zia, M.S., Najam-ur-Rehman, T.M., Rauf, H.T., Kadry, S.: A minority class balanced approach using the dcnn-lstm method to detect human wrist fracture. Life **13**(1), 133 (2023). https://doi.org/10.3390/life13010133
13. Senapati, B., Rawal, B.S.: Quantum communication with RLP quantum resistant cryptography in industrial manufacturing. Cyber Secur. Appl. **1**, 100019 (2023)
14. Soomro, A.M., et al.: Constructor development: predicting object communication errors. In: Proceedings of the 2023 IEEE International Conference on Emerging Trends in Engineering, Sciences and Technology (ICES&T), Bahawalpur, Pakistan, 9–11 January 2023, pp. 1–7 (2023)
15. Senapati, B., Rawal, B.S.: Adopting a deep learning split-protocol based predictive maintenance management system for industrial manufacturing operations. In: Hsu, C.-H., Mengwei,

Xu., Cao, H., Hojjat Baghban, A.B.M., Ali, S. (eds.) Big Data Intelligence and Computing: International Conference, DataCom 2022, Denarau Island, Fiji, December 8–10, 2022, Proceedings, pp. 22–39. Springer, Singapore (2023). https://doi.org/10.1007/978-981-99-2233-8_2

16. Sahin, M.E.: Image processing and machine learning-based bone fracture detection and classification using X-ray images. Int. J. Imaging Syst. Technol. **33**(3), 853–865 (2023). https://doi.org/10.1002/ima.22849
17. Naeem, A.B., Biswaranjan Senapati, Md., Sudman, S.I., Bashir, K., Ahmed, A.E.M.: Intelligent road management system for autonomous, non-autonomous, and VIP vehicles. World Electr. Veh. J. **14**(9), 238 (2023). https://doi.org/10.3390/wevj14090238
18. Sabugaa, M., Senapati, B., Kupriyanov, Y., Danilova, Y., Irgasheva, S., Potekhina, E.: Evaluation of the prognostic significance and accuracy of screening tests for alcohol dependence based on the results of building a multilayer perceptron. In: Silhavy, R., Silhavy, P. (eds.) Artificial Intelligence Application in Networks and Systems. CSOC 2023. LNNS, vol. 724. Springer, Cham (2023). https://doi.org/10.1007/978-3-031-35314-7_23
19. Moutsinas, G.A., Esponda-Pérez, J.A., Senapati, B., Sanyal, S., Patra, I., Karnaukhov, A.: Application of virtual reality in education. In: Silhavy, R., Silhavy, P. (eds.) Software Engineering Research in System Science. CSOC 2023. LNNS, vol. 722. Springer, Cham (2023). https://doi.org/10.1007/978-3-031-35311-6_33
20. Soomro, A.M., et al.: In MANET: an improved hybrid routing approach for disaster management. In: 2023 IEEE International Conference on Emerging Trends in Engineering, Sciences and Technology (ICES&T), Bahawalpur, Pakistan, pp. 1–6 (2023). https://doi.org/10.1109/ICEST56843.2023.10138831
21. Soomro, A.M., et al.: Constructor development: predicting object communication errors. In: 2023 IEEE International Conference on Emerging Trends in Engineering, Sciences and Technology (ICES&T), Bahawalpur, Pakistan, pp. 1–7 (2023). https://doi.org/10.1109/ICEST56843.2023.10138846
22. Senapati, B., Talburt, J.R., Naeem, A.B, Batthula, V.J.R.: Transfer learning based models for food detection using ResNet-50. In: 2023 IEEE International Conference on Electro Information Technology (eIT), Romeoville, IL, USA, pp. 224–229 (2023). https://doi.org/10.1109/eIT57321.2023.10187288
23. Senapati, B., Rawal, B.S.: Adopting a deep learning split-protocol based predictive maintenance management system for industrial manufacturing operations. In: Hsu, CH., Xu, M., Cao, H., Baghban, H., Shawkat Ali, A.B.M. (eds) Big Data Intelligence and Computing. DataCom 2022. LNCS, vol. 13864. Springer, Singapore (2023). https://doi.org/10.1007/978-981-99-2233-8_2

Improving Weeds Detection in Pastures Using Illumination Invariance Techniques

Ali Hassan Alyatimi[1,2], Thair Al-Dala'in[3], Vera Chung[1], Ali Anaissi[1(✉)], and Edmund J. Sadgrove[4]

[1] School of Computer Science, The University of Sydney, Camperdown, Australia
aaly3310@uni.sydney.edu.au, {vera.chung,Ali.Anaissi}@sydney.edu.au

[2] Computer Tech, Jazan College of Technology, Vocational Training Corporation (TVTC), Jizan, Saudi Arabia

[3] Western Sydney University, Sydney City Campus, Penrith, Australia
t.aldalain@city.westernsydney.edu.au

[4] School of Science and Technology, University of New England, Armidale, NSW 2351, Australia
esadgro2@une.edu.au

Abstract. Computers have various applications in relation to the classification of weeds, including computer vision. This paper demonstrates the use of illumination invariance techniques and shadow reduction in images to improve the accuracy of machine learning (ML) models using support vector machines. The paper's main aim is to identify the benefits of image optimisation utilising adjusting dark images. More specifically, the paper uses brightness and contrast adjustment to fix images and then compares the results of a dataset that underwent image pre-processing and a dataset that did not. Ensuring the clearness of an object in an image is essential if a ML model is to identify it accurately. Many issues within image datasets can hinder the accuracy of ML classification models, for example, illumination invariance and shadowed images, which entail underexposed dark pictures being projected onto the target in the absence of light sources. The paper uses several techniques and technologies to analyse the data, including cross-validation, a confusion matrix, the pre-processing technique, the TensorFlow framework and training conducted in both the central processing unit and graphics processing units. The results of these analyses show that the brightness has significantly enhanced the accuracy of the ML model. In addition, applying image pre-processing to the shadow has resulted in a slight improvement of 1% in this regard. In conclusion, this paper presents evidence concerning ML-based solutions for improving the accuracy of classification models by enhancing images of weeds using pixel brightness transformations.

Keywords: Machine Learning · Computer Vision · Support Vector Machine algorithm · Pre-processing Image Techniques · Weeds

K. Daimi and A. Al Sadoon (Eds.): ACR 2024, LNNS 956, pp. 70–82, 2024.
https://doi.org/10.1007/978-3-031-56950-0_7

1 Introduction

The identification and control of weeds in fields of crops have remained challenging among agricultural researchers and farmers for decades in Australia [1]. This has significantly lowered crop production, jeopardising food security. For a long time, weed identification has been done physically by pinpointing visible characteristics that distinguish weeds and crops. This method has been inaccurate and unreliable since some weeds have unique features that require special technology for identification and management practices to control effectively [2]. Besides, farmers have been using conventional methods to control weeds, such as mechanically removing them using hand, chemical, and biological techniques. However, they have recently started embracing technology by using computers to establish and control weeds which have proven more reliable and accurate. Generally, computers play a fundamental role in classifying weeds, whereas computer vision technology uses images of fields as fit data for training machines. Moreover, the techniques used to process digital images have led to the exploration of illumination invariance and its impact on the accuracy of model training [3]. This section explores the problem of weed identification, illumination invariance, and shallow images to elucidate the background of the present research.

Due to their adaptability and capacity to flourish in various environments, weeds constitute one of the most challenging issues in agriculture [3]. Uncontrolled weeds pose a problem to the environment, society, shared lands, and essential production industries. Indeed, they can harm and destroy natural landscapes and agricultural lands by eliminating natural species, contributing to land deprivation, and decreasing soil fertility and forest cover. Consequently, Australia has invested significant resources in dealing with weeds to shield ecosystems and protect production. According to the Australian Centre for Invasive Species Solution [4], Australia is home to 398 weed species, with weed infestation being monitored by creating management profiles containing management information, distribution data, images, and links to critical documents and literature. However, farmers continue to experience problems related to weed infestation and hence need assistance to identify and control weeds using a new and holistic technological approach.

The paper's main issue is investigating how adjustments in brightness and contrast of images impact the accuracy of SVM models for weed detection. The concept of illumination invariance will explain how the amount of light falling on an object determines its appearance and positioning of light in a digital image. Illumination invariance refers to the effect of light on a given image subject with minimal or no changes resulting from the image's properties [5]. This means that the appearance of such images solely depends on how the light shines on the image regardless of the image's positioning, scale, or rotation. Illumination quality falls in a spectrum between over-exposure and or low illumination, necessitating correcting techniques [6]. The shallow concept determines the amount of light that falls on the object, while illumination determines how much light is reflected. Images used in machine learning (ML) classification contain illumination robustness and adequate shadow to ease identification. For instance, localising, mapping, and classifying autonomous vehicles require using images whose essential aspects remain constant despite the amount of lighting available [7]. Therefore, machine learning uses illumination invariants with varying colour spaces to enhance image similarity throughout the day.

Furthermore, using the appropriate shallow helps capture the most identifiable aspects of a material's properties, thus, easing recognition. For example, after remapping images taken through illumination invariant colour space on a greyscale image, the identifiable aspects remain the same, regardless of further changes in illumination [8]. Therefore, machine learning classification of images requires illumination and invariance to create images that machines can accurately correlate with pre-existing input data.

Support Vector Machines (SVMs) will be used since they have a track record of success in binary classification tasks. Due to their capacity for handling high-dimensional data, which is the situation when working with detailed photographs of agricultural landscapes, SVMs are suited for weed detection [9–11]. The technique also gives structural risk minimisation a solid mathematical foundation, which helps generalise its use and avoid overfitting. SVMs can tackle non-linear problems using various kernel functions, increasing their applicability for identifying the complex patterns seen in photos of weeds and crops [12,13]. The ability to refine picture pre-processing methods will enable us to develop more precise and dependable weed identification models, leading to better crop management and ultimately enhancing food production and security.

1.1 Motivations and Objectives

The research paper delves into the classification of illumination challenges, particularly two types. The first type pertains to underexposed dark images taken without adequate light sources, while the second type relates to overexposed bright images captured in sunlight. Our main goal is to optimise images by adjusting the brightness of dark images to match that of light images. It also aims to evaluate our results using a support vector machine (SVM) in machine learning. Additionally, our sub-goals consist of:

- Develop an algorithm to detect images in shadow.
- Apply contrast adjustment to improve lighting consistency throughout the image set on dark images.
- Apply an efficient machine learning algorithm that can be used on a microprocessor more readily.
- Benchmark the algorithm provides result comparisons between shadow and contrast-adjusted datasets.

1.2 The Data Description

The dataset in this research paper was taken from previous research conducted by [1], in Robotic weed control, detailed in Table 1. It can classify Chinese apple weed and Lantana weed from the loaded dataset. There are 1000 images in each class, listed in Table 1. However, when images are manually divided into sunlight and shadow images, the number of images will be 500 for each category.

Table 1. Dataset description

No	Class Weed Name	No. of Images	Dimensions
1	Chinese apple	1000	100 × 100
2	Lantana	1000	100 × 100

2 Methodology

In the process of building a machine learning (ML) model, there are several vital steps to take, including data collection, data preparation, training, and model evaluation. This research study focused on identifying an ML model that works effectively with our particular dataset, and we have outlined two methods for achieving this. Furthermore, we explored image thresholding and pre-processing techniques that can enhance the image quality utilized in the model. Lastly, we presented a framework that leverages two training sets to tackle a large image dataset, reduce computing time for the Support Vector Machine (SVM), and evaluate two distinct validation models (cross-validation and confusion matrix) for each process.

2.1 Methods

Selecting images from the dataset has been managed in two methods in this research paper:

- Select images manually into two groups, those in shadow and those in direct sunlight.
- Select images automatically using Python code to aspirate images with shadow and sunlight.

It was, firstly, selecting images manually. This method created four folders of image categories in the workplace dataset Table 1, as follows:

- The first folder is for images with shadows only.
- The second folder is for images with shadows and sunlight.
- The third folder is for images with sunlight only.
- The fourth folder is for images with sunlight and enhanced images in shadow.

All images with shadows were selected manually and put in the research paper folder dataset. The dimensions of images have been set to size 100 × 100 and cropped by using the XnView tool, which is Freeware for private, non-commercial or educational use. XnView is a stable, easy-to-use, and comprehensive photo editor. It is a versatile and powerful photo viewer, image management, image resizer, and most common picture and graphics formats are supported [14].

The second method is selecting images automatically. This method determines the image's brightness level. It selects which images are in shadow or sunlight by finding an average light intensity using thresholding, the most common segmentation technique in computer vision. Pseudo-code (1) explains the code flow.

Algorithm 1. pseudo-code , the sampling images automatically with shadow and daylight.

Input: (images, determined brightness level)
Output: (classify images (shadow, sunlight))
Loop: ($image\ dataset \geq 1$)
($threshold \geq 35$)
$- -\ image_d ataset$
$Select(thebrightenimage, storeinfolder)$
$- -\ imagedataset$
$Select(thedarkimage, storeinfolder)$
(End loop)
Exit()

2.2 Image Thresholding Technique

Thresholding is the pixel intensity value or the grey level of the image. According to [15], in his article, Python libraries have many uses for image manipulation tasks, for example, sci-kit-image, NumPy, SciPy, Pil/Pillow, OpenCV, SimpleCV, Mahoyas, SimpleITK, and Pycairo. These libraries implement an easy and spontaneous way to convert images and use their data. Pil/Pillow library has been used in this research paper. It is a free library using Python code that supports image utilization in many different formats. Therefore, in this research paper, the examination of pixel values aimed to distinguish between images in shadow or sunlight. An object was used to return the image's pixel values and getdata().

2.3 Pre-processing Technique

Image enhancement enhances the quality of specific content from original data before processing, such as changing the contrast and brightness of an image. According to article published at [16], image enhancement techniques can be classified into two general sections. Firstly, a spatial domain enhancement occurs within each pixel in a mage according to the spatial coordinates with a specific resolution. Another category is the frequency domain enhancement gained by implementing the Fourier Transform to the spatial domain. Nevertheless, Python OpenCV has been used, which is one of the spatial domain tools. Furthermore, this research paper has processed brightness and contrast adjustment enhancement. The process is to access each pixel in the image, operate with BGR image values, and improve the brightness of images in shadow to be in the same level of sunlight. The outcome of the Python code appears as the original image on the left (a) and the enhancement image on the right (b) Fig. 3 (Fig. 1):

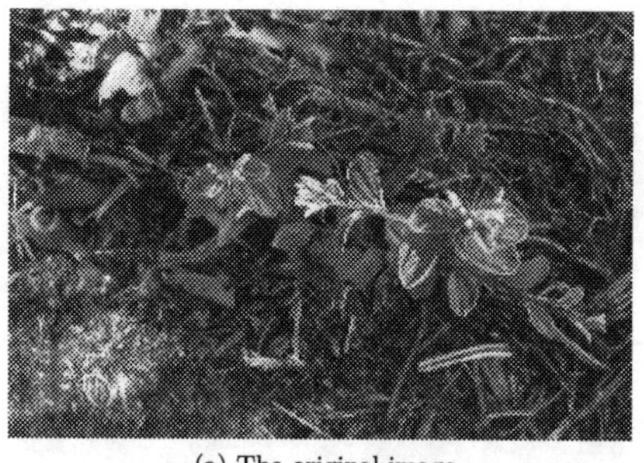
(a) The original image

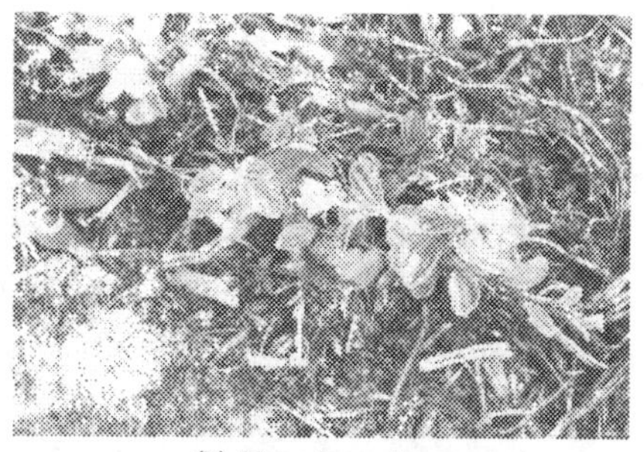
(b) The enhance image

Fig. 1. The outcome of Preprocessing technique

2.4 Framework

TensorFlow has been used in this research for many reasons. Firstly, large-scale training and inference can be supported in this environment. Moreover, fast training can be done because TensorFlow can enable multiple or single GPU servers and efficiently trains different models on several platforms. Additionally, it ranges from large distributed clusters in a data centre and can run locally on mobile devices. Finally, it is flexible, which can promote experimentation and study into new machine learning models and system-level optimisations [17]. In other words, TensorFlow is a combination of workflows that can develop and train models using Python, and it is manageable for people to create machine learning models.

2.5 Training

Four training processes were conducted in this research paper. School of Science & Technology, University of New England, has two servers capable of machine learning training and testing sets. The first server, the Bourbaki, has one GPU and uses a confusion matrix for validation. The second server is Engelbart, which has two GPUs and uses cross-validation to validate the dataset. It is summarised in Table 3. Here is more information about training and testing sets hardware in Table 2.

Table 2. Hardwar information

	Bourbaki	Engelbart
Memory	125.65 GiB RAM	94.26 GiB RAM
GPU	NVIDIA GV100GL [Tesla V100 PCIe 16 GB]	Device-2: NVIDIA GK210GL [Tesla K80], Device-3: NVIDIA GK210GL [Tesla K80]
Processor	bourbaki: 16 × 64 bit Intel Xeon (Skylake IBRS) 2394 MHz	16× Single Core model: Intel Core (Haswell IBRS), 2497 MHz
Operating system	Rocky Linux release 8.4 (Green Obsidian)	CentOS Linux release 7.9.2009 (Core)

Table 3. Training sets summary

Number of trainings	Method used	Pre-process (data)	Platform
3	Manually	No	Bourbaki
1	Manually	Yes	Bourbaki
3	Automatically	No	Engelbart
1	Automatically	Yes	Engelbart

2.6 The Support Vector Machine (SVM) Algorithm

Classification accuracy is a topic highlighted in this research. For example, classifying several classes of dates using images. Therefore, SVM is a supervised ML algorithm used in classifying data and was chosen in this research paper for many reasons [18]. According to [19], SVM has displayed reliability as a classification method in their study. Furthermore, it can achieve high accuracy and provide robust performance with a specific data type that includes different characteristics, shapes, textures, and colours [20]. In short, it can be fast in training and testing and has an excellent classification rate.

2.7 Cross Validation

Cross-validation is a resampling process used to evaluate machine learning models on a dataset. It divides the training data into several k-fold in equivalent size. Each k-fold is selected to test the dataset model, whereas the remaining k-fold is used as the training data. This process will continue until the last k-fold; the prediction accuracies across all blinded tests are combined to give an overall performance estimate [21]. Cross-validation can follow some steps, as Brownlee [22] mentioned: Firstly, the dataset will be shuffled randomly. After that, it will split into K groups which are ten groups in this research. Each K-C group will also take a test dataset, and the remaining K-C will be taken as a training dataset. Finally, record the evaluation score for each K-C. The klearn.model_selection was imported in this research paper and used a cross_val_score function to show accuracy [23].

2.8 Confusion Matrix

A confusion matrix is a tool used to analyse and normalise the accuracy of multiclass classifications. Moreover, it is a table layout that provides visualisation of a supervised learning algorithm. Each matrix column shows the predicted class, while each row outlines the actual class. Further, the correct predictions are located along the table's diagonal such that any non-zero values outside the diagonal can easily visualise errors [24]. Table 4 is based on [25] as a confusion matrix with two different classes.

Table 4. The confusion matrix for two-class classification

	Predicted Negative	Predicted Positive
Actual Negative	a (the number of correct)	b (the number of incorrect)
Actual Positive	c (the number of incorrect)	d (the number of correct)

Table 5. SVM training sets results (1)

No	Description	No. of classes	No. Images	Training Time/second(s)	Accuracy
1	Images exposure Sunlight & Shadow	2	1000	10.26	0.9025
2	All images with enhancing & exposure sunlight	2	1000	7.58	0.9125
3	Images with sunlight only	2	1000	9.15	0.955
4	Images with shadow only	2	1000	11	0.895

Table 6. SVM training sets results (2)

No	Description	No. of classes	No. Images	Training Time/second(s)	Accuracy
1	Images exposure Sunlight & Shadow	2	1000	9.66	0.89
2	All images with enhancing & exposure sunlight	2	1000	9.86	0.90
3	Images with sunlight only	2	1000	18.73	0.93
4	Images with shadow only	2	293	48.36	0.80

According to [26], the prediction accuracy and classification error can be calculated as follows:

$$Accuracy = \left(\frac{(a+d)}{(a+b+c+d)}\right)$$

$$Error = \left(\frac{(b+c)}{(a+b+c+d)}\right)$$

Where (a) is true positive (tp), (b) is false positive (fp), (c) is false negative (fn) and (d) is true negative (tn).

3 Results

Evaluating various images taken in different circumstances, such as sunlight or shadow, can affect computer vision algorithms' accuracy. Therefore, this research paper has conducted two group examinations, and the results are illustrated as follows.

Firstly, the training results were obtained using the Bourbaki server, as summarised in Table 5, and the validation technique employed the confusion matrix shown in Fig. 3. Second, the training results were implemented in the Engelbart server, which is summarised in Table 6, and the validation approach utilised a k-fold cross-validation, which is shown in Table 7. Figure 4 depicts the difference between both training model results, which reveals slightly different (Fig. 2).

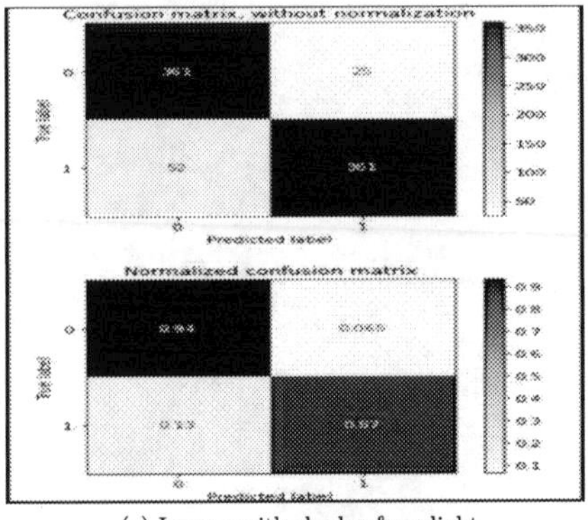

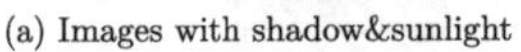

(a) Images with shadow&sunlight

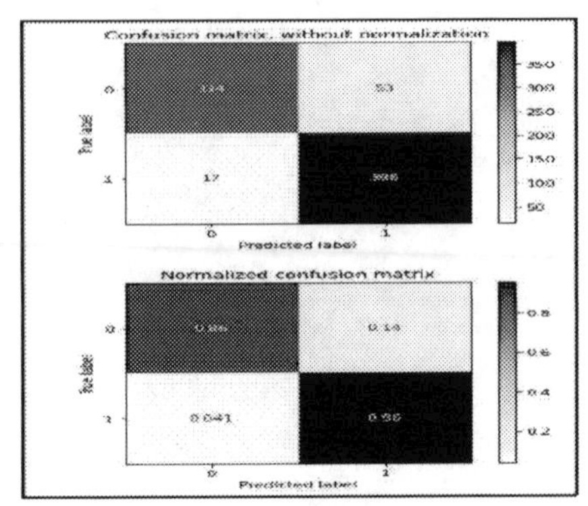

(b) All images with enhancing & sunlight

Fig. 2. The outcome of Preprocessing technique

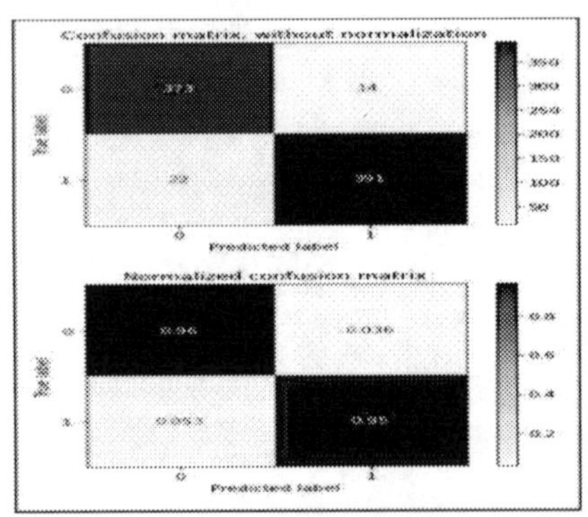

(a) Images with sunlight only

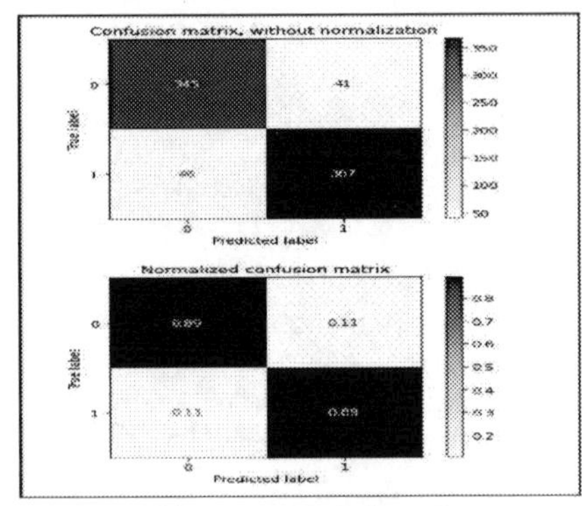

(b) Images with shadow only

Fig. 3. The outcome of Preprocessing technique

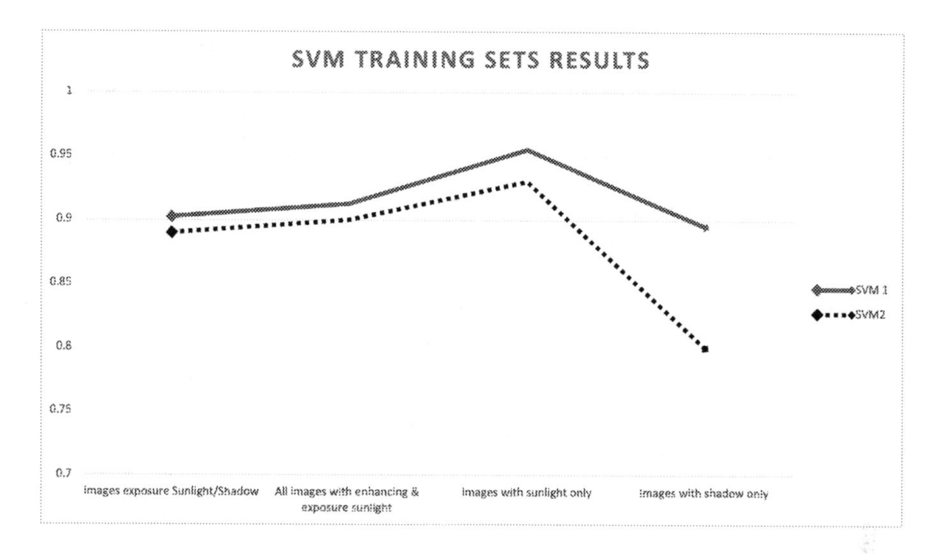

Fig. 4. SVM training sets results (1)

Table 7. Cross validation K-10, SVM training sets results (2)

No	Description	KC_1	KC_2	KC_3	KC_4	KC_5	KC_6	KC_7	KC_8	KC_9	KC_{10}	**AVG**
1	Images exposure Sunlight& Shadow	0.69	0.71	0.70	0.76	0.68	0.77	0.78	0.73	0.74	0.72	0.73
2	All images with enhancing&exposure sunlight	0.69	0.66	0.65	0.72	0.75	0.73	0.73	0.77	0.75	0.76	0.72
3	Images with sunlight only	0.69	0.77	0.74	0.74	0.72	0.73	0.67	0.74	0.65	0.76	0.72
4	Images with shadow only	0.65	0.65	0.65	0.65	0.62	0.68	0.61	0.67	0.67	0.69	0.65

4 Discussion

Experiment outcomes show that the module considerably enhances image quality. The abundance of sunlight has severely impacted the accuracy of the machine learning models used in this work in some images. For instance, Tables 5 and 6 display the results indicating the highest accuracy, around 93%; the two weed class images were each 1000 in size. In contrast, achieved roughly 80% accuracy was achieved in training images consisting entirely of shadows. Further, the machine learning module's accuracy drops when employing traditional and manual approaches to datasets, whether those datasets are noisy or influenced by light or shadow. For illustration, the images within shadow and sunlight in training No.1 Tables 5 and 6 show an accuracy percentage between 89% to 90%. Therefore, image pre-processing is essential in enhancing machine learning model accuracy. Through the implementation of the pixel brightness transformations (PBT) technique, we were able to achieve a 1% improvement over our prior results.

The Confusion Matrix and Cross-Validation are essential components in evaluating SVM machine learning image classification. Cross-Validation gives reliable performance estimations and assists with generalisation, while the

Confusion Matrix is useful for evaluating the model's forecasts. Because of these tools, we are able to evaluate and improve the accuracy of the image classification model, in addition to its resilience and general efficacy. Figure 3b displays that the accuracy of the Confusion Matrix in class [1] has increased to 96%. However, the accuracy of the dataset with training that does not include images of pre-processing techniques is 87%. Table 7 shows the results of the cross-validation, which identifies the lowest average rate in 65% of the images located within the shadow, while the remaining validations are approximately 72%. The results of the F-10 cross-validation are presented in Table 7 for each of the four dataset images.

Overall, research results demonstrate an improvement in the accuracy of images that use the image pre-processing approaches before training. This might help achieve the high accuracy of ML models in many various types of studies conducted in a variety of sectors, such as agricultural [27], medical imaging [28], document image [29,30], and undersea [31] research. In addition, a crop categorisation system has been developed to assist farmers and agricultural experts in controlling weed infestation on the land [32].

4.1 Future Work

In this research paper will plan to get more improvement in many ways. Firstly, increasing the accuracy will require more image pre-processing techniques, for example, image filtering, segmentation, and geometric transformations. According to Barui et al. [27], their research results determined a satisfying result by using the image segmentation technique. Unluckily, due to lack of time, this research could not examine these techniques. Additionally, developing an interface system could benefit people who have less knowledge of ML technology, such as weeds websites or smartphone apps.

5 Conclusion

To sum up, the research paper investigated machine learning (ML)-based solutions for improving classification model accuracy by enhancing weed images using the pixel brightness transformations (PBT) and the support vector machine (SVM) algorithm. The trained models were evaluated with four datasets using image selection methods, such as selected by hand or automatically. Based on the results presented in the result section, the accuracy was affected after image pre-processing. Finally, the future investigation will apply different image pre-processing techniques and design a social interface system such as websites or smartphone apps.

References

1. Olsen, A., et al.: Deepweeds: a multiclass weed species image dataset for deep learning. Sci. Rep. **9**(1), 2058 (2019)
2. Esposito, M., Crimaldi, M., Cirillo, V., Sarghini, F., Maggio, A.: Drone and sensor technology for sustainable weed management: a review. Chem. Biol. Technol. Agric. **8**(1), 1–11 (2021)
3. Westwood, J.H., et al.: Weed management in 2050: perspectives on the future of weed science. Weed Sci. **66**(3), 275–285 (2018)
4. CISS. Weeds australia is managed through the centre for invasive species solutions (ciss). Website article (2021). https://weeds.org.au/weeds-profiles/page/5/
5. Wan, X., Liu, J., Yan, H., Morgan, G.L.K.: Illumination-invariant image matching for autonomous UAV localisation based on optical sensing. ISPRS J. Photogram. Remote Sens. **119**, 198–213 (2016)
6. Wang, R., Zeng, L., Shiqian, W., Cao, W., Wong, K.: Illumination-invariant feature point detection based on neighborhood information. Sensors **20**(22), 6630 (2020)
7. Ramaiah, N.P., Ijjina, E.P., Mohan, C.K.: Illumination invariant face recognition using convolutional neural networks. In: 2015 IEEE International Conference on Signal Processing, Informatics, Communication and Energy Systems (SPICES), pp. 1–4. IEEE (2015)
8. Maddern, W., Stewart, A., McManus, C., Upcroft, B., Churchill, W., Newman, P.: Illumination invariant imaging: applications in robust vision-based localisation, mapping and classification for autonomous vehicles. In: Proceedings of the Visual Place Recognition in Changing Environments Workshop, IEEE International Conference on Robotics and Automation (ICRA), Hong Kong, China, vol. 2, p. 5 (2014)
9. Tang, J.-L., Chen, X.-Q., Miao, R.-H., Wang, D.: Weed detection using image processing under different illumination for site-specific areas spraying. Comput. Electron. Agric. **122**, 103–111 (2016)
10. Anaissi, A., Goyal, M.: Svm-based association rules for knowledge discovery and classification. In: 2015 2nd Asia-Pacific World Congress on Computer Science and Engineering (APWC on CSE), pp. 1–5. IEEE (2015)
11. Anaissi, A., et al.: Adaptive one-class support vector machine for damage detection in structural health monitoring. In: Kim, J., Shim, K., Cao, L., Lee, J.-G., Lin, X., Moon, Y.-S. (eds.) PAKDD 2017. LNCS (LNAI), vol. 10234, pp. 42–57. Springer, Cham (2017). https://doi.org/10.1007/978-3-319-57454-7_4
12. Anaissi, A., Khoa, N.L.D., Rakotoarivelo, T., Alamdari, M.M., Wang, Y.: Self-advised incremental one-class support vector machines: an application in structural health monitoring. In: Liu, D., Xie, S., Li, Y., Zhao, D., El-Alfy, ES. (eds.) ICONIP 2017, vol. 24, pp. 484–496. Springer, Heidelberg (2017). https://doi.org/10.1007/978-3-319-70087-8_51
13. Anaissi, A., Khoa, N.L.D., Rakotoarivelo, T., Alamdari, M.M., Wang, Y.: Adaptive online one-class support vector machines with applications in structural health monitoring. ACM Trans. Intell. Syst. Technol. (TIST) **9**(6), 1–20 (2018)
14. XnView MP. Image management the enhanced image viewer for (windows/macos/linux) version 0.99.6. Website article (2021). https://www.xnview.com/en/xnviewmp/#features
15. Pandey, P.: 10 python image manipulation tools. Website article (2019). https://opensource.com/article/19/3/python-image-manipulation-tools

16. Dynamsoft. Image processing 101 chapter 2.2: Image enhancement. Website article (2019). https://www.dynamsoft.com/blog/insights/image-processing/image-processing-101-image-enhancement/
17. Abadi, M., et al.: {TensorFlow}: a system for {Large-Scale} machine learning. In: 12th USENIX Symposium on Operating Systems Design and Implementation (OSDI 2016), pp. 265–283 (2016)
18. Manavalan, B., Shin, T.H., Lee, G.: PVP-SVM: sequence-based prediction of phage virion proteins using a support vector machine. Front. Microbiol. **9**, 476 (2018)
19. Scholten, M., Dhingra, N., Lu, T.T., Chao, T.H.: Optimization of support vector machine (svm) for object classification. In: Optical Pattern Recognition XXIII, vol. 8398, pp. 42–50. SPIE (2012)
20. Alzu'bi, AR., Anushya, E.H., Al Sha'ar, E.A., Vincy, B.S.: Dates fruits classification using SVM. In: AIP Conference Proceedings, vol. 1952. AIP Publishing (2018)
21. Kerbaa, T.H., Mezache, A., Oudira, H.: Model selection of sea clutter using cross validation method. Procedia Comput. Sci. **158**, 394–400 (2019)
22. Brownlee, J.: A gentle introduction to k-fold cross-validation. In: Machine Learning Mastery 2019 (2018)
23. Scikit-learn developers. Cross-validation: evaluating estimator performance. Website article (2020). https://scikit-learn.org/stable/modules/cross_validation.html
24. Patro, V.M., Patra, M.R.: Augmenting weighted average with confusion matrix to enhance classification accuracy. Trans. Mach. Learn. Artif. Intell. **2**(4), 77–91 (2014)
25. Szűcs, G.: Multiclass classification by min-max ecoc with hamming distance optimization. Visual Comput. **39**, 1–13 (2022)
26. Visa, S., Ramsay, B., Ralescu, A.L., Van Der Knaap, E.: Confusion matrix-based feature selection. Maics **710**(1), 120–127 (2011)
27. Loddo, A., Di Ruberto, C., Vale, A.M.P.G., Ucchesu, M., Soares, J.M., Bacchetta, G.: An effective and friendly tool for seed image analysis. Visual Comput. **39**(1), 335–352 (2023)
28. Zhu, H., Zhu, Z., Wang, S., Zhang, Y.: COVC-REDRNET: a deep learning model for covid-19 classification. Mach. Learn. Knowl. Extract. **5**(3), 684–712 (2023)
29. Miok, K., Corcoran, P., Spasić, I.: The value of numbers in clinical text classification. Mach. Learn. Knowl. Extract. **5**(3), 746–762 (2023)
30. Anaissi, A., Khoa, N.L.D., Rakotoarivelo, T., Alamdari, M.M., Wang, Y.: Smart pothole detection system using vehicle-mounted sensors and machine learning. J. Civil Struct. Health Monit. **9**, 91–102 (2019)
31. Dinakaran, R., Zhang, L., Li, C.-T., Bouridane, A., Jiang, R.: Robust and fair undersea target detection with automated underwater vehicles for biodiversity data collection. Remote Sens. **14**(15), 3680 (2022)
32. Werth, J.A., Preston, C., Roberts, G.N., Taylor, I.N.: Weed management practices in glyphosate-tolerant and conventional cotton fields in Australia. Aust. J. Exp. Agric. **46**(9), 1177–1183 (2006)

Credit Card Batch Processing in Banking System

Samir Poudel[1(✉)], Movinuddin[1], Sanjana Gutta[1], Revanth Kumar Kommu[1], Jiblal Upadhyay[2], Md Nahid Hasan[2], and Khem Poudel[1]

[1] Department of Computer Science, Middle Tennessee State University, 37132 Murfreesboro, TN, USA
spoudel04@gmail.com, {m2b,sg6t,rk4y}@mtmail.mtsu.edu, khem.poudel@mtsu.edu

[2] Computational and Data Science, Middle Tennessee State University, 37132 Murfreesboro, TN, USA
{ju2i,mh2ay}@mtmail.mtsu.edu

Abstract. Batch payments, involving a single transaction to multiple recipients via a single bank account, offer an efficient alternative to individual payments. This method condenses multiple payments into a single debit entry on bank statements, accelerating payment processing and enhancing business efficiency. Utilizing bank wire transfers is a prevalent means of initiating batch payments.

In contrast to real-time processing, where transactions are handled immediately, batch processing entails aggregating authorized credit card transactions by merchants for submission to their credit card processors at the close of each business day or at scheduled intervals [1]. Merchant-authorized credit card transactions are compiled and sent to customers' banks, seeking authorization. Upon approval, funds are transferred to the business's bank account.

Our objective is to identify fraudulent credit card transactions to safeguard credit card customers from erroneous charges for unauthorized purchases. The model employed aims to be both swift and adept at detecting anomalies, swiftly classifying potentially fraudulent transactions.

The study involved the evaluation of multiple classifiers such as Gradient-Boosted Tree (GBT) and Random Forest, revealing that while the GBT classifier exhibited exceptional precision, the Random Forest classifier emerged as the preferred choice for our dataset. The selection was based on practical considerations, including efficiency and ease of implementation.

Keywords: Anomaly Detection · Authorization Codes · Bank Wire Transfer · Batch Payment · Batch Processing · Credit Card Transactions · Fraudulent Transactions · Payment Processing

K. Daimi and A. Al Sadoon (Eds.): ACR 2024, LNNS 956, pp. 83–96, 2024.
https://doi.org/10.1007/978-3-031-56950-0_8

1 Introduction

This Method Used to Process Credit Card Payments to comprehend batch payments, it's essential to understand the working of credit card payments. This process can be segmented into three parts: authorization, processing, and settlement, although the steps may vary based on the payment processing provider chosen.

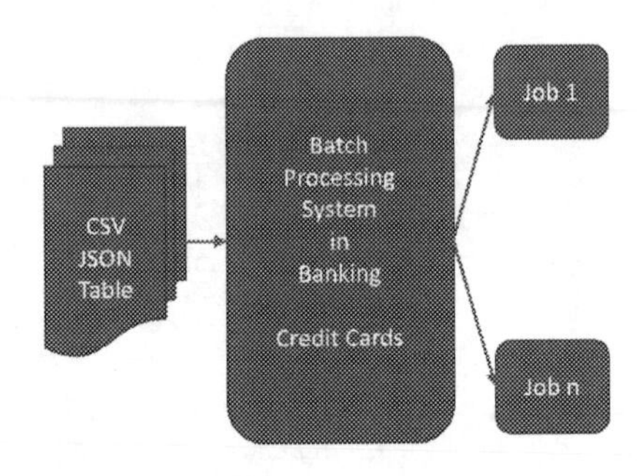

Fig. 1. Batch Processing

- **Authorization:**
  The initial step involves the authorization of a credit card transaction. When utilizing batch payment , customers make payments using their credit cards for merchant services. The Point of Sale (POS) transmits credit card details and transaction amounts to the credit card issuer (e.g., Mastercard, Visa).
  In essence, the POS checks if the card is stolen, real, and if sufficient money is available for the transaction. A hold is placed on the card for the transaction amount if it appears legitimate. Even if the transaction isn't completed, the funds are reserved.
- **Processing:**
  Next comes the processing of credit cards. The authorization hold transfers the customer's funds to the merchant account.
- **Settlement:**
  Settlement takes place when the payment processor instructs the bank to transfer funds between accounts. Upon reaching the seller's account, the transaction is settled, known as closing the transaction (Figs. 1, 2 and 3).

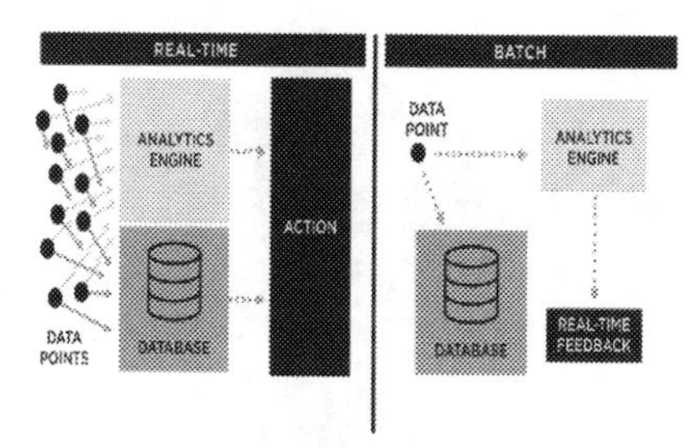

Fig. 2. Real Time vs Batch

1.1 Batch Processing

Batch processing refers to a computer executing a collection of tasks as a group. This method is completely automated and doesn't require human intervention. It's synonymous with workload automation (WLA) and job scheduling [2]. Business scenarios ideal for batch processing include:

- Processes not requiring immediate attention and real-time information
- Handling large data volumes
- Utilizing idle time on a computer or system
- Repetitive processes not requiring human input

An excellent example of batch processing is how credit card companies handle billing. Customers receive a consolidated bill for the entire month, processed on a specified date [3]. Information collected throughout the month is processed collectively at once.

1.2 Credit Card Transaction

The steps involved in a credit card transaction include:

- Customer's initial credit card usage for the transaction.
- Stacking of the transaction in the merchant's database.
- End of day (EOD), submission for authorization.
- Submission of transaction information to the gateway by the merchant.
- Transmission of transaction information to the merchant's bank processor by the credit card gateway.

1.3 Customer Profile Analyzer/Database

The merchant's bank submits the transaction to a network connected to the customer's bank. The customer's bank analyzes the payment using various scenarios and checks the customer's database to accept or decline the payment.

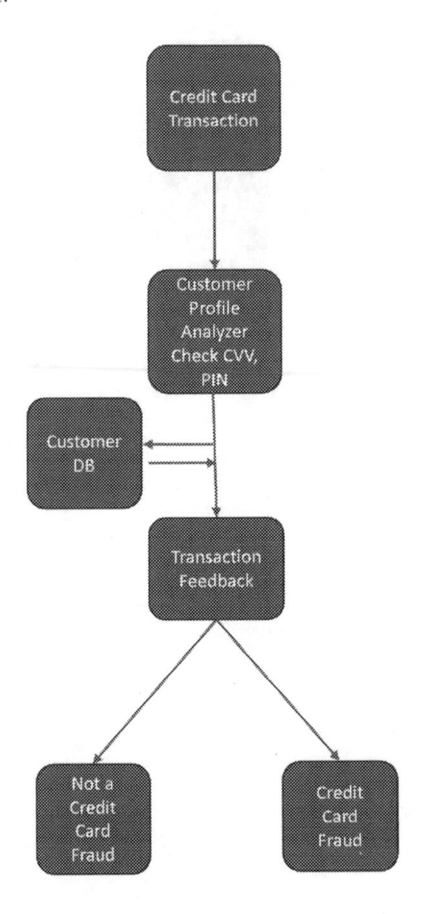

Fig. 3. Credit Card Fraud Detection Block diagram

2 Literature Review

Recent discussions on fraud trends have highlighted several key shifts in fraudulent activities. These include the use of automation by fraudsters, a transition in tactics from third-party devices to on-device fraudulent activities, and an increased focus on AI and machine learning in financial institutions for fraud prevention. Moreover, emerging trends shaping the fraud landscape, comprehensive analyses of significant fraud trends with protective insights, and discussions around machine learning and AI applications in fraud detection underscore the multifaceted and rapidly evolving nature of modern fraudulent practices, urging adaptive and technology-driven countermeasures.

A recent meeting convened by Susan Herbst-Murphy and the Payment Card Center with senior MasterCard officials facilitated information sharing on the clearing and settlement functions within MasterCard's services. The clearing function involves transferring card transaction details, while the payment function facilitates the exchange of monetary value between the cardholder's bank and the bank that accepts the card, as summarized in this document [1].

In another study, Niels Martin, Marijke Swennen, and colleagues discussed the concept of batch processing, wherein a resource performs specific operations on multiple instances either concurrently or sequentially. The study highlights the significant impact of batch processing on process performance and emphasizes its relevance in modeling business processes for performance evaluations [2].

Moreover, Luise Pufahl and Mathias Weske propose an innovative approach to define batch operations, deviating from a single-process model to centrally define batch operations in the data object lifecycle. Their work extends the data object lifecycle by incorporating batch conversion, focusing on data-driven business processes and centralized definition of data operations allowed by process operations for the data object class [3]. This approach redefines the lifecycle by introducing batch operations in the data-driven context.

3 Key Findings and Context

3.1 Credit Card Fraud and Recent Trends

Credit card fraud is a type of identity theft that occurs when someone other than you uses your credit card or bank account information to make unauthorized charges. Fraud can result from stolen, lost, or counterfeit credit cards. Additionally, with the rise of online retail, card fraud and the use of credit card numbers in e-commerce have become more common.

In the United States, credit card fraud has been the most common form of identity theft in four of the last five years. The United States is the country with the most fraud incidents, accounting for more than one-third of global card fraud losses. It is important to be knowledgeable about credit card fraud and identity theft so that you can practice good money habits and awareness in your daily life.

Key Credit Card Theft Findings: According to compiled key findings from the Federal Trade Commission's (FTC) Annual Data Book of 2020 to keep you informed about the frequency and severity of credit card fraud, as well as identified statistics about the populations who are most vulnerable to fraud:

- The most frequent payment method identified out of all fraud reports was credit cards.
- Credit card fraud made up a total of 459,297 reported instances of fraud and identity theft combined in 2020.
- 66,090 cases of reported fraud
- 393,207 cases of reported identity theft
- In identity theft cases, people ages 30–39 reported the most instances of credit card fraud while those age 80 and older reported the least.
- Instances of identity theft by credit card fraud increased by 44.6 percent from 271,927 in 2019 to 393,207 in 2020.
- Identity theft by new credit card accounts increased by 48 percent in 2020.

3.2 Pyspark and Apache Airflow

A Python API for Apache Spark. Apache Spark is an analytical processing engine for large-scale powerful distributed data processing and machine learning applications.

- PySpark is a general-purpose, in-memory, distributed processing engine that allows you to process data efficiently in a distributed fashion.
- Applications running on PySpark are 100x faster than traditional systems [4].
- You will get great benefits using PySpark for data ingestion pipelines. Using PySpark, we can process data from Hadoop HDFS, AWS S3, and many file systems [5].
- PySpark is also used to process real-time data using Streaming and Kafka. Using PySpark streaming, you can also stream files from the file system and from the socket.
- PySpark natively has machine learning and graph libraries (Fig. 4).

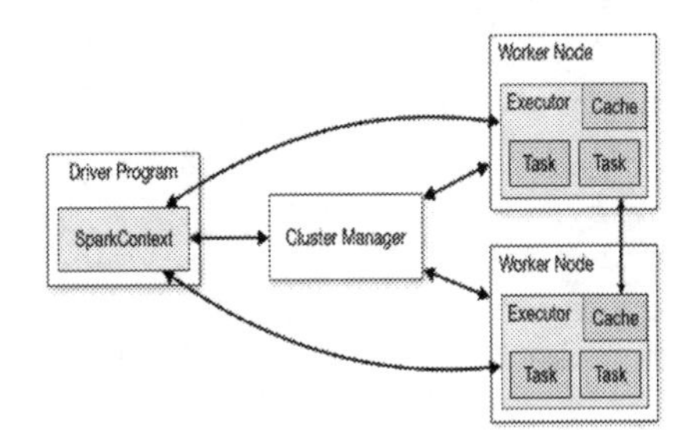

Fig. 4. PySpark Architecture

- Apache Spark works in a master-slave architecture where the master is called the "Driver" and the slaves are called "Workers".
- When you run a Spark application, the Spark Driver creates a context that is an entry point to your application, and all operations (transformations and actions) are executed on worker nodes, and the resources are managed by the Cluster Manager.

Apache Airflow: Apache Airflow is already a commonly used tool for scheduling data pipelines. Airflow uses the Python programming language to define the pipelines. Users can take full advantage of that by using for loops to define pipelines, executing bash commands, using any external modules like pandas, sklearn, GCP, or AWS libraries to manage cloud services, and much, much more [6].

Workflows can be created, scheduled, and monitored programmatically using Apache Airflow. Data engineers utilize it as one of the most reliable platforms for orchestrating workflows or pipelines. You can quickly see the dependencies, progress, logs, code, trigger tasks, and success status of your data pipelines. Users of Airflow can create workflows as task-based Directed Acyclic Graphs (DAGs). With Airflow's sophisticated user interface, it's simple to visualize pipelines that are currently in use, keep track of their progress, and address problems as they arise. When a task succeeds or fails, it can send an alert via email or Slack and links to different data sources. Given its distributed architecture, scalability, and flexibility, Airflow is a good choice for orchestrating complicated business logic.

Why Airflow? Airflow is a batch workflow orchestration platform. The Airflow framework includes operators that connect to many technologies and can be easily extended to connect to new technologies. If your workflow has a definite start and end and runs regularly, you can program it as an Airflow DAG (Fig. 5).

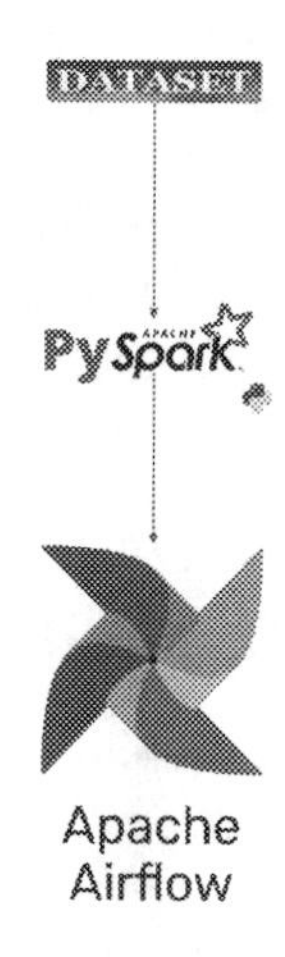

Fig. 5. Technology Flow: Dataset → PySpark → Airflow

If you'd rather code than click, Airflow is the tool for you. Workflows are defined as Python code. This means:

- Workflows can be saved in version control so you can revert to previous versions [6].
- Workflows can be developed by multiple people simultaneously.
- You can write tests to verify functionality.
- Components are extensible and can be built on a wide collection of existing components.

Extensive scheduling and execution semantics make it easy to define complex pipelines that run at regular intervals. Backfilling allows you to (re)run pipelines on historical data after changing logic. Also, sub-pipelines can be rerun after bug fixes, maximizing efficiency.

Airflow's user interface provides both a detailed view of pipelines and individual tasks, as well as an overview of pipelines over time. The user interface allows you to view logs and manage tasks, e.g., repeat the task if an error occurs.

Airflow's open-source nature ensures that we work on components that are developed, tested, and used by many other companies around the world.

DAGs: In Airflow, a DAG (Directed Acyclic Graph) is a collection of all tasks to execute, organized to reflect their relationships and dependencies.

A DAG is defined in a Python script that represents the DAG structure (tasks and their dependencies) as code. For example, a simple DAG might consist of three tasks: A, B, and C. You might say that A must run successfully before B runs, but C can always run. We can say that task A expires after 5 min and B can be restarted up to 5 times if it fails. It could also mean that the workflow runs every night at 10:00 PM, but is not scheduled to start until a certain date.

This is how a DAG describes how a workflow should run. A, B, and C can be anything. Perhaps A is preparing data for her B to analyze while C is sending emails. Alternatively, A can monitor your location so that B can open the garage door and C can turn on the house lights. The point is that the DAG doesn't care what its composition tasks do. Their job is to ensure that everything they do happens at the right time, in the right order, or with the right handling of unexpected problems. DAGs are defined in standard Python files placed in Airflow's DAGS FOLDER. Airflow runs the code in each file to dynamically create DAG objects. You can have any number of DAGs, each describing any number of tasks. In general, each should correspond to a single logical workflow.

Scope: Much like how a blockchain network consolidates transaction blocks [7], Airflow consolidates DAG objects, ensuring their operability within a unified context. Specifically, just as specific volatile cryptocurrencies undergo a standardized consolidation process to maintain transaction security, Airflow requires DAGs to be handled under a cohesive global environment. This consolidation approach is similar to safeguarding Airflow's functionality by defining SubDag-Operators within a confined local space, preventing potential fragmentation concerns in the workflow structure.

Dataset: Credit card fraud detection data set, from Kaggle (https://www.kaggle.com/datasets/mlg-ulb/creditcardfraud). This dataset contains credit card transactions from European cardholders for September 2013. This dataset represents transactions made within two days, with 492 frauds out of 284,807 transactions. The dataset is highly imbalanced, with the positive class (fraud) making up 0.172 percent of all transactions.

This includes only numeric input variables that are the result of PCA transformations. Unfortunately, due to confidentiality reasons, we are unable to provide detailed background information on the original features and data. Features V1, V2, ... V28 are the main components obtained by PCA and the only features that are not transformed by PCA are 'Time' and 'Magnitude'. The Time property contains the elapsed seconds between each transaction and the first transaction in the record. The property 'Amount' is the transaction amount. This property can be used, for example, for cost-aware learning. The characteristic "class" is the response variable and takes the value 1 if it is incorrect and 0 otherwise.

Classification Models: Classification model is created in pyspark, which will be later used to predict if a transaction is fraud or not [8]. From the new data, we spilt the data further for training and testing. The train/test split taken is 80/20. Random forest classifier is used to create the model.

Also, other different classification models have been used to find the best classifier for the given data.

- Gradient-boosted tree classifier (GBT)
- Decision tree classifier
- Random forest classifier
- Linear support vector machine
- Naïve bayes classifier

Metrics to Compare ML Models:

- Accuracy: Percentage of results correctly classified
- Precision: percentage of the results which are relevant
- Recall: percentage of total relevant results correctly classified (Fig. 6).

Classification Model	Accuracy	Precision	Recall
GBT Classifier	93.88	0.94	0.94
Decision Tree Classifier	94.90	0.89	0.95
Random Forest Classifier	94.90	0.89	0.95
Linear Support Vector Machine	94.90	0.89	0.95
Naïve Bayes Classifier	94.90	0.89	0.95

Fig. 6. Comparison of Different ML Models

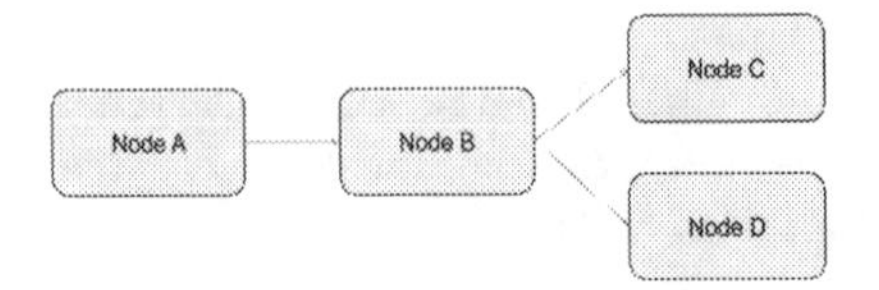

Fig. 7. Valid DAG Structure

Apache Workflow Characteristics:

- Dynamic: Airflow pipelines are configured as Python code, allowing for dynamic pipeline generation.
- Extensible: The Airflow framework contains operators to connect with numerous technologies. All Airflow components are extensible to easily adjust to your environment.
- Flexible: Workflow parameterization is built-in.

If the workflows have a clear start and end, and run at regular intervals, they can be programmed as an Airflow DAG.

Airflow DAG: DAG or a Directed Acyclic Graph - is a collection of all the tasks you want to run, organized in a way that reflects their relationships and dependencies. DAG is a graph with nodes, directed edges and no cycles. A DAG is defined in a Python script, which represents the DAGs structure (tasks and their dependencies) as code (Figs. 7 and 8).

DAG Run: DAG run is a physical instance of a DAG, containing task instances that run for a specific execution date. A DAG run is usually created by the Airflow scheduler but can also be created by an external trigger. Multiple DAG runs may be running at once for a particular DAG, each of them having a different execution date (Figs. 9, 10 and 11).

Tasks: A Task defines a unit of work within a DAG. It is represented as a node in the DAG graph, and it is written in python. Each task is an implementation of an Operator, for example, a PythonOperator to execute some python code, or a BashOperator to run a bash command [9].

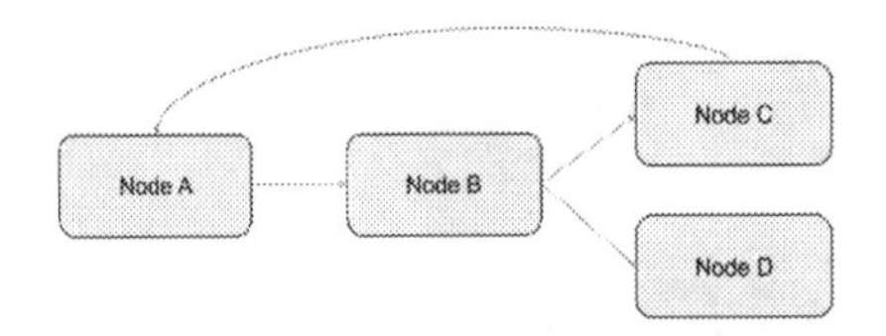

Fig. 8. Invalid DAG Structure

Task Lifecycle: The happy flow consists of the following stages:

- No status (scheduler created empty task instance)
- Scheduled (scheduler determined task instance needs to run)
- Queued (scheduler sent task to executor to run on the queue)
- Running (worker picked up a task and is now running it)
- Success (task completed)

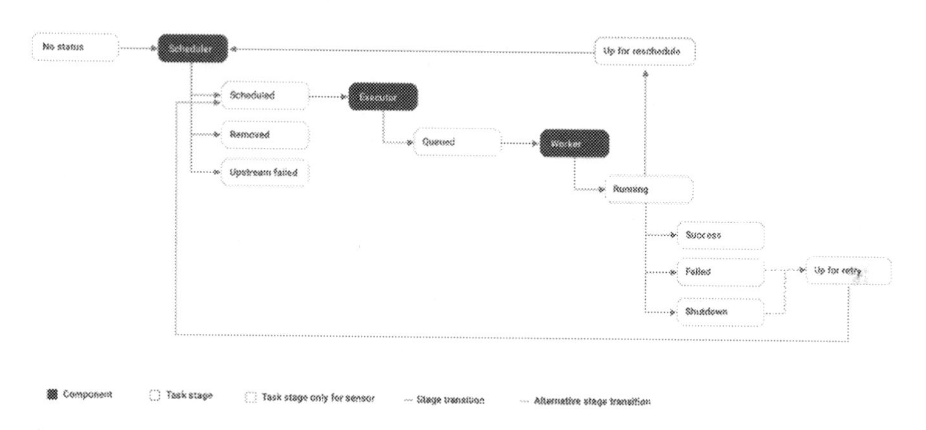

Fig. 9. Task Lifecycle

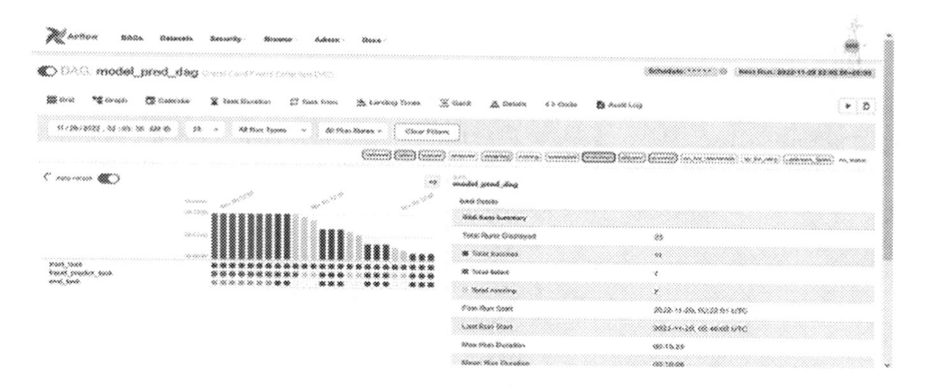

Fig. 10. Airflow Credit Card Fraud Detection DAG

Operators: While DAGs describe how to run a workflow, Operators determine what gets done by a task. An operator describes a single task in a workflow. Operators are usually (but not always) atomic, meaning they can stand on their

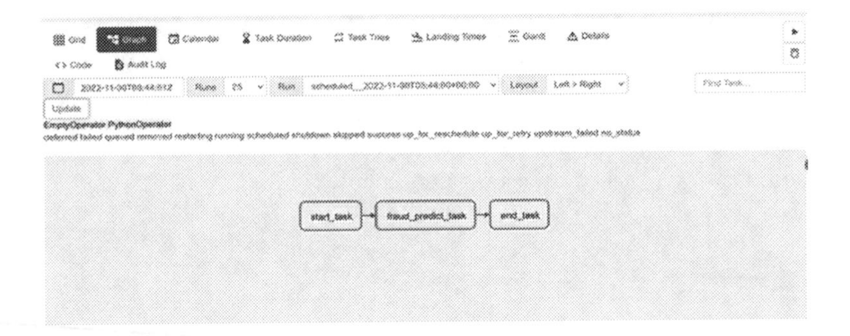

Fig. 11. Airflow Graph

own and don't need to share resources with any other operators[9]. If two operators need to share information, like a filename or a small amount of data, you should consider combining them into a single operator. Airflow provides operators for many common tasks, including:

- BashOperator: executes a bash command
- PythonOperator: calls an arbitrary python function
- EmailOperator: sends an email
- SimpleHttpOperator: sends an HTTP request
- MySqlOperator: executes a SQL command
- Sensor: an Operator that waits (polls) for a certain time, file, database row, S3 key, etc.

4 Result and Discussion

The Python ML code prints out the number of credit card frauds detected in the given dataset where class \$0 means the transaction was determined to be valid and \$1 means it was determined as a fraud transaction. This is used to calculate the accuracy score and precision of the algorithms. The results along with the classification report for the random forest algorithm are given in the output as follows:

$$\text{Total Transactions Checked} : 284,807 \text{transactions}$$
$$\text{Fraud Transactions Detected} : 513 \text{transactions}$$

The classification report provides insights into the performance of the Random Forest algorithm:

$$\begin{aligned} \text{Accuracy Score} &: \text{Indicates overall correctness of predictions} \\ \text{Precision} &: \text{Ratio of correctly predicted fraud to total predicted fraud} \\ \text{Other Metrics (Recall, F1-score)} &: \text{Further insights into the model's performance} \end{aligned}$$

The reported results indicate the Random Forest algorithm's effectiveness in identifying fraudulent transactions from a vast dataset of credit card transactions. However, optimizing the algorithm's precision, particularly in reducing false positives, remains crucial in the context of fraud detection. This might involve fine-tuning model parameters or exploring alternative methodologies to enhance precision without compromising overall accuracy.

5 Conclusion

In conclusion, our analysis of various classifiers has provided valuable insights into their performance. With the exception of the Gradient Boosting Tree (GBT) classifier, all other classifiers yielded nearly identical results, which could be attributed to the relatively limited size of our dataset.

Remarkably, the GBT classifier demonstrated a significantly higher precision compared to the other classifiers, suggesting its ability to accurately identify true positive cases. However, when examining accuracy and recall, the GBT classifier performed similarly to the other models.

Considering these findings, one might argue that, based on the data generated, the GBT classifier could be considered the optimal choice, particularly if precision is of utmost importance. However, it's essential to note that we ultimately opted for the Random Forest classifier for our specific dataset. This choice may have been influenced by several factors, including computational efficiency, model interpretability, or project-specific requirements.

In summary, while the GBT classifier excels in precision, the Random Forest classifier was selected for our dataset due to various practical considerations. The choice of classifier should be made with a holistic view of project objectives and constraints, ensuring that it aligns with the broader context and goals of the analysis.

References

1. Herbst-Murphy, S.: Clearing and Settlement of Interbank Card Transactions: A MasterCard Tutorial for Federal Reserve Payments Analysts. Federal Reserve Bank of Philadelphia (2013). https://www.philadelphiafed.org/payment-cards-center/
2. Martin, N., Swennen, M., Depaire, B., Jans, M., Caris, A., Vanhoof, K.: Batch Processing: Definition and Event Log Identification. Hasselt University, Agoralaan Building D, 3590 Diepenbeek, Belgium (2015)

3. Pufahl, L., Weske, M.: Batch processing across multiple business processes based on object life cycle (extended abstract). ResearchGate (2015). https://doi.org/10.13140/RG.2.1.4335.9120
4. Bandi, R., Jayavel, A., Karthik, R.: Machine learning with PySpark - review. Indon. J. Electr. Eng. Comput. Sci. **12**(1), 102–106 (2018). https://doi.org/10.11591/ijeecs.v12.i1.pp102-106
5. Oluwasakin, E., et al.: Minimization of high computational cost in data preprocessing and modeling using MPI4Py. Mach. Learn. Appl. **13**, 100483 (2023). https://doi.org/10.1016/j.mlwa.2023.100483
6. Shukla, S.: Creating data pipelines using apache airflow. Zenodo (2022). https://doi.org/10.5281/zenodo.6828344
7. Poudel, S.: Cryptocurrency price and volatility predictions with machine learning. J. Mark. Anal. (2023). https://doi.org/10.1057/s41270-023-00239-1
8. Manem, C., Arya, P., Shekhar, H., Acheadeth, L.: Imbalance multi-label Classification in Pyspark (2023)
9. Hasan, M.N., Hamdan, S., Poudel, S., Vargas, J., Poudel, K.: Prediction of length-of-stay at intensive care unit (ICU) using machine learning based on MIMIC-III database. In: 2023 IEEE Conference on Artificial Intelligence (CAI), Santa Clara, CA, USA, pp. 321–323 (2023). https://doi.org/10.1109/CAI54212.2023.00142

Irregular Frame Rate Synchronization of Multi-camera Videos for Data-Driven Animal Behavior Detection

Enkhzol Dovdon(✉), Manu Agarwal, Yanja Dajsuren, and Jakob de Vlieg

Mathematics and Computer Science Department,
Eindhoven University of Technology, Eindhoven, The Netherlands
{e.d.dovdon,m.agarwal,y.dajsuren,j.d.vlieg}@tue.nl

Abstract. Deep learning and camera-based monitoring play a pivotal role in effective farm management. However, reliable data availability remains essential for successful deep-learning applications. Cameras are the primary data sources for computer vision deep learning models. For effective farm management, a multi-camera setup is often used. In a multi-camera farm setup, the input dataset for deep learning is prepared by combining the records of the cameras installed on many sides of the farm. However, an irregular frame rate of various cameras in a multi-camera setup can cause issues such as drift. Therefore, the data from different cameras must be in sync before feeding it to a deep learning model. In this work, we present a method for frame rate synchronization that leverages the timestamp information on the video and achieves high accuracy. Our method addresses a critical use case where the frame rate synchronization is performed post-video recording. Its effectiveness is demonstrated in real-world animal behavior detection scenarios, where precise synchronization is vital. Via this work, we contribute to robust deep-learning models for farm management and livestock analysis by addressing frame rate irregularities.

Keywords: Frame rate synchronization · Multi-camera video synchronization · Optical character recognition · Feature extraction · Precision livestock farming

1 Introduction

In precision livestock farming, Information and Communications Technology improves the livestock farming process [9]. In particular, data-driven measures play a vital role in improving the well-being of animals on the farm as well as improving the production efficiency of the farming process. Data-driven measures involve collecting digital data from the farms and applying data analytics and machine learning to combat efficiency-related problems, innovative farm interventions, and profitability of agriculture [14]. For instance, via a continuous video-based stream from an animal housing facility, the farm managers can check the living conditions of animals and take corrective actions in case of a negative interaction among animals, such as tail biting in pigs. In addition, machine

K. Daimi and A. Al Sadoon (Eds.): ACR 2024, LNNS 956, pp. 97–112, 2024.
https://doi.org/10.1007/978-3-031-56950-0_9

learning and deep learning models can be used to study the behavior of animals, enabling phenotyping that can be potentially used for genetic selection and to perform the social network analysis in large groups of animals [10]. Machine vision has been used for assessing animal behavior [19], but the manual analysis of these videos is time-consuming and may introduce human error [4,5]. A computer vision-based deep learning analysis is increasingly being used to derive useful information from videos, e.g., automated detection of animal behaviors [11].

For deep learning analysis, access to high-quality data is crucial. In the case of automated detection of animal behavior on a farm, observation cameras are used as data collection devices. The deep learning-based object detection and tracking systems are being used extensively for animal welfare and behavior studies [9,10]. These systems are greatly affected by visual attributes, such as light effects, blur, and the temporary visibility of the object, depending on the camera's location. Tracking using multi-camera-based detection provides comprehensive information on the object's movement from multiple angles, solving problems associated with a single camera [16,27]. Therefore, multi-camera systems have received considerable attention in recent years, particularly in surveillance, tracking, image recognition, image sensing, and computer vision [20].

The performance of a multi-camera deep learning system depends heavily on how the video data from different cameras is synchronized precisely at the frame level. For instance, inconsistencies in the frame rate of multiple videos may cause issues, such as data drift. Therefore, video data from different cameras must be synchronized at the frame rate level before feeding this data to the machine learning model. This paper presents a novel methodology synchronizing each video stream's frame rate (measured in frames/sec) in a multi-camera setup. Although we demonstrate our work via a two-camera setup, this work can be used to correct the irregular frame rate in a multi-camera setup. We showcase the application of the proposed methodology in the context of IMAGEN and SmartTurkeys projects.

In the IMAGEN [18] and SmartTurkeys [3] project, a data platform [1] for automated phenotype detection is being built on the Dutch National HPC Surf [6]. Our proposed irregular frame rate synchronization method is implemented on this data platform via data pipelines.

This paper is organized as follows: Sect. 2 reviews the existing multi-camera video synchronization methods as well as their applicability in the case of irregular frame rate problem in pre-recorded videos. In Sect. 3, we propose an irregular frame rate synchronization method based on timestamp information extracted from the video files. In addition, we present the results of applying the proposed method in a case study. Finally, Sect. 4 concludes the paper and discusses future work.

2 Related Work

This section reviews the literature on frame-level synchronization of multi-camera videos, a challenging and well-studied problem with various solutions.

We classify the current methods into two broad categories: software-based and hardware-based. The Software-based methods use image features and/or audio signals to align the video frames from multiple cameras, while hardware-based methods rely on external devices or network protocols to synchronize the cameras. We further divide these categories into subcategories based on the specific techniques used by different researchers.

2.1 Software-Based Methods

Feature-Based Methods: To align the multi-camera videos temporally, Bo-Song et al. [12] propose a method that relies on feature point matching and refinement. Their method combines a SIFT (Scale Invariant Feature Transform) based SURF (Speed-Up Robust Feature) algorithm with Random Sample Consensus (RANSAC). The method extracts feature points from each video and applies a matching algorithm to find corresponding points across different cameras at different distances and views. The rate of detecting keyframes was 96%. Darshana Mistry and Asim Banerjee [17] present a comparative analysis of two widely used feature detection methods in computer vision: SIFT and SURF. The performance of these methods is evaluated in terms of accuracy, robustness, and computational efficiency under various conditions. The results show that SIFT outperforms SURF in detecting features across different scales, while SURF is faster and more robust to rotation, blur, warping, and RGB noise. Both methods have similar effects on feature detection under illumination changes. Karami et al. [13] also compare the performance of SIFT, SURF, Binary Robust Independent Elementary Features (BRIEF), as well as Oriented FAST and Rotated BRIEF (ORB) techniques on matching accuracy and computational efficiency metrics. They found that SIFT achieved the highest matching accuracy but was computationally expensive.

Feature Trajectory Matching: Ahmed Elhayek et al. [8] propose a method to synchronize videos from different viewpoints for multi-video analysis in general scenes. The method tracks and matches feature trajectories in each video. The matches are used to estimate the spatial and temporal parameters between the videos, such as the fundamental matrix, the offset, and the frame rate ratio. The method combines feature tracking, matching, and RANSAC for video synchronization. Sato et al. [23] propose a method to synchronize the two videos from the same scene using object and motion features. They combine static features from work objects and dynamic features from hand motions with adaptive weights based on alignment quality. They calculate inter-frame distances and match frames optimally by dynamic programming.

Rao et al. [21] propose a method to align two videos based on 3D epipolar geometry and dynamic time warping. The method uses a rank constraint of corresponding points to measure the similarity between trajectories and avoids the computation of the fundamental matrix. The method can synchronize videos of different individuals, times, and viewpoints and has applications in video synthesis, action recognition, and computer-aided training.

Shrestha et al. [24] present a novel approach to synchronizing multiple camera recordings based on audio and video features. They compare three realizations of their approach using flashes, audio fingerprints, and onsets. Furthermore, they evaluate these three realizations on a common data set and discuss their applicability and robustness. The onset-based realization is the most successful and reliable for synchronization. Also, according to their work, the realization choice depends on the application type and the availability of audio and flashes.

Machine Learning: Wieschollek et al. [26] propose a combination of deep neural networks and path-finding algorithms for synchronizing videos by approximating the similarity of frame pairs based on the feature embedding by a deep convolutional neural network. Utilizing the transitivity of matching tours, the complexity of the input data is gradually increased, thus allowing us to synchronize videos months apart under different conditions in a robust way.

2.2 Hardware-Based Methods

Kim Hyuno and Masatoshi Ishikawa [15] proposed a frame synchronization technique for a camera network using a linearly oscillating light spot. The approach projected a light spot on the scene and captured the videos using multiple cameras with different frame rates. The technique was tested using a comprehensive experimental setup and showed promising results in accuracy and robustness.

For synchronizing multi-camera videos, it is possible to use a timecode generator, a device or software that produces a timecode signal, and a series of numerical codes representing the time information of each video or audio frame. Timecode synchronizes multiple recordings or tracks and identifies specific points or events in a recording [22].

2.3 Summary of Literature Studies

The hardware-based solutions require deploying relevant hardware solutions before recording the scene. Thus, the scope of hardware-based solutions is limited in the case of pre-recorded videos. On the other hand, the software-based solution relies on the changes in the scene under observation to find the matching frames in multi-camera recordings. However, in the case of pre-recorded videos with significantly fewer or no changes in the consecutive frames, the existing approaches are not very helpful. For instance, in our scenario, the animals in the enclosure are not always active for all the moments. Our experimentation with SIFT-based similarity matching for such scenarios shows that it doesn't yield any suitable match. In other words, the existing approaches are not very helpful for correcting the irregular frame rates in pre-recorded videos with significantly fewer changes in the consecutive frames.

3 Proposed Irregular Frame Rate Synchronization Method for Pre-recorded Multi-camera Videos

The section proposes a method that solves the irregular frame rate problem in pre-recorded multi-camera videos. The section is organized as follows: Subsection A overviews our multi-camera video setup and discusses the problem of irregular frame rate in such a setup. In subsection B, we showcase an experiment using the SIFT method for irregular frame rate synchronization of videos. Furthermore, we discuss why the SIFT-based approach falls short in such use cases. In subsection C, we introduce our method that leverages timestamp information for precise frame rate synchronization at each second level. Finally, subsection D discusses the results of applying our proposed method in the IMAGEN project's camera recordings.

3.1 Overview of Our Multi-camera Video setup and Irregular Frame Rate Problem

The video data collected from a pig farm consists of recordings from two to three cameras installed in one pen. Each camera captures the behavior and activity of the pigs in the pen from different angles. These cameras are connected to a Network Video Recorder (NVR) as shown in Fig. 1. The NVR is programmed to start recording at a specific time and with a preset frame rate (frames/sec). In addition, the NVR also stores the recordings in files of one-hour duration for each camera stream attached to it. Each recorded file is approximately 110 MB, and the total length of the video data for one day is about 5.2 GB.

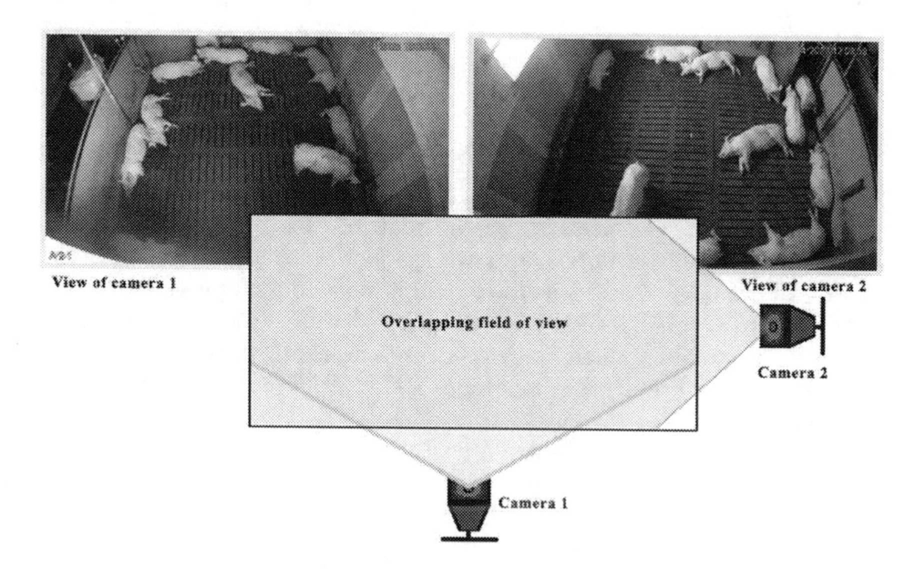

Fig. 1. Multi-camera setup in a pig pen.

For developing animal tracking and behavior detection AI models, these multi-camera video recordings are the base data sources. However, the irregular frame rates among the different camera recordings of the same scene lower the quality of the input dataset. The problem of irregular frame rate arises when the actual frame rate of each recorded video file varies slightly from the configured or preset frame rate at the NVR. For instance, for a preset frame rate of 15 Frames Per Second (FPS), the video stream from camera 1 might have an actual frame rate of 15.014 FPS, while the video stream from camera 2 might have an actual frame rate of 15.022 FPS. This means some seconds contain more or less than 15 frames, which causes a cumulative error in frame rate over time.

To further elaborate on how the irregular frame rate can cause errors in the multi-camera dataset for deep learning, we share here our findings based on a one-hour recording of Camera 1 from timestamps 19:00:00 to 19:59:59. We found that the video had four extra frames at the beginning, with a timestamp of 18:59:59. This indicated that the video started earlier than expected. Moreover, we observed that the video had 9 to 10 extra frames at each 10-minute interval, which suggested that the video had a slightly higher frame rate than the nominal 15 FPS. Conversely, the video had only ten frames at the last second, with a timestamp of 19:59:59. This indicated that the video ended earlier than expected. Therefore, the video had a total of 54059 frames and a duration of 1 h 0 min 0 s 601 ms, instead of the expected 54000 frames and 1 h 0 min 0 s.

For developing robust deep learning models for animal tracking and behavior detection, it was imperative that the issues caused by irregular frame rate and consequent data drift are addressed. Therefore, we needed to come up with a frame rate synchronization method for multi-camera video, considering the following requirements: (1) the ability to synchronize pre-recorded videos from multiple cameras with irregular frame rates, (2) the assurance that the synchronized data for training the multi-camera deep learning model is accurate at each camera level (3) the preservation of the original video quality.

3.2 SIFT-Based Synchronization Experiment

Based on literature reviews, we experimented using the SIFT method as a feature extraction and matching method for synchronizing the irregular frame rate of two videos of the same scene. The idea was as follows: Given the recordings from Camera 1 and Camera 2, align the frames of both recordings at each second level via the similarity-based methods. For instance, if we can pair the most similar frames at each second level in both video recordings, the drift caused by irregular frame rates can be solved. The following paragraph discusses our experiment around this idea and our findings.

To experiment with the similarity-based method, we made the first frame of the first second of Video 1 as the reference frame. We then sampled the first two seconds from Video 2, starting from frame #1, as the target frames. We applied the SIFT method to find the best matching frame among the target frames with the most similar features to the reference frame. The best matching frame is shown in Fig. 2.

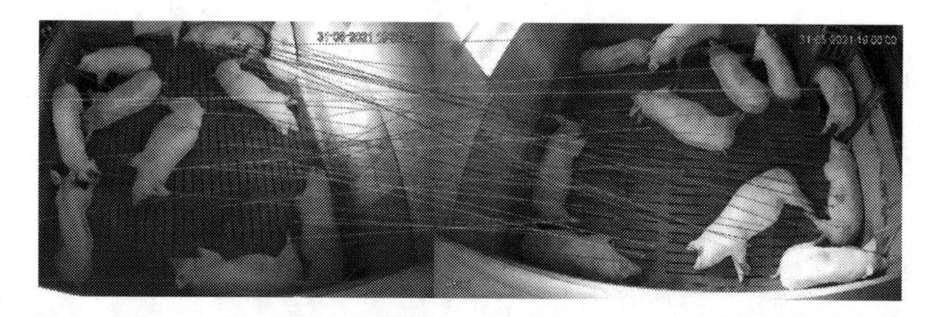

Fig. 2. SIFT matching frame, each match is shown as a line

Table 1. Results of SIFT method on a single frame of video #1 and first two seconds of video #2

Video #1	Video #2	Average matches distance
Frame_1	Frame_1	164.01
Frame_1	Frame_*	...
Frame_1	Frame_12	162.25
Frame_1	Frame_*	...
Frame_1	Frame_19	**154.93**
Frame_1	Frame_*	...
Frame_1	Frame_30	163.30

Based on the results of the SIFT algorithm in Table 1, the frame that matches the most with Frame_1 is Frame_19 from the next second of the video. Frame_19 has the lowest average distance (154.93). This showed that the similarity matching fails to find the best matches in the exact second because, in a few seconds, there are no significant changes in the videos. This results in very similar frames and limits the usage of such similarity-based synchronization methods, particularly in the animal behavior detection domain. Therefore, to achieve the frame-level synchronization of multi-camera videos, we propose a method that corrects the irregular frame rate at each second level by using the timestamp information in each video. This ensures that the deep learning models are fed with the multi-camera data synchronized at each second level.

3.3 Proposed Timestamp-Based Irregular Frame Rate Synchronization

In Fig. 3, we showcase our proposed timestamp-based irregular frame rate synchronization method. Our method has three phases, with various steps in each phase. The input to our method is a video recording with an irregular frame rate. The method's output is the reconstructed video with a consistent frame rate. For instance, in the case of a preset frame rate of 15 FPS, the output video of our method will have precisely 15 frames during each second.

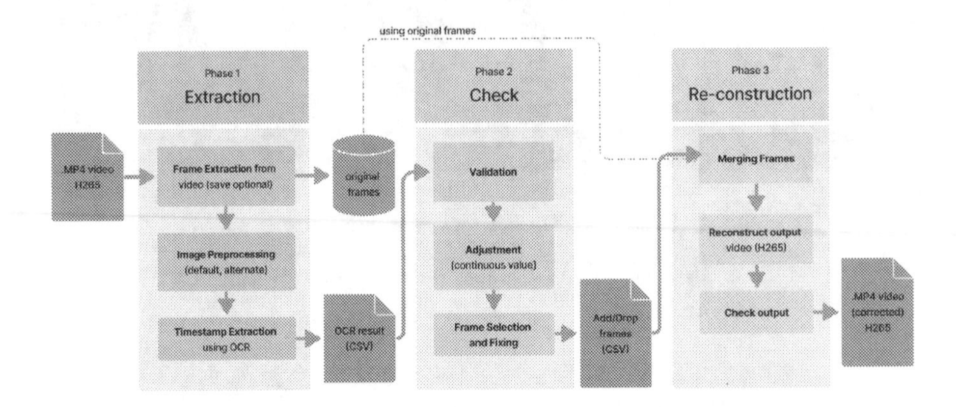

Fig. 3. Workflow of irregular frame rate synchronization of multi-camera video.

Phase 1: Extraction. This phase has three steps as follows:

1. *Frame Extraction:* The first step during the extraction phase involves extracting the frames from the input video and storing them in a directory for further analysis. The total number of frames in a video can be calculated by multiplying the preset frame rate and the duration of the input video (in seconds).

$$Total\ number\ of\ frames = PresetFrame\ rate \times Duration \tag{1}$$

2. *Image Preprocessing:* In the case of input video with irregular frame rate, the total number of frames are not equal to the total number of frames calculated via Eq. 1. Therefore, for synchronizing the frame rate at each second level, it is essential to know which seconds have additional or missing frames. For this purpose, we relied on the timestamp information present in each frame.
   Hence, the next step during the extraction phase was to extract the timestamp at each frame's top-right corner. We used Optical Character Recognition (OCR) to extract the timestamp information from each frame. However, due to different lighting conditions in specific frames, as shown in Fig. 4, it was very challenging to recognize the timestamp correctly via the OCR engine. Therefore, before applying an OCR on the cropped image region containing the timestamp, we performed several image-processing steps to enhance the accuracy of the OCR system. These steps included converting the image to Binarization, Grayscale, Filter, Upscale, Conversion, and Structure & Dilate [6]:
   (a) Binarization step converts the cropped image region containing the timestamp into a binary image, where each pixel is black or white. This is done

by applying a threshold value, determining whether a pixel is foreground or background. The equation for binarization is:

$$B(x,y) = \begin{cases} 0, \; if \; (I(x,y) < T) \\ 255, \; otherwise \end{cases} \tag{2}$$

where $B(x,y)$ is the binary image, $I(x,y)$ is the original image, and T is the threshold value.

(b) The grayscale step converts the binary image into a grayscale image, where each pixel has a value between 0 and 255. The equation for grayscale conversion is:

$$G(x,y) = 255 \cdot B(x,y) \tag{3}$$

where the grayscale image $G(x,y)$ is calculated by multiplying the binary image by 255 (the maximum intensity value for an 8-bit grayscale image), and $B(x,y)$ is the binary image, where (x,y) are the pixel coordinates.

(c) The filter step applies a Gaussian blur filter to the grayscale image, which smooths out any sharp or jagged edges. This is done using a radius value, determining how much the neighboring pixels are averaged. The equation for Gaussian filtering is:

$$F(x,y) = \frac{1}{2\pi\sigma^2} \int_{-\infty}^{\infty} \int_{-\infty}^{\infty} G(u,v) e^{-\frac{(x-u)^2+(y-v)^2}{2\sigma^2}} dudv \tag{4}$$

where $F(x,y)$ is the filtered image, $G(u,v)$ is the grayscale image, and σ is the standard deviation of the Gaussian kernel.

(d) The upscale step enlarges the filtered image by a factor of 5, using the nearest neighbor interpolation method. This is done by resizing the image dimensions by multiplying them by 5. The equation for nearest neighbor interpolation is:

$$U(x,y) = F(\lfloor x/5 \rfloor, \lfloor y/5 \rfloor) \tag{5}$$

where $U(x,y)$ is the upscaled image, and $F(\lfloor x/5 \rfloor, \lfloor y/5 \rfloor)$ is the nearest pixel in the filtered image to $(x/5, y/5)$.

(e) The structure & dilate step applies a morphological operation on the upscaled image. This operation expands the white regions in the image and shrinks the black regions. This is done using a kernel, a small matrix that defines how each pixel is affected by its neighbors. The equation for dilation is:

$$D(x,y) = \max_{(i,j)\in K} N(x+i, y+j) \tag{6}$$

where $D(x, y)$ is the dilated image, $N(x+i, y+j)$ is a grid-like format representation of the upscaled image from Eq. 5, and K is the kernel.

3. *Timestamp Extraction:*
After the image processing step, the final step in the extraction phase is to extract the timestamp from each frame using the OCR technique. We considered different clock formats for recognizing the timestamp information from the image, such as hh:mm:ss, mm:ss, and ss. The number of digits can affect the accuracy of the OCR system, as more digits may increase the chance of misrecognition or confusion. Therefore, through multiple tests, we decided to adopt the "ss" clock format. This choice significantly improved the accuracy of the OCR system in detecting and recognizing the timestamp digits.
Applying an OCR for detection on the cropped image region is expressed as:

$$T = E(C(F(V))) \tag{7}$$

where T is the extracted timestamp, E is the OCR function, C is the cropping function, F is the frame extraction function, and V is the video.

Phase 2: Check. This phase consists of the following steps:

1. *Validating and Adjusting the Extracted Timestamp:* Once the timestamp was extracted using an OCR, we validated its accuracy. A valid timestamp (i.e., "ss" clock format) ranges from 0 to 59. If the extracted timestamp was not valid, appropriate adjustments were made, such as comparing the invalid timestamp with neighboring timestamps and then do the necessary corrections.
2. *Frame Selection and Fixing:* In this step, we fixed the irregular frame rate at each second level. This step ensures that there is a consistent frame rate in the final output video. For instance, if the frame rate exceeds the desired value (such as 15 FPS) in a given second, additional frames are discarded to reduce it. Conversely, if the frame rate is lower than the desired value, frames are duplicated to increase it. Furthermore, a CSV log containing the information about which frames were selected and fixed, such as their index, timestamp, and status, was created during this step.

Phase 3: Re-construction. During the re-construction phase, the output video with a consistent frame rate at each second level was created by combining the stored original frames with the CSV log from the last phase. Equation 10 formulates this process as:

$$V' = E(R(F, L)) \tag{8}$$

where V' is the output video, E is the encoding function, R is the reconstruction function, F is a list of original frames, and L is a CSV log.

3.4 Results and Discussion

In this subsection, we discuss our findings when applying our method for correcting the irregular frame rate problem in the IMAGEN project. As OCR-based timestamp detection plays a vital role in the success of our method, we detail the performance of various OCR approaches in our use case. Furthermore, we detail: 1) How different OCRs perform when detecting the "SS" digits in a "HH:MM:SS" based timestamp in the image, 2) The effect of the image processing step on the performance of OCR, and 3) How "validating and adjustment" step corrects the OCR detection errors. We conclude this subsection by showcasing how the output video is reconstructed after fixing the irregular frame rate at each second level in the input video.

1) Performance of different OCRs: We evaluated EasyOCR, PyTesseract,and KerasOCR for timestamp extraction. We applied these OCRs on various numbers of frames and recorded the failure rates for each recognizer. The results are summarized in Table 2, showing failure rates of 0.1% on 54,000 frames for EasyOCR, 9.1% on 27,000 frames for PyTesseract, and 1.5% on 9,000 frames for KerasOCR. Based on the evaluation results, EasyOCR emerged as the most reliable option. Thus, we decided to utilize EasyOCR for timestamp extraction from the frames.

Table 2. OCR analysis

Recognizer	Support	Frames used for testing	Failure rate (SS)
EasyOCR [2]	70 languages *(digits, letters, symbols)*	54000	0.1
Pytesseract [25]	100 languages *(digits, letters, symbols, punctuation)*	27000	9.1
KerasOCR [7]	English and Arabic *(digits, letters)*	9000	1.5

2) The effect of the image processing step on the performance of OCR: The aim of our OCR was to extract the last two digits of the timestamp, which indicate the seconds (SS) from the cropped region of each video frame. However, as the frames had different backgrounds and lighting conditions that affected the visibility of the digits, our OCR recognizer faced challenges in detecting the digits correctly. Figure 4 shows how the background and lighting varied across the frames. Some frames had a wall as the background, while others had a rail. Some frames were bright, while others were dark. These factors influenced the performance of the OCR system.

To address these challenges, we applied various processing steps to the image. As mentioned in Subsection C, the processing consisted of steps such as binarization, grayscale, filtering, upscaling, as well as structure & dilate. Figure 5 depicts these step.

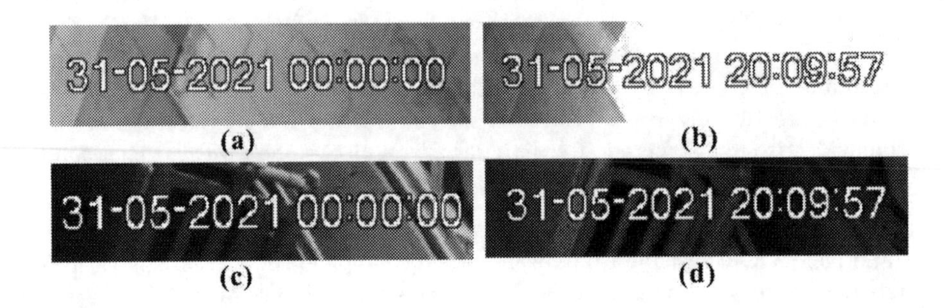

Fig. 4. Different backgrounds and lighting instances: a) wall b) bright c) rail d) dark

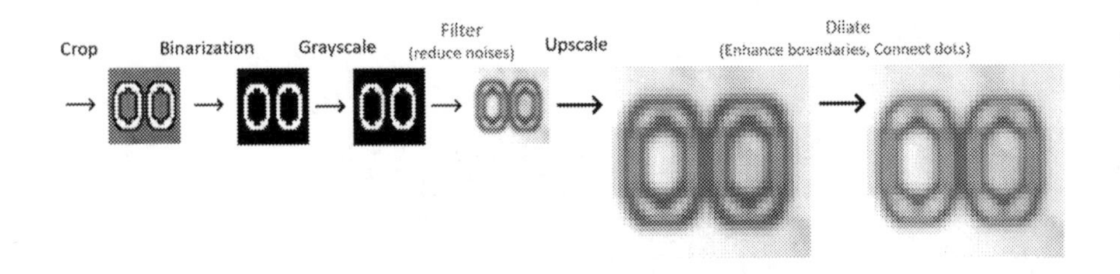

Fig. 5. Results of image processing steps

We found that applying these steps in different orders produced different results. For instance, applying binarization before grayscale resulted in a better contrast than using grayscale before binarization. Adjusting the threshold value in the binarization step was crucial for dealing with frames with extremely white backgrounds, such as those with sunlight or light reflection. The default threshold value was 200, close to the average of the image RGB values. However, we increased the threshold value to 230 or 240 for brighter images, which made more pixels in the digit region white and more distinguishable against the black background. In addition, when the background is darker than average, the threshold value is 150. After that, EasyOCR successfully detected the digit in a frame.

3) Correcting the OCR detection errors via the "validating and adjustment" step: As shown in Table 2, the EasyOCR had a failure rate of 0.1%. Therefore, to correct the EasyOCR errors in 0.1% of the frames, we designed an "validation and adjustment" algorithm that evaluates the OCR results based on predefined rules and assigns a confidence score to the OCR result. The algorithm evaluates an OCR results under the following rules:

- The format of the OCR result: It should consist of exactly two digits, not letters or symbols.
- The range of the OCR result: Because "SS", i.e., seconds, can have a value only between 00 to 59. The OCR result should be within the range of 00 to 59, inclusive.
- The continuity of the OCR result: 1) It should differ from the previous result by either zero or one, **AND** 2) It should match the majority of the neighboring results within a certain window size.

Based on these rules, the algorithm assigns a confidence score to the OCR result. If the confidence score is below a certain threshold, the algorithm corrects the OCR result by replacing it with the most probable value based on these rules.

Table 3. OCR result with incorrect result example

Filename (frame)	Value (SS)	Confidence score	Verification
4497.png	59	0.999999	correct
4498.png	59	0.999999	correct
4499.png	58	0.752233	incorrect
4500.png	59	0.999999	correct
4501.png	0	0.971225	correct

For instance, Table 3 shows an incorrect OCR result for filename 4499.png, with a low confidence score of 0.75. The algorithm corrects this result by changing 58 to 59, which matches the previous, current, and neighboring results.

Creating the Output Video: After completing the OCR-based timestamp extraction and necessary validation and adjustments, we identified the frames needing to be deleted or duplicated to achieve a constant frame rate. This information is recorded in a CSV log file. Later, the output video is reconstructed using the original frames and this CSV log file.

Figure 6 depicts this whole process. The created output video is always 60 min long with 54000 frames and a constant frame rate of 15 FPS. The quality and accuracy of the output video are evaluated by comparing it with the original videos. In particular, we measured the output videos on the following metrics:

- Resolution: The resolution of our output video was the same as the original videos, which was 1280×720 pixels. Thus, the proposed method did not affect the image quality or clarity of the output video.
- Irregular Frame rate: The output video had a consistent frame rate of 15 FPS. The method improved the temporal alignment and consistency of the output video frames.

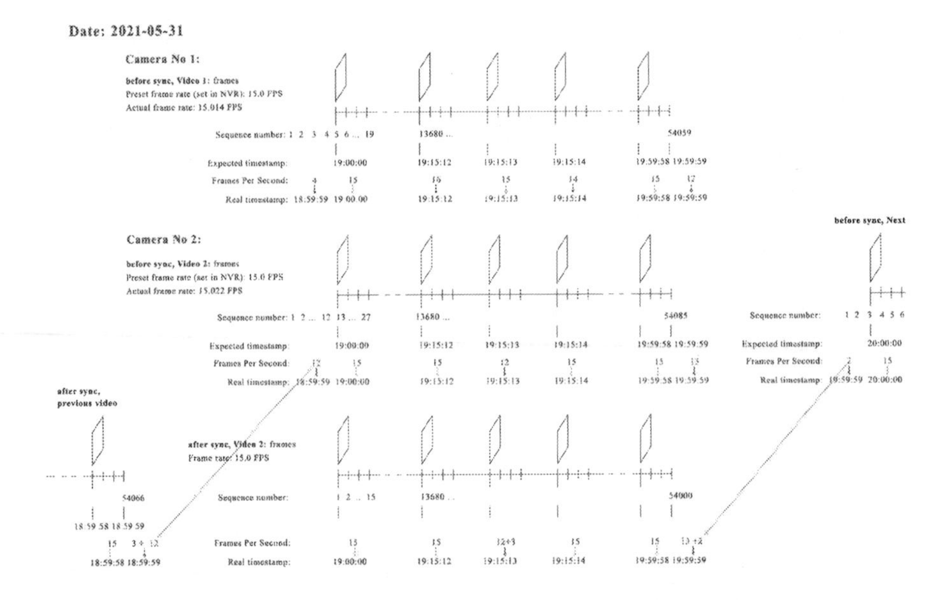

Fig. 6. Representation of synchronization method for irregular frame rate of video.

- Visual quality: The visual quality of the output video was similar to the original videos. This method did not introduce noticeable artifacts or distortions in the output video.
- Robustness: The method's robustness was high for different lighting conditions, camera angles, and movements, and it could handle these scenarios very well.
- Scalability: The scalability of our method was moderate for a different number of cameras, frame rates, and resolutions.

4 Conclusions and Future Work

The irregular frame rates in multi-camera video recordings can cause issues such as data drift. Therefore, it is imperative that the video data from different cameras be synchronized precisely at the individual frame level before feeding it to a deep learning model.

In this paper, we propose an innovative method for synchronizing irregular frame rates of multi-camera videos. As our method works well for already recorded videos, it does not require any hardware modifications. In addition, it can handle scenarios where SIFT-based similarity methods are not viable owing to fewer changes in the scene within a few seconds. Our method is robust for lighting conditions, camera angles, and movements.

As our method employs OCR technology for extracting the timestamp from the images, we also evaluated three OCRs, EasyOCR, PyTesseract, and KerasOCR in our use case. Our results showed that EasyOCR outperformed the other two OCRs. While these OCRs are general-purpose and can recognize letters, numbers, and characters in many languages, we only need to recognize digits (seconds) in our case. The use of general-purpose OCR leads to increased computation costs. Therefore, as future work, we believe using a specially trained machine learning model can improve the computational cost of using these OCRs.

Acknowledgements. This work is supported by the Dutch NWO project IMAGEN [P18-19] of the research program Perspectief. Topigs Norsvin, the Netherlands, offered data from the Volmer facility in Germany. The authors would like to thank EngD Software Technology trainees from the Eindhoven University of Technology for assisting in implementing our method as data pipelines on the IMAGEN Data Analytics Platform.

References

1. Agarwal, M., Dovdon, E., Barge, L.R., Dajsuren, Y., de Vlieg, J.: A HPC-based data analytics platform architecture for data-driven animal phenotype detection. In: 2023 IEEE 6th International Conference on Cloud Computing and Artificial Intelligence: Technologies and Applications (CloudTech), pp. 1–6. IEEE (2023)
2. Baek, Y., Lee, B., Han, D., Yun, S., Lee, H.: Character region awareness for text detection. In: Proceedings of the IEEE/CVF Conference on Computer Vision and Pattern Recognition, pp. 9365–9374 (2019)
3. Breed4Food: Smart turkeys, NWO open technology program (2023). https://www.breed4food.com/affiliate-projects/item/23-smart-turkeys-nwo-open-technology-program. Accessed 28 Sep 2023
4. Brito, L.F., et al.: Large-scale phenotyping of livestock welfare in commercial production systems: a new frontier in animal breeding. Front. Genet. **11**, 793 (2020)
5. Catarinucci, L., et al.: An animal tracking system for behavior analysis using radio frequency identification. Lab. Anim. **43**(9), 321–327 (2014)
6. Russ, J.C.: The Image Processing Handbook. CRC Press (2006)
7. Deng, Y., Kanervisto, A., Ling, J., Rush, A.M.: Image-to-markup generation with coarse-to-fine attention. In: International Conference on Machine Learning, pp. 980–989. PMLR (2017)
8. Elhayek, A., Stoll, C., Kim, K.I., Seidel, H.-P., Theobalt, C.: Feature-based multi-video synchronization with subframe accuracy. In: Pinz, A., Pock, T., Bischof, H., Leberl, F. (eds.) DAGM/OAGM 2012. LNCS, vol. 7476, pp. 266–275. Springer, Heidelberg (2012). https://doi.org/10.1007/978-3-642-32717-9_27
9. Garcia, R., Aguilar, J., Toro, M., Pinto, A., Rodriguez, P.: A systematic literature review on the use of machine learning in precision livestock farming. Comput. Electron. Agric. **179**, 105826 (2020)
10. Guo, Q., et al.: Enhanced camera-based individual pig detection and tracking for smart pig farms. Comput. Electron. Agric. **211**, 108009 (2023)
11. Hofstra, G., Roelofs, J., Rutter, S.M., van Erp-van der Kooij, E., de Vlieg, J.: Mapping welfare: location determining techniques and their potential for managing cattle welfare a review. Dairy **3**(4), 776–788 (2022)
12. Huang, B.S., Shen, D.F., Lin, G.S., Chai, S.K.D.: Multi-camera video synchronization based on feature point matching and refinement. In: 2019 IEEE/ACIS 18th International Conference on Computer and Information Science (ICIS), pp. 136–139. IEEE (2019)

13. Karami, E., Prasad, S., Shehata, M.: Image matching using sift, surf, brief and orb: performance comparison for distorted images. arXiv:1710.02726 (2017)
14. Kawamura, T., Katsuragi, T., Kobayashi, A., Inatomi, M., Oshiro, M., Eguchi, H.: Development of an information research platform for data-driven agriculture. Int. J. Agric. Environ. Inf. Syst. (IJAEIS) **13**(1), 1–19 (2022)
15. Kim, H., Ishikawa, M.: Sub-frame evaluation of frame synchronization for camera network using linearly oscillating light spot. Sensors **21**(18), 6148 (2021)
16. Liu, T., Liu, Y.: Moving camera-based object tracking using adaptive ground plane estimation and constrained multiple kernels. J. Adv. Transp. 2021 (2021)
17. Mistry, D., Banerjee, A.: Comparison of feature detection and matching approaches: sift and surf. GRD J. Glob. Res. Dev. J. Eng. **2**(4), 7–13 (2017)
18. Nederlandse Organisatie voor Wetenschappelijk Onderzoek (NWO): Animal group sensor - integrating behavioural dynamics and social genetic effects to improve health, welfare and ecological footprint of livestock (IMAGEN) [p18-19] (2023). https://www.nwo.nl/onderzoeksprogrammas/perspectief. Accessed 28 Sept 2023
19. Oczak, M., Ismayilova, G., Costa, A., Viazzi, S., Sonoda, L.T., Fels, M., Bahr, C., Hartung, J., Guarino, M., Berckmans, D., et al.: Analysis of aggressive behaviours of pigs by automatic video recordings. Comput. Electron. Agric. **99**, 209–217 (2013)
20. Olagoke, A.S., Ibrahim, H., Teoh, S.S.: Literature survey on multi-camera system and its application. IEEE Access **8**, 172892–172922 (2020)
21. Rao, G.S.: View-invariant alignment and matching of video sequences. In: Proceedings Ninth IEEE International Conference on Computer Vision, pp. 939–945. IEEE (2003)
22. Ratcliff, J.: Timecode A User's Guide: A User's Guide. CRC Press, Boca Raton (1999)
23. Sato, T., Shimada, Y., Taniguchi, Y.: Temporal video alignment based on integrating multiple features by adaptive weighting. In: 2018 International Workshop on Advanced Image Technology (IWAIT), pp. 1–5. IEEE (2018)
24. Shrestha, P., Barbieri, M., Weda, H., Sekulovski, D.: Synchronization of multiple camera videos using audio-visual features. IEEE Trans. Multimedia **12**(1), 79–92 (2009)
25. Smith, R.: An overview of the tesseract OCR engine. In: Ninth International Conference on Document Analysis and Recognition (ICDAR 2007), vol. 2, pp. 629–633. IEEE (2007)
26. Wieschollek, P., Freeman, I., Lensch, H.P.: Learning robust video synchronization without annotations. In: 2017 16th IEEE International Conference on Machine Learning and Applications (ICMLA), pp. 92–100. IEEE (2017)
27. Xiao, S., et al.: Multi-view tracking, re-id, and social network analysis of a flock of visually similar birds in an outdoor aviary. Int. J. Comput. Vision **131**(6), 1532–1549 (2023)

Increasing the Accuracy of a Deep Learning Model for Traffic Accident Severity Prediction by Adding a Temporal Category

Luis Pérez-Sala, Manuel Curado(✉), Leandro Tortosa, and Jose F. Vicent

Department of Computer Science and Artificial Intelligence, University of Alicante, Alicante, Spain
{lpg95,manuel.curado,tortosa,jvicent}@ua.es

Abstract. Artificial Intelligence become a tool widely used in the context of urban mobility and road safety applications. This paper focuses on predicting the severity of traffic accidents, from the point of view of the need for assistance, using general features that can be easily and quickly collected. We propose a deep learning model based on a convolutional neural network that compares, in performance, to several machine learning models for predicting the severity of traffic accidents. Our proposal modifies a previous model by refining the categorizing of the accident, implementing an area filter to address the imbalance data, reorganizing dataset into different features based on their nature, and discretizing the time of accidents using sine and cosine functions. This work demonstrates superior performance over six machine learning models, achieving an important improvement in the prediction of the two categories analyzed (accidents with and without requiring assistance). Datasets from two cities in the United Kingdom were analyzed, obtaining an improvement in the F1-score of 4.6% and 13.2% for attended and unattended accidents in the Liverpool dataset and 3.1% and 17.2% in the Southwark dataset.

Keywords: deep learning · convolutional neural networks · traffic · genetic algorithms · severity accidents prediction

1 Introduction and Related Work

1.1 Introduction

Artificial Intelligence (AI) has become an integral part of our lives, with applications spanning healthcare, transportation or sustainability, between others. In the context of urban mobility and road safety, the pressing issue of traffic accidents has garnered significant attention. Research efforts have explored the causes and severity of accidents through statistical models and machine-learning

K. Daimi and A. Al Sadoon (Eds.): ACR 2024, LNNS 956, pp. 113–124, 2024.
https://doi.org/10.1007/978-3-031-56950-0_10

approaches. While statistical models often make assumptions about data distribution, machine learning models offer flexibility and strong performance without such assumptions. Various models, including decision trees and logistic regressions, have been applied to classify accident severity, with distinctions made between property damage-only accidents and injuries, as well as between slight and serious injuries. This paper proposes a deep learning model based on a convolutional neural network to predict traffic accident severity, considering different factors or categories, such as environmental conditions or important data about the vehicle or personal characteristics of the implied people. Moreover, we implement an area filter to address the imbalance data, reorganizing dataset into different features based on their nature, and highlighting the discretization of the temporality information (i.e. date, day of the week and hour of the accident) using sine and cosine functions.

The research is structured as follows: the study reviews related work in Sect. 1.2, details the methodology (Sect. 2), presents experimental results in Sect. 3, and offers conclusions, addressing the complex challenge of accident prediction from different angles, in Sect. 4.

1.2 Related Work

The study of traffic accident prediction has been a well-explored area in recent years. Various methodologies have been applied, including genetic algorithms and fuzzy classifiers with evolutionary programming to solve this problem. Some approaches combine these methods with artificial neural networks (ANN) and multilayer perceptrons to increase the performance of the prediction and find relevant characteristics and relationships in accident data [1,2]. Other works use evolutionary techniques to help in optimization input hyperparameters, such as Support Vector Classifier (SVC) parameters. These methods are useful to optimize the input hyperparameters from external models to apply them to the severity of traffic accidents [3].

Other approaches focus on data visualization and pattern analysis to identify important accident characteristics, such as the age of the vehicle or the state of the road [4,5]. Equally, game theory has been used to model traffic interactions, although this kind of methods do not reflect the dynamics of the traffic daily [6].

From a machine learning perspective, particularly neural networks, there are applications, with focus on deep learning models, as convolutional neural networks (CNN), such as [7,8]. These techniques have been widely studied in fields like image recognition, computer vision, and speech recognition. In the area of traffic accident severity prediction, CNNs have been applied, but challenges include low-quality datasets and data imbalance issues [9,10].

In [11], a new model is presented to predict the severity of traffic accidents from a set of features such as environmental situations or driver gender, where the data has to be classified into different categories to help characterise the model using relevant information. This information is transforming from qualitative data into numerical matrices to feed evolutionary methods for hyperparameter optimization in two CNN architectures, both one- and two-dimensional.

However, data is imbalanced (there are few fatal accidents with respect to the remaining categories), and important characteristics such as temporality (day of the week and date) are not taken into account. This kind of data is very relevant. In [12] shows that in a tourist city in Spain, the geo-located mobility on working days (Monday to Friday) is similar but at weekends decreases on Saturdays and Sundays the 16% and 33%, respectively. Moreover, mobility is significantly high early in the morning during the week.

For that, in this paper we propose a model for predicting the need for medical assistance in traffic accidents from a set of different characteristics, highlighting temporality data, aiming for generalizability across cities in real-time. It employs a two-dimensional convolutional neural network with an optimized architecture to address these challenges.

2 Methodology

In a previous work [11], a methodology was presented for predicting accident severity specifically tailored to the city of Madrid. This approach centered on predicting three distinct levels of severity for accident victims: fatal, severe, and minor. However, a notable limitation of this methodology surfaced in its generalization capabilities, primarily attributed to the data imbalance issue. This imbalance resulted from a disproportionate representation of fatal accidents compared to severe and minor accidents due to their varying frequencies.

In response to this challenge, our current methodology introduces a novel approach aimed at mitigating these issues. Specifically, we simplify the victim's injury severity into two broad classes: 'Needed Assistance' and 'Slight'. We also implement a new filtering process designed to address the imbalance between these two classes. Additionally, we augment the dataset with new features, enriching the input data for our proposed model. These enhancements collectively empower our model with a richer information landscape, ultimately leading to improved performance in predicting accident severity.

2.1 Dataset

The dataset is under the ownership of the Department for Transport of the United Kingdom's government, as referenced in [13]. It encompasses a multitude of features, 81 in total, which meticulously delineate the mode and circumstances surrounding every recorded accident across the United Kingdom. Within the scope of this article, we have elected to focus on data corresponding to the subsequent cities: Liverpool and Southwark.

To ensure the inclusion of only valuable features in our dataset, those with a correlation coefficient less than 0.42 have been systematically excluded. It is well-established that a subset of features exhibiting high correlation can detrimentally impact model training. Furthermore, we have prioritized features that are readily available in accident datasets from various international locales. This approach aligns with our overarching goal of establishing a methodology with broad applicability across diverse urban contexts.

The resulting characteristics go through a categorisation process, where those characteristics that share the same nature are grouped into the same category. The resulting categories after grouping the variables are six: i) Location and Scale of Accident, encompassing details about accident location and magnitude; ii) Driving Limitations, encompassing road conditions and legal constraints; iii) Environmental Features, focusing on climatic aspects, particularly light conditions; iv) Vehicle Features, related to accident vehicles, including weight and age; v) Victim Features, concerning individuals involved, such as age and role; and vi) Temporal Features, involving accident timing, including specific time, day of the week, and week of the year.

2.2 Pre-processing Data

The initial phase of the methodology involves data Pre-processing and preparation. This entails performing a cleansing process, wherein duplicate records are removed, those with missing values in the selected features are filtered out, and outliers are addressed. Subsequently, discretization is applied, where qualitative variables are translated into numeric ones, as Machine Learning models inherently operate with numerical data. This discretization process is executed by assigning a numerical value (ranging from 0 to N) based on the significance of each value within each variable, resulting in a numeric dataset that can be comprehended by the models.

The subsequent phase involves the application of a novel filtering process aimed at mitigating the disproportion between Assistance and Slight accidents, which adversely affects model training and, consequently, their generalization to unseen accident inferences. To achieve this, the urban areas of each city have been divided into grids, and accidents have been projected onto these grids. In order to reduce the imbalance between Slight and Assistance accidents from the original dataset, areas where both types of accidents coexist have been selected. As a result, the resulting filtered dataset exhibits a considerably less noticeable imbalance than the original, yielding greater variability in the features that differentiate these two classes. The size of the grid areas for each city has been determined through experimental results.

At this juncture, the data is split into a training set (80%) and a test subset (20%). Once the training dataset is available, a data resampling technique using Borderline SMOTE-II [14] is applied. This method generates new samples for the minority classes around the boundary region that separates the two classes, aiming to create a balanced dataset by modifying the values of minority samples. This resampled dataset will be used for model training.

2.3 Temporal Features

As a significant enhancement to the previous methodology, we introduce the incorporation of a novel temporal category, reclassifying the initial five categories from the previous study into six distinct categories. This new category encompasses attributes related to the temporal information surrounding the accident, incorporating additional descriptors such as the day of the week, the week in the year, and the exact time of the incident. Furthermore, we employ a refined transformation process for the accident's timestamp. In contrast to the previous study's binary classification of day and night accidents, we adopt a more precise approach, representing the exact hour of the accident through two components based on sine and cosine functions. This phenomenon arises due to the considerable temporal gap between a data point occurring 5 min prior to and 5 min subsequent to the time division. Such a temporal distance is, in practice, quite substantial and undesirable. For instance, it is imperative for our machine learning model to accurately recognize that the time instances of 23:55 and 00:05 are merely 10 min apart. However, under the old representation, these timestamps would erroneously appear to be separated by a duration of 23 h and 50 min. This discrepancy can significantly impact the model's ability to discern temporal relationships accurately [15]. To execute this procedure, we commence by converting the hour and minute of each accident occurrence into seconds and calculating the number of total seconds in a day to create a normalized temporal feature set. Subsequently, we employ the ensuing mathematical expressions upon the temporal data in seconds to portray the accident occurrence time as two distinct sinusoidal and cosinusoidal components:

$$\sin((2 \cdot \pi \cdot DaySeconds)/SecondsInDay)$$
$$\cos((2 \cdot \pi \cdot DaySeconds)/SecondsInDay)$$

In this context, sine and cosine functions serve as faithful representations of the temporal progression This representation aims to capture the cyclic nature of accident occurrence throughout the day.

2.4 Post-processing Data

The subsequent stage of our methodology is dedicated to preparing input data for the proposed convolutional model. This entails a transformation from tabular data into a matrix format, a requisite since the 2D Convolutional Neural Network (CNN-2D) operates on data presented in matrix structures. Consequently, we employ a strategic mapping approach to allocate each data feature, initially organized in row format, to a specific position within a two-dimensional matrix.

To construct these matrices, two stages are applied:

- The first stage involves calculating feature importance by searching for a Boosting model based on decision trees that is optimized using a genetic algorithm. This process begins with the initial training of N-boosting models, each initialized with a different set of hyperparameters that will be optimized over successive generations through a genetic algorithm. The optimization of these models is based on the heuristic function derived from each model, specifically the F1 score achieved on the validation set belonging to the original dataset. Once the best Boosting model is obtained, the importance of each feature is calculated based on its relevance during the training of the best model found.

- The second phase involves calculating the indices where each feature will be positioned based on its importance. This process will make use of the categories mentioned in Sect. 2.1. Each of these six categories will be associated with a specific row in the new matrix, while the features will be positioned in each of the columns within their respective category rows, resulting in a matrix with dimensions of 6×5. The category row is calculated based on its importance, which will be the result of the importance of the features it contains. Thus, the most relevant category will be assigned the central position, the second most important will be positioned in the row immediately above, and the next will be in the row immediately below, following the same process for the remaining categories. Once the categories are positioned, it is time to position the features within their categories, where the most important feature will be placed in the center, the second most relevant immediately to its left, and the next immediately to the right, and so on. This meticulous feature organization ensures that the matrix structure captures the significance of each element effectively resulting in a 6×5 matrix.

2.5 New CNN-2D Model

The new proposed model features a convolutional architecture comprising four 2D layers, each with a 3×3 kernel and ReLU activation function. Batch normalization is applied to the output of each convolutional layer. The first layer consists of 64 kernels, followed by 512 in the second, 128 in the third, and 256 in the fourth.

The output of each convolutional layer manifests as feature maps, outcomes of filter multiplication on the input data with a stride of 1. Convolution padding is employed to accommodate cases where filter multiplication extends beyond matrix boundaries by adding zeros at the limits.

The feature maps from the final layer undergo flattening, transforming data to a single dimension post-convolutions. These flattened data points interconnect with 256 nodes in a dense (Fully Connected) layer. Ultimately, the dense layer connects to a final layer with a Softmax activation function, yielding probabilities for each new sample's classification into one of the two classes.

2.6 Comparison Metrics

To compare the results of the new convolutional model with state-of-the-art models, we consider widely used metrics in the Machine Learning literature.

- **Precision:** Accuracy measures the proportion of correctly classified instances in a classification task. It assesses the overall correctness of a model's predictions.
- **Recall:** Recall quantifies the model's ability to correctly identify all positive instances in a dataset. It measures the proportion of actual positives correctly predicted as positive by the model.

- **F1-Score:** The F1 Score is a single metric that balances precision and recall. It provides a holistic assessment of a model's performance, particularly valuable in situations with imbalanced datasets or when false positives and false negatives carry significant implications. This is the metric that will be used to compare the performance of the models.

2.7 Comparison Models

In this section, we introduce the six state-of-the-art models against which the new CNN-2D model proposed in this article will be compared based on the defined metrics: Naive Bayes (NB), Support Vector Classifier (SVC), K-Nearest Neighbors (KNN), Random Forest (RF), Logistic Regression (LR), and Multi-Layer Perceptron (MLP). NB relies on Bayes' theorem and is suitable for high-dimensional data. SVC is a versatile method for classification and regression tasks, particularly effective in high-dimensional spaces. KNN leverages data similarity for classification and regression, offering non-parametric flexibility. RF builds an ensemble of decision trees for classification and regression, providing a robust and user-friendly option. LR employs statistical analysis to predict binary outcomes based on independent variables. MLP represents a common neural network model with input, hidden, and output layers for complex learning tasks.

3 Results

In this section, we present the outcomes of the proposed CNN-2D convolutional model, conducting a thorough comparative analysis against six state-of-the-art models. We will showcase the Precision, Recall, and F1-Score metrics obtained from the validation dataset for each model, evaluated independently for each city under investigation. This rigorous evaluation serves to elucidate the model's performance in predicting traffic accident severity, with a focus on its precision, recall, and F1-Score metrics. In Table 1 we can observe, for each coordinate axis, the size and the resulting total number of areas for city of Liverpool.

Table 1. Area distribution for Liverpool and Southwark.

City	Axis	Areas Number	Areas Size
Liverpool	X	2107	12
Southwark	Y	717	21

It is important to point out that, for both cities, we have divided the dataset into subsets. The model is trained and evaluated ten times, using a different fold as the validation set each time. The model generalization performance metric, shown in this section, is the average of the resulting metrics for each subset.

3.1 Liverpool

The original number of accidents in the Liverpool dataset is 49, 291 in Slight and 5, 161 in Assistance. After filtering by areas we obtain 3, 640 light and 1, 192 more serious and, finally, the data resulting from the application of the Borderline SMOTE-II algorithm are 2, 554 and 2, 554 respectively.

In Table 2, we can observe the results obtained for the city of Liverpool.

Table 2. Liverpool models metrics. The analysis reveals that our proposed model consistently attains impressive F1-Score values, approximately 95% for Slight-type accidents and around 85% for Assistance-type accidents. These metrics significantly outshine the performance of state-of-the-art models included in the comparative assessment.

		Train			Test		
Model	Severity	Precision	Recall	F1	Precision	Recall	F1
NB	Slight	0.716	0.424	0.533	0.872	0.412	0.560
	Assistance	0.591	0.832	0.691	0.283	0.794	0.417
SVC	Slight	0.883	0.852	0.867	0.917	0.818	0.865
	Assistance	0.857	0.887	0.872	0.545	0.745	0.630
KNN	Slight	0.797	0.642	0.711	0.912	0.631	0.746
	Assistance	0.700	0.836	0.762	0.386	0.792	0.519
RF	Slight	0.723	0.690	0.706	0.901	0.631	0.742
	Assistance	0.703	0.735	0.719	0.377	0.763	0.504
LR	Slight	0.672	0.745	0.706	0.889	0.737	0.806
	Assistance	0.714	0.636	0.672	0.432	0.685	0.530
MLP	Slight	0.964	0.941	0.952	0.932	0.888	0.910
	Assistance	0.943	0.964	0.953	0.671	0.779	0.721
CNN2D	**Slight**	0.993	0.991	0.992	0.960	0.953	**0.956**
	Assistance	0.988	0.966	0.977	0.843	0.863	**0.853**

It is evident that the CNN-2D, the newly proposed model, exhibits the best generalization performance for Slight and Assistance accidents following the F1-Score metric, obtaining a 95,6% and 85%respectively, with an improvement of 4.6% and 13.2% compared to the next best-performing model on the validation set, the MLP. In terms of Precision, our model exhibits values of 96% and 84.3%, marking an improvement of 2.8% and 17.2% for Slight and Assistance accidents, respectively, over the next best model, MLP. Regarding Recall, our novel model achieves 95.3% for Slight-type accidents, enhancing performance by 6.5% compared to the next best model, MLP. Additionally, it attains an 86.3% Recall rate for Assistance-type accidents, surpassing the NB model by 6.9%.

3.2 Southwark

It is appropriate to highlight the number of elements in the Southwark dataset. Then, the original number of accidents is 27,105 in Slight and 3,109 in Assistance. After filtering by area we get 4,251 for minor accidents and 1,256 for more serious accidents and finally the data resulting from the application of the Borderline SMOTE-II algorithm is 2,973 for both types of accidents.

Table 3. Southwark models metrics. The comparative analysis unequivocally showcases the superior performance of the proposed model, achieving an approximate F1-Score of 96% for Slight-type accidents and 88% for Assistance-type accidents. These results significantly outstrip the performance of all other models considered in the study.

		Train			Test		
Model	Severity	Precision	Recall	F1	Precision	Recall	F1
NB	Slight	0.726	0.397	0.513	0.861	0.356	0.504
	Assistance	0.585	0.850	0.693	0.266	0.803	0.400
SVC	Slight	0.896	0.768	0.827	0.928	0.744	0.826
	Assistance	0.797	0.911	0.850	0.477	0.803	0.599
KNN	Slight	0.757	0.527	0.622	0.909	0.508	0.652
	Assistance	0.637	0.831	0.721	0.328	0.825	0.469
RF	Slight	0.728	0.506	0.597	0.893	0.409	0.561
	Assistance	0.621	0.811	0.704	0.290	0.831	0.430
LR	Slight	0.610	0.635	0.622	0.844	0.614	0.711
	Assistance	0.620	0.594	0.607	0.315	0.608	0.415
MLP	Slight	0.978	0.947	0.962	0.941	0.892	0.916
	Assistance	0.948	0.979	0.963	0.686	0.809	0.743
CNN2D	**Slight**	0.998	0.994	0.996	0.972	0.956	**0.964**
	Assistance	0.994	0.998	0.996	0.858	0.904	**0.881**

In Table 3, the inference metrics for the models are once again observed, this time for the city of Southwark. Comparing the F1-Score metric, the newly proposed CNN-2D model again demonstrates the best results for Slight and Assistance accidents, achieving an improvement of 4.8% and 13.8%, respectively, compared to the next best-performing model (MLP) for both types of accidents. In terms of Precision, our model exhibits a metric of 97.2% for Slight-type accidents and 85.8% for Assistance-type accidents, surpassing the MLP model, the next best performer in both cases, by 3.1% and 17.2%, respectively. Concerning Recall, the newly proposed model achieves 95.6% for Slight-type accidents and 90.4% for Assistance-type accidents, demonstrating a 6.4% improvement over MLP in the former case and a 7.3% improvement over RF, the next best performer in the latter metric.

3.3 Comparison Summary

To comprehensively assess the advancement realized by our novel proposed model, this section introduces a visual representation that juxtaposes the outcomes of our state-of-the-art models with those of the newly introduced CNN-2D convolutional model.

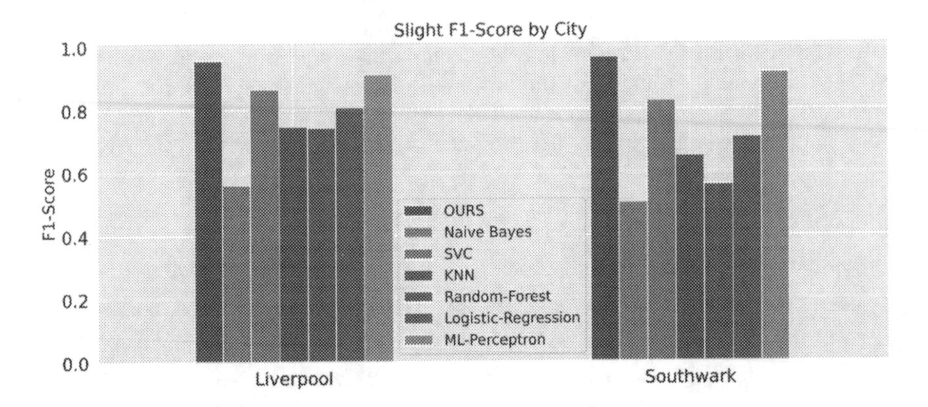

Fig. 1. Models Slight F1-Score by city on Slight accidents. Graphical representations clearly depict the superiority of our proposed model for Slight-type accidents in both Liverpool and Southwark cities, exhibiting a maximum improvement of 4.8% and a minimum of 4.6% over the next-best MLP model in the comparison.

The assessment is conducted based on the F1-Score metric applied to the test dataset containing accident instances, thereby elucidating the performance of the models across both urban settings.

As depicted in Fig. 1, an illustrative presentation of the model outcomes is provided for accidents categorized as "Slight," while Fig. 2 elucidates the corresponding results for incidents of the "Assistance" category.

In these graphs, the significant difference in performance of the proposed new CNN-2D model compared to the rest is visually evident. There is a notable improvement, particularly in accidents of the Assistance class, while the improvement in the case of Slight-type accidents is relatively more modest, it remains noteworthy and indicative of the model's adaptability across diverse accident scenarios.

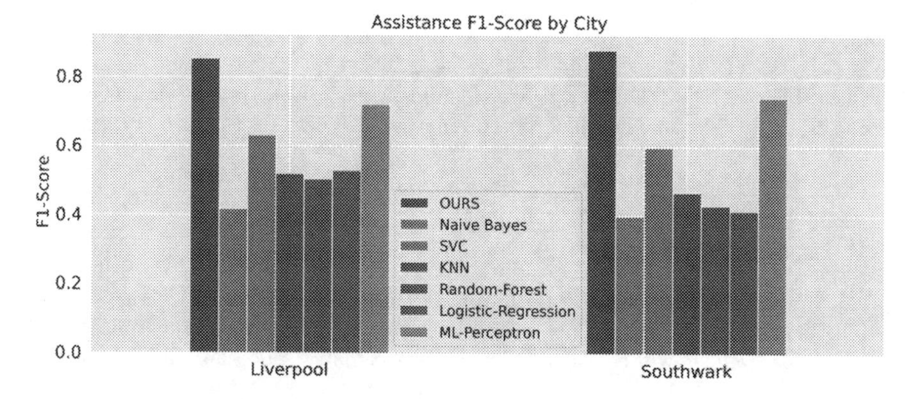

Fig. 2. Models Assistance F1-Score by city. Graphical representations depict the superior performance of the proposed Assistance-type accident model compared to all other models in both Liverpool and Southwark cities, with a maximum improvement of 13.8% and a minimum of 13.2% over the next best MLP model.

4 Conclusions

This work introduces a novel CNN-2D convolutional model for traffic accident severity prediction, demonstrating superior performance over six state-of-the-art models, achieving a minimum improvement of 4.6% on slight accidents prediction and 13.2% on accidents requiring assistance prediction. These enhancements were achieved by refining the previous methodology, specifically by categorizing accident severity into two classes (Needed Assistance and Slight), implementing an area filter to address the disproportion between Slight and Assistance accidents (data imbalance), reorganizing dataset features into different categories based on their nature, and cyclically representing the time of accidents (initially on 24 h format) use of sine and cosine functions and addition of new functions such as week in year and day in week. The primary future work for this research involves applying the proposed CNN-2D model to other cities with readily available data to observe its performance.

References

1. Hashmienejad, S.H.A., Hasheminejad, S.M.H.: Traffic accident severity prediction using a novel multi-objective genetic algorithm. Int. J. Crashworth. **22**(4), 425–440 (2017)
2. Beshah, T., Ejigu, D., Krömer, P., Plato, J., Abraham, A.: Learning the classification of traffic accident types. In 2012 Fourth International Conference on Intelligent Networking and Collaborative Systems, pp. 463–468. IEEE (2012)
3. Amiri, A.M., Sadri, A., Nadimi, N., Shams, M.: A comparison between artificial neural network and hybrid intelligent genetic algorithm in predicting the severity of fixed object crashes among elderly drivers. Accid. Anal. Prev. **138**, 105468 (2020)
4. Ezenwa, A.O.: Trends and characteristics of road traffic accidents in Nigeria. J. R. Soc. Health **106**(1), 27–29 (1986)

5. Li, K., Xu, H., Liu, X.: Analysis and visualization of accidents severity based on LightGBM-TPE. Chaos, Solitons Fractals **157**, 111987 (2022)
6. Chen, L., Sun, J., Li, K., Li, Q.: Research on the effectiveness of monitoring mechanism for "yield to pedestrian" based on system dynamics. Phys. A **591**, 126804 (2022)
7. Mao, Q., Dong, M., Huang, Z., Zhan, Y.: Learning salient features for speech emotion recognition using convolutional neural networks. IEEE Trans. Multimed. **16**(8), 2203–2213 (2014)
8. Rawat, W., Wang, Z.: Deep convolutional neural networks for image classification: a comprehensive review. Neural Comput. **29**(9), 2352–2449 (2017)
9. Liu, Y., Wu, C., Wen, J., Xiao, X., Chen, Z.: A grey convolutional neural network model for traffic flow prediction under traffic accidents. Neurocomputing **500**, 761–775 (2022)
10. Wenqi, L., Dongyu, L., and Menghua, Y.: A model of traffic accident prediction based on convolutional neural network. In: 2017 2nd IEEE International Conference on Intelligent Transportation Engineering (ICITE), pp. 198–202. IEEE, September 2017
11. Pérez-Sala, L., Curado, M., Tortosa, L., Vicent, J.F.: Deep learning model of convolutional neural networks powered by a genetic algorithm for prevention of traffic accidents severity. Chaos, Solitons Fractals **169**, 113245 (2023)
12. Estudio de la movilidad con Big Data en España. Ministerio de Transportes, Movilidad y Agenda Urbana. https://www.mitma.gob.es/ministerio/proyectos-singulares/estudio-de-movilidad-con-big-data
13. Department for Transport. Reported road collisions, vehicles and casualties tables for Great Britain. https://www.gov.uk/government/statistical-data-sets/reported-road-accidents-vehicles-and-casualties-tables-for-great-britain
14. Han, H., Wang, W.-Y., Mao, B.-H.: Borderline-SMOTE: a new over-sampling method in imbalanced data sets learning. In: International Conference on Intelligent Computing (2005)
15. Encoding cyclical continuous features - 24-hour time. Ian London. https://ianlondon.github.io/blog/encoding-cyclical-features-24hour-time/

2ARTs: A Platform for Exercise Prescriptions in Cardiac Recovery Patients

Andreia Pereira[1], Ricardo Martinho[2], Rui Pinto[3], Rui Rijo[2], and Carlos Grilo[4](✉)

[1] ESTG, Polytechnic of Leiria, Leiria, Portugal
2210627@my.ipleiria.pt

[2] INESCC-DL, ESTG, Polytechnic of Leiria, Leiria, Portugal
{ricardo.martinho,rui.rijo}@ipleiria.pt

[3] ciTechCare, ESSLei, Polytechnic of Leiria, Leiria, Portugal
rui.pinto@ipleiria.pt

[4] CIIC, ESTG, Polytechnic of Leiria, Leiria, Portugal
carlos.grilo@ipleiria.pt

Abstract. Due to limited access, increasing costs and an ageing population, the global healthcare system faces significant coverage problems that call for innovative approaches. Health professionals are actively seeking alternative methods to provide care to an increasingly needy population, without increasing human effort and associated costs. eHealth platforms, which use technology to provide patient care, are emerging as transformative solutions for addressing these problems. This study is centered on the demand for a Decision Support System (DSS) in cardiology to enable doctors to prescribe individualized care inside Cardiac Rehabilitation Programmes (CRPs). The 2ARTs project's main objective is to include a cardiac rehabilitation platform with a DSS within the hospital infrastructure. This DSS uses models to classify patients into different groups, delivering crucial information to assist with decisions regarding treatment. Regarding the DSS, Principal Component Analysis (PCA) emerged as a standout technique for dimensionality reduction, due to its interoperability with clustering algorithms and superior evaluation metrics. The most appropriate clustering technique was determined to be the K-means algorithm, which was supported by the experts analysis. In accordance with the goals of the 2ARTs project, this integration of PCA and K-means provides meaningful insights that improve reasoned decision-making.

Keywords: Cardiac Rehabilitation Programmes · Clustering Algorithms · Data Analytics in Healthcare · Decision Support System · Machine Learning · Pervasive Healthcare · Predictive Models

1 Introduction

The global healthcare sector faces many challenges such as accessibility, affordability, quality of care and an ageing population. Solutions must balance the demands of cost and quality, taking into account factors such as financial constraints, distant locations and limited resources [1], which restrict access to healthcare and the reach of cardiac

K. Daimi and A. Al Sadoon (Eds.): ACR 2024, LNNS 956, pp. 125–136, 2024.
https://doi.org/10.1007/978-3-031-56950-0_11

rehabilitation programmes. Limitations on physical resources, including equipment and facilities, the lack of post-hospital follow-up and support systems disrupt continuity of care [2], preventing eligible individuals from participating in programmes. Innovative eHealth platforms, such as wearables, remote monitoring, telemedicine, mobile health applications, electronic health records (EHRs), AI-based information and health information exchanges (HIEs), bridge the gaps in care [3]. These technologies improve efficiency, engagement and outcomes, while addressing exclusions and require cooperation between technology, policy and healthcare stakeholders. Challenges in specialized fields, such as cardiac rehabilitation, reflect wider healthcare concerns, highlighting the need for comprehensive solutions that address specific and general barriers to healthcare delivery.

CRPs face challenges in patient participation and adherence, with around a third dropping out and adherence decreasing over time due to factors such as lack of referrals, medical conditions, reimbursement processes and geographical restrictions. Contextual differences, such as Portugal's low CRP enrollment rate of 8% compared to Europe and the US, highlight the impact of institutional support and regional infrastructures [4]. The integration of technology into CRP, including monitoring devices and remote platforms, increases the convenience and effectiveness of remote progress monitoring and personalized guidance. However, technology integration, such as clinical decision support systems (CDSS), poses both ethical concerns and technical challenges that require innovative solutions. Despite the benefits of digital healthcare, the effective analysis of vast patient data remains a challenge. CDSS act as digital assistants [5], providing crucial data for informed decision-making without replacing doctors, improving pattern identification and predictive modeling. Advanced analytics and machine learning have the potential to transform healthcare by predicting disease outcomes, detecting trends and estimating results based on historical data, enabling proactive risk assessment, patient monitoring and adaptive treatment strategies.

The objective of this project is to integrate a CDSS with the 2ARTs eHealth digital platform, aiming to empower healthcare professionals with tools for comprehensive cardiac rehabilitation patient progress monitoring, data analysis, and informed decision-making. This involves designing a user-friendly health platform that integrates with a patient-used mobile app, streamlining data management and communication between healthcare providers and patients. The CDSS architecture has been developed to facilitate effective decision support within the health platform by leveraging patient biomedical data for generating predictive models and actionable insights.

The rest of the document is organized as follows: Sect. 2 introduces fundamental related work, providing context and identifying research gaps. Section 3 outlines the methodology used for platform development and research study. Section 4 details the practical steps taken to deploy the proposed health platform. Section 5 explains the development of the decision support system model. Finally, Sect. 6 provides a discussion of the proposed platform, conclusions and future work.

2 Related Work

This section provides insights into the approach we took to discover relevant research papers and their connection to the field of cardiac rehabilitation. The retrieved articles from this search cover a range of DSS applications along with AI application examples, spanning from examples of machine learning to more detailed discussions on cardiac rehabilitation, highlighting advancements and innovations within this domain. To integrate AI into decision support systems (DSS), there are current on-going approaches in order to transform patient monitoring. These AI-driven methods enable continuous data analysis and proactive healthcare interventions. For example, Machine Learning (ML) algorithms offer the potential to continuously monitor patients' physiological data, allowing early detection of critical changes [6] and personalized care recommendations. Furthermore, AI has proven effective in interpreting various medical data, such as echocardiograms (ECG), contributing to precise diagnoses and treatment suggestions for cardiac diseases [7].

The authors in reference [8] proposed a comprehensive model featuring a DSS coupled with a chatbot for user feedback, capable of understanding text and speech, including emotions, feelings, trust, and motivation. The model is integrated with a data-driven dashboard and a cloud-based analytics platform. The authors conducted 10 independent experiments comparing their model to a randomized one whereas the results indicate that their model achieves, on average, a 43% higher success rate in finding optimal therapy plans, making it more effective for therapy planning.

In [9], the authors used a rule-based approach to process the data in their DSS for the patient's guidance in an unsupervised exercise-based rehabilitation program, with the supplementation of smart devices such as mobile phones, smart sensors and smartwatches, using a virtual coach for cardiac rehabilitation exercises at home. The evaluation involved a simulation and real-world study, considering two metrics: a) Recovery from low heart rate (HR) events, with results reaching 83% and 93% in 2-min and 3-min windows, respectively, and b) Recovery from low movement accuracy events, with results reaching 85% and 100% in 1-min and 2-min time windows, respectively.

Another significant aspect involves the development of CDSS for CRPs. These CDSS are designed to guide patients in personalized exercise-based rehabilitation programs [9]. Smart devices, including mobile phones and smart sensors, are integrated into these systems to monitor and assist patients during their exercise routines.

The articles mentioned earlier primarily concentrate on tackling individual issues in isolation. Consequently, there is not a consolidated platform capable of simultaneously emphasizing the significance of exercise and diet in cardiac rehabilitation and assisting doctors in analyzing the extensive patient data generated through a Decision Support System (DSS). In the developed platform, the primary emphasis lies in providing phenotypes related to each patient's health level, alongside addressing nutritional and medication aspects related to each. Additionally, it assists doctors in compiling comprehensive patient information, enabling them to prescribe treatments that are more personalized and uniquely suited to each patient's specific needs.

3 Methodology

In this section, we explore the methodologies for developing the 2ARTs digital platform and CDSS, adapting the CRISP-DM framework for the latter.

For the 2ARTs digital platform, we employed an agile software development methodology, combining Scrum and Kanban principles. Scrum structured the software development process into sprints, ensuring effective feature-focused development, while daily stand-ups and sprint reviews facilitated collaboration and feedback. Kanban, supported by a Trello board, managed task flow efficiently, maintaining transparency and addressing bottlenecks.

As for the CDSS, we adapted the CRISP-DM [10] framework to fit our research objectives and requirements. Our adaptation maintains six major stages: the Business Understanding stage, where we clarified research goals, identified challenges in cardiac rehabilitation, and aimed to enhance decision-making tools; Data Understanding, where we explored different datasets; Data Preparation which involved cleansing, transformation, and iterative improvements to ensure quality data on the chosen dataset for the next step; Modeling, in which we include testing with four methods in order to find the best accuracy; Evaluation in which we identified cluster traits and patterns by evaluating model performance using measures like WCSS and Silhouette Coefficient and, lastly, Deployment which involved implementing our model in a decision support system on the 2ARTs digital platform, enhancing personalized patient care. This iterative approach enhances project relevance and optimizes data quality.

Importantly, this academic adaptation of CRISP-DM is iterative, allowing for stage refinements based on later insights and enabling an evolving research process.

In Sect. 4, we provide an overview of the development process of each CRISP-DM phase described above, unravelling the details and methodologies that underlie them, as well as an analysis of the post-execution results and the significance of the outcomes achieved in these stages.

4 The Classification Model

It is essential to understand the dataset attributes and variances, as they will guide our decision-making regarding the methods and solutions chosen for the subsequent phases of data cleaning and pre-processing. It is crucial that we select methods and solutions that are adapted to the attributes and challenges presented by this dataset, ensuring that the data is cleaned and prepared for further analysis.

This section outlines the steps in building a classification model: dataset description, modelling approach where we delve into the specifics of techniques, algorithms, and parameters chosen and evaluation metrics.

4.1 The Dataset, Data Cleaning and Pre-processing

During our research, we collaborated with experts in the area to select an appropriate dataset for the development of the mentioned CDSS. This led us to select the Myocardial Infarction Complications Database [11]. This dataset contains data from

1700 patients, encompassing 123 attributes, including 111 related to clinical phenotypes and 12 associated with potential myocardial infarction complications (MI). Despite presenting analytical challenges and having 7.6% of null values, this extensive dataset offers a comprehensive representation of clinical data in the cardiology domain.

The dataset underwent multiple techniques to address common data quality issues and boost its integrity. Collaborating with the domain experts, we pruned irrelevant features, retaining 108 attributes (79 binary, 17 categorical, 12 numerical). The data cleaning and pre-processing operations undertaken were the following:

- **Null Value Handling:** Columns with over 60% null values were discarded, and for the rest, missing values were imputed using appropriate methods. Numerical features with normal distributions were replaced with means, skewed features with medians, and categorical nulls with modes, ensuring imputed values aligned with the data distribution. After this step, 104 columns remained.
- **Correlation Matrix and PCA:** A correlation matrix allowed us to identify highly correlated features and drop one of them. To address multicollinearity, PCA was employed. PCA transforms correlated features into uncorrelated principal components [12], effectively reducing dimensionality.
- **Scaling:** Numerical feature scaling standardization enhanced consistency and comparability, removing magnitude differences. Scaling enabled unbiased interpretation across features with distinct measurement scales.
- **One-Hot Encoding:** Categorical features were one-hot encoded, creating binary variables to facilitate model interpretation and integration.

4.2 Modeling

The purpose of this research is to provide doctors with the ability to classify patients into a set of phenotypes which will then allow them to prescribe exercise and diet according to the identified phenotype/category. However, the dataset we used lacked the labels corresponding to the phenotypes. As such, we applied (unsupervised) clustering algorithms to the data, with the phenotypes being assigned to the resulting clusters by experts in the field. The experts team was composed of two cardiologists, one physiologist and a clinical practice doctor with a degree in Data Science.

In order to achieve this goal, we explored two alternative approaches: Feature Reduction and Feature Selection. Feature Reduction involves reducing the number of features used in a dataset. The goal is to simplify the dataset while retaining its relevant information, which can lead to more efficient modeling and improved model performance. Feature Selection, on the other hand, involves selecting a specific subset of the most relevant features from the original set, discarding the less important ones, aiming to improve model performance, reduce overfitting, and enhance interpretability.

Feature Reduction

We tested two Feature Reduction methods: PCA and Factor Analysis of Mixed Data (FAMD). The purpose of PCA is to simplify complex datasets by transforming them into a new set of orthogonal variables called principal components, which capture the most significant variation in the original data, reducing noise and redundancy. In order to obtain the maximum variance of the data, we calculated the Cumulative Explained

Variance to decide how many components would be kept, determining the point at which adding more components would result in diminishing returns in terms of capturing the variability of the data set. The results show that the first two components accounted for at least 85% of the variance [12], therefore, we have used these 2 components.

To determine the optimal number of clusters, k, to apply to the chosen clustering algorithm, we employed the Elbow Method and Silhouette Scores. The Elbow Method, as shown in Fig. 1, helps determine the optimum number of clusters by looking for a "curve" in the sum-of-squares graph within the cluster, while the Silhouette scores assess how well the data points are grouped by measuring their similarity to their own cluster versus neighbouring clusters. Higher scores indicate better cluster quality. Based on the results (Fig. 1, left), k was set to 3 when using data reduced with PCA.

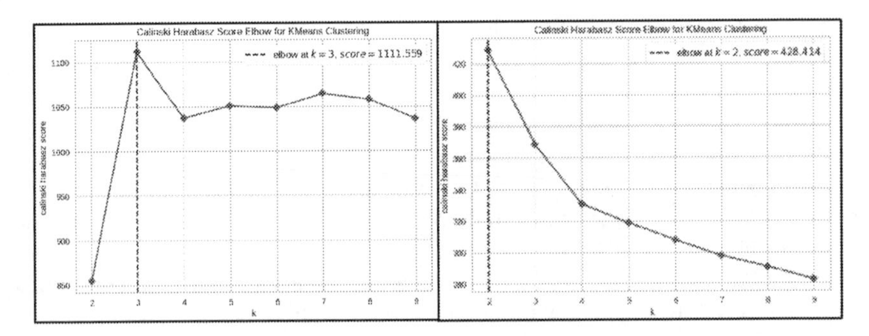

Fig. 1. PCA's (left) and FAMD's (right) Elbow Method.

For optimal component retention in FAMD, we considered the variance explained by each component. Conducting FAMD with up to 10 components, we calculated cumulative variance percentage to balance dimensionality reduction with meaningful data retention, which led us to keep seven components, ensuring at least 80% variance explained. To ascertain the best cluster count in the transformed data, we employed the two already mentioned techniques: the Elbow Method, shown in Fig. 1 (right) above and Silhouette Score, determining an optimal 2-cluster arrangement.

For clustering, we have used the K-Means algorithm. To evaluate the results, we used the Within-Cluster Sum of Squares (WCSS) and Silhouette Coefficient metrics. WCSS calculates the sum of the squared distances of the data points to their respective cluster centers, whereas the latter quantifies how similar each data point is to its own cluster compared to other clusters. A lower WCSS value indicates more compact and well-separated clusters, and a higher Silhouette Coefficient value indicates better-defined clusters. Table 1 below shows that PCA has better results for the two metrics. Furthermore, according to the experts, two clusters, as obtained with the components generated with the FAMD method, are not enough to group the phenotypes.

Feature Selection

We tested two different feature selection methods: the Variance Threshold method and one we will refer to as Experts Selection method, where experts were engaged to select highly relevant features based on their insights, focusing the analysis on meaningful

Table 1. Feature Reduction Methods' Evaluation.

	PCA	FAMD
WCSS	4754.24	45060.39
Silhouette Coefficient	0.3772	0.2255

elements. The Variance Threshold method was used with a threshold of 0.25 to retain features with significant variability, resulting in 17 selected features.

Regarding the optimum number of clusters, the Elbow Method metric (Fig. 2 – left picture) and Silhouette Scores prescribe two clusters. Due to the experts' opinion that two clusters are not enough, we also used the Gap Statistics method which compares the total intracluster variation for different values of k with their expected values under null reference distribution of the data (i.e., a distribution with no obvious clustering) [13]. This metric gave us a result of four clusters, as seen in Fig. 2 (right picture), which we decided to stick with for further analysis after discussing it with the experts.

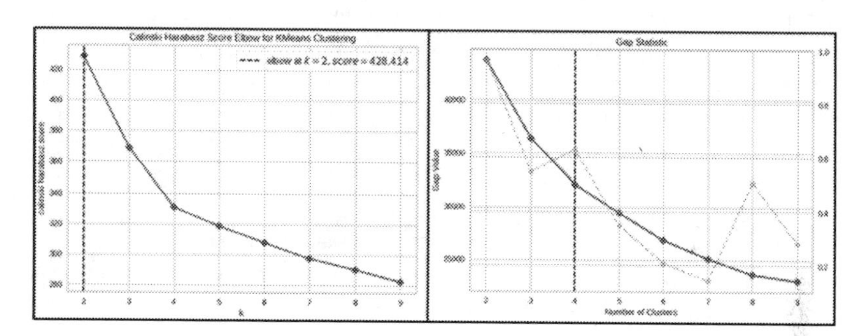

Fig. 2. Expert's Selection Elbow Method and Gap Statistics.

For the Experts' Selection, we started with the 108 initial features, narrowing them down to 16 based on relevance. We excluded three features with substantial null values (included in the 4 features removed in the data cleaning process) and applied one-hot encoding to six categorical features. Because we were still left with a few features to work with, we had to appeal again to some dimensionality reduction techniques like PCA or FAMD because we could not input them all in a clustering algorithm. We then opted for PCA due to its alignment with the experts' advice. Three PCA components were selected, capturing around 60% of the total variance. The optimal cluster count, determined through the Elbow Method and Silhouette Score as before, was three clusters. Subsequently, we assessed clustering quality using the WCSS and SC metrics. Table 2 below shows that the Expert's Selection presented better WCSS results (lower), however, that did not happen with the Silhouette Coefficient values even though they are very close between both methods.

Table 2. Feature Selection Methods' Evaluation.

	Feature Selection Methods	Experts' Selection
WCSS	538953.114	6230.614
Silhouette Coefficient	0.2280	0.1764

4.3 Evaluation

In this section, we delve into the analysis of CDSS outcomes, concentrating on cluster results, phenotype identification, and model performance. Summarizing the results across different modeling approaches, PCA emerged as the top-performer, yielding lower WCSS values and higher Silhouette Coefficient values, indicative of well-defined and distinct clusters. The Experts' Selection method also demonstrated favourable results, particularly in terms of lowering WCSS values. Therefore, we concentrate our analysis on these two methods.

Starting with the PCA method, t-tests were employed to analyze the relevance of numerical features to the definition of the generated clusters, highlighting significant differences that define distinct phenotypes. Based on those differences in the numerical features by cluster, and according to the experts, Cluster 0, with symptoms of pulmonary edema and cardiogenic shock, represents a "Congestion" phenotype, Cluster 1 exhibits characteristics associated with a "Non-Ischemic" phenotype, including the absence of exertional angina, no history of infarction, and absence of angina symptoms and, finally, Cluster 2, consists of intermediate-age patients with prior infarctions and severe Coronary Artery Disease (CAD), corresponding to an "Ischemic" phenotype.

To assess the quality and accuracy of these clusters, we also sought the experts' input and requested their evaluation of a representative sample from each cluster, ensuring a minimum of 10% coverage for each cluster. The experts were asked to determine whether the samples were appropriately positioned within their respective clusters. The results are shown in Table 3. These results validate the effectiveness of the clustering approach in capturing meaningful patterns and grouping similar samples.

Table 3. Accuracy of each cluster (PCA).

Cluster	Accuracy
0	91%
1	71%
2	91%

On the other hand, despite the Expert's Selection approach attempting to capture key features for cluster differentiation, this approach yielded high p-values in the t-student table, indicating limited statistical significance. As a result, this approach fell short in achieving the same reliability as the PCA method, since the experts were not able to match useful phenotypes to the generated clusters.

5 Development of the 2ARTs Digital Platform

This section focuses on the development of the 2ARTs digital platform, a crucial monitoring platform for doctors working with cardiac rehabilitation patients. The information provided by this platform to physicians and nutritionists about patient progress and possible outcomes is vital. It serves as physicians' and nutritionists' main interface, providing a variety of functions to make it easier to monitor and evaluate patients' heart health throughout rehabilitation. The clinical study behind this platform as been submitted and approved by the competent ethics committee, carried out in adults over 18 years which gave their informed consent to be included in the study. In the next sections, we outline the technologies employed in the back-office module, discuss its available features, and detail its integration with the DSS model.

5.1 Main Software Features

The platform features were designed to facilitate communication, patient progress monitoring, and individualized care. Platform administrators oversee health professionals, patients and biomedical data, while physicians tailor exercise prescriptions to patients' unique needs, as shown in Fig. 3 in the left picture. Nutritionists offer personalized nutrition plans and monitor dietary intake, collaborating with other doctors for comprehensive care (also depicted in Fig. 3 in the right picture). Cardiologists assess patients' medical data, prescribe medications, and provide specialized recommendations, including via group chat for real-time insights. Both these roles (physicians and nutritionists) can input biomedical data (as well as the patient) and review prescription histories. This empowers doctors to collect and monitor diverse patient information, spanning medical test results, diagnostic assessments, body measurements, and vital signs. The group chat feature fosters direct communication between patients and the healthcare team, promoting informed decision-making and collaborative care where patients can engage with all doctors simultaneously, sharing progress and seeking guidance.

5.2 AI Model and Digital Platform Integration

The AI clustering model was integrated in the health platform, allowing patients to be assigned to specific clusters based on their characteristics, as seen in the example of Fig. 4. These clusters' phenotypes offer insights for informed decisions and personalized treatment. This empowers doctors to tailor prescriptions and interventions according to the assigned group, promoting personalized care and improved patient outcomes.

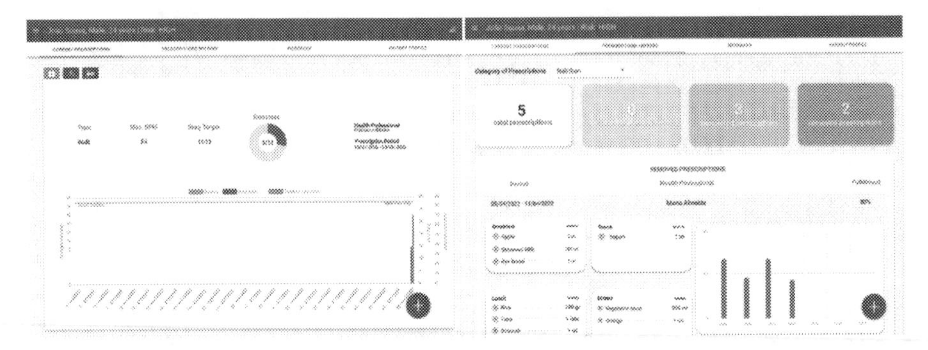

Fig. 3. History of Nutrition Prescriptions and Active Exercise Prescription.

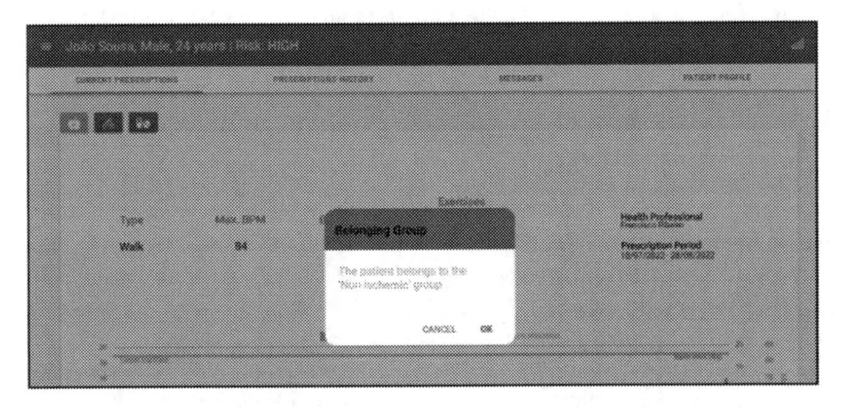

Fig. 4. Patient's predicted outcome in the platform.

6 Discussion and Conclusion

In this closing chapter, we will summarize the key findings of the research in comparison to the objectives and research goals, discussing their value and contribution. At the same time, we will discuss possible future work of the study. On a related note, we conducted tests on a dataset to classify patients for Cardiac Rehabilitation Programmes using clustering models, which were then integrated into a platform that could enhance decision-making by providing personalized recommendations, improving the quality of patient care. Essentially, this work has harnessed data-driven information to transform cardiac rehabilitation, offering tools and knowledge in order to help doctors make informed decisions such as, for example, the necessary amount of exercise or adequate diet in the prescriptions for each patient. Our work involved a comprehensive dataset, data analysis, the use of feature reduction and selection methods to build clusters that ultimately resulted in the generation of clusters that led to the identification of distinct clinical phenotypes identified by experts in the area.

Out of all the techniques used for data selection/reduction, the PCA method was the one showing the best results, effectively capturing underlying data variability and enabling the identification of distinct phenotypes - Ischemic, Non-Ischemic, and Congestion. These phenotypes serve as vital indicators for tailored patient management, enhancing the effectiveness of cardiac rehabilitation. Experts' evaluations further validated PCA's ability to group similar samples and uncover meaningful patterns, underscoring its robustness in achieving the study's goals.

The experts' insights played a crucial role in guiding the evaluation of both PCA and Expert's Selection, the ones that performed better out of the four methods tested, ultimately highlighting the superiority of the PCA approach in capturing relevant patterns and insights. These insights are vital as they enable the platform to offer crucial information about a patient's health group, empowering doctors to make more informed decisions when prescribing exercise and dietary plans tailored to each individual's unique needs.

For future work, incorporating historical prescription data into our Decision Support System (DSS) model has the potential to significantly improve its predictive capabilities, providing a deeper understanding of patient profiles for various phenotypes. Consequently, this would lead to better conclusions and recommendations, increasing the system's ability to guide doctors in optimizing patient treatment approaches.

Another promising avenue for further exploration involves subjecting the collected data to a rigorous validation process using microneurography. This advanced technique involves inserting fine electrodes into peripheral nerves, allowing direct recording and analysis of neural activity, thereby establishing a direct link between predicted clinical phenotypes and actual physiological responses in the patient population. This validation would provide a greater measure of confidence in the accuracy and applicability of the DSS predictions, reinforcing the reliability and real-world relevance of our research findings, as well as the potential to advance our understanding of the intricate interaction between clinical phenotypes and neural activity.

Acknowledgments. This work was financially supported by Project 2ARTS - Acesso ao Controlo Autonómico em Reabilitação Cardíaca (PDTC/EMD-EMD/6588/2020), funded by Fundação para a Ciência e a Tecnologia.

References

1. Levesque, J.-F., Harris, M.F., Russell, G.: Patient-centred access to health care: conceptualising access at the interface of health systems and populations. Int. J. Equity Health **12**(1), 18 (2013)
2. Gavic, A.M.: Addressing the problem of cardiac rehabilitation program distribution. J. Cardiopulm. Rehab. **25**(2), 85–87 (2005)
3. Ben-Assuli, O.: Electronic health records, adoption, quality of care, legal and privacy issues and their implementation in emergency departments. Health Policy (New York) **119**(3), 287–297 (2015)
4. Abreu, A., et al.: Mandatory criteria for cardiac rehabilitation programs: 2018 guidelines from the Portuguese society of cardiology. Rev. Port. Cardiol. **37**(5), 363–373 (2018)
5. Moreira, M.W.L., Rodrigues, J.J.P.C., Korotaev, V., Al-Muhtadi, J., Kumar, N.: A comprehensive review on smart decision support systems for health care. IEEE Syst. J. **13**(3), 3536–3545 (2019)

6. Ojha, S.: Recent advancements in artificial intelligence assisted monitoring of heart abnormalities and cardiovascular diseases: a review. Lett. Appl. NanoBioSci. **12**(3), 89 (2022)
7. Lopez-Jimenez, F., et al.: Artificial intelligence in cardiology: present and future. Mayo Clin. Proc. **95**(5), 1015–1039 (2020)
8. Ishraque, M.T., Zjalic, N., Zadeh, P.M., Kobti, Z., Olla, P.: Artificial intelligence-based cardiac rehabilitation therapy exercise recommendation system. In: 2018 IEEE MIT Undergraduate Research Technology Conference, pp. 1–5 (2018)
9. Triantafyllidis, A., et al.: Computerized decision support for beneficial home-based exercise rehabilitation in patients with cardiovascular disease. Comput. Methods Programs Biomed. **162**, 1–10 (2018)
10. Rahman, M., Karim, M.: Designing a model to study data mining in distributed environment. J. Data Anal. Inform. Process. **9**(1), 23–29 (2021)
11. Golovenkin, S.E., et al.: Myocardial infarction complications database. Univercity of Leicester (2020). https://doi.org/10.25392/leicester.data.12045261.v3
12. Hair, J., Black, W., Babin, B., Anderson, R.: Multivariate data analysis: a global perspective. Pearson (2014)
13. Tibshirani, R., Walther, G., Hastie, T.: Estimating the number of clusters in a data set via the gap statistic. J. R. Stat. Soc. Ser. B Stat Methodol. **63**(2), 411–423 (2001)

Understanding Consumers Attitudes Towards Sustainability

Ali Anaissi[1(✉)], Maria P. Mandiola[1], Sabreena Zoha Amin[2], and Widad Alyassine[1]

[1] School of Computer Science, The University of Sydney, Camperdown, Australia
{ali.anaissi,widad.alyassine}@sydney.edu.au, Mpmandio@uc.cl
[2] School of Business, Western Sydney University, Sydney, Australia
s.amin@uws.edu.au

Abstract. Adopting Sustainable Brand Strategies is a 'must' and not a 'should' anymore in the Business Industry. Traditional academic knowledge on how to define Brand Strategy based in the STP process (Segmentation, Target and Positioning) has been worldwide adopted by data-driven Brand Managers. However, incorporation of Sustainability motivations of consumers in this methodology is a task where little literature can be found about. This project aims to incorporate this emerging topic of Sustainability on the classic Market Segmentation approach for Brand Strategy formulation. Focused on the Chilean market case, through a data-set collected by the researcher from a own-designed survey, an Unsupervised Clusterization Model plus other Machine Learning techniques will be applied to achieve this objective. The expected outcome is on one side, finding Meaningful Consumers Clusters able to guide companies in their path to combine profitability with sustainability in an optimal way. Additionally, a Sustainable Brands Ranking across all industries of the Chilean market is expected to be the output of a Sustainable Index Score creation, sorted in descendent order. This Index will evaluate a selected list of the most important brands of the country, based on several Brand Value Rankings published by different consolidated and worldwide known Market Research companies. Further investigation is required to have in-deep analysis by industries, as each of them has unique characteristics and hence, different consumer behaviour and motivations. Enlarging the sample size and fine tuning the data collection process would also be desired for future research on this topic. Updated questionnaires based on data driven findings learned from this project can be applied for future investigations.

Keywords: Sustainability · Brand Strategy · Clustering · Tensor Decomposition

1 Introduction

Sustainability, as a term, has certain ambiguity within its' definitions, or at least on how the can be interpreted. This sometimes may lead to confusion when it is

K. Daimi and A. Al Sadoon (Eds.): ACR 2024, LNNS 956, pp. 137–150, 2024.
https://doi.org/10.1007/978-3-031-56950-0_12

used in different contexts or with distinct purposes. Consequently, it is necessary to set our understanding of this concept before any other context for this research is provided.

In 1987, the United Nations defined sustainability as *"meeting the needs of the present without compromising the ability of future generations to meet their own needs"* [22]. This is, therefore, how we will understand and use this concept on the present research.

The impact that humanity have on this planet and on our society is unarguable nowadays. The recent report of IP-CC released on August 9 2021 was protagonist of countless newspapers headlines claiming Climate Change was 'unequivocally' caused by human activities [9]. This is a categorical statement on a topic that have been subject of discussions that were -until now- based mostly on beliefs, due to the lack of evidence. A topic that is a 'golden key', because it determines whether we, as humans, should take actions towards Sustainability or not.

Business have included Sustainability in their agendas since many years using terms that have been evolving over the time and progressively acquiring higher demands as well. However, this is a topic that probably still remains in a development phase. Stakeholder's management, Corporate Social Responsibility (CSR), Sustainability Governance Models, Business Purpose, are just a few of the concepts that have, in different ways, approached this conception about the responsibilities companies have, beyond the generation of profits.

Brands, as protagonists on Business and Consumers interactions (B2C), have been an active entity on this evolution. This can be appreciated on the evolving way how they relate to consumers through their Marketing Mix, but nowadays more deeper, on how they define their whole Brand Strategy; from Brand Positioning to the more tactic marketing activity they make.

This project aims to guide Brands on this last issue; their Brand Strategy formulation, acknowledging that Sustainability must, without doubt, be the core of the formula. This will be addressed through the Chilean market case across all market industries, as a general overview.

Chile is a 19 million people [5] country of South America that has been many times labelled as the most prosperous country of the region [13]. However, as the World-Bank mentioned on April 2021, "The stagnation of growth and productivity in the last decade has raised questions over the sustainability of the country's growth trajectory and the type of reforms needed" [6]. This is why the case of study applied to this country takes more relevance than ever before, and may be a concrete tool that helps, or even encourages Chilean companies to move forward on the world's sustainability needs.

Moreover, a recent study of the Chilean Market found that 29% of consumers belong to a conscious segment who believe that brands have a role in society and have the power to change the world [8]. This estimation means there are around 5.5 million people in the country that can be addressed in a more optimal way if we had a deeper understanding of their motivations.

On the following chapter, the Research Question the project intends to investigate will be clearly stated. The scope of the project and its' boundaries will be delimited, so the reader now exactly what to expect. Objectives, and how their complexion will be measured will also be explained on this section.

The main objective of this work is to understand consumers attitudes towards the different set of sustainability actions that brands can take to make social and/or environmental positive impact while generating economic benefits for themselves. Our aim is to develop and implement a Machine Learning model which is able to guide and encourage brands to commit with sustainability in the more optimal possible manner, providing specific data-driven guidelines to brand managers on their path to improve the world where we live in a profitable way. The contribution of the work in this study is twofold.

1. Data driven Market Segmentation of consumers attitudes towards sustainability.
2. Sustainability Index Score which evaluates Brands sustainability comitment based on consumers perceptions.

2 Related Literature

On the following section, the most relevant previous research and findings about Brand Strategy methodologies, consumers approaches to sustainability and previous related works are exposed. The examination of these three topics is needed, and essential to the project, because they establish the basis where this project leans.

The review of previous related work confirms which are the spaces of improvements on sustainable motivations research, supporting the significance this project has itself. In the source literature is difficult to find segmentation criteria referring to sustainability motivations within consumers [19], and there are no published studies taking Latin America's market, and therefore, the Chilean consumers into account.

The exposed previous literature in next sections was selected considering relevance to the subject, reliability of the source and analytical quality (inferred from the expressed methodology description of each article). A wide range of dates has been included in this gathering, as this particular project combines both classical Branding and Statistical methods with contemporary Machine Learning processes and Consumer Behaviour trends.

2.1 Brand Strategy Methodology

The Segmentation-Targeting-Positioning (STP) process is the foundation of all marketing strategy [12]. In 1997, Kotler proposed this methodology where demographic segmentation of consumers (Sex, Age, geographics, etc.) where integrated with attitudinal features resulting in a clear and complete framework for data-driven CMOs aiming to define solid and optimal Marketing Strategies for their brands portfolios (Fig. 1).

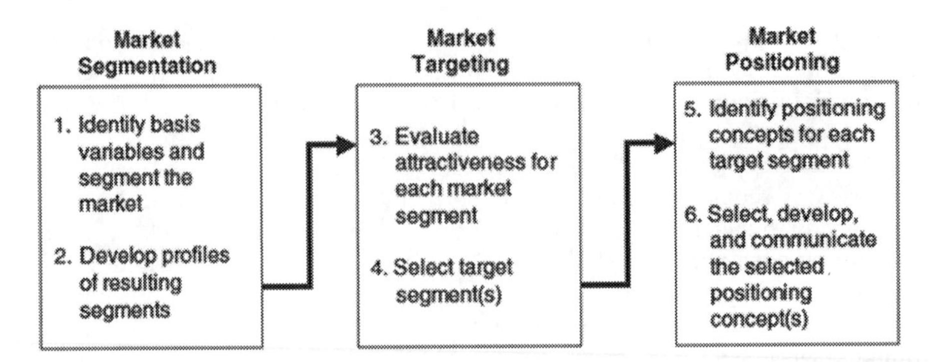

Fig. 1. The STP Process. *(Source: Desarbo et al. 2009, Modified from Kotler 1997)*

Desarbo et al. 2009 [12], classifies empirical modeling approaches in the STP area in two forms:

The more traditional approaches have employed the sequential use of multidimensional scaling (MDS) and cluster analysis. One of the methodological problems of this approach, as discussed by DeSarbo et al. (2008) is that each type of those analysis typically optimize different loss functions. (In fact, many forms of cluster analysis optimize nothing.) Furthermore, they state there is little a priori theory to suggest the most appropriate methodological selection for a marketing application. As well, the various combinations of types of MDS and cluster analyses typically render different results. Lastly, as noted by Holman (1972), the Euclidean distance metric utilized in many forms of MDS is not congruent with the ultra-metric distance formulation metric utilized in many forms of hierarchical cluster analysis.

The second approach is an evolution of the first one, through the parametric finite mixture or latent class MDS models. (cf. DeSarbo, Manrai, and Manrai 1994; Wedel and DeSarbo 1996). In these models, usually estimated applying Maximum Likelihood Method, the number of hyper-parameters is significantly reduced relative to individual-level models.

Hajibaba et al. 2020 [15] propose a methodology that combines k-means method with the variable selection proposed by Brusco (2004) and the Global Stability Analysis introduced by Dolnicar and Leish on 2010. They discuss the vulnerability that traditional cluster analysis methodologies presents in terms of the arbitrary selection of the hyper-parameters defined as an input of the algorithms.

2.2 Sustainability in Business

The idea that business should go beyond their own interests (say, generating profits for their shareholders) is not new. In 1759, Adam Smith, father of capitalism, noted in The Theory of Moral Sentiments that the individual is *"sensible too that his own interest is connected with the prosperity of society,* and that the happiness, perhaps the preservation of his existence, depends on its preservation." (Sneader et al. 2021). However, it has been left to the goodwill of the owners and managers how much that individual-society connection was applied to the objectives of the company.

On January 2016, 193 countries included in their agendas the 17 SDGs (Sustainable Development Goals) defined by the United Nations [23]. This worldwide document has been adapted to the business industries, providing clear guidelines for companies to direct their strategies to create positive impact [14]. This global initiative have had great impact, as they have boosted the incorporation of sustainability to the core of business strategies, which is meaningful progress for the business industry in this matters.

A study run in United States both in 2019 and 2021, showed that 60% of consumers say they are willing to pay more for sustainable brands [7]. This is evidence of the increasing importance of joining business and sustainability into one integrated topic, as the present project aims to do. On this same study, the top 3 issues that consumers expected from companies to focus on where: 1) Providing fair compensation to their employees, 2) Ensuring worker safety, 3) Creating positive work environment with life-work balance. However, Gen Z showed a clear inclination to be more worried about civil inequality, human rights and climate change over economic stability and inequality.

Nevertheless, in general, sustainable values applied by consumers in their purchasing decisions are rarely taken into account in consumer segmentation [19].

2.3 Related Works

There are not many similar research connecting Market Segmentation process with consumers' sustainability motivations on the previous academic literature. The most similar previous work found after the literature review dates on 2011, from Hanss et al. [16] They asked themselves how important various sustainable products attributes are for consumers, and raised their own data-set in Bergen, Norway through in-deep interviews. This was a small qualitative study, where PCA and factor analysis were applied to a sample of 123 students focused in two industries: groceries and cosmetics. They found 3 factors that were the same for both industries: Factor 1 comprises attributes that relate to the protection and distribution of resources. Factor 2 involves the ones that relate to natural pureness and animal protection and Factor 3 represents economic attributes.

On the private side, however, we can find more similar research obectives and good benchmarks for the present project. The Natural Marketing Institute (NMI) has been carrying on a Cluster Analysis of American consumers in relation to sustainability, published as the LOHAS Market Report since 2001 [24]. LOHAS stands for Lifestyles of Health and Sustainability and is a market segment that represents conscious consumers who care more about brand values than the physical benefits they offer. The New York Times called it "the biggest market you have never heard of" [11] and on 2010 they expanded the study to Asia [20].

The NMI's unique and proprietary segmentation model applies k-means defining center as dense regions in the multivariate space of attitudinal variables, tested using T-tests to identify the significal differences between segments [24].

Regarding to Europe, SB-Insight is driving the agenda of the deep understanding of sustainable consumers motivations since 2011 [26]. They have released every year a market segmentation regarding to sustainability attitudes of currently 8 european countries. They have found 4 meaningful groups of consumers which they have labelled under the names of "Ego", "Moderated", "Smart" and "Dedicated" [1].

On 2017, an academic report applying LOHAS logic to the Hungarian market was published [27]. They applied CATPCA (Categorical Principal Components Analysis) on Likert Scale dimensions as a pre-processing step, and then compared Ward's hierarchical clustering method and Mac-Queen's K-means clustering algorithm with 3–6 clusters each and applying different linkage and distance methods. Based on the applied quality indices (Silhouette, Calinski-Harabasz, Dunn), K-means clustering with 5 clusters proved to be the appropriate configuration. The largest cluster was the one containing LOHAS segment, but other type of consumers too. So a second clusterization to this largest cluster was done, until the specific LOHAS segment was found and its size was estimated as 8.7% of Hungarian population as a whole.

A similar study was run on 2019 by Maciejewski et al. on the Polish Market [19]. They focused on the coffee industry and conducted a survey collecting a sample of 800 people, and searched for segments that could describe the market in a more manageable way for marketers. They also applied PCA and factor analysis to the data and later compared both Ward's hierarchical cluster method and k-means.

Kamil and Navrátil, 2019 [25] also applied factor analysis plus Ward's hierarchical clustering to identify the relationship between the consumer's affiliation with a LOHAS segment and its buying behaviour, where 3 LOHAS segments were found with rmANOVA test.

In this paper, we are analyzing Chilean consumers across all industries, in a general overview. As this is a wide spectrum, we are focusing this particular study only on the biggest brands of the country, based on the most important brand studies previously run on this location.

The selection of brands included in this work is listed in Table 1. This selection was based on the biggest Brand Rankings available on the market, provided by consolidated Research Market companies in the country. The public rankings took as input for the listed selections were:

- BrandZ (Kantar)
- Chile 3D (GFK)
- Marcas Ciudadanas (Cadem)
- Meaningful Brands (Havas)
- BAV (Prolam Y&R)
- i-Creo (Almabrands)

3 Methodology

3.1 Data Collection

Survey Design. The questionnaire was designed by the authors during the second quarter of the year 2022. Prior to the research, the survey was pilot

Table 1. Brand list selected based on public ranking

Brand List			
Brand Name	Q7	Q8	Q9
Colun	x	x	x
Nestle	x	x	x
Carozzi	x	x	x
Soprole	x	x	x
Sodimac	x	x	x
Falabella	x	x	x
Dr. Simi	x	x	x
Coca-Cola	x	x	x
Paris	x	x	x
Lider		x	
Nido		x	
CCU	x	x	
Easy		x	
Confort		x	
Jumbo		x	
Entel		x	
Copec		x	
Lipigas		x	
Calo		x	
Watt's		x	
Ripley		x	
WOM		x	
Unimarc		x	
Luchetti		x	
Danone		x	
Mega		x	
Bilz & Pap		x	
Cristal		x	
Latam		x	
Banco de Chile		x	
Unilever	x	x	

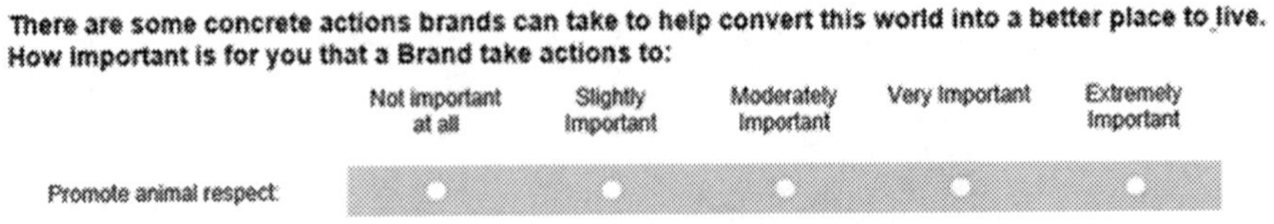

There are some concrete actions brands can take to help convert this world into a better place to live. How important is for you that a Brand take actions to:

	Not important at all	Slightly Important	Moderately Important	Very Important	Extremely Important
Promote animal respect	○	○	○	○	○

Fig. 2. Q4 Example: One of the 23 prompts

run to mitigate possible errors of the data collection process, assess its clarity ensuring questions and instructions are easy to understand and guarantee its' suitability to achieve the objectives of this project.

The complete survey is composed of 10 questions exploring consumers attitudes towards sustainability actions brands can take. The questions were formulated in the form of open, closed, and semi-closed questions using Single and Multiple choice and Likert scales. On the present study, we are focusing on Q4-Q5 for contribution 1. and Q7-Q9 for contribution 2. *(See Sect.* 1).

- Q4 is a Matrix-type question, containing a set of 23 sub-questions, each of them designed with the exact same structure, corresponding to a unique-choice type of question, between 5 ordinal evaluations designed as a Likert-scale. To help a clear comprehension for the reader, the literal question, and 1 of the 23 prompts (sub-questions) randomly picked is provided on Fig. 2. The complete list of prompts of this question is given in Table 2.
- Q5 is a extension of Q4, as it takes in account which of the 23 prompts are the most important for the respondent. This complements the analysis helping us discriminate better when respondents tend to evaluate too many features as the same, and then, improve our understanding of the relative importance of each sentence.

Q7-Q9 cover the brands performance from a different point of views:

- Q7 captures which are the most preferred brands within consumers. It covers a subset of the total list of brands *(See Table* 1, column Q7).
- Q8 explores 5 general statements across the complete list of brands given in Table 1.
- Q9 covers how much the 23 prompts of Q4 are associated to a subset of the brands listed in Table 1 *(See column Q9).*

Table 2. Complete list of prompts Q4 and Q9

1	Support entrepreneurs or start-ups
2	Reduce unemployment rate
3	Improve people's nutrition
4	Enhance and improve education
5	Enhance conscious water consumption
6	Enhance recycling or reusing of products
7	Promote consumption reduction
8	Offer good labour conditions to their employees
9	Impulse local economies
10	Foster positive impact innovation
11	Foster race/origin equality
12	Encourage socio-economic equality
13	Promote social security
14	Minimize environmental contamination
15	Promote peace and social harmony
16	Promote animal respect
17	Promote economic growth and development
18	Reduce poverty
19	Promote a healthy lifestyle
20	Foster gender equality
21	Apply environmental caring production process
22	Promote protecting oceans and beaches
23	Protect ecosystems and eco-diversity
24	Other: (OPTIONAL)

Domain. The study was conducted through an online panel provided by a subcontractor (a worldwide market research specialized company) during May 2022. The target sample size was reached within a week, and 309 valid answers where obtained. Length of Interview (LOI) was 20 min average per person for the whole survey. The panel is composed by regular citizens between 16 and 75 years old that have been recruited to answer questions. As a best practice, random test questions checking the respondent ability to answer the survey were implemented. These were simple questions, i.e., what is the current year, that allow us safeguard the reliability of the data field collection process.

3.2 Data Overview

The 309 respondants of the database are distributed on a representative way, based on the Chilean population distribution [10] in terms of sex, age, socio-economic level (SEL) and district zone. Table 4 shows the demographic composition of the

Table 3. Full list of Socio-Demographic distribution of the sample.

Variable	Labels	National Distribution (%)	Database (%)	Database (count)
GENDER	Male	49%	49%	151
	Female	51%	51%	158
AGE	0–15	20%	0%	0
	16–24	15%	16%	50
	25–34	16%	21%	66
	35–44	14%	20%	61
	45–54	14%	17%	52
	55–64	11%	14%	44
	65–74	7%	12%	36
	75+	4%	0%	0
SEL	AB	1%	2%	5
	C1a	6%	7%	21
	C1b	6%	6%	20
	C2	12%	13%	40
	C3	25%	25%	76
	D	37%	28%	88
	E	13%	19%	59
DISTRICT	Tarapacá	2%	2%	6
	Antofagasta	3%	3%	10
	Atacama	2%	2%	5
	Coquimbo	4%	4%	13
	Valparaiso	10%	10%	31
	O'Higgins	5%	5%	16
	Maule	6%	7%	21
	Bío Bío	9%	9%	29
	Araucanía	5%	5%	16
	Los Lagos	5%	4%	13
	Aysén	1%	1%	2
	Magallanes	1%	1%	3
	Metropolitana	40%	40%	125
	Los Ríos	2%	2%	7
	Arica y Parinacota	1%	1%	4
	Ñuble	3%	3%	8

database, compared with the national distribution of Chile. To see the complete table including SEL and District distribution, please refer to Table 3.

Table 4. Demographic distribution of the sample.

Variable	Labels	National Distribution (%)	Database (%)	Database (count)
GENDER	Male	49%	49%	151
	Female	51%	51%	158
AGE	0–15	20%	0%	0
	16–24	15%	16%	50
	25–34	16%	21%	66
	35–44	14%	20%	61
	45–54	14%	17%	52
	55–64	11%	14%	44
	65–74	7%	12%	36
	75+	4%	0%	0

3.3 Tensor-Based Clustering Method

The proposed approach to address the exposed Research Question is to perform a Cluster Analysis. This means we will be applying Unsupervised Machine Learning techniques to analyse the data, as we will be dealing with an unlabelled class feature.

On a pre-processing phase, Tensor Decomposition will be applied to the data, treating Q4, Q5 and Q7-Q9 as matrices (or *slices*) contained in a higher order tensor (i.e. N-way arrays with $N \geq 3$) [3,4]. This technique has not been applied before in consumer segmentation research, thus this project is contributing to the technical approach in terms of how Data Science advances can be applied to the social sciences in the Market segmentation field through the exploration of this approach.

A tensor is a multidimensional or N-way array that have applications in many sciences, being psychometrics one of them [2,18,21]. There are many tensor decomposition's, in this project the Canonical Polyadic (CP), known as

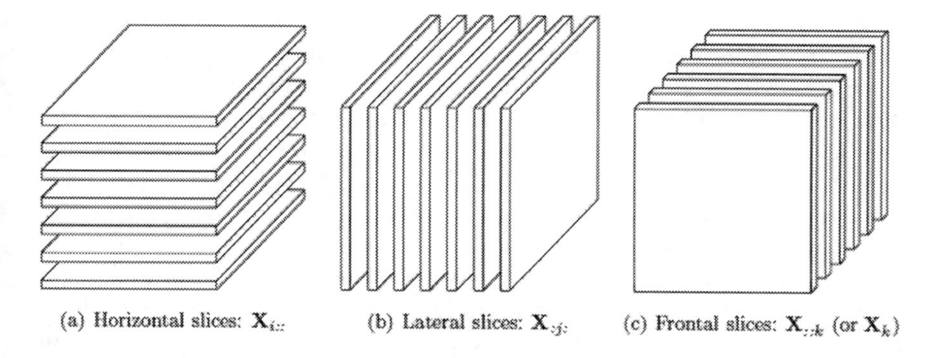

(a) Horizontal slices: $\mathbf{X}_{i::}$
(b) Lateral slices: $\mathbf{X}_{:j:}$
(c) Frontal slices: $\mathbf{X}_{::k}$ (or $\mathbf{X}_k$)

Fig. 3. Slices of a 3rd-order tensor. *(Source: Kolda and Bader, 2009)*

CANDECOMP/PARAFRAC will be explored [17]. This method is an extension of the matrix singular value decomposition, as it decomposes a tensor as a sum of rank-one tensors. Figure 3 shows how this *slices* can be visualized on a third-order tensor.

On a parallel way, Exploratory Factor Analysis and PCA will be applied in order to achieve a dimensional reduction applying data mining to our database. Confirmatory Factor Analysis will be run afterwards and reduction of dimensions will be evaluated to secure a proper basis for the further Machine Learning model implementation. The output of this approaches will be analyzed and compared to decide which one will be selected to advance to the second phase of the analysis.

The Unsupervised Clusterization Problem must be addressed through at least two different methodologies and each of them shall be run with a grid of hyper-parameters to ensure the results come from the best suited model selection. Grid Search with Cross Validation approach will be implemented for this hyper-parameter tuning purpose in terms of scanning every possible combination of number of clusters and distance measure. Based on the previous literature, the two approaches that will be applied to find the consumer segments will be Ward's Hierarchical clustering and K-means approach.

Finally, a Multivariate Regression will be run and contrasted with the Factor loading's obtained in the pre-processing step, in order to generate a Composed Index Score for the evaluated brands on the data set using Q7, Q8 and Q9 information.

3.4 Results

The present Clusterization problem has no true label, so there is no absolute solution to measure how the analysis performed. We cannot evaluate the performance with an External Index as Homogeinity, Completeness and V-Measure.

Moreover, the deep true indicator of how much the objectives of this study were achieved is the interpretability of the clusters, and how much they make sense to the investigator. Hence, human interpretation of the output will be undeniably, the key criterion to evaluate the accomplishment of this project goals.

However, we do have numeric measures that indicates the quality of our clusters, as the Sum of Squared Errors (SSE), also called Inertia, and the Silhouette Coefficient. Percentile Boostrap does not apply here neither, as we lack the condition of having a minimum of 1,000 samples to be an accurate evaluation. We are looking for lower Inertia, the lower the better, and higher Silhouette Score, as the ideal is the closest to 100%. Nevertheless, to confidently state which model is better, statistically significance must be tested.

To compute statistical significance, Paired T-Test will be applied, comparing p-value between the two best scored methods. The reason this type of test is chosen is we are comparing between the same group of observations, but under two different scenarios. Standard deviations are equal and Gaussian distribution is expected. The hypothesis setting goes as follows:

H0: *The two methods have similar performance.*
H1: *The two methods have different performance.*

A minimum of 95% of confidence will be demanded to consider statistical significance on the comparison of the models score.

4 Conclusion

The output of this project has the potential to profoundly change Brand Strategies, from their core. The understanding of consumers segmentation with this new look through the lenses of Sustainability leaves the stage for Brands to define their Brand Purpose, and consequently, re-define their whole strategy and subsequent marketing activities in a Data-Driven way.

The Sustainable Brands Ranking may have a big impact as it is a public mirror for Brands and consumers about how well are brands performing in terms of *being* and *being-seen* as Sustainable Brands. This should encourage Brands to take action, adding pressure to move on this path of transcending beyond their own interests, caring more about the planet and/or environment. It is also a public recognition for Brands that have been pioneers in this matter and gives them stage to be seen and hopefully inspire the others.

This article attempt to fill the research gap found in terms of project scope, as it was found there is no similar research diving deeply within sustainable consumers motivations within the Chilean market and no deep dive either in any country in a cross-industry overview. Furthermore, methodological contribution is being shared with the application of Tensor Decomposition Analysis as a key previous step, challenging the classical market segmentation approaches to level up the analytic techniques that can be applied.

References

1. AB, S.I.: Official report 2020 - Europe's largest brand study on sustainability, July 2020
2. Anaissi, A., Suleiman, B., Alibasa, M.J., Truong, H.: Multi-contextual recommender using 3d latent factor models and online tensor decomposition
3. Anaissi, A., Suleiman, B., Alyassine, W., Zandavi, S.M.: A fast parallel tensor decomposition with optimal stochastic gradient descent: an application in structural damage identification. Int. J. Data Sci. Anal. 1–13 (2023)
4. Anaissi, A., Suleiman, B., Zandavi, S.M.: Online tensor-based learning model for structural damage detection. ACM Trans. Knowl. Disc. Data (TKDD) **15**(6), 1–18 (2021)
5. The World Bank. Chile (2021). https://data.worldbank.org/country/CL/. Accessed 7 Sept 2021
6. The World Bank. The world bank in Chile, April 2021. https://www.worldbank.org/en/country/chile/overview. Accessed 3 Sept 2021
7. Barkley, J.G.: The purpose action gap: The business imperative of ESG, LLC, August 2021

8. Cadem: Marcas ciudadanas en clave COVID-19, June 2020
9. Carrington, D.: Climate crisis 'unequivocally' caused by human activities, says un IPCC report. The Guardian, Manchester, NH (2021)
10. National Statistics Institute of Chile. Population and inhabitants census 2017 (2017). https://www.ine.cl/estadisticas/sociales/censos-de-poblacion-y-vivienda/poblacion-y-vivienda
11. Cortese, A.: Business; they care about the world (and they shop, too). New York Times (July 2003), 3rd Paragraph. Accessed 4 Sept 2021
12. DeSarbo, W.S., Blanchard, S.J., Atalay, S.: A new spatial classification methodology for simultaneous segmentation, targeting, and positioning (STP analysis) for marketing research. In: Review of Marketing Research, vol. 5, pp. 75–103. Emerald Group Publishing Limited (2009)
13. Democratic Republic of the Congo, Economic of the OECD. OECD economic surveys: Chile 2021, p. 7, February 2021 (1st paragraph)
14. U.N.G.C.U. Global Reporting Initiative (GRI), W.B.C. for Sustainable Development (WBCSD). SDG compass - the guide for business actions of the SGDS (2015)
15. Hajibaba, H., Grün, B., Dolnicar, S.: Improving the stability of market segmentation analysis. Int. J. Contemp. Hosp. Manage. (2019)
16. Hanss, D., Böhm, G.: Sustainability seen from the perspective of consumers. Int. J. Consum. Stud. **36**(6), 678–687 (2012)
17. Khoa, N.L.D., Anaissi, A., Wang, Y.: Smart infrastructure maintenance using incremental tensor analysis. In: Proceedings of the 2017 ACM on Conference on Information and Knowledge Management, pp. 959–967 (2017)
18. Kolda, T.G., Bader, B.W.: Tensor decompositions and applications. SIAM Rev. **51**(3), 455–500 (2009)
19. Maciejewski, G., Mokrysz, S., Wróblewski, Ł: Segmentation of coffee consumers using sustainable values: cluster analysis on the polish coffee market. Sustainability **11**(3), 613 (2019)
20. McTigue, L.: Lohas gaining in Asia (2014). https://www.packagingdigest.com/smart-packaging/lohas-gaining-asia. Accessed 8 Sept 2021
21. Naji, M., Anaissi, A., Braytee, A., Goyal, M.: Anomaly detection in x-ray security imaging: a tensor-based learning approach. In: 2021 International Joint Conference on Neural Networks (IJCNN), pp. 1–8. IEEE (2021)
22. United Nations. Sustainability (2021). https://www.un.org/en/academic-impact/sustainability. Accessed 16 Aug 2021
23. United Nations. The sustainable development agenda, January 2016. https://bit.ly/2YKD7sv. Accessed 18 Aug 2021
24. Natural Marketing Institute (NMI). Understanding the Lohas market text trademark report, March 2008
25. Pícha, K., Navrátil, J.: The factors of lifestyle of health and sustainability influencing pro-environmental buying behaviour. J. Clean. Prod. **234**, 233–241 (2019)
26. SB-Insight: About. https://www.sb-insight.com/about. Accessed 5 Sept 2021
27. Szakály, Z., Popp, J., Kontor, E., Kovács, S., Pető, K., Jasák, H.: Attitudes of the lifestyle of health and sustainability segment in Hungary. Sustainability **9**(10), 1763 (2017)

Enriching Ontology with Named Entity Recognition (NER) Integration

Nabila Khouya(✉), Asmaâ Retbi, and Samir Bennani

Rime Team, Mohammadia School of Engineers (EMI), Mohammed V University in Rabat, Rabat, Morocco
nabila_khouya@um5.ac.ma, {retbi,sbennani}@emi.ac.ma

Abstract. Our work focuses on the development of an innovative search and annotation system for arXiv, a platform renowned for its advanced capabilities in exploring research articles, with a particular emphasis on machine learning. Our approach, which enhances content through contextual annotations, goes beyond traditional categorizations. This involves a thorough exploration of machine learning works on arXiv, complementing the existing search features of the platform such as categories, authors, dates, affiliations, etc. The aim is to transcend simple domain categorization by incorporating specific annotations like sub-domains of machine learning, algorithms used, and other relevant information. In this study, we implemented transformer-based natural language processing models to identify and annotate named entities in machine learning articles on arXiv. BERT, in particular, proved to be exceptionally effective, offering high precision in annotation. The methods used and the results obtained highlight the efficiency of these advanced models in enriching academic resources, thus contributing to the creation of an informative and contextual tool for the academic community.

Keywords: Named Entity Recognition · Transformers · Machine Learning · arXiv API · academic research

1 Introduction

In the field of academic research, the quantity of scientific literature, articles, and documents available is simply enormous [1]. This abundance of resources creates a major challenge in terms of efficient management, search, analysis, and collaboration within the scientific community [2, 6]. ArXiv [5] emerges as an indispensable beacon, providing researchers with a plethora of advanced search features. These powerful tools enable a meticulous exploration of the vast expanse of scientific literature, offering categorization by domain through features such as category search, author search, title search, date search, and much more. ArXiv's categories encompass various fields such as computer science, mathematics, physics, quantitative biology, economics, and many others, thus providing a clear and precise organization of research articles.

However, our quest for enrichment goes beyond simple categorization. Our work is part of an innovative approach that involves extracting machine learning articles

K. Daimi and A. Al Sadoon (Eds.): ACR 2024, LNNS 956, pp. 151–159, 2024.
https://doi.org/10.1007/978-3-031-56950-0_13

[16] from arXiv and providing them with more specific annotations [7], surpassing the traditional categories offered by the platform.

While category-based searching on arXiv provides an initial classification, our ambition is to provide more targeted and relevant annotations for the field of machine learning. We have identified crucial but often missing annotation axes, such as specific subdomains within machine learning, the algorithms used, relevant statistics, referenced URLs, types of data utilized, evaluation metrics, and other valuable information.

Our approach, which we term enriching annotology, aims to supplement the information available on arXiv by adding layers of specific annotations [7] to machine learning. This tailored approach will enable us to transcend the boundaries of general categories, providing a more in-depth and contextual understanding of machine learning articles.

Our work is rooted in a vision of advanced exploration and enhancement of existing knowledge on arXiv, providing annotations not only specific to the fields of machine learning but also relevant to the technological and conceptual advancements in this constantly evolving discipline. As for the choice of machine learning, it stems from its central and growing role in contemporary research, making our approach relevant and targeted. Specific annotation within this domain will facilitate a better understanding of nuances and developments within the machine learning community.

2 Related Work

A recently published work has highlighted the creation of EduNER [16], a Chinese NER dataset dedicated to education. Emphasizing the crucial importance of high-quality data for Named Entity Recognition (NER) in the educational domain, this initiative compiled information from various educational sources over a decade. The team defined the educational NER schema and annotated EduNER through a collaborative platform, forming a dataset with 16 types of entities and over 11,000 sentences. It underwent in-depth statistical analysis and was compared to eight other NER datasets. Sixteen state-of-the-art models were employed to validate NER tasks [8, 10], positioning EduNER as a valuable resource for developing NER models focused on education.

Simultaneously, our work, focused on enriching research articles in machine learning on arXiv with specific annotations [7], shares similarities with the EduNER study. While the goals differ, these two initiatives converge towards the creation of domain-oriented datasets. While EduNER aims to develop NER models for education in Chinese, our work aims to provide an in-depth perspective on machine learning articles by adding contextual annotations. These approaches contribute to the creation of specialized resources for advanced analysis and understanding tasks in their respective domains.

Another initiative related to our research on Named Entity Recognition (NER) [11] in the academic context involves the creation of a course recommendation system based on Natural Language Processing (NLP) [17] for the fields of computer science and information technology (IT) [7]. In the rapidly growing technological sector, our research, focused on enriching research articles in machine learning on arXiv with specific annotations, could draw inspiration from this approach. While the mentioned study utilizes Named Entity Recognition (CSIT-NER) to extract skills and entities related to technology, our approach also involves annotating machine learning articles to provide a more detailed perspective. This convergence toward the use of NER in academic contexts can contribute to a more in-depth exploration and efficient utilization of available resources, benefiting both students and researchers in the field of machine learning on arXiv.

3 Methodology

In the context of our methodology, we have meticulously detailed the crucial steps implemented to develop and evaluate our three Natural Language Processing (NLP) [17] models based on transformers [19], namely BERT [12], DistilBERT [13], and RoBERTa [16]. Initially, we conducted a careful selection of arXiv articles related to the field of machine learning. This filtering phase aimed to selectively extract relevant documents from the extensive arXiv collection, covering areas such as physics, mathematics, computer science, quantitative biology, quantitative finance, statistics, electrical engineering, systems science, and economics. Subsequently, we introduced specific entities, particularly sub-domain categories, to effectively structure the extracted articles. This approach aims to facilitate navigation within this abundance of documents and provide a more in-depth understanding, with a particular emphasis on the sub-domain of machine learning. Simultaneously, each article was meticulously annotated with detailed information such as the specific sub-domains explored, the machine learning algorithms used, extracted statistics, referenced URLs, identified authors' email addresses, employed evaluation metrics, as well as the types of data, tools, and specific libraries mentioned in the articles.

This combined methodology of targeted filtering, sub-domain categorization, and detailed annotations aims to provide a thorough and specific perspective on the content of arXiv articles in the field of machine learning, thereby enhancing the relevance and value of the extracted information.

3.1 Entity Selection Process

In defining the entities to be recognized in our study, we considered the diverse features offered by arXiv for article search, with a particular emphasis on the sub-domains of machine learning. This platform provides an extensive variety of categories covering various academic fields such as computer science, mathematics, physics, quantitative biology, etc. Users can refine their search by category, author, or even by title, facilitating the location of specific articles.

Our choice of entities to include in the study aims to provide added value to researchers in the field of machine learning. Beyond the traditional categories offered by arXiv, we sought to explore more specific and often overlooked aspects of articles. Thus, our selection of entities includes precise sub-domains of machine learning, details about the algorithms used, relevant statistics, referenced URLs, authors email addresses, evaluation metrics, types of data, as well as tools and libraries mentioned in the articles.

By adopting such a comprehensive and specifically sub-domain-oriented approach to machine learning, our goal is to enhance the understanding of the content of arXiv articles, providing detailed and specific information to support research and development in this constantly evolving field. This approach aims to complement the advanced search features of arXiv by offering detailed annotations beyond general categories, allowing for a more in-depth and contextual exploration of scientific articles related to machine learning. Thus, not only can each domain category be explored for specific machine learning research, but also the concept of machine learning sub-domains is integrated for a finer and more targeted exploration. Among these sub-domains are supervised learning, unsupervised learning, reinforcement learning, natural language processing (NLP), deep neural networks, and other specific areas.

3.2 Dataset

To construct our dataset, we used a Python script specifically designed to automate the search, download, and backup of research articles from arXiv. The process was streamlined through this script, allowing us to target specific articles in the field of machine learning. By defining a search query, namely machine learning", and setting a maximum limit of 100 articles to extract, the dataset's final composition consists of a total of 55,000 sentences. The decision to set a maximum limit of 100 articles to extract in each run of this script was motivated by several considerations. Firstly, this limit provides control over the scope of the search, enabling us to specifically target articles relevant to our area of interest, namely machine learning. By defining a precise search query, "machine learning" in this case, we ensure that the extracted articles are directly related to this thematic focus.

Additionally, this approach ensures efficient resource management, both on the side of our script and arXiv's server. By avoiding overloading the server with a large number of requests, we optimize the efficiency of the data collection process while adhering to the API usage policies.The limit of 100 articles also aligns with our analysis objectives, offering a manageable quantity of data for initial exploration and analysis. This approach facilitates the processing of extracted information while preserving the quality of the results.

The script communicates with the arXiv API by sending HTTP requests and then analyzes the responses in XML format using BeautifulSoup. This step allows us to extract essential information, such as links to articles and their unique arXiv identifiers. By downloading the articles in PDF format from these links, the script then stores them in a dedicated directory on Google Drive, facilitating access and management of our research resources.

Displaying progress messages throughout the process and managing errors ensure a smooth and reliable user experience. Ultimately, this script played a fundamental role in constructing our machine learning research dataset by efficiently automating the tedious tasks associated with collecting and organizing relevant articles from arXiv.

In the ongoing processing flow, we start by generating a list of PDF files present in the specified directory. Then, for each PDF file in the list, we extract the corresponding text. Text cleaning is performed to eliminate excessive line breaks and unnecessary spaces, enhancing readability. A crucial step in this process is cutting the text into predefined-sized segments. This cutting is essential to ensure that text segments do not exceed a specified limit. This limitation is due to the performance and memory constraints that the Spacy library [20] may encounter when processing very long texts.

3.3 Data Preprocessing

Once the content of the PDF files has been successfully extracted, our process continues with several key steps. First, we segment the text into sentences to divide the content into discrete units of meaning, facilitating its processing and analysis. Next, we implement an entity identification process aimed at spotting specific information in the text. These entities encompass various categories, including precise subdomains of machine learning, details about the algorithms used, relevant statistics, referenced URLs, authors' email addresses, evaluation metrics, types of data, as well as tools and libraries mentioned in the articles. Recognizing these entities is crucial for extracting essential information from the PDF documents stored on the ArXiv platform.

To accomplish this task, we use a predefined extraction method that enables us to identify these different key entities in the text. Once these entities have been identified, we structure and organize all this information into a specific data structure called a DataFrame. This DataFrame plays a central role in our process, as it provides a structured presentation of the extracted information. It contains the words extracted from the text, their corresponding entity labels, and associated sentence identifiers, allowing for a clear and organized overview of this information.

The dataset structured in the DataFrame serves as a starting point for our subsequent analyses. The collected data is thus prepared to be used as input in our models. This step is crucial as it ensures the quality and readiness of the data, representing a critical step to take before embarking on any in-depth text analysis. In summary, our comprehensive process of extracting and structuring the content of PDF documents aims to rigorously and efficiently prepare the data for further analyses.

3.4 BERT

The domain of Natural Language Processing (NLP) has achieved a noteworthy milestone with the advent of BERT (Bidirectional Encoder Representations from Transformers) [12], signaling the dawn of a new era in NLP. BERT stands as a cutting-edge model constructed on various breakthroughs within the NLP community.

Much like the encoder in Transformers, BERT deeply processes an input sequence of words. Each layer applies self-attention, conveys its outcomes to a feedforward network, and subsequently transmits them to the next encoder. The training of a stack of encoders poses a intricate challenge that BERT addresses by incorporating the "Masked LM" (Masked Language Model) [18] concept. This process entails randomly selecting 15% of input tokens, masking 80% of them by substituting 10% with another entirely random token (a different word), and leaving the remaining 10% unchanged. The objective is for the model to accurately predict the modified original token (via cross-entropy loss). Consequently, the model is compelled to uphold a contextual distributional representation of each input token (Fig. 1).

The outputs of BERT are hidden-size vectors, which can be utilized for various tasks [9], including named entity recognition.nommées [11].

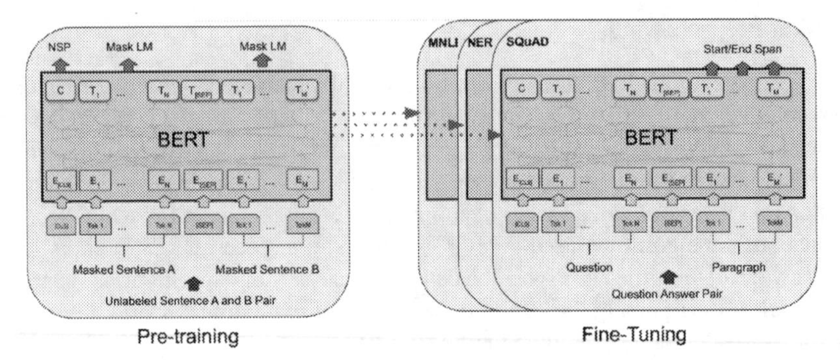

Fig. 1. BERT architecture.

3.5 DistilBERT

The smaller and lighter DistilBERT (distilled version of BERT) [13] is a Transformer model based on the BERT (Bidirectional Encoder Representations from Transformers) architecture designed for natural language processing (NLP). This downsized version of BERT aims to enhance the efficiency of NLP operations. DistilBERT's approach is centered on knowledge distillation during the pre-training phase, reducing the model size while preserving much of its language comprehension capabilities. The model is faster, more cost-effective to pre-train, and retains the inductive biases acquired by larger models through a triple loss combining language modeling, distillation, and cosine distance losses. Overall, DistilBERT provides a lighter and less resource-intensive solution for NLP, suitable for applications with limited computational resources.

3.6 RoBERTa

RoBERTa (A Robustly Optimized BERT Pretraining Approach) [14] represents an advanced evolution of the BERT model, specifically designed for deep analysis and processing of natural language. This model stands out due to significant advancements: it's trained on larger datasets, benefits from an extended learning period, omits the task of predicting successive sentences, employs dynamic masking, and utilizes larger batch sizes.

These improvements endow RoBERTa with an enhanced ability to understand and process natural language, making it highly effective for a range of linguistic processing tasks, such as text classification, automatic translation, and question answering. Moreover, RoBERTa demonstrates remarkable adaptability, delivering excellent results even with relatively limited datasets. This versatility arises from advanced training methods that optimize the use of each piece of data. Consequently, RoBERTa emerges as a robust and adaptable solution, effective in a multitude of scenarios, regardless of the size or nature of the data processed.

4 Results and Discussion

After preparing our dataset, we set the key parameters for a Named Entity Recognition (NER) task using three language models. Initially, we focused on data preparation, renaming dataset columns, converting labels to uppercase, and splitting the data into training and test sets using scikit-learn. Then, we defined learning parameters for the NER model, including setting the number of training epochs to 5, the learning rate to 1e-4, and the batch size to 32, among others. The NER models were constructed using BERT, RoBERTa, and DistilBERT architectures with previously identified NER labels. These models were then trained and their effectiveness was evaluated on the test set data. The "eval_model" method was used to assess performance, encompassing metrics like accuracy, precision, recall, F1 score, and others, depending on the specific NER task. Model performances were primarily evaluated based on their ability to accurately identify named entities in the text.

Table 1 below presents the results obtained for three different models: BERT, RoBERTa, and DistilBERT, in the context of Named Entity Recognition (NER). Each of these models was evaluated using accuracy, precision, recall, F1 score and Eval-loss metrics.

Table 1. Results for Named Entity Recognition (NER)

Metrics	Accuracy	Precision	recall	F1-score	Eval-loss
BERT	**0,895397**	0.808583	**0.804217**	**0.806394**	**0.419967**
DistilBERT	0,884194	**0.811903**	0.798541	0.805167	0.441549
RoBERTa	0,881903	0.808507	0.797338	0.802884	0.436638

It is noteworthy that BERT stands out for having the lowest evaluation loss, scoring 41.9967%, which suggests superior performance in minimizing errors on the validation data for this specific dataset. In terms of precision, DistilBERT shows a slight edge with a score of 81.1903%, indicating a higher acuity in correctly identifying named entities, hence better distinguishing true positives from false positives.

BERT proves to be more adept in recall, achieving a high score of 80.4217%, demonstrating its ability not to miss out on true positives, a critical quality for named entity recognition tasks. With all models exhibiting close recall scores, this demonstrates their collective capacity to effectively retrieve most relevant entities.

The F1 score, which balances precision and recall, is led by BERT with a result of 80.6394%, suggesting that it maintains the best balance between these two essential metrics. In terms of accuracy, BERT continues to shine with an impressive score of 89.5397%, indicating it makes fewer overall classification errors on the test dataset compared to the other models.

Despite the close performance metrics, BERT demonstrates a marginal lead in evaluation loss, recall, and accuracy, as illustrated by Fig. 2. However, DistilBERT and RoBERTa stand as highly competitive alternatives, particularly when factoring in DistilBERT's reduced complexity and diminished computational resource demands. This analysis not only emphasizes the effectiveness of these advanced language model architectures in executing named entity recognition tasks but also underlines the critical need for careful selection of the model that aligns with the unique constraints and objectives of the work at hand.

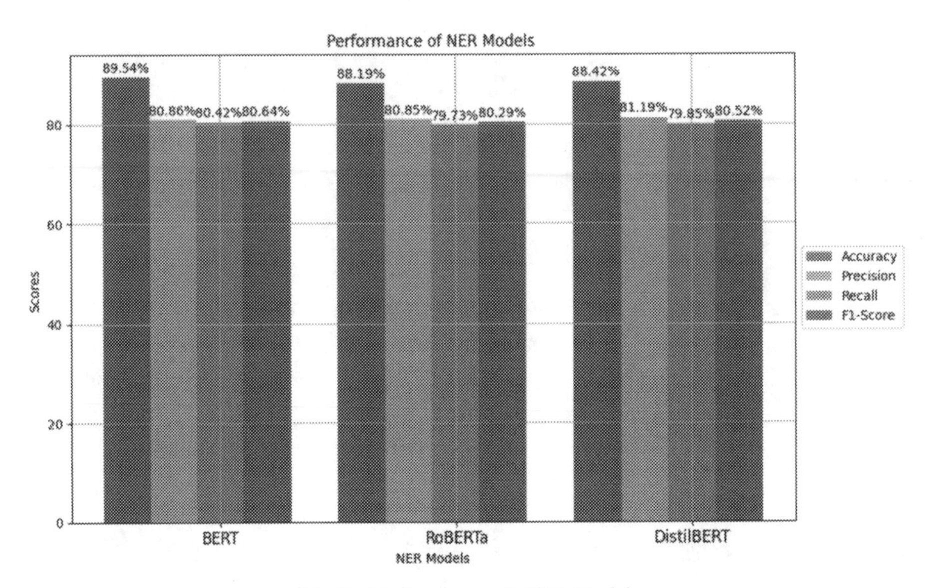

Fig. 2. Performance of NER Models

5 Conclusion and Future Work

In the specific context of our machine learning-focused study, our approach has centered on the exploration and utilization of three natural language processing models based on transformers [19]: BERT [12], DistilBERT [13], and RoBERTa [14]. These models were intentionally chosen for their excellence in contextual and semantic understanding, making them particularly well-suited for analyzing complex academic documents.

The central objective was to develop a Named Entity Recognition (NER) system specifically tailored to the academic research context in machine learning. Using these state-of-the-art models, our approach aimed to accurately and contextually capture relevant entities specific to the field of machine learning present in arXiv articles.

After meticulously examining the results of our experiments, it became evident that BERT [12] stands out for its ability to make precise and reliable predictions for the task of Named Entity Recognition (NER).

For future work, we plan to extend our system beyond machine learning to encompass a broader range of research domains. This expansion aims to enhance the versatility and utility of our system across various academic disciplines. Simultaneously, we intend to dynamize the annotations to adapt to rapidly evolving fields by employing machine learning mechanisms to identify and integrate emerging sub-domains. Additionally, we will develop an intuitive user interface, enabling easier exploration within these new sub-domains. This interface will feature filtering options based on sub-domain categories and will include detailed documentation to enable users to contribute to the system's evolution. These initiatives will ensure that our tool remains current, accessible, and user-friendly, providing a valuable resource for the entire academic community.

References

1. Leonelli, S.: La recherche scientifique à l'ère des Big Data : Cinq façons dont les Big Data nuisent à la science et comment la sauver, Histoires belges (2019)
2. Pochet, B.: Comprendre et maîtriser la littérature scientifique, Gembloux (Belgium) (2015)
3. Distilbert-base-casedHugging Face, huggingface.co/distilbert-base-cased. 2022/11/03
4. Bourdois, L.: Illustration of BERT (lbourdois.github.io). 2019/12/06
5. ArXiv:arXiv.org e-Print archive
6. Goyal, A., Gupta, V., Kumar, M.: Recent named entity recognition and classification techniques: a systematic review. Comput. Sci. Rev. **29**, 21–43 (2018)
7. Vo, N.N., Vu, Q.T., Vu, N.H., Vu, T.A., Mach, B.D., Xu, G.: Domain-specific NLP system to support learning path and curriculum design at tech universities. Comput. Educ. Artif. Intell. **3**, 100042 (2022)
8. Li, J., Sun, A., Han, J., Li, C.: A survey on deep learning for named entity recognition. IEEE Trans. Knowl. Data Eng. **34**(1), 50–70 (2020)
9. Lan, Z., Chen, M., Goodman, S., Gimpel, K., Sharma, P., Soricut, R.: Albert: a lite BERT for self-supervised learning of language representations (2019). arXiv preprint arXiv:1909.11942
10. Naseer, S., et al.: Named entity recognition (NER) in NLP techniques, tools accuracy and performance. Pakistan J. Multidiscip. Res. **2**(2), 293–308 (2021)
11. Shelar, H., Kaur, G., Heda, N., Agrawal, P.: Named entity recognition approaches and their comparison for custom NER model. Sci. Technol. Libr. **39**(3), 324–337 (2020)
12. Devlin, J., Chang, M.W., Lee, K., Toutanova, K.: Bert: Pre-training of deep bidirectional transformers for language understanding. arXiv preprint arXiv:1810.04805 (2018)
13. Sanh, V., et al.: DistilBERT, a distilled version of BERT: smaller, faster, cheaper and lighter. arXiv preprint arXiv:1910.01108 (2019)
14. Liu, Y., et al.: RoBERTa: a robustly optimized BERT pretraining approach. arXiv preprint arXiv:1907.11692 (2019)
15. Li, X., et al.: EduNER: a Chinese named entity recognition dataset for education research. Neural Comput. Appl. 1–15 (2023)
16. Yang, Y., Chen, W., Li, Z., He, Z., Zhang, M.: Distantly supervised NER with partial annotation learning and reinforcement learning. In: Proceedings of the 27th International Conference on Computational Linguistics, pp. 2159–2169 (2018)
17. Khurana, D., Koli, A., Khatter, K., Singh, S.: Natural language processing: state of the art, current trends and challenges. Multimed. Tools Appl. **82**(3), 3713–3744 (2023)
18. Song, K., Tan, X., Qin, T., Lu, J., Liu, T.Y.: Mass: masked sequence to sequence pre-training for language generation. arXiv preprint arXiv:1905.02450 (2019)
19. Kitaev, N., Kaiser, Ł., Levskaya, A.: Reformer: the efficient transformer (2020). arXiv preprint arXiv:2001.04451
20. Honnibal, M., Montani, I.: spaCy 2: natural language understanding with Bloom embeddings, convolutional neural networks and incremental parsing. **7**(1), 411–420 (2017)

Data Transfer Methods and Strategies: Unified Replication Model Using Trees

Alberto Arteta(✉), Sai Sharan Karam, Vanga Ritesh Reddy, and Sontireddy Ranjith Reddy

Troy University, Troy, AL 36081, USA
{aarteta,skaram,rvanga,rsontireddy}@troy.edu

Abstract. We propose integrating binary tree-based and AVL tree-based CRDTs with the MD-Replica protocol to achieve scalability, strong consistency, high throughput, and low latency in a distributed system. Both the binary tree-based CRDT and the AVL tree-based CRDT represent data hierarchically, but the AVL tree-based CRDT is balanced. Numerous copies in parallel can efficiently update both data representations. Optimizing data storage and updating can also improve tree-based CRDT performance. The integrated approach replicates every binary tree, AVL tree, and tree-based CRDT node across multiple distributed system replicas. This keeps data current. The MD-Replica protocol ensures that all copies of a node reflect changes and voting resolves disagreements. The binary tree and tree-based CRDT's hierarchical structure partitions data, increasing the system's scalability. Inherently balanced AVL trees improve update and query effectiveness and conflict totals.

Keywords: data transfers · replication · binary tree · AVL tree · backup strategies

1 Introduction

Distributed applications require high availability. That is why redundant solutions such as RAID or Automated backups/restore strategies on separate servers are done. This is how availability is achieved [1]. The pressure to achieve low latency, fast response, minimal downtime, and high throughput is constantly under research [2].

Primary-Backup Replication (PBR) [2] provides ideal conditions to minimize downtime. However, the primary ends up being a bottleneck because it has more computing and communication overhead than the backups [3]. The Chain Replication (CR) sorts out those redundant clusters to be used in case of need [4]. However, selecting the replicas is not a linear process, and therefore consumes a considerable amount of time [5]. In addition, the overhead costs for the middle replicas are lower than those for the head and tail replicas.

Moreover, numerous replication protocols have been developed over the years to remove the bottleneck caused by PBR without compromising the system's high level of consistency [6]. However, they increase the cost, most notably in the form of increased latency. Unidirectional Replication (UR) seems to enhance the throughput and latency

K. Daimi and A. Al Sadoon (Eds.): ACR 2024, LNNS 956, pp. 160–171, 2024.
https://doi.org/10.1007/978-3-031-56950-0_14

of PBR and CR while retaining a high level of consistency. In UR, the resulting states are propagated in parallel, like PBR, but with fewer messages [7]. In later sections, we will study and contribute with an update that suggests that the proposed solution can show promising results when pursuing, low latency and high availability systems.

1.1 Primary-Backup Replication (PBR)

PBR, a format that is utilized by Apache One of the replicas in the cluster will be selected by Kafka to serve as the primary, while the remaining replicas will serve as backups [2]. The primary database oversees ordering the read and write requests that are sent in by clients, and the backup databases reflect the ordering that is decided by the primary. When the primary receives a written request, the following steps take place:

(1) It processes the request and produces a state, adds the resulting state to its speculative history, which stores the initial resulting states, and propagates it to the backups; (2) the backups add the resulting state to their speculative histories and inform the primary that they have added it to their speculative histories; and (3) the primary adds the resulting state to its stable history, which stores the initial resulting states. As can be seen in Fig. 1, when the primary receives a read request, it will respond to the client only after the backups have acknowledged all of the write requests that were received before the read request.

1.2 Chain Replication (CR)

CR, which is employed across the Google File System Amazon Simple Storage Service Distributed File System Cosmos Amazon The origin of the names FAWN, Hibari, and Ray is PBR [5]. It then forms a chain with the linearly ordered replicas, where the head, which is the first replica in the chain, processes write requests, the tail, which is the last replica in the chain, handles read requests, and the replicas in the between are used as backups. The read request is processed by the tail as it is received, and the tail then makes use of its consistent history to quickly reply to the client.

Figure 2 depicts the processes that are carried out in CR to handle a write request and a read request. m1, m2 and m3 are messages that imply, respectively, "The result is added to the speculative history," "Add the result to the speculative history," and "Add the result to the stable history.

1.3 Unidirectional Replication (UR)

The fail-stop model is assumed to be followed by replicas in the sense that a replica will follow the protocol's specifications until it fails; if it fails, it will not take any action; a replica failure will be reliably detected by every live replica in the cluster; and no replica will be suspected of having failed until it fails. If we define n as the replication factor, then UR can withstand up to $(n - 1)$ failures before it is forced to reduce its availability [3]. In what follows, we will proceed under the assumption that there is always at least one live replica. Additionally, we assume that replicas communicate with one another using trustworthy first-in-first-out links [8].

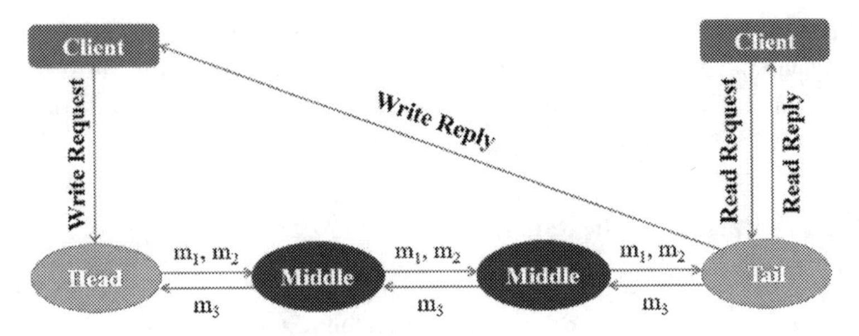

Fig. 1. Handling a write request and a read request in CR

UR makes use of a process known as the master to both establish a cluster and deal with the failure of a replica [9]. The master is presumed to be implemented in a single, infallible server. We make this assumption even if it is not based on reality to make the exposition easier to understand.

The Procedure in Its Normal Form

As illustrated in Fig. 3, when a client sends a read request, it is routed to the tail, where it is processed, and the tail then instantly responds to the client by utilizing its stable history.

Because the reply to any kind of request is generated by the tail, a point of serialization can be said to exist there [11]. This ensures that a high level of uniformity is upheld.

Even though write requests are sent to each replica in the cluster, the computation that leads to the creation of a new state is only carried out once at the head node. When the final state is sent to the witnesses and the tail, those nodes merely store the object difference, which is a more cost-effective operation than the original computation [4]. Read requests, on the other hand, just entail a single replica, therefore they are quite inexpensive to process.

1.4 Dealing with the Failure of a Replica

The objective of UR is to be able to withstand fail-stop failures, and the fail-stop model assumes that failures can be consistently recognized. If the master detects a problem in one of the replicas, the cluster will be reconstructed to remove the faulty replica by considering one of the following three scenarios: (1) head failure; (2) witness failure; and (3) tail failure.

In the event of a head failure, the master sends a message to the witnesses and the tail, informing them of the failure and requesting the lengths of their speculative histories; each replica then replies to the master; the master sends a message to the witnesses and the tail, informing them of the identity of the new head, which is the replica with the longest speculative history; if there is more than one candidate, one of the replicas, other than the candidate with the longest history,

There is always the possibility that the head will try to include a consequent state in its speculative history but will be unsuccessful in doing so before trying to propagate the information to the witnesses and the tail [12]. In this scenario, the resulting state is lost; nevertheless, this does not pose an issue since after some time has passed, the client resends its write request to the new head and retries (Figs. 4, 5 and 6).

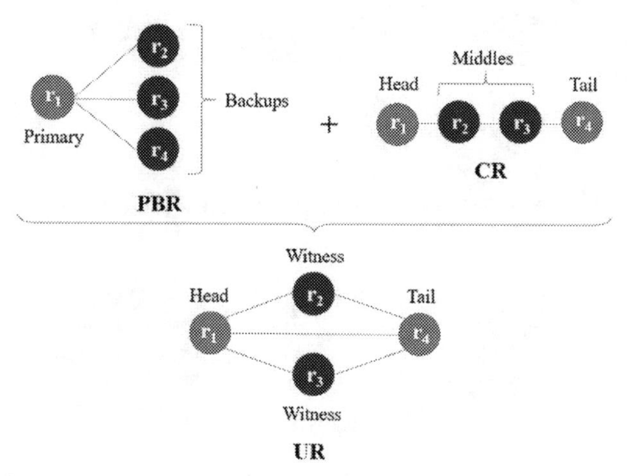

Fig. 2. Merging PBR and CR into CR in an example of a cluster of four replicas

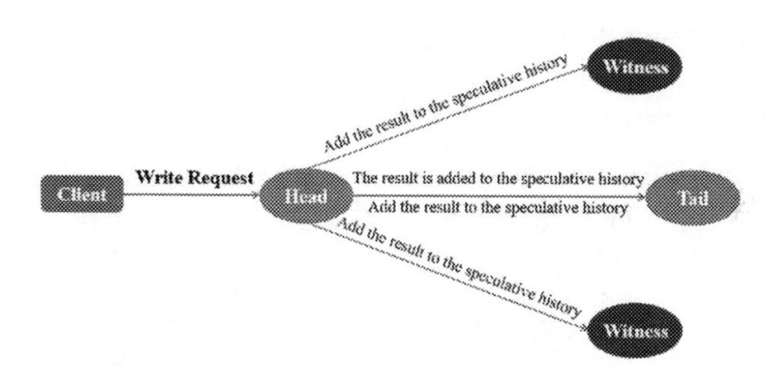

Fig. 3. Handling a write request in UR (step 1)

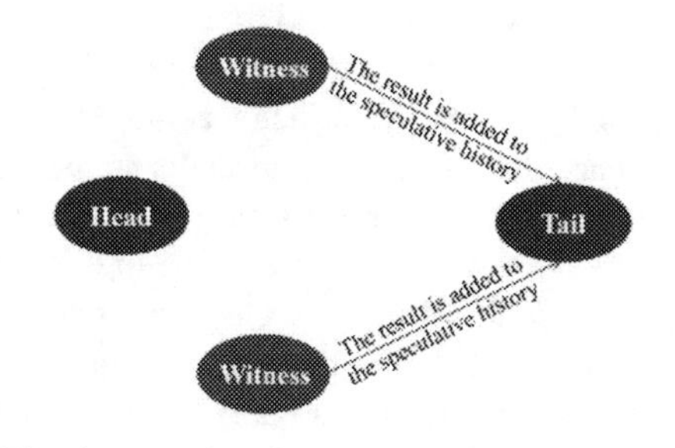

Fig. 4. Handling a write request in UR (step 2)

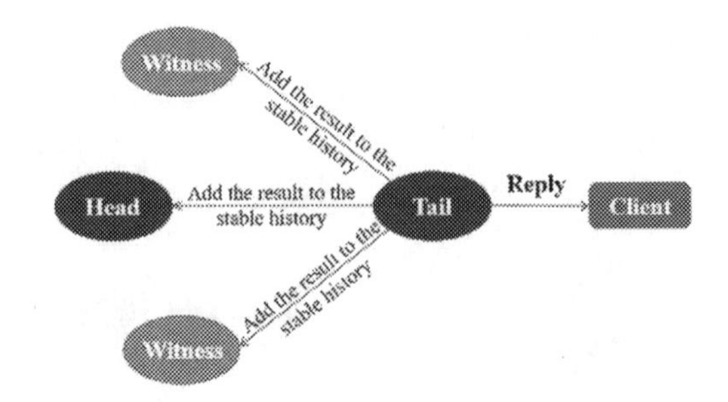

Fig. 5. Handling a write request in UR (step 3)

Fig. 6. Handling a read request in UR

2 Proposed Enhancement

2.1 Using Binary Trees in Unified Replication

A distributed data replication strategy, the Unified Replication model ensures that all copies of data are kept up to date in a unified and effective fashion. In this method, the information is kept in the form of a binary tree, with each node standing in for a different iteration of the information. Data versions before and after the current one are represented as offspring of each node in the graph. Since it has no sibling nodes, the root node stands in for the most recent data version. The data versions represented by the tree's leaves are the oldest ones; they have produced no offspring.

The Unified Replication model employs a two-phase commit technique to guarantee data integrity between copies. The initial step is for the update to be broadcast to all replicas, after which each replica will decide whether it will commit or roll back the change locally. In the second step, the coordinator compiles all the votes and decides whether to commit or roll back the update. The update is applied to the local replica and then broadcast to the other replicas if the decision is to commit. Updates and queries may be executed quickly thanks to the Binary tree structure. When new versions of the data are made, they are appended to the existing one as offspring. In doing so, a new version representing the fork system call in the tree is created. When a replica receives an update, it determines if it is compatible with the data it has on hand. If the change is good, a new version of the data is made and added as a sibling to the existing one. The Unified Replication model employs a conflict resolution technique that considers both the version of the data and the timestamps of the updates to address conflicts that emerge from concurrent updates. If two updates have conflicting timestamps, the one with the latter one is used.

Garbage collection of obsolete data is also facilitated by the Binary tree structure. When a version is no longer supported, it and all its offspring are removed from the family tree. This keeps the tree in equilibrium and reduces the amount of storage space it needs.

Example:

let's consider an example to illustrate how updates are propagated in the Unified Replication model with a Binary tree structure. Suppose we have three replicas R1, R2, and R3, and the current state of the system is as follows.

```
        R1 (a)

        |

        (b)

        / \

R2:(c)  R3:(d)

/ \      /\

(g) (f) (e) (i)
```

where (a), (b), (c), (d), (e), and (f) represent the values stored in the nodes of the binary tree. In this example, R1 is the root replica, and (a) is the head.

Now, let's say a client updates the value of (e) to (g). This update is first propagated to R1, which then forwards it to R2 and R3. Since R1 is the root replica, it sends two separate messages to R2 and R3, one for each child of (b):

```
R1

|


a

|

b

/ \

/\

R2:(c)     R3:(d)

/ \         / \

(e) (f) (e) (f)
```

R2 and R3 update their local tree copies

R1

|

a

|

b

/ \

/ \

R2:(c) R3:(d)

/ \ / \

(g) (f) (e) (f)

Lastly, R2 and R3 send an acknowledgment message to R: Update successful.

R1

|

a

|

b

/ \

/ \

R2:(c) R3:(d)

/ \ / \

(g) (f) (e) (f)

\ /

(h) (h)

This is how updates are propagated in the Unified Replication model with a Binary tree structure. The heads and tails model can be used to optimize the propagation of updates and reduce the overhead of maintaining multiple copies of.

2.2 Using AVL Trees in Unified Replication Structure

As a method for duplicating data in distributed systems, Multidirectional Replication (MDR) enables high throughput, low latency, and excellent consistency. The Unified Replication (UR) model is one method for implementing MDR; it depicts the system as a directed graph. In this study, we offer an alternative to MDR based on AVL trees, which simplifies and optimizes the process of managing replication.

2.3 Using a Replicated AVL Tree

In our suggested method, the replication structure is represented as an AVL tree, where each node is either a head or a tail. The tree's trunk represents the system's central authority, while its branches and leaves stand in for individual client copies. An update from a client replica is always sent first to its parent node, which may be the network's head or its tail. In either case, the parent node will combine the update with its local state before sending the result to its other child node. The AVL tree is traversed from top to bottom, beginning at the root and ending at the leaves.

2.4 Tree-Based Replication Using AVL has Many Benefits

Effective dispute resolution is one benefit of this method. The AVL tree's balancing algorithm can detect and resolve conflicting updates. AVL trees are binary search trees that automatically rebalance themselves after an update is done to ensure peak performance. Updates in the UR model can be propagated in either direction, which can slow down and complicate dispute resolution.

2.5 Effective Replication Using AVL Trees for Updates

The AVL tree-based method also facilitates speedy updates, which is a clear plus. By using AVL trees, we can be guaranteed that changes are distributed reliably and quickly. Only one copy of an update is sent up the AVL tree before it is sent down to the affected replicas. This can increase system performance by lowering the necessary quantity of network traffic.

Example:

Let us have we have a three-node AVL tree, with a root and two offspring nodes. An update from a replica has been sent to one of the child nodes. Whenever a child node's value changes, it notifies its parent node via a message. The message is sent to the parent node, which then modifies its value.

After the update, the parent node discovers that the imbalance factor has changed.

The parent node then executes the necessary rotation(s) to restore equilibrium to the tree.

Due to the rebalancing, the tree's structure is updated to its root.

To equilibrium the tree, the root node can also perform rotations if necessary.

All replicas will always have the most up-to-date data if the changes are made at the root node and then "trickle down" to the other nodes.

Even in the face of failures and network partitions, the AVL tree topology guarantees that changes are efficiently and reliably transmitted across all copies.

Representation:

Root Node

/ \

Child Node 1 Child Node 2

/ / \

Grandchild Grandchild Grandchild

Node 1 Node 2 Node 3

Update received at Grandchild Node 1:

Root Node

/ \

Child Node 1 Child Node 2

/ / \

Grandchild. Grandchild Grandchild

Grandchild Node 1 sends an update to Child Node 1:

Root Node

/ \

Updated Child Child Node 2

Node 1

/ \

/ Node 2 Node 3

Grandchild

Node 1

Child Node 1 sends the update to the Root Node and rebalances it.

Root Node

/ \

Updated Child 2 Updated Child 1

/ / \

Node 2 Grandchild Node 1 Node 3

Updated Child 1 sends the update to all children:

Root Node

/ \

Updated Child 2 Updated Child 1

/ / \

Node 2 Grandchild Node 1 Node 3

All replicas will have the latest version of the data in the AVL tree structure.

3 Comparison and Results

We'll look at the pros and cons of each method and how they affect the unified replication model's implementation to determine which is best. Self-balancing: AVL trees are automatically rebalanced whenever a node is added or removed, keeping the tree's overall height to a minimum. This keeps the tree stable and speeds up searches for specific keys. However, since binary trees aren't self-balancing, their height can grow much more rapidly than AVL trees, which can slow down the search process. Because AVL trees need extra space for balancing information, binary trees use less memory overall. Each node in a binary tree can only produce two offspring, but in an AVL tree, that number can be any multiple of three. utilizing AVL trees to achieve the unified replication model is more complicated than utilizing binary trees. This is because keeping an AVL tree balanced after each insertion and deletion requires a more complex balancing procedure. While the insertion and deletion algorithms for binary trees are simpler, rebalancing the tree may require additional code [1].

In terms of performance, AVL trees have an insertion, deletion, and search time complexity of O(log n). The worst-case time complexity of a search in a binary tree is also O(log n), but updates can take up to O(n) time. This means that, especially with larger datasets, AVL trees perform better than binary trees [2]. For large-scale applications, where scalability is a need, AVL trees are preferable. This is because they are self-balancing, which keeps the tree at a manageable height and shortens the amount of time needed for searches. If the number of nodes in a binary tree gets too high, the tree can become unbalanced, which can slow down searches.

In conclusion, the unified replication model can be implemented using either AVL trees or binary trees. However, binary trees are better suited for smaller datasets where space efficiency and ease of implementation are more important than performance and scalability, while AVL trees are more appropriate for large-scale applications.

4 Case Study and Discussion

4.1 Implementing an AVL Tree (Case Study 1)

Picture a social network that wants to organize its users' profiles following the Unified Replication model and AVL trees. In the AVL tree, each user profile is a node, and the top-level node represents the most important user (e.g., the one with the most followers). For redundancy and stability, user profiles are stored on several different machines.

Suppose a user modifies aspects of their profile, like their image or bio. The user's primary profile copy stored on a particular server will have this change made to it first. The modified user profile is subsequently distributed to the cluster's other servers' replicas.

The AVL tree construction keeps the tree balanced and the user's profile available even if one of the servers housing a replica copy of the profile fails. To keep the tree uniform and well-balanced, the AVL executes rebalancing operations like rotating and removing nodes automatically.

When it comes to user profiles on the social media site, the AVL tree solution provides good consistency and fault tolerance overall. In the case of a server or network failure, users' profiles will still be available and up-to-date.

4.2 Implementing a Binary Tree (Case Study 2)

Now imagine a web store that plans to use a binary tree structure based on the Unified Replication model for its product catalog. Each product is represented by a leaf node in the binary tree, with the most popular option at the tree's root.

Each new item in the catalog becomes a child node in the binary tree. Multiple servers are used to store the same product data in case of server failure. With the binary tree structure in place, data about products can be accessed even if a server in the cluster housing a replica copy of the data goes down.

Any changes made to a product's description or price are first reflected in the master copy of that product's data stored on a single server. The replicated product data on the other nodes in the cluster is then updated to reflect the change.

A server failure during update propagation does not prevent the update from being distributed to the rest of the cluster because of the binary tree topology. The number of network queries needed to retrieve product information can be reduced by the use of caching methods, making the binary tree structure more suitable for low latency and high throughput.

In sum, the binary tree implementation guarantees high reliability and fault tolerance for the online store's product catalog. It provides quick access times for users exploring the product catalog and assures that product information is accessible and up-to-date even in the event of server failures or network challenges.

5 Conclusion

The Unified Replication model can be implemented with either the AVL tree or the binary tree data structure. There are, however, some distinctions between the two methods. Faster convergence and better consistency are made possible by the AVL tree structure, which allows for more efficient balancing of the tree during updates and replica failures. However, the binary tree structure is better suited for low-power devices and resource-constrained environments due to its ease of implementation and low computational requirements.

Both architectures scale well in terms of scalability, accommodating a large number of replicas without sacrificing consistency or latency. However, the AVL tree structure's efficient balancing mechanism may make it a better fit for extremely large-scale rollouts. Ultimately, factors like the number of copies, available computational resources, and required consistency and latency levels should guide the decision between the AVL tree and binary tree designs.

References

1. Gilbert, L.N.: Brewer's conjecture and the feasibility of consistent, available, partition-tolerant web services. Assoc. Comput. Mach. **33**(2), 51–59 (2002)
2. Van Renesse, F.B.: Chain replication for supporting high throughput and availability. OSDI **4**, 91–104 (2004)
3. Bezerra, V.R.: Scalable state-machine replication. In: 2014 44th Annual IEEE/IFIP International Conference on Dependable Systems and Networks, pp. 331–342 (2014)
4. Terrace, J.M.: Object storage on CRAQ: high-throughput chain replication for read-mostly workloads (2009)
5. Oki, B.M.: Viewstamped replication: a new primary copy method to support highly-available distributed systems. In: Proceedings of the Seventh Annual ACM Symposium on Principles of Distributed Computing, pp. 8–17 (1988)
6. Alsberg, D.J.: A principle for resilient sharing of distributed resources (1998)

7. Lamport, L.: The part-time parliament. In: Concurrency: The Works of Leslie Lamport, pp. 277–317 (2019)
8. Shvachko, C.R.: The Hadoop distributed file system. In: 2010 IEEE 26th Symposium on Mass Storage Systems and Technologies (MSST), IEEE, pp. 1–10 (2010)
9. Enes, S.P.: State-machine replication for planet-scale systems. In: Proceedings of the Fifteenth European Conference on Computer Systems, pp. 1–15 (2020)
10. Ganesan, R.H.: Strong and efficient consistency with consistency-aware durability. ACM Trans. Storage (TOS) **1**(17), 1–27 (2021)
11. Flocchini, P., Prencipe, G., Santoro, N.: Distributed Computing by Oblivious Mobile Robots. Springer, Cham (2022). https://doi.org/10.1007/978-3-031-02008-7

Optimized Vehicle Repair Cost by Means of Smart Repair Distribution Model

Franck van der Sluis[1,3(✉)], Cristian Rodriguez Rivero[1,2], and Joris Hooi[3]

[1] University of Amsterdam, Science Park, 1098XH Amsterdam, XH, The Netherlands
mail.franck@proton.me

[2] Cardiff Metropolitan University, Cardiff, Wales CF52YB, UK
crodriguezrivero@cardiffmet.ac.uk

[3] Openclaims, Amsteldijk 10, 1074HP Amsterdam, HP, The Netherlands
jorishooi@openclaims.com

Abstract. The distribution of vehicle damages to bodyshops is not cost-effective. Every damage is unique, and every bodyshop has its specialization(s). Currently, the distribution of damages to bodyshops is predominately based on the distance between the customer and the bodyshop. This paper provides a method to optimize the distribution of vehicle damages to bodyshops in a way that the repair is executed by the most cost-effective bodyshop available for a particular damage based on damage and context characteristics. Three machine learning models have been evaluated to determine which is most suitable for predicting the cost of repair for one particular damage for each bodyshop available. The neural network produced the best results with an average error of €383. In order to apply this approach to real-world problems, we highlight the use of data from visual assessment of the damages using computer vision technology and onboard vehicle data in order to yield the biggest improvement in the average prediction error.

Keywords: Neural Network Regression · Vehicle Repair Cost Optimization · Car Repair Cost Optimization · Repair Costs Reduction · Vehicle Insurance · Vehicle Leasing · Car Lease

1 Introduction

Vehicle insurance portfolios in the Netherlands are loss-making. In 2018, for every euro made, the cost was €1.22 [30]. The total cost of vehicle repair for risk carriers and leasing companies in the Netherlands is estimated at €2.9 billion annually in 2018 [30]. It is the biggest cost these parties have and therefore affects their business case. Due to macroeconomic developments, the cost of vehicle repair increased even further in 2022 [34]. This research is focused on the Dutch market due to the available data. However, this problem is not limited to the Dutch market. A similar trend is visible in the United Kingdom where vehicle repair costs increased 40% over the period 2018–2022 [35]. Distribution of vehicle repairs to bodyshops is not optimized in a way that vehicles are repaired by the

K. Daimi and A. Al Sadoon (Eds.): ACR 2024, LNNS 956, pp. 172–183, 2024.
https://doi.org/10.1007/978-3-031-56950-0_15

most cost-efficient bodyshop. It is solely based on the location of the customer in relation to bodyshops. Because the distribution of repairs to bodyshops is not optimized based on other factors, this results in an unnecessarily high total cost of repair. Exploratory data analysis shows that the average repair cost per bodyshop differs heavily from one to another. The difference between the cheapest and most expensive bodyshop is more than €2000 while the average vehicle repair cost for the market is €1359 [31]. The average repair cost for one specific brand at one bodyshop compared to the same brand at another bodyshop differs over 50% on multiple occasions. These differences are unexplained. Because of this, there is a demand in the market coming from insurance and leasing companies to optimize the distribution of vehicle repairs in a way that cost reduction is effectuated. This research explores three machine learning models, finding the best performing model to predict the cost optimal bodyshop for a specific repair. Repair cost-based ranking data is not available because one damage is always repaired by one bodyshop. Therefore, the problem is approached as a supervised regression problem. Predicting the cost of repair for one individual damage for multiple bodyshops. The cost of repair is a continuous label, which makes it a regression problem [11] Approaching it with a supervised method offers the ability to estimate the true prediction error of the used models to assess the model's generalization ability and to prevent overfitting [4]. A machine learning model is proposed that can predict the cost of repair for a vehicle damage per bodyshop based on case characteristics. In the experimental setup, the model only used contextual data. The proposed approach will benefit majorly from adding actual collision data that is collected onboard in modern vehicles and data from visual assessment of the damage using computer vision based on pictures of the damage. Furthermore, this paper addresses how this model is developed and what actions are needed to put this approach into practice. The main research question being addressed is: *How can the assignment of vehicle damages to bodyshops be optimized in a way that the repair is executed by the most cost-efficient bodyshop available?* This research question is divided into the following sub-questions.

RQ1 How can factors that influence the cost of vehicle repair be identified?
RQ2 What model is suitable to assign repairs to bodyshops in a way that the repair is assigned to the most cost-efficient bodyshop available for each specific repair?

This research was conducted at Openclaims, a SaaS (software) provider in the insurance and lease industry. Openclaims' software is used by vehicle insurance- and leasing companies to manage vehicle repairs. Due to the uniqueness of the main research question, little to no literature has been found that covers this topic specifically. In addition, there has been a search for literature regarding the ranking of firms based on their financial performance on specific tasks. Also, on this broader and more generic topic, no literature has been found. The problem being addressed is a new field of research. However, for the subquestions, literature has been found that describes how parts of the problem that was researched can be addressed. The most important literature for each subquestion is described below. In essence, **RQ1** is being addressed by assessing the association between the independent variables and the cost of repair. Khamis (2018) [16] describes various methods to assess the associations between the following six variable combinations. 1. continuous-continuous 2. continuous-ordinal 3. continuous-nominal 4. ordinal-ordinal 5. ordinal-nominal 6. nominal-nominal For **RQ2**, Mirkin (2019) [20] describes the most generic and popular methods to learn correlations between two or more variables. Four of the described methods can be used when there is a continuous target variable. Those methods are linear regression, canonical correlation analysis, neural network regression, and regression tree. Nor Mazlina and Izah Mohd (2009) [1] describe the successful application of both methods in predicting bank performance. In this research, the neural network performed better than the linear regression. Another paper, by Osita and Desmond (2013) [3], also addresses the application of the same two regression techniques for a different problem. In this case, the techniques were used to predict the performance measures of firms. In a third research, the neural network outperformed linear regression described by Jahn (2018) [13]. For instance, the K-Nearest Neighbor approach was successfully implemented in an economic forecasting problem by Bafandeh Imandoust and Bolandraftar (2013) [12]. Based on the gathered literature, three regression techniques have been identified that provide a solid base to approach this research question.

2 Methodology

This section provides an overview of the data available for this research, and describes the methods used to answer the research questions. Furthermore, it explains how three baseline models have been set up and what model from the baseline setup has been selected to continue the experiments with, and how it was further optimized.

The dataset contains data about vehicle repairs, specifically passenger car [36] damages, that have been repaired by bodyshops (not dealerships). Vehicles that are a total loss are not included because these vehicles are not repaired but recycled and/or destroyed. The average cost of repair is €1367. The maximum cost of a single repair was €52359. The minimum was €7. Because this variable can only have a positive value, the distribution is right-skewed. This is visible in Fig. 1. It shows the distribution for the cost of repair for all repairs in the dataset, excluding the repairs with a repair cost higher than €10k. Figure 2 shows that it is clear that it can not be assumed that the differences between the bodyshops are solely caused by the individual bodyshop's performance. The differences are so big that it should be assumed that the differences are also caused by other factors independent of the bodyshop itself. The five datasets used were joined together on individual damage level. The result of this step is a single large dataset where every record represents one damage. The dataset has been deduplicated based on the unique identifier of the damage. If duplicates are found, the newest record is kept. The dataset is filtered to include only bodywork repairs. Total loss cases (non-repairs) are filtered out of the dataset as well. The dependent variable (cost of repair) has been checked for obviously incorrect data. For example negative values or values of zero. These records are cleaned from the dataset.

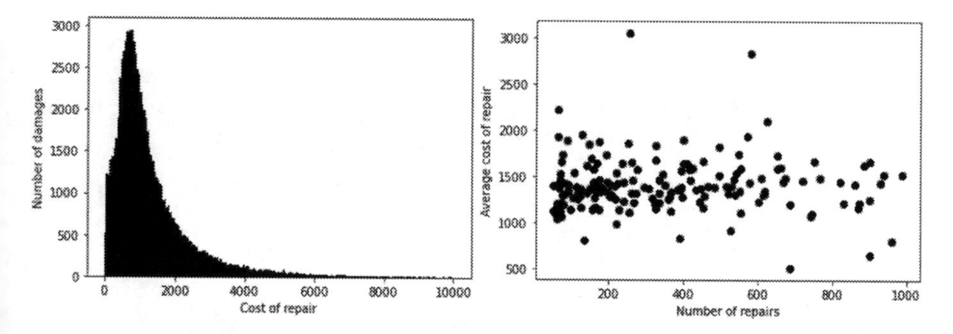

Fig. 1. Histogram of cost of repair - frequency of repairs per damage amount

Fig. 2. Average cost of repair and number of repairs per bodyshop

Feature Selection. As described in Sect. 1, the proposed model should be able to predict which bodyshop will perform a repair the most cost-efficient for a specific damage based on case characteristics. This means that when the model is operationalized, all features that were used to train the model should be potentially available when the model needs to predict the cost of a repair. Potentially here means that Openclaims can make this data available in the process of assigning a damage to a bodyshop, e.g. a feature that indicates if a damage is complex or cosmetic could be generated based on a picture of the damage using computer vision or collision data collected in the onboard computer of the vehicle. Features like the number of hours spent on a repair are therefore excluded from the model. Furthermore, features are selected by assessment of the association between the independent variables and the dependent variable, the cost of repair. In the dataset, there are two types of variables available as follows.

Continuous - Continuous. As a measure of association between two continuous variables, the Pearson correlation coefficient has been used. This measure indicates the strength of association between two variables with a value between -1 and 1. -1 indicates a strong negative relationship and $+1$ a strong positive relationship. 0 would indicate that there is no relationship.

Categorical - Continuous. As a measure of association between categorical variables and the independent continuous variable, the point-biserial correlation coefficient has been used. Robert Tate (1954) [28] describes how the Pearson correlation coefficient can be applied to categorical variables. Categorical variables are converted into binary variables (0/1). Each level of a categorical variable is converted to a binary variable. The Pearson correlation coefficient is then calculated with the binary variables. This is referred to as the Point-biserial correlation coefficient.

Significance. All features with a significant Pearson correlation coefficient have been selected as features that are used in both the baseline and experimental setup of the research. Significance is tested using a two-sided p-value, which should be ≤ 0.05 to be considered significant.

Input data. All features that were tested as significant, are fed to the input of the models in the baseline and experimental setup. Table 1 shows these features in a categorized way along with some key features as example.

Table 1. Input data for models

Category	Example features
Damage context	Cause & date
Driver	Age & location
Contract	Duration & kilometers
Bodyshop	Name & location
Vehicle	Brand & age
Calculation	Cost of repair

Table 2. Baseline neural network model architecture

Layer	Input	Output	Function
Input	–	1491	–
Fully con	1491	128	ReLu
Output	128	1	Linear

Validation. Khamis et al. (2005) [15] found that extreme values negatively impact Neural Network generalization abilities. It is hard to determine what should be considered as extreme values in this research. All vehicle repairs are actual executed repairs by bodyshops. The variance in the dataset is so high that it is hard to determine what can be considered an extreme value and what not. For instance, a €4k repair on a Tesla is not extreme while it is on a Volkswagen. It is also fair to say that the model should be able to perform good on 95% of the distribution and not on the extreme values. Therefore, the extreme values have been determined per vehicle brand. For instance, the cap for Tesla is €5k while for Volkswagen it is €3.6k. In this research, the extreme cases have been filtered out of both the training set and the validation set. This decision was made because it's simply not interesting how well the model performs on extreme cases. Including them in the input data in any way would negatively impact the generalization abilities of the model for the interesting 95% of the distribution, which has the most potential for optimization. So these are all disregarded from the research. One of the most popular methods to validate supervised learning methods is cross-validation [4]. The size of the training/validation split is 80% of the available data for the training set and 20% for the validation set, as recommended by Raschka (2018) [23].

Evaluation Metrics. We proposed to use Mean Square Error (MSE), Root MSE (RMSE), Mean Absolute Error (MAE) and Mean Absolute Percentage Error (MAPE) as regression evaluation metrics via surveys [5]. As MAPE is a timeseries forecasting evaluation metric, and this research does not entail a timeseries forecasting problem, it is disregarded from this research. RMSE and MAE are the remaining evaluation metrics that was focused on. The definition of MAE and RMSE [7] are shown below in equation one and two, respectively.

$$MAE = \frac{1}{n}\sum_{i=0}^{n}|e_i| = \frac{1}{n}\sum_{i=0}^{n}|y_i - \hat{y}_i| \tag{1}$$

$$RMSE = \sqrt{\frac{1}{n}\sum_{i=0}^{n}e_i^2} = \sqrt{\frac{1}{n}\sum_{i=0}^{n}(y_i - \hat{y}_i)^2} \tag{2}$$

There is a noteworthy amount of literature available that states that RMSE is superior over MAE and vice versa. In this project [7], MAE was selected as the main evaluation metric over RMSE because of three reasons. First, RMSE is sensitive to extreme residual values because the residuals are squared before taking the average. Because of this, the effect on the evaluation would be magnified. As shown in Fig. 1, the distribution has a long tail all the way to €52359. Because of this, there are many outliers which cause large residual values. For this specific model, large residual values on outliers are not particularly undesired, as most of the optimization potential for the cost of damage repair lies on the left side of the distribution. Therefore, RMSE is not the most robust evaluation metric to evaluate the model. The second reason is that RMSE is not suitable for inter-comparisons of average model performance on different datasets because it is a function of the average error (MAE). The third reason is that MAE is simple to interpret [32] because the evaluation result is the average residual value. In this research, MAE is used as the main metric and RMSE is used alongside to identify potential issues.

2.1 Experimental Setup

In the baseline setup, three different models have been trained. Linear regression, K-nearest neighbors, and a neural network. Another baseline K-nearest neighbors model was trained using every number between 1 and 100 for K. K is the number of neighbors used to determine the predicted value with. It's the hyperparameter of the K-nearest neighbor model. Lastly, neural network model has been trained using a learning rate of 0.01. The architecture and other hyperparameters of this model are shown in Sect. 3, Table 2. The model with the best baseline results has been selected for further improvement and optimization. The baseline results are described in Sect. 3. As both in the literature and in the baseline setup the neural network achieved the best baseline results, this model has been selected for further experimenting. The next steps describe what optimization steps have been experimented with to optimize the neural network. The learning algorithm that is used for optimizing the neural network's weights is called stochastic gradient descent, as described by Kingma and Ba (2015) [17]. The neural network has many hyperparameters that can be tuned. The most important are the number of hidden layers, the number of neurons per layer, the learning rate used by the learning algorithm and a potential drop-out layer to prevent overfitting [26]. There is no literature available that specifies what hyperparameters are best. It is 100% dependent on the dataset and therefore unique for every situation. The best combination of hyperparameters is found experimentally. In this research, this process was automated using Keras tuner [29]. In Table 3 the search space used in this research is shown.

Table 3. Keras tuner search space

Hyperparameter	Boundaries	Step
Number of layers	1–20	1
Width per layer	128–1536	128
Dropout layer	0.0–0.1	0.02
Learning rate	0.01–0.0001	0.0002

The algorithm used by the Keras tuner is Bayesian optimization [25]. This algorithm was chosen because it adjusts the hyperparameters based on how the previous combinations performed. This way it is faster than trying combinations of hyperparameters at random. If the best performing model found has a hyperparameter that is exactly on a boundary as specified in Table 3, the tuner reports that the boundaries should be moved further to potentially find a better model. Important note: it became clear rather quickly that a learning rate of approximately 0.001 consistently led to the best result. From that point, the learning rate was removed from the search space. This did not have an impact on finding the best learning rate because the learning rate was further optimized during training, as will be shown in Sect. 3. To enable the neural network to learn non-linear effects, non-linear activation functions have to be added to the hidden layers. The most widely used activation function for this purpose is ReLu. Sharma et al. (2020) [24] point out that ReLu gives the best results in most of the cases. Additional methods should be experimented with if ReLu does not give satisfactory results. To prevent the model from overfitting, a regularization method called Early Stopping was used while training the neural network [6]. With this method, the performance on the validation set is monitored every epoch. If the performance on the validation set does not improve anymore, the learning algorithm stops updating the model's parameters to prevent overfitting.

3 Results and Discussion

3.1 Feature Selection

As described in Sect. 2, continuous variables have been tested using the Pearson correlation coefficient and categorical variables have been tested using the point-biserial correlation coefficient. Table 4 shows five (rounded) results that were generated using this method. 37 continuous variables and 25 categorical variables were tested as significant. (1,491 variables when counting one for each category).

Table 4. Output correlation test

Significance	Variable	Coeff.	P-value
Significant	List price	0.0562	0.0000
Significant	Airbag popped	0.1187	0.0000
Significant	Sill damaged	0.2830	0.0000
Insignificant	Province Limburg	0.0012	0.7727
Insignificant	First color yellow	0.0010	0.8005

The three selected models have been trained in the baseline setup. The worst performing model is K-nearest neighbors. It performed best with the hyperparameter set to K = 93. The second best-performing model is the linear regression. The best-performing baseline model is the neural network. The architecture of this model is shown in Table 2. This model has 190,976 trainable parameters. The results for all models, including baseline, are summarized in Table 5. The parameters of a neural network are trained iteratively. The optimum of the model was reached at 4427 epochs. As the best-performing baseline model, the hyperparameters of the neural network were further optimized according to the methods as described in Sect. 2. As shown in Fig. 3, the MAE of the baseline neural network showed large spikes during the training of the neural network. This indicates that the learning algorithm would benefit from a smaller learning rate. The learning rate for the advanced neural network was set to 0.001 and was decreased by 10% every time the MAE did not improve after 50 epochs. The architecture of the advanced neural network is shown in Table 6. This model has 1,354,368 trainable parameters.

Table 5. Model evaluation results

Type	Model	MAE	RMSE
Baseline	K-NN	691	975
Baseline	Lin. Regression	445	633
Baseline	Neural Net.	424	644
Advanced	Neural Net.	383	600

Table 6. Advanced neural network model architecture

Layer type	Shape in	Shape out	Activation
Input	–	1491	–
Fully con.	1491	512	ReLu
Fully con.	512	1152	ReLu
Output	1152	1	Linear

As described, the learning rate was decreased by 10% every time the MAE did not improve for 50 epochs. Figure 3 shows the MAE after each epoch for the advanced neural network. The learning rate for each epoch is shown in Fig. 4.

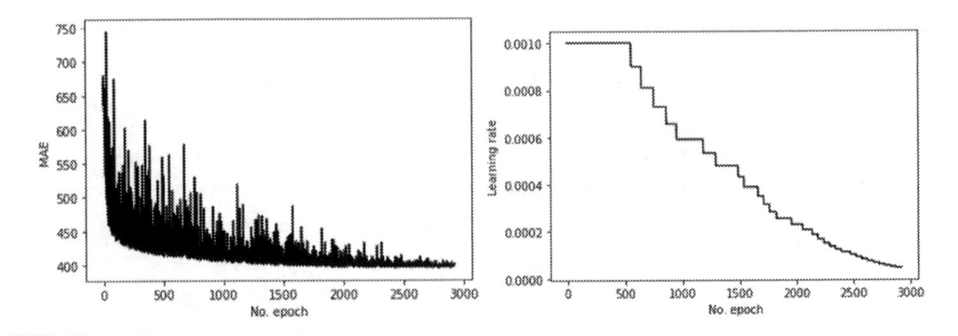

Fig. 3. Advanced neural network learning curve

Fig. 4. Advanced neural network learning rate per epoch

3.2 Interpretation

In the baseline setup, K-nearest neighbors, linear regression, and a neural network were evaluated. The baseline neural network outperformed both K-nearest neighbors and the linear regression without any tweaking or optimizing of the network. The neural network performed best on the main evaluation metric, MAE, but performed slightly worse than the linear regression on RMSE. This means that the neural network performed better on most of the data, but had a higher frequency of extreme residual values. The best architecture for the model was found within the determined boundaries of the search space. The width per layer was optimized using steps of 128 nodes for the sake of saving time. A better-performing architecture likely exists within the steps of 128. It is therefore recommended to optimize the width of the layers using steps of 1 instead of 128. The model's performance would benefit majorly from extending the dataset with additional sources of actual damage data. Features have been selected by testing all independent variables for their association with the dependent variable, the cost of repair. This has been done independently of each other. One observation from the validation set was used to demonstrate how the model's output can be used. The real cost of the repair for this observation was €1135.23. The model was used to predict the cost of the repair for three bodyshops. These predictions are shown in Table 7.

Based on these predictions, the repair would be assigned to the one with the lowest predicted cost of repair, which in this case is bodyshop 3.

Table 7. Model predictions for three bodyshops

Bodyshop	Prediction
Bodyshop 1	€949.734
Bodyshop 2	€1065.7368
Bodyshop 3	€945.39484

Explainability. When vehicle damages are assigned to bodyshops based on a machine learning model, there will likely be a demand in the market to explain the model in detail. The reason for this is that it has a financial impact on stakeholders. The best-performing model, the neural network, is much harder to explain to the market because it's a "black box". It has millions of parameters that are determined by a learning algorithm. Yang (2019) [33] proposes a "hybrid" version of the neural network, xNN, in which architecture constraints have been added to achieve the perfect balance between model performance and interpretability. This could be considered as a solution in case the market demands better explainability of the model.

4 Conclusions

This research provides a method to optimize the assignment of vehicle damages to bodyshops in a way that the repair is executed by the most cost-efficient bodyshop available. Firstly, the key factors for the cost of vehicle repair have been identified using the Pearson Correlation Coefficient for continuous variables and the Point-biserial Correlation Coefficient for categorical variables. Secondly, based on the identified factors, multiple models have been trained to predict the cost of a repair. The neural network has shown the best performance to predict the cost of a repair for each bodyshop based on the input data with an average error of €383 which was evaluated using unseen evaluation data. From the models that was experimented with, it is the most suitable model to predict the cost of repair for an individual damage per bodyshop. These predictions can be input for a system to select the bodyshop with the cheapest prediction. In future work More features in general make the neural network more likely to overfit and perform worse on the evaluation data than it potentially could. As discussed, it is also advisable to experiment with Lasso regularization and Ridge regularization at this stage.

References

1. Bakar, N.M.A., Tahir, I.M.: Applying Multiple Linear Regression and Neural Network to Predict Bank Performance. Int. Bus. Res. 2 (2009). https://doi.org/10.5539/ibr.v2n4p176
2. Adnan, N., Ahmad, M., Adnan, R.: A comparative study on some methods for handling multicollinearity problems. Matematika **22**, 109–119 (2006)
3. Predicting performance measures using linear regression and neural network: a comparison **1**, 84–89 (2013)
4. Berrar, D.: Cross-Validation (2018). https://doi.org/10.1016/B978-0-12-809633-8.20349-X
5. Botchkarev, A.: A new typology design of performance metrics to measure errors in machine learning regression algorithms. Interdiscipl. J. Inf. Knowl. Manag. **14**, 045–076 (2019). https://doi.org/10.28945/4184
6. Caruana, R., Lawrence, S., Giles, C.: Overfitting in neural nets: backpropagation, conjugate gradient, and early stopping. Adv. Neural. Inf. Process. Syst. **13**, 402–408 (2000)

7. Chai, T., Draxler, R.R.: Root mean square error (RMSE) or mean absolute error (MAE)?- Arguments against avoiding RMSE in the literature. Geosci. Model Dev. **7**(2014), 1247–1250 (2014). https://doi.org/10.5194/gmd-7-1247-2014
8. ControlExpert. [n.d.]. https://www.controlexpert.com/. Accessed 23 Jun 2021
9. Daoud, J.I.: Multicollinearity and regression analysis. J. Phys: Conf. Ser. **949**, 12009 (2017). https://doi.org/10.1088/1742-6596/949/1/012009
10. Dave, V., Shah, K.: Comparative analysis of regularization techniques in arteficial neural networks (2019). https://doi.org/10.1729/Journal.22756
11. Hurwitz, J., Kirsch, D.: Machine Learning for Dummies. Wiley, Hoboken (2018)
12. Imandoust, S.B., Bolandraftar, M.: Application of K-nearest neighbor (KNN) approach for predicting economic events theoretical background. Int. J. Eng. Res. Appl. **3**, 605–610 (2013)
13. Jahn, M.: Artificial neural network regression models: predicting GDP growth. HWWI Research Papers 185. Hamburg Institute of International Economics (HWWI) (2018)
14. Jayawardena, S.: Image-Based Automatic Vehicle Damage Detection. Ph.D. Dissertation (2013)
15. Khamis, A., Ismail, Z., Khalid, H., Mohammed, A.: The effects of outliers data on neural network performance. J. Appl. Sci. **5**, 1394–1398 (2005)
16. Khamis, H.: Measures of association: how to choose? J. Diagnostic Med. Sonography **24**(2008), 155–162 (2008). https://doi.org/10.1177/8756479308317006
17. Kingma, D.P., Ba, J.: Adam: a method for stochastic optimization (2017). arXiv:cs.LG/1412.6980
18. KPMG. Automotive Data Sharing (2020). https://assets.kpmg/content/dam/kpmg/no/pdf/2020/11/Automotive_Data_Sharing_Final%20Report_SVV_KPMG.pdf
19. McKinsey. Connected car, automotive value chain unbound. Technical Report (2014)
20. Mirkin, B.: Core Data Analysis: Summarization, Correlation, and Visualization. Springer, Cham (2019). https://doi.org/10.1007/978-3-030-00271-8
21. Obite, C., Olewuezi, N., Ugwuanyim, G., Bartholomew, D.: Multicollinearity effect in regression analysis: a feed forward artificial neural network approach. Asian J. Probabil. Stat. 22–33 (2020). https://doi.org/10.9734/ajpas/2020/v6i130151
22. Potdar, K., Pardawala, T., Pai, C.: A comparative study of categorical variable encoding techniques for neural network classifiers. Int. J. Comput. Appl. **175**, 7–9 (2017). https://doi.org/10.5120/ijca2017915495
23. Raschka, S.: Model evaluation, model selection, and algorithm selection in machine learning. CoRR abs/1811.12808 (2018). arXiv: http://arxiv.org/abs/1811.12808
24. Sharma, S., Sharma, S., Athaiya, A.: Activation functions in neural networks. Int. J. Eng. Appl. Sci. Technol. **4**(12), 310–316 (2020)
25. Snoek, J., Larochelle, H., Adams, R.P.: Practical Bayesian optimization of machine learning algorithms. In: Pereira, F., Burges, C.J.C., Bottou, L., Weinberger, K.Q. (eds.) Advances in Neural Information Processing Systems, Vol. 25. Curran Associates, Inc. (2012). https://proceedings.neurips.cc/paper/2012/file/05311655a15b75fab86956663e1819cd-Paper.pdf
26. Srivastava, N., Hinton, G., Krizhevsky, A., Sutskever, I., Salakhutdinov, R.: Dropout: a simple way to prevent neural networks from overfitting. J. Mach. Learn. Res. **15**, 1929–1958 (2014)
27. Statsmodels.org. Patsy: Contrast Coding Systems for categorical variables (2021). https://www.statsmodels.org/dev/contrasts.html#sum-deviation-coding. Accessed 25 May 2021

28. Tate, R.: Correlation between a discrete and a continuous variable point-biserial correlation. Ann. Math. Stat. **25**(3), 603–607 (1954)
29. Keras team. Keras Tuner documentation (2021). https://keras-team.github.io/keras-tuner/. Accessed 26 May 2021
30. van Dijk, M., Harnam, I., Koudijs, D., Botden, M.: Visie door Data - Moving forward in Mobility. Technical Report (2018)
31. Vermeulen, I.: Gemiddeld schadebedrag boven 1.300 euro-grens (2020). https://automotive-online.nl/management/laatste-nieuws/schade/27000-arbeidsloon-en-hogere-onderdelenkosten-zorgen-voor-stijgend-schadebedrag. Accessed 5 Mar 2021
32. Willmott, C.J., Matsuura, K.: Advantages of the mean absolute error (MAE) over the root mean square error (RMSE) in assessing average model performance. Clim. Res. **30**, 79–82 (2005). https://doi.org/10.3354/cr030079
33. Yang, Z., Zhang, A., Sudjianto, A.: Enhancing Explainability of Neural Networks through Architecture Constraints (2019). arXiv:stat.ML/1901.03838
34. Peys, R.: Noodklok over sterk gestegen kosten schadeherstel (2022). https://www.automobielmanagement.nl/autoschadeherstel/2022/09/12/noodklok-over-sterk-gestegen-kosten-schadeherstel/. Accessed 12 Jan 2024
35. Gareth Roberts. 40% rise in vehicle repair costs over past five years (2023). https://www.fleetnews.co.uk/news/fleet-industry-news/2023/03/22/40-rise-in-vehicle-repair-costs. Accessed 12 Jan 2014
36. eurostat. Glossary:Passenger car. https://ec.europa.eu/eurostat/statistics-explained/index.php?title=Glossary:Passenger_car. Accessed 16 Jan 2024

Classification of Eye Disorders Using Deep Learning and Machine Learning Models

Manal El Harti[1](✉), Saad Zaamoun[2], Said Jai Andaloussi[1], and Ouail Ouchetto[1]

[1] Department of Mathematics and Computer Science, Faculty of Science Ain Chock, Hassan II University, Casablanca, Morocco
elhartimanal94@gmail.com, {said.jaiandaloussi, ouail.ouchetto}@etu.univh2c.ma

[2] Faculty of Juridical, Economic and Social Sciences Ain-Chock, Hassan II University, Casablanca, Morocco
s.zaamoun@gmail.com

Abstract. Early diagnosis and screening of eye disorders are crucial for effective treatment. However, with the increasing prevalence of these conditions and a shortage of ophthalmic specialists, it is imperative to employ automated image evaluation methods to ensure consistent diagnoses and address this growing concern. Previous studies have focused on identifying eye conditions such as glaucoma, diabetic retinopathy, and cataracts using a single computer vision pipeline. In our research, we propose a hybrid approach that combines a classical neural network with four machine-learning models to classify these ophthalmic disorders. Our approach uses the pre-trained VGG16 model from the ImageNet dataset as a feature extractor. We then utilize the extracted features as input for the machine-learning models. To carry out this research, we harnessed a publicly available Kaggle database comprising images from various sources, including the Indian Diabetic Retinopathy Image Dataset, Oculur recognition, retinal datasets, and others. Finally, we conducted a comprehensive comparison of the results obtained with those from the top-rated deep learning models, to select the optimal model for diagnosing dry eye disease, which is our ultimate goal.

Keywords: Dry Eye Disease · Glaucoma · Cataract · Diabetic Retinopathy · Deep Learning · Machine Learning

1 Introduction

Given the growing usage of visual display terminals for long periods, an aging population, pollution, unhealthy lifestyles, and other issues, eyes become more prone to illness and could experience functional issues [1, 2]. In this paper, we selected four common ocular disorders to discuss, and they are as follows: Diabetic retinopathy (DR), Glaucoma, Cataract, and Dry eye disease (DED). DR is a worldwide chronic eye disease that is caused by long-term diabetes. It affects blood vessels in the retina and is considered a primary and increasing cause of vision loss and blindness in people with diabetes [3]. By 2040, DR will affect over 200 million people worldwide [4, 5]. Glaucoma is a

K. Daimi and A. Al Sadoon (Eds.): ACR 2024, LNNS 956, pp. 184–194, 2024.
https://doi.org/10.1007/978-3-031-56950-0_16

chronic neurodegenerative disease of the eye that leads to irreversible blindness [6]. It is asymptomatic in its early stage and eventually affects 3.54% of the population aged 40–80 years around the world. The prevalence of glaucoma is expected to reach 111.8 million in 2040 [7]. A cataract is an eye condition where the typically clear lens becomes opaque, obstructing the flow of light. It is the leading cause of treatable blindness, resulting in moderate or severe vision impairment in an estimated 52.6 million people worldwide [8]. This burden is expected to increase substantially due to rapidly aging populations. DED is a multifactorial ocular surface disorder. It is characterized by a loss of the tear film homeostasis causing blurred vision [9]. DED affects somewhere between 5% and 34% of the world's population [10] and it is most common in women and increases with age [11].

Effective care for these diseases depends on well-established screening programs for early detection and timely treatment to prevent vision loss. Automated algorithms that can assess images and provide quick referral alternatives are necessary to address the dearth of ophthalmic knowledge. Artificial intelligence (AI) has recently attracted a lot of attention for its capacity to automatically and objectively evaluate images and provide consistency in diagnosis, notably in the field of ophthalmology. Many studies have been undertaken in this field thus far using various methods and technologies, yielding promising results in identifying and treating eye conditions.

Several convolutional neural networks (CNN) based models have been used to extract the representation from retinal fundus pictures utilizing publicly available datasets for DR diagnosis purposes. Case in point: using the Kaggle dataset, multiple CNN configurations were examined in [12], with VGGNet achieving the highest experiment-level accuracy. Besides, for the sake of detecting multiple classes of DR on the Messidor-2 dataset, [13] proposed a VGGNet-based model achieving a high sensitivity of 96.8% on referable DR. Furthermore, using an Inception-based architecture, [5] was able to identify referable DR and attained a sensitivity of 96.8% and a specificity of 87.0%.

On the other hand, considerable advancements have been made in deep learning (DL) research for glaucoma, employing a variety of imaging modalities. To automatically identify glaucoma from the online retinal fundus image database for glaucoma analysis and research (ORIGA) and Singapore Chinese Eye Study (SCES) datasets, [14] have developed a CNN architecture reaching the area under the curve (AUC) values of 0.8321 and 0.887, respectively. In [15], the authors used various feature extraction techniques to identify glaucoma eye condition using deep feed-forward neural network (FNN), combined with machine learning (ML) classifiers, such as random forest (RF), gradient boosting (GB), and support vector machine (SVM). The algorithm employed achieved an AUC value of 92.5%. Therefore, new methods for screening, diagnosing, and monitoring changes may be introduced for early glaucoma detection [16–18].

To address the shortage of ophthalmologists in rural areas in China, [19] have developed a six-level method for grading cataracts based on multi-feature fusion. They extracted high-level features from ResNet18 and textural features from the gray-level co-occurrence matrix (GLCM). The proposed method's average accuracy is up to 92.66%. In addition, [20] proposed CataractNet, a revolutionary deep neural network for automatic cataract identification in fundus images. The proposed method surpassed current approaches with an average accuracy of 99.13%.

So far, several research studies have been conducted for the application of artificial intelligence in DED diagnosis, [21]. Furthermore, [22] employed the SVM model to classify dry eye types utilizing interference fringe color images of the tear film. When compared to expert ophthalmologists' diagnosis, there was a high level of inter-rater agreement (kappa coefficient = 0.820). [23] compared the efficacy of VGG19 in DED diagnosis to that of other diagnostic approaches. The autonomous model was substantially more accurate than other techniques in classifying anterior segment optical coherence tomography (AS-OCT) images, with an accuracy of 84.62%.

In this paper, we introduce a hybrid approach that combines a classical neural network with well-established machine-learning models to classify three ophthalmic disorders: diabetic retinopathy, glaucoma, and cataracts. To conduct this research, we utilized a publicly available Kaggle database with four classes, each comprising approximately 1,000 images. We employed the ImageNet pre-trained weights in conjunction with the VGG16 model for classification, utilizing transfer learning to extract features. These extracted features serve as input for the machine learning classifiers, which are trained to achieve the desired performance. Subsequently, a comprehensive comparison is conducted, assessing the results against those from top-rated deep learning models by calculating various evaluation metrics. Our main objective is to identify the optimal model for diagnosing dry eye disease in the future.

The rest of this paper is structured as follows: Part two provides an overview of DED, its types, and the diagnostic processes. Part three presents related works, part four explains our methodology and the experiments performed, part five discusses our findings, and finally, we conclude.

2 Dry Eye Disease Overview

2.1 Cause, Risk Factors, and Symptoms

Dry Eye Disease is an ophthalmological condition characterized by the loss of tear film homeostasis, which keeps the eye moist, smooth, and clear. The tear film comprises three layers: the lipid (oily) layer, the aqueous (watery) layer, and the mucus layer. Various factors can disrupt the tear film, leading to DED. These factors include medical conditions (e.g., Sjogren's syndrome), medications, and issues like corneal nerve sensitivity. Clogged meibomian glands can also contribute to DED by increasing tear evaporation [24]. Factors that lead to increased tear evaporation include meibomian gland dysfunction, eyelid problems, environmental conditions, and vitamin A deficiency. Certain demographics, such as age over 50, women undergoing hormonal changes, a diet lacking in omega-3 fatty acids, and a history of wearing contact lenses, are more likely to experience DED. DED can manifest through symptoms that impact health-related quality of life [21], like a scratchy sensation in the eyes, stringy mucus, light sensitivity, eye redness, contact lens discomfort, blurred vision, and watery eyes due to compensatory lacrimal gland response.

2.2 Dry Eye Disease Subtypes

The most common DED types are:

- Aqueous deficient dry eye (ADDE): which is characterized by aqueous tear deficiency. It occurs when the lacrimal glands don't produce enough watery components of the tear film.
- Evaporative dry eye (EDE): which is characterized by a deficiency in the oil layer of the tear film. EDE affects approximately 65% of dry eye patients. It is caused by Meibomian gland dysfunction (MGD) [25], which creates the glands responsible for producing the lipid component of tears, slowing the process of evaporation and keeping the tears stable. MGD is known as the most prevalent cause of hyperevaporative dry eyes [26].

Although dry eyes are mainly classified into these two categories, they are not mutually exclusive and can coexist. This is known as mixed dry rye (MDE).

2.3 Methods Used for DED Diagnosis

To accurately diagnose DED and determine its severity, the patient is submitted to a variety of examinations:

- Questionnaires: the subjects are asked to fill out a questionnaire so that the ophthalmologist can learn about their symptoms as well as their medical history [27].
- Eye exam: the ophthalmologist performs an eye exam to assess the health of both eyes and determine the source of symptoms.
- Clinical tests: many tests can be used to diagnose DED including a Slit lamp exam that analyzes the stability of the tear film and determines the number of tears produced by both eyes using a slit lamp microscope [28]. Schirmer's test is responsible for measuring tear production through a tiny piece of paper that is placed along the edge of the eyelid [23]. Tear breakup time (TBUT) checks how quickly the tears evaporate [29]. It measures the amount of time between the last blink and when the first dry area shows up on the cornea.

3 Related Work

Numerous studies have investigated the recognition of multiple eye diseases using artificial intelligence (AI). For instance, in reference [30], the focus was on identifying age-related eye disorders by analyzing retinal fundus images from an online dataset. They proposed a CNN-based multiple disease detection (CNN-MDD) model, achieving an impressive accuracy of 95.27%. Similarly, [31] introduced a deep learning-based classification method for four types of digital retinal images (DRI) using the Inception v4 model, which yielded a high accuracy rate of 96%. In another study, as cited in [32], the integrated detection of cataracts, diabetic retinopathy, and glaucoma was conducted via a single computer vision pipeline. This research employed eight SVM classifiers and twelve deep-learning models across three different pipelines. The Inception V3 normal model outperformed others, achieving an F1-Score of 99.39%. In [33], five diverse

Convolutional Neural Network architectures, including DenseNet, EfficientNet, Xception, VGG, and ResNet, were utilized to detect eye diseases. The dataset included 2,748 retinal fundus images from various disease groups, with the EfficientNet architecture demonstrating the highest classification performance at an accuracy rate of 94.88%. In addition, [34] presents an innovative multi-label classification system for the early detection of multiple retinal diseases using fundus images sourced from various platforms. The dataset is meticulously constructed and post-processed to ensure quality. A transformer-based model is employed for image analysis and decision-making. The system surpasses state-of-the-art methods, achieving a remarkable improvement of 7.9% and 8.1% in AUC scores for disease detection and classification, respectively.

4 Our Work

4.1 Data Source and Preprocessing

Eye disease retinal images is a publicly available dataset from Kaggle that includes retinal images of four different conditions: normal, diabetic retinopathy, cataract, and glaucoma, with roughly 1000 photos in each class. The dataset utilized consists of the resized Red Green Blue (RGB) color images with a resolution of 256×256 gathered from sources such as IDRiD, Oculur recognition, retinal dataset, and others. The data was loaded from a local directory, and the images underwent image preprocessing, where each image was resized to a uniform dimension of 224×224 pixels with RGB color channels, followed by the flattening process. Notably, no data augmentation or extensive preprocessing techniques were employed, as the aim was to directly assess the performance of the top-rated deep learning models and compare them with the hybrid method.

4.2 Experimentation

We conducted a simple test of the top-rated machine learning and deep learning models using the eye disease retinal images dataset. The objective was to assess these models' performance before deciding which one would be best to use for the diagnosis of dry eye disease. The experimentation proceeded as follows:

The first part involved the application of deep learning models. In this section, we begin by randomly partitioning the dataset into three parts: training (60%), validation (20%), and test set (20%). The training set is used to train the model, the validation set is used to tweak the model and limit the risk of overfitting and finally, the test set is used to report the success of the trained model. Besides, we utilized the transfer learning strategy, in which all models tested were initially trained on the ImageNet dataset. The experimented architectures were as follows: DenseNet169, InceptionV3, and VGG16.

The models are initialized with weights from the 'ImageNet' dataset and enhanced with feature adaptation layers, including global average pooling, a dense layer for feature learning, and dropout to mitigate overfitting. The final output layer consists of four neurons employing a SoftMax activation function for multi-class classification. Subsequently, the models are compiled using the Adam optimizer, categorical cross-entropy loss, and accuracy as the evaluation metric. These models undergo 30 epochs of training, with an early stopping mechanism in place to halt training if no improvement is observed over five consecutive epochs. This early stopping ensures that the model ceases training when its performance on the validation set no longer improves, guarding against overfitting.

In the second part, we proposed a hybrid classification technique that combines VGG16 with the following machine learning models: SVM, RF, K-Nearest Neighbor (KNN), and Decision Trees (DT). In addition, two ensemble learning algorithms: AdaBoost and XGBoost were used to combine the output of DT classifiers into a powerful classifier.

Feature extraction involves applying the VGG16 model to the training data, which results in the transformation of images into a feature vector. These extracted features are subsequently reshaped into the required format and employed for training the machine learning classifiers. In the case of SVM, a 10-degree polynomial kernel is utilized, along with a regularization parameter set to 10. Additionally, a specific independent term (coef0 = 2) is meticulously configured to fine-tune the model. Besides, the KNN classifier considers the 20 nearest neighbors to a data point when determining its class label. Furthermore, the Random Forest classifier is thoughtfully created with a specified random seed value (42) to ensure reproducibility in the results. For the Decision Tree classifier, a maximum depth of 100 levels is imposed, with a requirement of at least 10 samples in the leaf node. It's important to highlight that the ensemble learning process utilizes 100 Decision Trees, all configured in the same way. Combining VGG16 with traditional machine learning models provides several advantages. VGG16 is proficient at extracting meaningful image features and capturing complex hierarchical attributes. Through transfer learning, its pre-trained knowledge from ImageNet enhances traditional models, especially when working with limited data. These extracted features reduce data dimensionality, leading to improved efficiency and facilitating better generalization to new data. Finally, a comparison of the methods used was performed to select the best classifier for our future work.

4.3 Evaluation Metrics

To assess the performance of each machine learning model, we opt for the 10-fold cross-validation method due to our relatively small dataset. This choice aims to yield a more robust estimate of our model's performance by dividing the data into a greater number of subsets. The objective is to maximize the utilization of the available samples for both training and testing. Then, we use the confusion matrix, to calculate the following metrics for all the models used:

- Accuracy: the percentage ratio between the number of correct predictions and the total number of predictions. The accuracy is calculated using (1)

$$\text{Accuracy} = \text{TP} + \text{TN}/\text{TP} + \text{FP} + \text{TN} + \text{FN} \tag{1}$$

- Precision: the percentage ratio between the number of correct predictions and the total number of positive predictions. The precision is calculated using (2)

$$\text{Precision} = \text{TP}/\text{TP} + \text{FP} \tag{2}$$

- Recall: the percentage ratio between the number of correct predictions and the total number of positive samples. The recall is calculated using (3)

$$\text{Recall} = \text{TP}/\text{TP} + \text{FN} \quad (3)$$

- F1-score: This is the harmonic mean of precision and recall. F1-score is calculated using (4)

$$\text{F1} - \text{score} = 2 * (\text{Precision} * \text{Recall})/\text{Precision} + \text{Recall} \quad (4)$$

4.4 Results

This section presents the results of the tested algorithms. For each model, we calculated the evaluation metrics mentioned before, using the predictions of the test set to assess the performance.

Tables 1 and 2 show the obtained results using deep learning and machine learning models respectively, while Figs. 1 and 2 show a comparison of the tested DL and ML algorithms respectively:

Table 1. Results of the DL models experimentation

DL Models	Evaluation metrics			
	Accuracy	Precision	Recall	F1-score
DensNet169	90.28%	90.97%	89.34%	89.91%
InceptionV3	82.11%	83.70%	79.62%	81.53%
VGG16	85.43%	87.11%	84.12%	85.46%

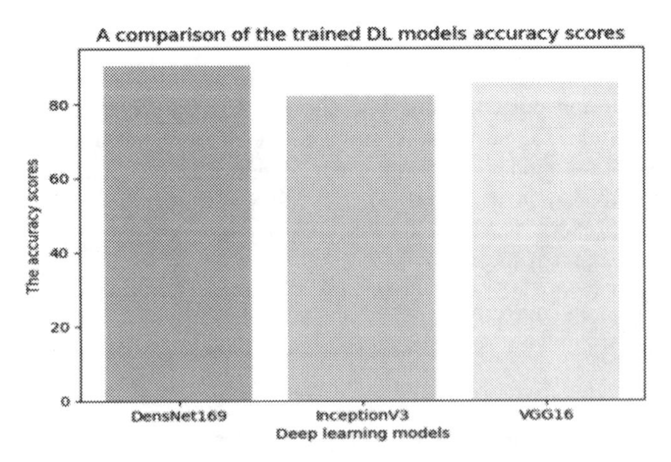

Fig. 1. A comparison of the trained DL models' accuracy scores

Table 2. Results of ML models experimentation

ML Models	Evaluation metrics				
	10-fold CV	Accuracy	Precision	Recall	F1-score
SVM	88.20%	88.74%	88.77%	88.74%	88.76%
RF	86.75%	87.09%	87.11%	87.09%	87%
DT	77.08%	78.55%	78.64%	78.20%	78.29%
KNN	77.59%	79.50%	81.17%	79.50%	77.95%
AdaBoost	87.37%	88.03%	88.06%	88.03%	87.98%
XGBoost	88.14%	88.63%	88.59%	88.62%	88.60%

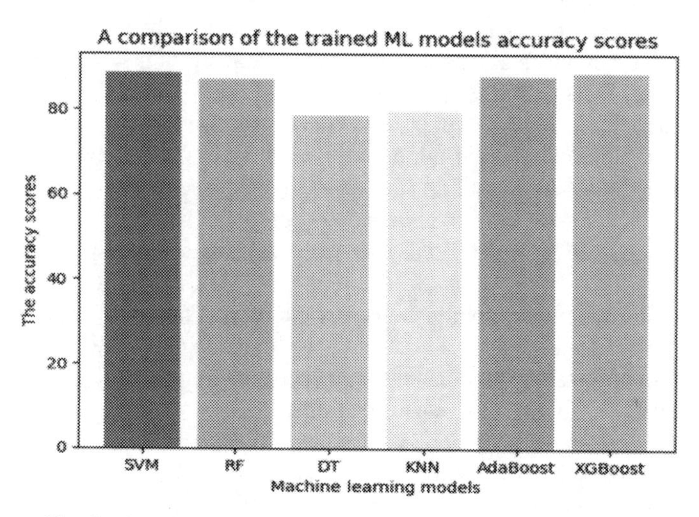

Fig. 2. A comparison of the trained ML models' accuracy scores

These results demonstrate that the VGG16 combined with the SVM model had the greater accuracy score for the machine learning methods, whereas the DT model had the lowest accuracy. Besides, when employing the two ensemble learning strategies, the accuracy of the DT model considered as a weak learner in our study is increased from 78.55% to 88.03% and 88.63% using AdaBoost and XGBoost respectively. Additionally, the use of the RF model produces positive outcomes with an accuracy of 87.09%.

Among the studied deep learning architectures, DenseNet169 has the greatest accuracy score of 90.28%, followed by 85.43% obtained by VGG16. The lowest accuracy score was obtained by InceptionV3.

The experimentation revealed that the effectiveness of hybrid and ensemble learning approaches for classification is on par with that of the top-rated deep learning techniques.

5 Discussion

Despite the disparity in the results obtained in our study compared to those in other works, it is plausible to assert that our findings are on par with state-of-the-art performance. This assertion is grounded in the fact that we exclusively employed the VGG16 model for feature extraction, in contrast to [32], which explored diverse approaches involving traditional computer vision techniques such as Histogram of Oriented Gradients (HOG) and Grey-Level Co-occurrence Matrix (GLCM). Additionally, our study placed less emphasis on the preprocessing stage and data augmentation (DA).

DA is regarded as a form of regularization approach to reduce the generalization error of the model and has grown in popularity as a way to expand the amount and variety of the training dataset. It is essential in industries where big datasets aren't frequently accessible and getting new pictures is costly and time-consuming, which is the case when working with medical imaging. This strategy has been applied by numerous researchers to increase the size of the data sample and to cut down on the number of useless features, and so far, the results are promising.

The researchers in [35, 36] demonstrated the efficacy of DA techniques. In the first paper, elastic transformation and perturbation have been used as two stages of data augmentation to triple the training data set and improve the model's accuracy. Elastic transformation generates a deformed version of an image while retaining its essential characteristics. In medical imaging, it is used to align and compare pictures from various patients.

Perturbation adds minor modifications to the training data to increase the diversity of examples and improve the robustness and generalization capabilities of models. The common perturbation techniques include geometric transformations, deformation, noise injection, and color and intensity transformations.

In the second paper, the dataset was expanded using the rotation and flip techniques, which increased the accuracy rate to 97%.

Rotation improves the variety of object orientations, strengthening models and enabling them to handle objects at various angles.

Flipping creates additional training examples with different perspectives by flipping the original images horizontally or vertically.

In addition to the DA approach and network configuration, numerous researches have demonstrated that non-architectural elements such as preprocessing, also have a significant effect on the model's performance enhancement. [37] evaluates how preprocessing methods affect the model's performance for different types of clinical applications.

In our future research, we should investigate the effects of preprocessing techniques as well as the data augmentation approach for early DED detection. Furthermore, we will apply the previously tested and chosen models in various configurations.

6 Conclusion

In this paper, we investigate a hybrid approach and compare it with various deep-learning techniques for classifying retinal images into four distinct groups. After a thorough evaluation of the top-performing methods, we identified the most suitable architecture for model training. The results of our experiments demonstrate that combining VGG16 and SVM as a machine learning model delivers results on par with the top-rated deep learning models. Notably, DensNet169 stood out as the most effective deep-learning model in our study. In future studies, we anticipate enhancing the accuracy of the top-performing algorithms evaluated for dry eye disease diagnosis.

References

1. Mandell, J.T., Idarraga, M., Kumar, N., Galor, A.: Impact of air pollution and weather on dry eye. J. Intern. Med. **9**(11), 3740 (2020)
2. Nichols, J.J., Ziegler, C., Mitchell, G.L., Nichols, K.K.: Self-reported dry eye disease across refractive modalities. Invest. Ophthalmol. Vis. Sci. **46**(6), 1911–1914 (2005)
3. Lee, R., Wong, T.Y., Sabanayagam, C.: Epidemiology of diabetic retinopathy, diabetic macular edema and related vision loss. Eye Vision **2**(1), 1–25 (2015)
4. Cheung, N., Mitchell, P., Yin Wong, T.: Diabetic retinopathy. Lancet **376**, 124–136 (2010)
5. Gulshan, V., et al.: Development and validation of a deep learning algorithm for detection of diabetic retinopathy in retinal fundus photographs. JAMA **316**(22), 2402–2410 (2016)
6. Hood, D.C., Raza, A.S., de Moraes, C.G.V., Liebmann, J.M., Ritch, R.: Glaucomatous damage of the macula. Prog. Retin. Eye Res. **32**, 1–21 (2013)
7. Tham, Y.C., Li, X., Wong, T.Y., Quigley, H.A., Aung, T., Cheng, C.Y.: Global prevalence of glaucoma and projections of glaucoma burden through 2040: a systematic review and meta-analysis. Ophthalmology **121**(11), 2081–2090 (2014)
8. Flaxman, S.R., et al.: Global causes of blindness and distance vision impairment 1990–2020: a systematic review and meta-analysis. Lancet Glob. Health **5**(12), 1221–1234 (2017)
9. Zeev, M.S.B., Miller, D.D., Latkany, R.: Diagnosis of dry eye disease and emerging technologies. Clin. Ophthalmol. **8**, 581–590 (2014)
10. Vicnesh, J., et al.: Thoughts concerning the application of thermogram images for automated diagnosis of dry eye–a review. Infrared Phys. Technol. **106**, 103271 (2020)
11. Matossian, C., McDonald, M., Donaldson, K.E., Nichols, K.K., MacIver, S., Gupta, P.K.: Dry eye disease: consideration for women's health. J. Women's Health **28**(4), 502–514 (2019)
12. Wan, S., Liang, Y., Zhang, Y.: Deep convolutional neural networks for diabetic retinopathy detection by image classification. Comput. Electr. Eng. **72**, 274–282 (2018)
13. Abràmoff, M.D., et al.: Improved automated detection of diabetic retinopathy on a publicly available dataset through integration of deep learning. Invest. Ophthalmol. Vis. Sci. **57**(13), 5200–5206 (2016)
14. Chen, X., Xu, Y., Wong, D.W.K., Wong, T.Y., Liu, J.: Glaucoma detection based on deep convolutional neural network. In: 2015 37th Annual International Conference of the IEEE Engineering in Medicine and Biology Society (EMBC), pp. 715–718. IEEE (2015)
15. Asaoka, R., Murata, H., Iwase, A., Araie, M.: Detecting preperimetric glaucoma with standard automated perimetry using a deep learning classifier. Ophthalmology **123**(9), 1974–1980 (2016)
16. Weinreb, R.N., Aung, T., Medeiros, F.A.: The pathophysiology and treatment of glaucoma: a review. JAMA **311**(18), 1901–1911 (2014)
17. Harwerth, R.S., Carter-Dawson, L., Smith, E.L., Barnes, G., Holt, W.F., Crawford, M.L.: Neural losses correlated with visual losses in clinical perimetry. Invest. Ophthalmol. Vis. Sci. **45**(9), 3152–3160 (2004)
18. Harwerth, R.S., Carter-Dawson, L., Shen, F., Smith, E.L., Crawford, M.L.J.: Ganglion cell losses underlying visual field defects from experimental glaucoma. Invest. Ophthalmol. Vis. Sci. **40**(10), 2242–2250 (1999)

19. Zhang, H., Niu, K., Xiong, Y., Yang, W., He, Z., Song, H.: Automatic cataract grading methods based on deep learning. Comput. Methods Programs Biomed. **182**, 104978 (2019)
20. Junayed, M.S., Islam, M.B., Sadeghzadeh, A., Rahman, S.: CataractNet: an automated cataract detection system using deep learning for fundus images. IEEE Access **9**, 128799–128808 (2021)
21. Storås, A.M., et al.: Artificial intelligence in dry eye disease. Ocul. Surf. **23**, 74–86 (2022)
22. Yabusaki, K., Arita, R., Yamauchi, T.: Automated classification of dry eye type analyzing interference fringe color images of tear film using machine learning techniques. Model. Artif. Intell. Ophthalmol. **2**(3), 28–35 (2019)
23. Chase, C., Elsawy, A., Eleiwa, T., Ozcan, E., Tolba, M., Abou Shousha, M.: Comparison of autonomous AS-OCT deep learning algorithm and clinical dry eye tests in diagnosis of dry eye disease. Clin. Ophthalmol. **15**, 4281–4289 (2021)
24. Phadatare, S.P., Momin, M., Nighojkar, P., Askarkar, S., Singh, K.K.: A comprehensive review on dry eye disease: diagnosis, medical management, recent developments, and future challenges. Adv. Pharm. **2015**, 1–12 (2015)
25. Shao, Y., et al.: Detection of meibomian gland dysfunction by in vivo confocal microscopy based on the deep convolutional neural network. Res. Square 1 (2021)
26. Nichols, K.K., et al.: The international workshop on meibomian gland dysfunction: executive summary. Invest. Ophthalmol. Vis. Sci. **52**(4), 1922–1929 (2011)
27. Okumura, Y., et al.: A review of dry eye questionnaires: measuring patient-reported outcomes and health-related quality of life. Diagnostics **10**(8), 559–567 (2020)
28. Hung, N., et al.: Using slit-lamp images for deep learning-based identification of bacterial and fungal keratitis: model development and validation with different convolutional neural networks. Diagnostics **11**(7), 1246–1251 (2021)
29. Su, T.Y., Liu, Z.Y., Chen, D.Y.: Tear film break-up time measurement using deep convolutional neural networks for screening dry eye disease. IEEE Sens. J. **18**(16), 6857–6862 (2018)
30. Glaretsubin, P., Muthukannan, P.: Optimized convolution neural network based multiple eye disease detection. Comput. Biol. Med. **146** (2022)
31. Raza, A., Khan, M.U., Saeed, Z., Samer, S., Mobeen, A., Samer, A.: Classification of eye diseases and detection of cataract using digital fundus imaging (DFI) and inception-V4 deep learning model. In: 2021 International Conference on Frontiers of Information Technology (FIT), pp. 137–142. IEEE (2021)
32. Orfao, J., van der Haar, D.: A comparison of computer vision methods for the combined detection of glaucoma, diabetic retinopathy and cataracts. In: Papież, B.W., Yaqub, M., Jiao, J., Namburete, A.I.L., Noble, J.A. (eds.) Medical Image Understanding and Analysis (MIUA 2021). LNCS, vol. 12722, pp. 30–42. Springer, Cham (2021). https://doi.org/10.1007/978-3-030-80432-9_3
33. Arslan, G., Erdaş, Ç.B.: Detection of cataract, diabetic retinopathy and glaucoma eye diseases with deep learning approach. Intell. Methods Eng. Sci. **2**(2), 42–47 (2023)
34. Rodríguez, M.A., AlMarzouqi, H., Liatsis, P.: Multi-label retinal disease classification using transformers. IEEE J. Biomed. Health Inform. **27**(6), 2739–2750 (2023)
35. de Raad, K.B., et al.: The effect of preprocessing on convolutional neural networks for medical image segmentation. In: 2021 IEEE 18th International Symposium on Biomedical Imaging (ISBI), pp. 655–658 (2021)
36. Prabhu, S.M., Chakiat, A., Shashank, S., Vunnava, K.P., Shetty, R.: Deep learning segmentation and quantification of Meibomian glands. Biomed. Signal Process. Control **57**, 101776 (2020)
37. Su, T.Y., Ting, P.J., Chang, S.W., Chen, D.Y.: Superficial punctate keratitis grading for dry eye screening using deep convolutional neural networks. IEEE Sens. J. **20**(3), 1672–1678 (2019)

Effects of Parallel and Distributed Learning on CNN Performance for Lung Disease Classification

Lara Visuña(✉), Javier Garcia-Blas, and Jesus Carretero

Computer Science and Engineering Department, University Carlos III of Madrid, Leganes, Spain
lvisuna@pa.uc3m.es, {fjblas,jcarrete}@inf.uc3m.es

Abstract. The development of Deep Learning applications has sped up by using Graphical Parallel Units (GPUs), but even the finite capacity of a single GPU could be a limitation for the Deep Learning progress. To cope with this problem, it is possible to develop parallel training phases by distributing the workload between several GPUs in single and multiple compute nodes. Thus, distributed learning implies not only a reduction of the time requirements but also, slight accuracy variations that could have huge implications in high-precision areas like medicine. This paper analyzed the performance and accuracy effects of distributed and parallel learning of a Convolutional Neural Network (CNN) developed for X-ray disease classification. For this aim, the paper presents a complete framework for X-ray diagnosis. Furthermore, a new database was built from several public datasets. This database includes chest X-rays split into 5 classes (COVID-19, viral pneumonia, bacterial pneumonia, tuberculosis, and healthy). The experiments show a speed-up of the training phase of 1.7 using two GPUs, reaching a speed-up upper to 2 using three GPUs. The results prove that parallel training does not imply a negative effect on the accuracy results, showing even an increase in the final accuracy for the models trained with two or more GPUs, these results contribute to the feasibility of the use of distributed learning.

Keywords: CNN · Deep Learning · Distributed Learning · X-Ray · Horovod

1 Introduction

In recent years, the use of Deep Learning has spread to very diverse areas, providing innovative solutions in multiple areas of expertise such as automotive, economics, and health. Despite its high potential, one of their major limitations is related to the time required for the training of the large number of parameters inherent to the neural networks, as well as the time needed for the analysis of the large databases managed.

The development of the Graphical Parallel Units (GPUs) promoted to manage and speed up the Deep Learning processes, like backpropagation operations. Therefore, GPU's capacity for massively parallel execution has outbreaks the use

K. Daimi and A. Al Sadoon (Eds.): ACR 2024, LNNS 956, pp. 195–205, 2024.
https://doi.org/10.1007/978-3-031-56950-0_17

and evolution of deep neural networks. But even the finite capacity of a single GPU could be a limitation for the development, and the time requirement of many projects [1].

To address this problem, it is possible to design parallel training for the distribution of the workload between different compute nodes. This training technique enables the simultaneous use of several GPUs or central processing units (CPUs) [2,3]. This is translated into speeding up the training and testing of neural networks thanks to distributed learning and inference.

The main challenge to face in distributed learning is the correct code modification that allows the proper training and node communication [2]. One of the well-known technologies for distributed learning is Horovod [4]. Horovod is an open-source framework, developed by the Uber team, it is available for algorithms developed in TensorFlow, Keras, and Pythorch. It uses the Message Passing Interface (MPI) model and the *ring-allreduce* algorithm for node communication, where every node communicates with two of its peers. One of the main advantages is their simple use at the user level, with a little code modification is possible to extend the training to one to multiple nodes. Some previous work has already stated the advantages of the speed-up for CNN training with Horovod [5].

Distributed learning has proven to be highly beneficial in the fields of healthcare and medicine. By speeding up the training process, Deep Learning models can be quickly adapted to new diseases and medical events, while facilitating research into new network configurations. The medical domain involves a vast and diverse range of data, including patient information, hospital records, and technological variables. Various studies have explored distributed learning solutions in the medical field. For instance, Chang et al. [6] proposed distributing non-parallel learning to prevent data sharing between institutions. However, this approach is less efficient than parallel learning.

Despite the advantages of parallel learning regarding time, it is also necessary to study other performance implications. The use of parallel GPUs can produce inconsistent accuracy results between runs [7]. Even the same Deep Learning model with the same hyperparameters might differ in terms of performance due to different training frameworks or hardware [8]. Mercy et al. [9] state the impact on the performance in image segmentation task for single vs multiple nodes. This slight performance difference has an important implication in the medical domain. The medical Deep Learning solutions look for the most accurate response due to the multiple implications of the errors, errors could imply the not treatment of a patient, their earlier medical discharge, or unnecessary surgery.

A previous work [7] has already established the impact of the use of different hardware types in deep neural network training but in a non-distributed setting The authors of this work state the importance of the analysis of distributed training stability.

Given this context, we propose analyzing the effects of the different hardware and its parallelization on the time and classification performance of pulmonary diseases. Previous works have already presented the capacity of CNN for lung diagnosis with X-ray [10,11]. In this novel work, we want to speed up the training phase of a well-known Deep Learning architecture VGG19 [12] with a Horovod framework in a heterogeneous GPU Cluster without accuracy loss. The main contribution of the paper are as follows:

- We present a complete framework for X-ray lung classification with the well-known VGG19. We establish a benchmark for time and accuracy for the classification of X-rays in a heterogeneous and imbalanced database.
- Creating and cleaning a large X-ray database of pulmonary diseases including COVID-19, tuberculosis, viral pneumonia, bacterial pneumonia, and healthy subjects. This Database can contribute to developing or validating new tools for lung diagnosis.
- We analyze the implications of the use of different GPU accelerators for training the CNN model in several metrics of time and performance. Also, we evaluated the implication of the distribution and paralleling of the training phase with Horovod.

The paper is organized as follows, Sect. 2 includes the material and methods implemented during the experimental tests. Section 3 presents the results and a discussion about them. Finally, the conclusion is introduced in Sect. 4.

2 Material and Methods

During this Section, we present the material and methods used to analyze the influence of parallel and distributed learning in a Deep Learning X-ray image classification tool performance. The experiments pipeline is shown in Fig. 1. First, we select a specific hardware to train the CNN model. The Deep Learning classificator is designed following the implementation details presented in Sect. 2.1. Then, the training data is loaded and preprocessed, in Sect. 2.2, are introduced all the details of the database used for the design and evaluation carried out during the paper. The third step includes all the training processes needed for the CNN architecture. Finally, the results and models are saved for post-evaluation. The same configuration and databases are used throughout all the experiments to ensure the results conscience.

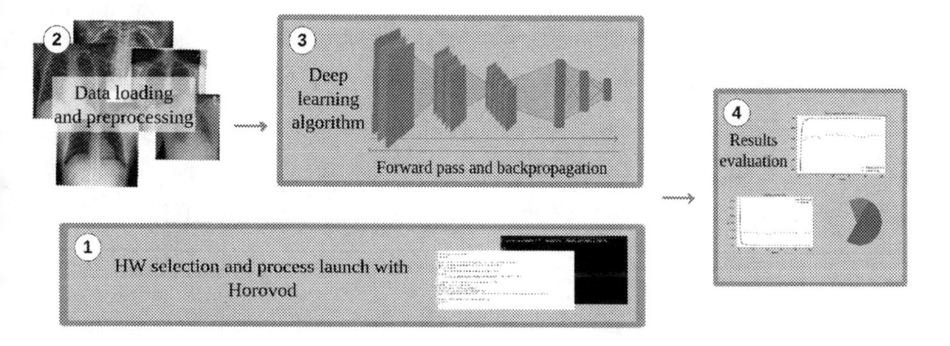

Fig. 1. Framework for parallel and distributed learning of a CNN diagnosis tool.

2.1 Convectional Neural Network

The Deep Learning classificator is designed with a Convolutional Neural Network and a dense neural network. As Convolutional Neural Network was selected the well-known VGG19, which we have already proved its efficiency in X-Ray classification tasks [13]. VGG19 is composed by 19 layers, 16 of them convolutional layers, it belongs to the very deep convolutional networks family. Following the CNN we add a dense network described in Table 1 (Left).

Table 1. Dense neural network configuration (left) and hyperparameter configuration (right).

Layer (type)	Rate	Units	Activation
GlobalAveragePooling2D	-	-	-
Flatten	-	-	-
Dense	-	128	Relu
Dropout	0.2	-	-
Dense	-	32	Relu
Dropout	0.2	-	-
Dense	-	5	Softmax

Hyperparameters set	
Learning rate	0.0001
Optimazer	Adam
Epochs	100
Batch size	32

The VGG19 is used with the weights of the previous training in the Imagenet dataset [14]. In order to fine tuning the network all the layers are frozen their training with the exception of the two last convolutional layers and the dense network. Table 1 (Right) presents all the hyperparameters for the network training. The hyperparameters were selected after carrying out several test runs with different configurations. The selected hyperparameters reported the maximum validation accuracy.

In order to improve the replicability and conscience in the several experiments, we force the determinism of the system to avoid the random initializations inherent to the training process of a CNN. Listing 1.1 shows the code employed for this task. This code allows major stability of the training framework, with the hardware of the only variance source utilized for the training phase.

```
1 import tensorflow as tf
2
3 tf.keras.utils.set_random_seed(123)
4 tf.config.experimental.enable_op_determinism()
```

Listing 1.1. Python code to allow determinism for the random processes.

2.2 Data Acquisition and Preprocesssing

For this experiment, a database composed of chest X-rays was built, 14,167 images were collected from public datasets. The database includes 3,615 images diagnosed with COVID-19 collected from [15]. Also, we include 1,493 X-rays diagnosed with viral pneumonia and 2,780 labeled as bacterial pneumonia, these images were collected also from a Kaggle dataset [16]. As another bacterial disease, there were included 2,780 images diagnosed with tuberculosis, these images are accessible at [17]. As the last category, we include 4,000 images without pathology to use this category as a control. We compose this category with 3,500 images from [15] and also 500 from [16] to avoid bias. The database was divided into 3 sets (train, validation, and test) with a hold-out cross-validation scheme. The division is shown in Table 2.

Table 2. Thoracic X-ray dataset breakdown, split into train, validation, and test.

	Train	Validation	Test	Total
COVID-19	2,169	542	904	3,615
Healthy	2,400	600	1,000	4,000
Viral Pneumonia	896	224	373	1,493
Tuberculosis	1,368	342	569	2,279
Bactarial Pnemonia	1,668	417	695	2,780
Total	**8,501**(60%)	**2,125**(15%)	**3,541**(25%)	**14,167**(100%)

The clean and assembled version of the dataset is provided at [18]. It is important to highlight that the dataset is not well-balanced, having fewer images of viral pneumonia and more labeled as healthy. The loss function (Categorical cross-entropy) is weighted regarding the dataset class distribution. The images are very heterogeneous, coming from different sources. During the database creation, the images with revealing watermarks, blurred or mistaken were deleted to avoid incorrect learning. All the images are in black and white, composed in a fake RGB (3-channel images) with the same information in every channel. For the training, all the images are reshaped into 256×256 to homogenize the input for the CNN. Also, all the X-ray images were normalized into 0–1 values.

3 Results and Discussion

In this section, we discuss the experimental results of the multi-GPU Deep Learning classificator. The hardware used to carry out the experiments consists of a 4-nodes cluster running Ubuntu 22.04. Each node is equipped with one Intel(R) Xeon(R) Gold 6212U CPU 24-Core processor and a clock speed per core of 2.4 GHz. Network topology is created with a fat-tree network at 10 Gbps. The experiments were conducted on compute nodes with the following software setup: Python 3.9.7, Tensorflow 2.14.0, and Keras 2.14.0. To test the framework with different hardware was carried out the experiments in compute nodes with different NVIDIA GPUs, including NVIDIA GTX 3070, GTX 3080 Ti, and GTX 3090. The CUDA version installed was 11.8 for all the compute nodes and, for the learning distribution, Horovod 0.28.1 was applied.

Table 3. Performance of the CNN model on single node and GPU training.

GPU	Time (hours)		Accuracy		
	Mean	σ	Train	Validation	Test
RTX 3070	3.24	0.0113	0.99	0.90	0.88
RTX 3080 Ti	2.87	0.0074	1.00	0.90	0.88
RTX 3090	2.81	0.0123	1.00	0.90	0.88

Table 4. Performance of the CNN model on multiple nodes and GPUs training.

# of GPU	Time (hours)		Accuracy		
	Mean	σ	Train	Validation	Test
2 (RTX 3070)	1.88	0.0045	1.00	0.89	0.89
2 (RTX 3090)	1.60	0.0047	1.00	0.91	0.88
3 (RTX 3070+3080Ti+3090)	1.40	0.0066	0.99	0.9	0.88

Table 3 shows the results for the traditional training of the neural network in a single GPU/node. The results show the highest speed of the RTX 3090, very near to the RTX 3080Ti performance. The accuracy results are equal for these two GPUs and have a slight decay for the RTX 3070, which also has a lower time performance.

During multiple runs the accuracy remain invariant, thanks to enable the training determinism, which allows the repeatability of the experiments. In terms of execution time, there is a slight variation, stated by the standard deviation of the sample (σ).

Table 4 presents the results with multiple GPUs, which implies a time reduction. The simultaneous use of two GPUs means a speed-up of 1.7 over a single GPU of the same kind. The experiments reach a speed-up upper to 2 with the use of 3 nodes. Figure 2 shows the different speed-up over the execution time in a single RTX 3070 (blue line) and a single RTX 3090 (orange line). The number of images analyzed per second by the framework is shown in Fig. 3, showing a peak of 168 images/sec.

The accuracy performance of distributed training differs slightly from traditional training results (single GPU). Figure 4 depicts the number of X-ray images of the test set correctly classified by the CNN. We demonstrate that the parallel training does not imply a negative effect on the accuracy results. The results show even an increase in the final accuracy for the models trained with two or more GPUs.

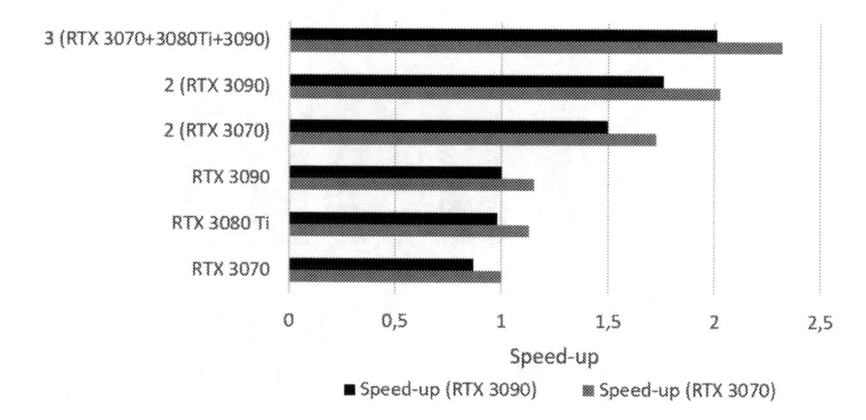

Fig. 2. Comparative analysis of speed-up over the different hardware configurations of the CNN training.

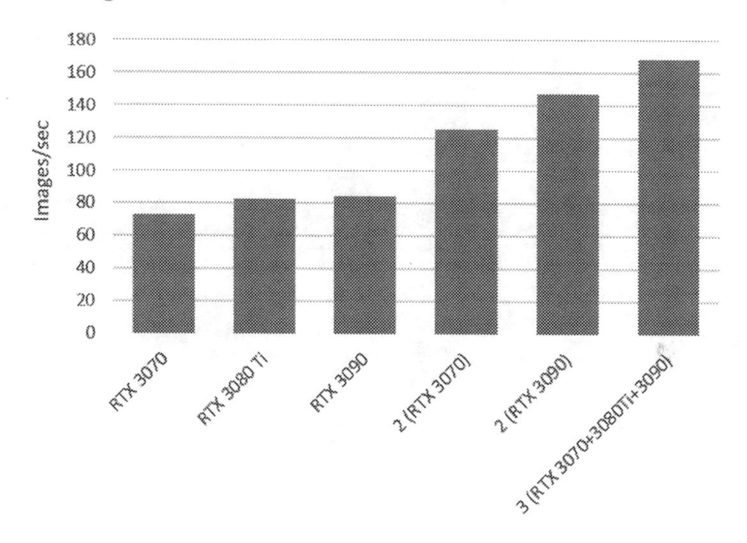

Fig. 3. Images analyzed per second over different hardware configurations of the CNN training.

As we are working on a multiclass environment, Table 5 provides the test confusion matrix for every trained model. The classes underrepresented are the more misclassified by all the systems. The models trained with a single GPU have a close behavior, with slight classification differences. Nevertheless, increasing the number of GPUs the behavior diverges. This picture the strong influence of the training hardware on the response of a deep-learning model.

Figure 6 contrasts the ROC and PR curves (micro-averaging) for the models trained on different hardware. The curves report close results on all hardware configurations. Nevertheless, the training using several GPUs manifests an

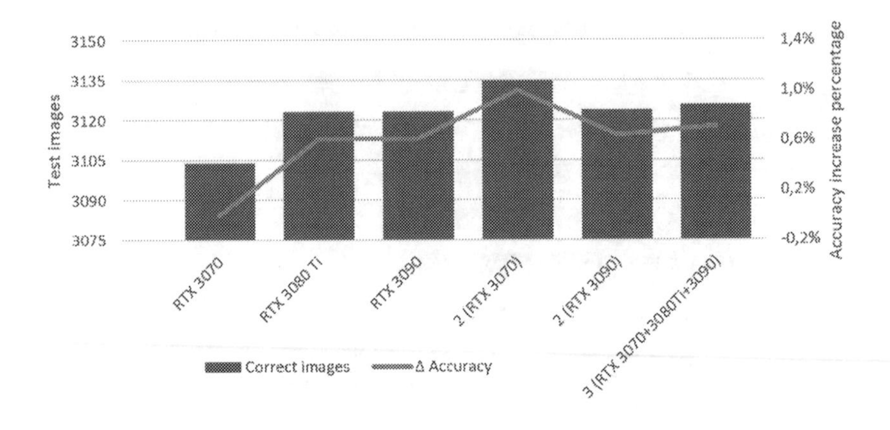

Fig. 4. CNN test accuracy performance variation through the different training hardware.

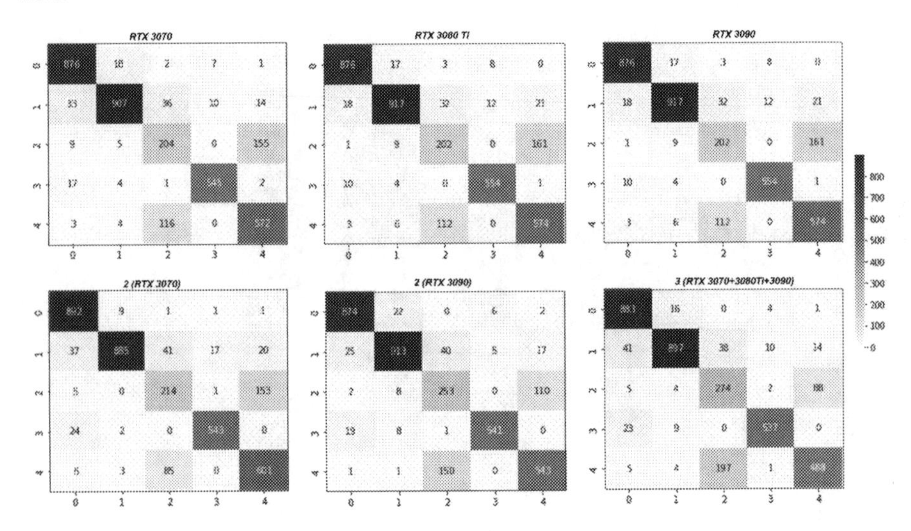

Fig. 5. Test confusion matrix on the different GPUs configurations (classes: 0-COVID-19, 1-Healthy, 2-Viral Pneumonia, 3-Tuberculosis and 4-Bacterial Pneumonia.)

increase in the area under the curve (AUC) and the area under the precision-recall curve (AP) versus the single GPU cases.

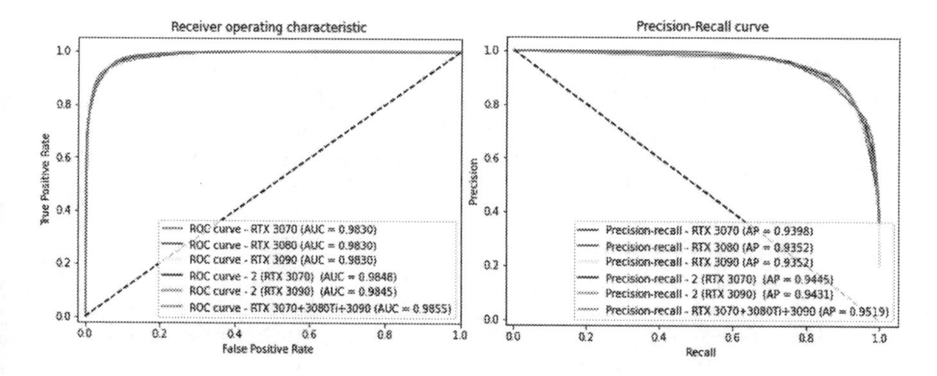

Fig. 6. Receiver operating characteristic (ROC) and precision-recall curve (PR) for the Deep Learning classificator on different Hardware (Test set).

4 Conclusions

In this paper, we have investigated the influence of different GPUs series and distributed learning configurations over a CNN model, focusing on time and accuracy metrics. The experiments were carried out with Horovod in a Deep Learning framework for lung X-ray disease classification. For this research, a new chest X-ray database with 14,167 images was built. Our experiments demonstrated a training speed-up of 1.7 using 2 GPUs and a speed-up upper of 2 with 3 GPUs. The training hardware is the only variance source during the training phase. While analyzing the accuracy fluctuation it was found that there was a slightly positive impact on the models trained with a distribution technique, increasing the test accuracy up to 1% with the same model and hyperparameter configuration.

Our results show the positive effects of the distributed training of a CNN with Horovod. Despite that, further investigation is required with other GPUs and learning frameworks, the experiments state the feasibility and positive impact of the use of distributed learning over time and accuracy metrics.

Acknowledgments. This work was supported by the Innovative Medicines Initiative 2 Joint Undertaking (JU) under grant agreement No 853989. The JU receives support from the European Union's Horizon 2020 research and innovation programme and EFPIA and Global Alliance for TB Drug Development non-profit organization, Bill & Melinda Gates Foundation and University of Dundee.

Disclaimer. This work reflects only the author's views, and the JU is not responsible for any use that may be made of the information it contains.

References

1. Farkas, A., Kertész, G., Lovas, R.: Parallel and distributed training of deep neural networks: A brief overview. In: 2020 IEEE 24th International Conference on Intelligent Engineering Systems (INES), pp. 165–170. IEEE (2020)
2. Gupta, K.G., Maity, S.K., Das, A., Wandhekar, S.: Performance analysis of different distribution of Python and TensorFlow to efficiently utilize CPU on HPC Cluster. In: 2021 International Conference on Electrical, Computer and Energy Technologies (ICECET), pp. 1–6. IEEE (2021)
3. Malik, A., Lu, M., Wang, N., Lin, Y., Yoo, S.: Detailed performance analysis of distributed Tensorflow on a gpu cluster using deep learning algorithms. In: 2018 New York Scientific Data Summit (NYSDS), pp. 1–8. IEEE (2018)
4. Sergeev, A., Del Balso, M.: Horovod: fast and easy distributed Deep Learning in TensorFlow. arXiv preprint arXiv:1802.05799 (2018)
5. Kavarakuntla, T., Han, L., Lloyd, H., Latham, A., Kleerekoper, A., Akintoye, S. B.: A Generic Performance Model for deep learning in a Distributed Environment. arXiv preprint arXiv:2305.11665 (2023)
6. Chang, K., et al.: Distributed Deep Learning networks among institutions for medical imaging. J. Am. Med. Inform. Assoc. **25**(8), 945–954 (2018)
7. Zhuang, D., Zhang, X., Song, S., Hooker, S.: Randomness in neural network training: characterizing the impact of tooling. Proc. Mach. Learn. Syst. **4**, 316–336 (2022)
8. Shi, S., Wang, Q., Chu, X.: Performance modeling and evaluation of distributed Deep Learning frameworks on GPUs. In: 2018 IEEE 16th International Conference on Dependable, Autonomic and Secure Computing, 16th International Conference on Pervasive Intelligence and Computing, 4th International Conference on Big Data Intelligence and Computing and Cyber Science and Technology Congress (DASC/PiCom/DataCom/CyberSciTech), pp. 949–957. IEEE (2018)
9. Ranjit, M. P., Ganapathy, G., Manuel, R.F.: Impact of distributed training on mask R-CNN model performance for image segmentation. In: 2020 International Conference on Emerging Trends in Information Technology and Engineering (ic-ETITE), pp. 1–7. IEEE (2020)
10. Ayan, E., Ünver, H.M.: Diagnosis of pneumonia from chest X-ray images using Deep Learning. In: 2019 Scientific Meeting on Electrical-Electronics & Biomedical Engineering and Computer Science (EBBT), pp. 1–5. IEEE (2019)
11. Rangarajan, A.K., Ramachandran, H.K.: A preliminary analysis of AI based smartphone application for diagnosis of COVID-19 using chest X-ray images. Expert Syst. Appl. **183**, 115401 (2021)
12. Simonyan, K., Zisserman, A.: Very deep convolutional networks for large-scale image recognition. arXiv preprint arXiv:1409.1556 (2014)
13. Visuña, L., Yang, D., Garcia-Blas, J., Carretero, J.: Computer-aided diagnostic for classifying chest X-ray images using deep ensemble learning. BMC Med. Imaging **22**(1), 178 (2022)
14. Russakovsky, O., et al.: Imagenet large scale visual recognition challenge. Int. J. Comput. Vision **115**, 211–252 (2015)
15. Rahman, T., et al.: COVID-19 Radiography DAtabase (2021). https://www.kaggle.com/tawsifurrahman/covid19-radiography-database
16. Kermany, D., Zhang k., Goldbaum M.: Chest X-Ray Images (Pneumonia) (2022). https://www.kaggle.com/datasets/paultimothymooney/chest-xray-pneumonia

17. Rahman, T., et al.: Tuberculosis (TB) Chest X-ray Database (2021). https://www.kaggle.com/tawsifurrahman/tuberculosis-tb-chest-xray-dataset
18. Visuña, L.: Chest X-ray images dataset of viral and bacterial pulmonary diseases. [Data set]. Zenodo (2023). https://doi.org/10.5281/zenodo.10084748

A Federated Learning Anomaly Detection Approach for IoT Environments

Basem Suleiman[1], Ali Anaissi[1](✉), Wenbo Yan[1], Abubakar Bello[2], Sophie Zou[1], and Ling Nga Meric Tong[1]

[1] School of Computer Science, The University of Sydney, Camperdown, Australia
{Basem.Suleiman,Ali.Anaissi,Wenbo.Yan,Sophie.Zou,ling.tong}@sydney.edu.au
[2] School of Social Sciences, Western Sydney University, Penrith, Australia
a.bello@westernsydney.edu.au

Abstract. The fast-growing development of smart home environments and the popularity of IoT devices have increasingly raised security concerns about anomalous behaviour and events. Traditional methods employ machine learning (ML) models that require sharing data collected from many IoT devices from smart homes so anomalous behaviour can be learned and detected. Such approaches introduce many problems in terms of privacy of sensitive IoT data to be shared over the network, models performance overhead, and scalability. We propose a novel Federated Learning Anomaly Detection (FLAD) approach for IoT smart home environments that address these problems. Our FLAD approach maintains the privacy of IoT data and faster training and detection performance by training several local models, instead of sharing it with a global model, on data collected from local devices. The local models require sharing only the learning parameter values with a global model which aggregates these values and sent them back to the local models to update their learning accordingly. Our experimental analysis of our FLAD approach on real IoT smart devices demonstrated very high accuracy (reaching over 99%) which is very comparable with the accuracy of the non-FL approach. Furthermore, our FLAD approach maintains the highest level of IoT privacy and faster model training time as it retains the IoT data within its local models and reduces network communication overhead, which has the potential to scale to a very large number of IoT devices.

Keywords: Federated Learning · IoT · Smart Home · Anomaly Detection · Deep Learning

1 Introduction

The use of Internet of Things (IoT) devices has considerably grown in smart home and smart city environments. Such IoT devices continuously sense data and monitor events to intelligent perform actions that create a convenient user experience. These IoT devices are often connected to the Internet so they can transmit

K. Daimi and A. Al Sadoon (Eds.): ACR 2024, LNNS 956, pp. 206–218, 2024.
https://doi.org/10.1007/978-3-031-56950-0_18

data and communicate with other devices and systems to perform desired functions. This, however, has significantly increased the vulnerability of such IoT devices and data to intrusion events through network traffic. As such, the need for detecting abnormal events or behaviours has become the main challenge and focus to prevent and protect the risks against anomalous activities.

One of the common security techniques to detect anomalous activities is using a network intrusion detection system (NIDS) [17,20,21]. The common practice in such NIDS is to monitor all the network traffic of IoT devices and send collected data to an algorithm running on a global model to identify anomalous behaviour. Data aggregated from different devices can help to identify anomalous patterns and thus improve detection accuracy. Such anomaly detection algorithms are often hosted in cloud environments where powerful computing resources can be used to perform timely analysis of a large volume of data aggregated from different devices. Although such detection methods are fundamental it increases privacy vulnerability concerns as it involves transmitting raw data collected from IoT devices over the network and storing it on a cloud server. Thus, one of the biggest challenges is how to detect anomalies in the smart home environment while preventing, or reducing, leakage of sensitive data and maintaining acceptable accuracy levels.

Recently, advanced machine and deep learning approaches such as [16,17] have been employed to enhance the performance of anomaly detection techniques. Examples of such well-known algorithms are the Deep Auto-encoder and KitNET. Both algorithms extract important features in well-structured architecture where the auto-encoder techniques show their merits in nonlinear and complex problems [16,17]. Furthermore, they classify the given observations as an anomaly by how they set up the auto-encoder to train the model.

In more recent studies [4,18,19,22], federated learning has been employed for anomaly detection. Studies such as [6,18] focus on intrusion detection but with focus on improving the speed of detection in smart buildings [19] and introducing case studies only [18]. Other studies such as [3,10,22] focus on multi-dimensional anomaly detection for in-vehicle networks to ensure driving safely. The approach in [2,7,12] attempts to detect anomalous behaviour of local models in terms of deviation from federated learning training and thus its adverse impact on the global model. To the best of our knowledge, none of the existing studies attempted anomaly detection in smart home IoT devices using a federated learning approach.

In this paper, we propose a Federated Learning Anomaly Detection (FLAD) approach for detecting an anomaly in smart home environments while preserving the privacy of data collected from IoT devices. Our approach is capable of precisely detecting anomalies (attacks on IoT devices) with accuracy similar to or higher than non-FL approaches. Moreover, our FLAD approach does not require transmitting data collected from IoT devices but rather using the data to train multiple local models and only transferring the learning coefficients. The global model as such shares the aggregated learning coefficients back with all local models to reflect on the learning shared by all models. Our FLAD approach can maintain privacy, and thus reduce the vulnerabilities, of the data collected from IoT devices and significantly reduce the amount of data that need to be transmitted over the network and stored.

The remainder of this paper is organized as follows. Section 2 introduces related literature in the area of anomaly detection in common deep learning and FL approaches. In Sect. 3, we present our FLAD for detecting anomalies in smart home environments. Section 4 presents the dataset collected from IoT devices and the data pre-processing and preparation. Our experiments and results using the IoT devices dataset are discussed in Sect. 5. Section 6 draw key conclusions and results and future work.

2 Related Work

Anomaly Detection in IoT applications has gained a lot of interest in recent years. It has been successfully applied in several application domains, such as intrusion attacks on computers and fraudulent activities in credit cards. In such applications, action is often required eagerly and in an online manner to detect any abnormal behaviour. Nevertheless, several authors have raised concerns about a large storage space which is often needed to handle the high-velocity of data traffic network [8,9]. In other words, consolidating this data in a centralized learning model can often be computationally complex and costly.

Therefore, the problem of training on decentralized data from IoT devices has become an important research direction due to the computational prohibitive and information security in the centralized learning model. [11,14,15] have firstly proposed the concept of Federated Learning (FL) in 2016 that to prevent leakage of private information by allowing each device to perform training locally and send the learning coefficient to the global model for ensuring privacy. Moreover, those papers introduce the Federated Averaging algorithm, which is computationally efficient but requires an immense number of rounds of training to generate well results, thus is robust to unbalanced and non-IID data distributions.

The effect of FL on anomaly detection has been studied by several authors that indicates the efficiency for demonstrations on simulated datasets such that the real data can be distributed evenly and preserved data privacy with using LSTM and DAE approach on IoT devices [5,12,13,22]. However, there still exist many challenges of federated learning in the IoT environment from the above studies. The main challenges are the heterogeneity that is from the device (high communication cost), statistical (non-IID data will result in weight divergence), and model (different types of devices may have different models).

To address this challenge, our proposed FLAD approach is aimed to maintain the highest level of data security and models performance as it does not require transferring network traffic data of IoT devices to a global ML model, often running on a cloud server, for model training and anomaly classification of continuously received data from various IoT devices. This can also reduce the amount of data that need to be transferred especially in real-time environments, and thus improve the performance of the ML model in predicting anomalous events.

3 Federated Learning Anomaly Detection (FLAD) Approach

Our FLAD approach consists of a number of local models (clients) and one global (central) model. We first introduce our proposed structure for the local models, then we present the overall architecture of our proposed FLAD approach including the global model. Each local model in our federated learning network employs a Deep Auto-encoder (DAE) Neural Network as an anomaly detection model. The rational idea of DAE is to force the network to learn a lower dimensional space for the input features, and then try to reconstruct the original feature space. In this sense, the main objective is to learn reproducing input vectors $\{x^1, x^2, x^3, \ldots, x^m\}$ as outputs $\{\hat{x}^1, \hat{x}^2, \hat{x}^3, \ldots, \hat{x}^m\}$.

Once we successfully train the DAE on the positive data, we compute the mean square error (MSE) and compute the anomaly threshold (atr) as shown in Eq. 1.

$$atr = \overline{MSE}_{positive\_atr} + std(MSE_{positive\_atr}) \tag{1}$$

This threshold will be compared to the reconstruction error (RE) for a new incoming sample to determine if its anomalous or not. Intuitively, the network will be able to reconstruct a new incoming positive data, while it fails with anomalous data. This will be judged based on the RE which is measured by applying the Euclidean norm to the difference between the input and output nodes as shown in Eq. 2.

$$RE(x) = \|x_i - \hat{x}_i\|^2 \tag{2}$$

The measured value of RE is used as an anomaly score for a given new sample. Intuitively, examples from the similar distribution to the training data should have low reconstruction error, whereas anomalies should have a high anomaly score. Figure 1 provides an overview of the whole process of anomaly detection by using the deep auto-encoder model locally.

3.1 Problem Formulation in Federated Learning

In FL setting, a set of K local models (devices) are connected to a global model to solve the following problem:

$$\min_{\omega \in \mathbb{R}^d} f(\omega) := \frac{1}{n} \sum_{i=1}^{n} f_i(\omega) \tag{3}$$

where f_i is the loss function corresponding to a local model k which defined as follows:

$$f(w) := \mathbb{E}[\mathcal{L}_i(\omega; x_i)] \tag{4}$$

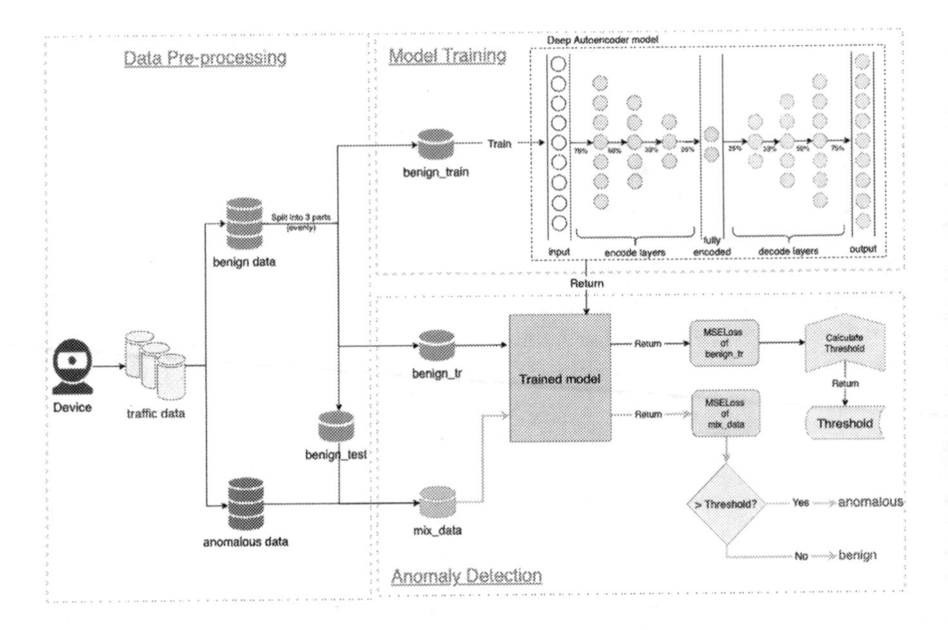

Fig. 1. Anomaly Detection with Deep Auto-encoder model

where $\mathcal{L}_i(\omega; x_i)$ measures the error of model ω given the input x_i defined in Eq. 2.

The stochastic gradient descent (SGD) method solves the above problem defined in Eq. 4 by repeatedly updates ω to minimize $\mathcal{L}(\omega; x_i)$. It starts with some initial value of $\omega^{(t)}$ and then repeatedly performs the update as follows:

$$\omega^{(t+1)} := \omega^{(t)} + \eta \frac{\partial \mathcal{L}}{\partial \omega}(x_i^{(t)}, \omega^{(t)}) \tag{5}$$

In FL, each local model performs a number of E epochs at each round to compute the gradient of the loss over its local data and send the model parameters ω_i^{t+1} to the global model. The global model aggregates these gradients and applies the global model parameters update by taking the average of the resulting models' parameters as follows:

$$\omega^{(t+1)} := \frac{1}{n} \sum_{i=1}^{n} \omega_i^{(t+1)}; \tag{6}$$

3.2 Anomaly Detection in Federated Setting

Based on the FL problem formulation and DAE model described above, we present our FLAD approach. Our DAE neural network uses the stochastic gradient descent algorithm to learn reconstructions $\hat{X}$ that is close to its original input X. At each round, each local model performs a number of E epochs to update the model parameters and report them to the global model. Once the

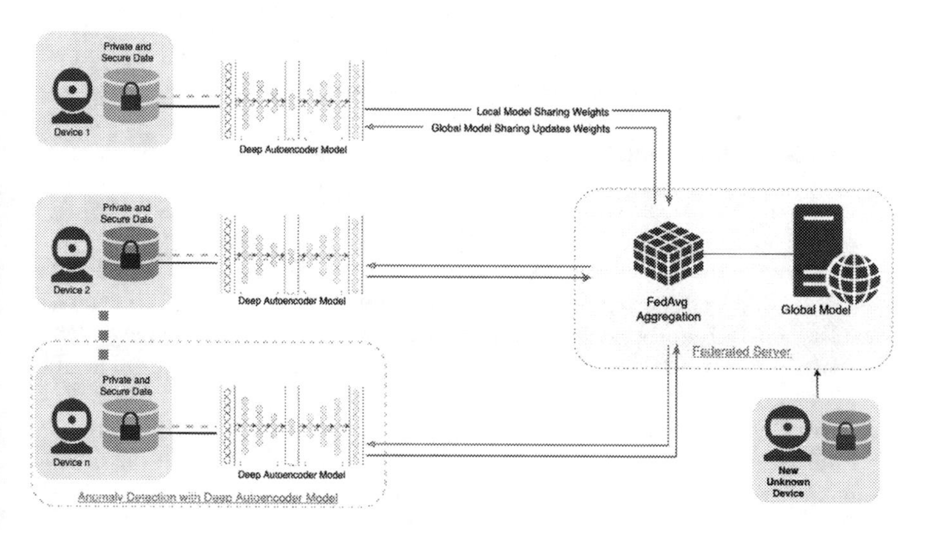

Fig. 2. Our Proposed Federated Learning Anomaly Detection with Deep Auto-encoder model

---

Algorithm 1 *FederatedAveraging.*The K local models (clients) are indexed by k;B is the local minibatch size, E is the number of local epochs, and η is the learning rate.

Global server:

initialize global model ω_0

for each round r = 1,2,... **do**

$m \leftarrow max(C \cdot K, 1)$ // Output the number of selected local models

$S\_r \leftarrow (random\ set\ of\ m\ localmodels)$ // Randomly select the local model from m

for each local model $k \in S\_r$ **do** in parallel

$\omega_{r+1}^k \leftarrow Local\ Model\ Update(k, \omega\_r)$

$\omega_{r+1} \leftarrow \sum_{K}^{k=1} \frac{n_k}{n} \omega_{r+1}^k$

Local Model Update(k, ω)**:** //Run on local model k

$\beta \leftarrow (split\ \rho_k\ into\ batches\ of\ size\ B)$

for each local epoch e from 1 to E **do**

for batch $b \leftarrow \beta$ **do**

$\omega \leftarrow \omega - \eta \nabla l(\omega)$

upload parameter to Global Model

---

updates are received, the global model will aggregate them using Eq. 6 and send them back to all local models as shown in Fig. 2. Algorithm 1 explains the learning phase in the FL setting.

Moreover, to improve the federated model efficiency and robustness, a partial selection mechanism has been involved in the federated model architecture. This means a random number of client devices would be chosen for the real training process in each communication round instead of using all of the client devices.

After the federated model is trained, the anomaly detection can be directly applied on both the client devices and any new devices.

4 Data Preparation

We evaluate our FLAD approach on a smart home dataset which is collected from several IoT devices (N-BaIoT dataset)[1]. The dataset contains 7,062,606 traffic data from nine devices, each belonging to one of the five types of IoT devices: thermostat, doorbell, baby monitor, webcam, and security camera. This dataset resembles non-IID real-world settings for IoT devices. Normally, when a device is functioning, it will generate normal traffic data, which is benign. The nine devices are attacked by ten types of Botnet attacks respectively, which leads to each device generating a large amount of anomalous traffic data. Figure 3 illustrates the overall number of benign traffic data is only 8% while the number of anomalous traffic data is 92%. Our exploratory analysis also shows that the distribution of benign and anomalous data for each device is extremely uneven (as shown in Fig. 4).

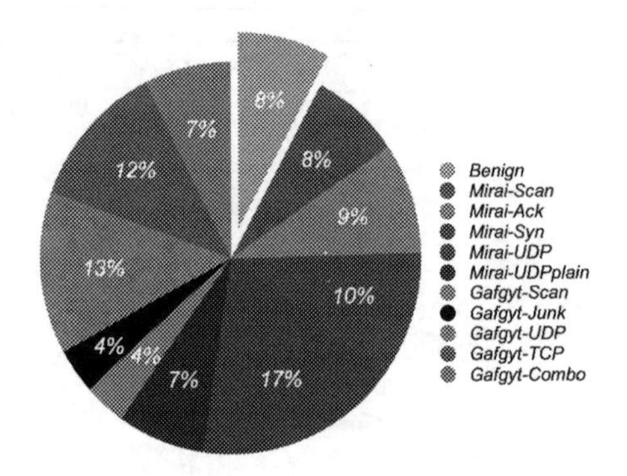

Fig. 3. Overall Distribution of Benign Data and Anomalous Data

There are 89 CSV files in total and more than six separate CSV files for each IoT device. To complete the following methodologies for anomaly detection, it is required to load all CSV files at the beginning, which is time-consuming and potential for making mistakes. Therefore, to prevent the possible risks and make the future detection process more easily, for each device, the separated CSV files that belong to the same IoT device have been combined into a single CSV file. There is a new feature added at the end called "type" to distinguish the traffic data is benign or attacked by which Botnet attacks. For instance, the type "enign"means the data is benign, whereas "m_scan" indicates the data is attacked by "Scan" of the Mirai Attacks and "g_combo" represents the data is attacked by "Combo" of the Gafgyt Attacks. Before the combination, the feature names and their order have been checked to ensure every CSV files are consistent. After the processing, the nine devices have a single CSV file with 116 features respectively.

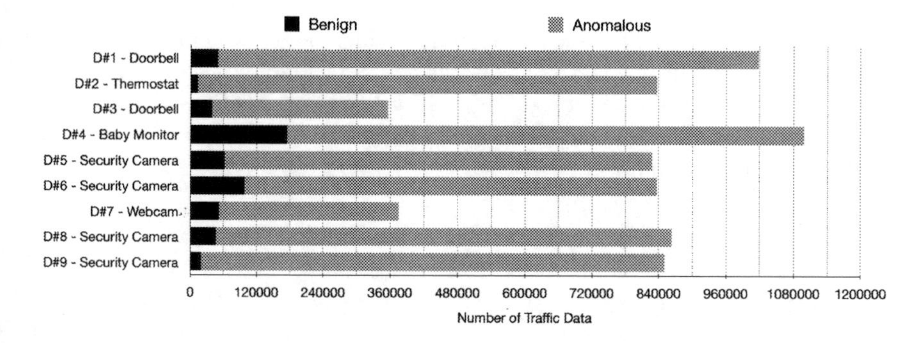

Fig. 4. Distribution of Benign Data and Anomalous Data among Nine Devices

Table 1. FLAD Local and Global Parameters

Parameters	Value	Meaning
lr	0.012	Learning rate for Deep Auto-encoder
num_clients	9	Number of clients
num_selected	3	Number of clients we choose for train each round
batch_size	128	the dataset size in each training iteration
num_rounds	100	Total number of communication rounds
epochs	5	For train local model
local_epochs	500	Only for the local deep auto-encoder training

5 Experiment and Results

We have conducted two sets of experiments. The first experiment set is by implementing our FLAD approach with the deep auto-encoder as local models. The second experiment set is the Non-FL learning model by using the deep auto-encoder model. We run the experiments on the smart home dataset to compare and analyse the performance of both experiment sets.

5.1 Experiment Setting

We implemented our proposed FLAD local and global models using Pytorch library on Google Colab virtual environment with Intel(R) Xeon(R) CPU and 69 GB memory. We have implemented the FedAvg aggregation algorithm and SGD with momentum as the optimizer. The other parameters we set up for our FLAD local and global models are summarised in Table 1. We initially set up the parameter values based on the experimental results reported in [16]. We then run a number of experiment combinations with the aim to optimize the parameters of each trained model so that the trained model maximizes the true positive rate and minimizes the false positive rate.

We split the training and testing data in our FLAD approach as illustrated in Fig. 1. Each IoT device has its local model which is trained using the device's training positive data. This results in nine local models (clients). Each local model shares its resulting learning parameters with the global model at each iteration. The global model then shares the aggregated learning values with all local models. Once the training is completed, we tested each local model with its corresponding test dataset.

5.2 Evaluation Metrics

To evaluate the performance of our model, we have used True Positive Rate (TPR), False Positive Rate (FPR) and F1 score. These metrics are common for evaluating the performance of anomaly detection tasks. In addition, we have recorded the training time to measure the model's computation resources cost.

5.3 Results and Analysis

We have conducted the experiments as explained in Sects. 5.2 and 5.1. Table 2 provides a comparative summary of the accuracy of our FLAD approach and the non-FL approach in terms of average TPR, average FPR, average F1 score, and the training time. Our FLAD approach achieved very similar accuracy compared to the non-FL approach. The model training process of our FLAD approach is much faster (requires %55 less training time) than the non-FL model, which is a huge superiority for building an instant anomaly detection model especially in real-time systems. A more detailed comparison of the accuracy of our FLAD approach and the non-FL for all the nine IoT devices is summarized in Tables 3, 4, and 5.

Table 2. FLAD model VS Non-FL model

Model type	Avg. TPR	Avg. FPR	Avg. F1 score	Time (mins)
FLAD model	**0.9009**	0.03525	93.073	**52.6**
Non-FL model	0.90076	**0.02232**	**93.095**	3109

Table 3. The TPR comparison for our FLAD and the non-FL model in nine devices

Method	Device Number								
	#1	#2	#3	#4	#5	#6	#7	#8	#9
FLAD model	**0.99999**	**1**	**0.35083**	0.99986	0.99992	0.99988	**0.9996**	**0.99991**	0.75814
Non-FL model	0.99988	0.99987	0.35081	0.99986	**0.99993**	0.99988	0.99918	0.99927	0.75814

Table 4. The FPR comparison for our FLAD and the non-FL model in nine devices

Method	Device Number								
	#1	#2	#3	#4	#5	#6	#7	#8	#9
FLAD model	**0.00702**	0.03409	0.00568	0.02412	0.10826	0.06928	0.01553	**0.04958**	0.00369
Non-FL model	0.09137	**0.00047**	**0.00445**	**0.02265**	**0.03195**	**0.03383**	**0.00754**	0.00559	**0.00307**

Table 5. The F1 score comparison for our FLAD and the non-FL model in nine devices

Method	Device Number								
	#1	#2	#3	#4	#5	#6	#7	#8	#9
FLAD model	99.993	99.991	51.934	99.917	99.850	99.840	99.938	99.948	86.242
Non-FL model	99.993	**99.994**	51.934	**99.922**	**99.953**	**99.919**	**99.939**	**99.958**	86.242

From the detailed experiments (Tables 3, 4, and 5), it can be observed that our FLAD approach achieved very comparable accuracy compared to the non-FL model in terms TPR, FPR and F1 score. In terms of the TPR, our FLAD model scored higher accuracy than the non-FL model, especially in Device #1 and #2, where our FLAD model achieved almost 100%. The non-FL approach, on the other hand, achieved slightly higher FPR and F1 score, especially in Device #2 and #5, where the non-FL model with low false alarm ratio.

In the context of the above experiments, it can be concluded that our FLAD approach achieved very comparable accuracy compared to the non-FL approach. Furthermore, the learning and detection of anomalous behaviour of our FLAD approach has its own unique advantages over non-FL approach. First, our FLAD model has very good generalizability as and the characteristics of different IoT devices can be learned by aggregating weights and other parameters of different local models corresponding to IoT devices. Second, our FLAD approach maintains a higher level of privacy as it does not require sharing the sensitive traffic data collected from IoT devices over the network (for storage and training one non-FL model). Unlike the non-FL model, collected data is fed to corresponding local models and only learning coefficients are shared with the global model. Third, the learning that happens at local models also improves the speed of model learning and anomaly detection as data are not transmitted over the network and our FLAD approach requires fewer training devices in each round, so it requires less training data. Sharing the coefficient values by the local models and the aggregated learning values from the global model back to the local models have much less network overhead, especially in real-time system settings. This was evident by the model training time resulted from our experiments with our FLAD approach which was 55% less than the non-FL approach.

Besides the above advantages, our FLAD approach is more practical and scalable than non-FL approaches. In reality, non-FL anomaly detection systems will require collecting IoT devices from multiple homes to train a model to achieve good performance, but the premise is that data collected from IoT devices of every smart home will need to be fed to the anomaly detection model. Besides, exposing sensitive and private data, such as camera and baby monitor devices, can be expensive in terms of network traffic and data storage. The non-FL model will need to process a large amount of aggregated data. In contrast, our FLAD model will send the local models' parameters to the global model for each communication round which avoids the direct data vulnerability problem.

6 Conclusion and Future Work

In this paper, we address the detection of anomalous behaviour that could arise from IoT devices in smart home environments. We have proposed a novel Federated Learning Anomaly Detection approach that overcomes the problems of traditional machine learning (non-FL) approaches. Our FLAD model comprising several local models each of which learns from data collected from corresponding IoT devices and a global model. The local models only share the learning values of their parameters with the global model which in turn aggregates the learning values and send it back to the local models so it can reflect it in its local learning. This demonstrated the ability of our FLAD model to capture and share the learning from IoT devices from different characteristics. Our experimental analysis on IoT smart home dataset with benign and botnet attacks demonstrated a very comparable accuracy when compared to the non-FL approach. Unlike non-FL, our FLAD model does not require transmitting the data collected from the IoT devices but only the learning values and thus it maintains the privacy of the sensitive IoT data and significantly improves the model training speed.

As future work, it could be interesting to investigate the performance of our FLAD model by training the local models on data combined from different IoT devices in each smart home (i.e., one local model per IoT device in one smart home). Also, it could be interesting to investigate training one local model on devices of similar functions or characteristics (e.g., security cameras and baby monitors).

Acknowledgment. We would like to thank Xia Wei and Ruijue Zou for assisting in data analysis and running some experiments.

References

1. Uci mchine learning repository: detection_of_iot_botnet_attacks_n_baiot data set. http://archive.ics.uci.edu/ml/datasets/detection_of_IoT_botnet_attacks_N_BaIoT
2. Anaissi, A., Khoa, N.L.D., Rakotoarivelo, T., Alamdari, M.M., Wang, Y.: Adaptive online one-class support vector machines with applications in structural health monitoring. ACM Trans. Intell. Syst. Technol. (TIST) **9**(6), 1–20 (2018)
3. Anaissi, A., Khoa, N.L.D., Rakotoarivelo, T., Alamdari, M.M., Wang, Y.: Smart pothole detection system using vehicle-mounted sensors and machine learning. J. Civ. Struct. Heal. Monit. **9**(1), 91–102 (2019)
4. Anaissi, A., Suleiman, B., Alyassine, W.: Personalised federated learning framework for damage detection in structural health monitoring. J. Civil Struct. Health Monit. 1–14 (2022)

5. Anaissi, A., Suleiman, B., Alyassine, W.: A personalized federated learning algorithm for one-class support vector machine: an application in anomaly detection. In: Groen, D., de Mulatier, C., Paszynski, M., Krzhizhanovskaya, V.V., Dongarra, J.J., Sloot, P.M.A. (eds.) ICCS 2022, pp. 373–379. Springer, Heidelberg (2022). https://doi.org/10.1007/978-3-031-08760-8_31
6. Anaissi, A., Suleiman, B., Naji, M.: Intelligent structural damage detection: a federated learning approach. In: Abreu, P.H., Rodrigues, P.P., Fernández, A., Gama, J. (eds.) IDA 2021. LNCS, vol. 12695, pp. 155–170. Springer, Cham (2021). https://doi.org/10.1007/978-3-030-74251-5_13
7. Anaissi, A., Suleiman, B., Zandavi, S.M.: Online tensor-based learning model for structural damage detection. ACM Trans. Knowl. Disc. Data (TKDD) **15**(6), 1–18 (2021)
8. Eskin, E., Arnold, A., Prerau, M., Portnoy, L., Stolfo, S.: A geometric framework for unsupervised anomaly detection: detecting intrusions in unlabeled data. Appl. Data Mining Comput. Secur. **6** (2002)
9. Hawkins, S., He, H., Williams, G., Baxter, R.: Outlier detection using replicator neural networks. In: Kambayashi, Y., Winiwarter, W., Arikawa, M. (eds.) DaWaK 2002. LNCS, vol. 2454, pp. 170–180. Springer, Heidelberg (2002). https://doi.org/10.1007/3-540-46145-0_17
10. Khoa, N.L.D., Anaissi, A., Wang, Y.: Smart infrastructure maintenance using incremental tensor analysis. In: Proceedings of the 2017 ACM on Conference on Information and Knowledge Management, pp. 959–967 (2017)
11. Konečný, J., McMahan, H.B., Ramage, D., Richtárik, P.: Federated optimization: distributed machine learning for on-device intelligence. arXiv preprint arXiv:1610.02527 (2016)
12. Li, S., Cheng, Y., Liu, Y., Wang, W., Chen, T.: Abnormal client behavior detection in federated learning. arXiv preprint arXiv:1910.09933 (2019)
13. Liu, Y., et al.: Deep anomaly detection for time-series data in industrial IoT: a communication-efficient on-device federated learning approach. IEEE Internet Things J. **8**(8), 6348–6358 (2020)
14. McMahan, H.B., Moore, E., Ramage, D., Arcas, B.A.: Federated learning of deep networks using model averaging. arXiv preprint arXiv:1602.05629 (2016)
15. McMahan, H.B., Moore, E., Ramage, D., Hampson, S., Arcas, B.A.: Communication-efficient learning of deep networks from decentralized data (2017)
16. Meidan, Y., et al.: N-baiot-network-based detection of IoT botnet attacks using deep autoencoders. IEEE Pervasive Comput. **17**(3), 12–22 (2018). https://doi.org/10.1109/mprv.2018.03367731
17. Mirsky, Y., Doitshman, T., Elovici, Y., Shabtai, A.: Kitsune: an ensemble of autoencoders for online network intrusion detection (2018)
18. Preuveneers, D., Rimmer, V., Tsingenopoulos, I., Spooren, J., Joosen, W., Ilie-Zudor, E.: Chained anomaly detection models for federated learning: an intrusion detection case study. Appl. Sci. **8**(12) (2018). https://doi.org/10.3390/app8122663. https://www.mdpi.com/2076-3417/8/12/2663
19. Sater, R.A., Hamza, A.B.: A federated learning approach to anomaly detection in smart buildings (2020)
20. Zandavi, S.M., Chung, V., Anaissi, A.: Accelerated control using stochastic dual simplex algorithm and genetic filter for drone application. IEEE Trans. Aerosp. Electron. Syst. **58**(3), 2180–2191 (2022). https://doi.org/10.1109/TAES.2021.3134751

21. Zandavi, S.M., Chung, V.Y.Y., Anaissi, A.: Stochastic dual simplex algorithm: a novel heuristic optimization algorithm. IEEE Trans. Cybern. **51**(5), 2725–2734 (2019)
22. Zhu, K., Chen, Z., Peng, Y., Zhang, L.: Mobile edge assisted literal multi-dimensional anomaly detection of in-vehicle network using LSTM. IEEE Trans. Veh. Technol. **68**(5), 4275–4284 (2019)

Taxonomy of AR to Visualize Laparoscopy During Abdominal Surgery

K. C. Ravi Bikram[1], Thair Al-Dala'in[2(✉)], Rami S. Alkhawaldeh[3], Nada AlSallami[4], Oday Al-Jerew[5], and Shahad Ahmed[6]

[1] Study Group Australia, Darlinghurst, Australia
[2] Western Sydney University, Penrith, Australia
t.aldalain@city.westernsydney.edu.au
[3] Department of Computer Information Systems, The University of Jordan, Aqaba, Jordan
r.alkhawaldeh@ju.edu.jo
[4] Computer Science Department, Worcester State University, Worcester, MA, USA
[5] Asia Pacific International College, Parramatta, Australia
[6] Department of Computer Science, The University of Duhok, Duhok, KRG, Iraq

Abstract. The augmented reality (AR) is the latest technology in laparoscopy and minimally invasive surgery (MIS). This technology decreases post-operative pain, recovery time, difficulty rate, and infections. The main limitations of AR systems are system accuracy, the depth perception of organs, and real-time laparoscopy view. The aim of this work is to define the required components to implement an efficient AR visualization system. This work introduces Data, Visualization techniques, and View (DVV) classification system. The components of DVV should be considered and used as validation criteria for introducing any AR visualization system into the operating room. Well-designed DVV system can help the end user and surgeons with a clear view of anatomical details during abdominal surgery. This study validates the DVV taxonomy and considers system comparison, completeness, and acceptance as the primary criteria upon which the proposed DVV classification is based upon. This work also introduces a framework in which AR systems can be discussed, analyzed, validated and evaluated. State_of_the_art solutions are classified, evaluated, validated, and verified to describe how they worked in the domain of AR visualizing laparoscopy during abdominal surgery in the operating room. Finally, this paper states how the proposed system improves the system limitations.

Keywords: Augmented reality (AR) · Minimally invasive surgery (MIS) · laparoscopy · 3D image · classification · Operating Room (OR)

1 Introduction

AR visualization has become a promising technology in the medical field for surgical guidance, training, diagnosis and planning [1,13]. Introducing AR to laparoscopic surgery proved to be a feasible solution to reduce intervention which

K. Daimi and A. Al Sadoon (Eds.): ACR 2024, LNNS 956, pp. 219–229, 2024.
https://doi.org/10.1007/978-3-031-56950-0_19

causes loss of direct vision and tangible feedback on the spot for the surgeons. The main purpose of the technology is to help the surgeon eliminate most of the shortcomings of open surgery like proper depth perception, less operating time, real-time laparoscopic view and high-quality image during surgery [11]. This is typically achieved by proper registering pre-operative datasets like CT images, MRI, X-ray, etc. to intraoperative datasets and the patient in the operating room (OR) [16]. Due to the use of AR in image-guided surgery, and in pre and intra-operative surgical plans, the patient's anatomical representation and graphical models of the surgical instruments are localized in real-time which guides the surgeons during surgical procedures [2,13]. In abdominal surgery where non-rigidity of abdominal tissues and organs remains challenge, the AR visualization system provides the surgeon more extensive view beyond the visible anatomical surface of the patient thereby reducing patient's trauma and improving clinical outcomes. Thus, the researcher has to focus on DVV components of AR systems to achieve high-quality visualization during abdominal surgery that helps surgeons in operation room [13]. Numerous AR systems and visualization techniques have been proposed but few systems are occasionally used for image-guided surgery and even fewer are developed for commercial use. Previous AR visualization classification and framework have usually focused on only one or two aspects of the visualization [14]. *The primary objective of this study is to present a novel framework to visualize Laparoscopy during Abdominal Surgery. The framework builds upon the work conducted by* [13], *which focuses on the analysis, validation, and evaluation of the components of an Augmented Reality (AR) system. By utilizing this framework, we aim to introduce a comprehensive approach that enhances Laparoscopic procedures in abdominal surgery. It allows a better comparative understanding of the most relevant and important components and sub-components of this technology. It also shows how the system accuracy, image quality and real-time view can be improved in AR visualization systems.*

The remaining of this paper is organized as follows: The literature survey is given in Sect. 2. In Sect. 3, we have introduced the components of the DVV system. We evaluate and validate the DVV classification in Sect. 4 and Sect. 5 gives the discussion and explores the components which are not explained clearly in the chosen publications and point out future research efforts. Finally, conclusions are given in Sect. 6.

2 Literature Review

Bernhardt et al. [2] explained the primitive AR visualization technique used in laparoscopy during abdominal surgery known as surface rendering. The technique displays the surface representing the interfaces between two separate structures like lung/air or vessel/lumen using different methods like marching cubes, statistical atlases, geometrical priors and random forest. It helps to enhance the realism with a frame rate of 10 f/s or 25 f/s for continuous motion perception and ease interpretation of the surface with an average latency of 250 m at that time. But it miserably fails to visualize complete surface reconstruction, invisible and inner critical structures, high resolution of the organs and tissues and could not produce a reliable result which affects the accuracy of the system. Rowe, et al. [14] proposed a complex lighting model to produce the photorealistic image considering CT images, eliminating the shadowing effect. it helps to visualize complex anatomy and soft tissues during surgery differentiating the operative organs, vacuum and other organs in terms of opacity. But, the image quality was affected by noise interference reducing the efficiency of the system. Cheung et al. [5] proposed a new algorithm other than the primitive one known as the intraductal dye injection technique with an indocyanine green (ICG) fluorescence imaging system using a camera head to detect a bile leak and bile duct during the liver and adrenal gland surgeries. The proposed system reduces the complication rate to 15%, and survival and accuracy were increased to 90% but were time-consuming and cumbersome which fail to explain the distribution variation of covariates among individuals. Zhao, et al. [15] proposed 3D reconstruction algorithm for accurate and real-time measurement of intra-operative data into 3D geometric CAD model and 3D mesh patient model for clear visualization of the abdominal organs during surgery. The system recognized the deformation distance using the root mean square of the coordinates, spot detection higher than 0.99 mm and image quality to 0.9 f/s, and finally increasing the accuracy of the system. But failed to increase image quality in overexposed areas or distortion of normal anatomy. Bourdel, et al. [3] explained the use of AR software to view a tumor in the kidney and uterus. The AR approach provides a clear orthographic projection of a tumor with high accuracy of resection with less difficulty level (0.87). Zou, et al. [17] proposed a spectral imaging technique using deformable modelling on the animal model. The system uses image detection to reduce the processing time and refreshment rate with high accuracy but they are not sure that the same output can be maintained if the system is applied to humans. Kenngott, et al. [17] proposed marker based visualization system using CT image registration on liver resection preventing blood clots using a hand port or trocar. The system helped for good visualization of the liver (2.8 mm) and bleeding point (minimal) from the CT image providing better tactile feedback. Ganni, et al. [9] proposed a markerless AR visualization system where the 2D operative image (CT images) obtained from angular movement by endoscope are superimposed on the 3D autostereoscopic image. The false discovery rate (0.04 s), the relative distance between the operative organ(0.1 mm), and the false negative rate (0.08 s) were reduced, increasing the true positive rate (0.9 s) and positive predictive value (0.85 s) by the system. But the operative organ detection in bright light reduces the system efficiency. Chen, et al. [4] proposed a novel simultaneous localization and mapping algorithm (SLAM) based on all data stages (input datasets, analytical abstraction, visualization abstraction and view) and transformation operators (data transformation, visualization transformation and visualization mapping transformation) that maps data between all stages. The algorithm superimposed 2D intra-operative images (i.e. CT images and MRI) on the 3D autostereoscopic image considering tissue deformation without changing data structures at any stage of the process. Chen's algorithm helps in-depth perception and error variation using root mean square distance through coordinate points which is based on the surface area of operative abdominal organs. This method provides a good result; 90% accuracy in organ recognition and 0.1 mm RMSD, but real-time processing was high (0.6 s).

3 Proposed System Components

Based on our literature review and prior knowledge of the technology and domain, we believe in increasing system accuracy, giving a clear depth perception during the surgery, and having a real-time laparoscopy view. Therefore, first, we must find out what available data must be used in the surgery. Second, we must figure out how these related data can be effectively merged and visualized. Lastly, we must know how the analyzed data can be displayed. This information helps the end user in successful abdominal surgery. The main components of robust AR system for visualizing laparoscopy during abdominal surgery are data, visualization techniques and view [13]. Table 1 summarizes the features of the selected research on three components.

Data: The purpose of using data as part of classification is to pinnacle the significance of determining which accessible data should be displayed to the end user. Different type of data is presented, but we considered only a few data classes to lessen viewer or end user confusion. Only the raw data obtained from the sensor or endoscopic camera or endoscope is considered which helps to produce the analyzed imaging data that combines with prior knowledge to form derived imaging data [13].

Majority of the paper describes the surface representation of the modality data. Kenngott et al. [12], Cheung et al. [5], and Bernhardth et al. [2] used a simple representation of the surfaces using CT images. Volume data were used in some of the systems like Rowe, et al. [14], Bourdel et al. [3], and Ganni, et al. [9]. Image intensity is defined in all the paper that uses volumetric data which helped in processing speed and depth perception. Rowe, et al. [14] used a cinematic rendering technique and Bourdel, et al. [3] used AR software to calculate the image intensity. Whereas, Ganni, et al. [9] used 3D reconstruction algorithm, volumetric rendering, spectral imaging technique and motion tracking to determine the image quality of the data. Bernhardt et al. [2] and Christiansen et al. (2018) used both surface and volume models, whereas Zhao et al. [15] used 3D mesh patient model using mesh data and Zou, et al. [17] used point patient model to increase the image quality of the output. Bernhardt et al. [2], Bourdel et al. [3], Bernhardth et al. [2], and Chen et al. [4] described the visualisation of prior knowledge data that too in terms of tool depiction. Bernhardt et al. [2], Chen et al. [4], and Zhao et al. [15] described the visualization of derived data. The image quality of the output is mostly determined by this data in these systems.

Visualization Techniques: The visualization techniques component highlights the proficiency of using the data to provide the foremost statistical information for a specific task at a given surgical step. The primary purpose of using visualization techniques as part of classification is to determine which techniques are used to analyse the data. With help of visualization techniques, the analyzed imaging data, derived data, and prior knowledge data are transformed into visually processed data that interact with the interaction tools of the view to give the output to the viewer using display devices [13].

Most visualization techniques have dealt with the visualisation of anatomical data. Recent papers have used 3D imaging techniques whereas intraoperative images are transformed into 3D models for the visualisation process. Bernhardt et al. [2] system described surface and volume rendering techniques. Bourdel et al. [3], and Cheung et al. [5] described AR software as visualization techniques. Ganni et al. [9], and Kenngott et al. [12] described different visualization techniques which are motion tracking, video-based techniques, marker-based algorithm, Monochrome channel filtering algorithm and spectral imaging techniques. However, chen, et al. [4] described a new markerless visualization technique known as simultaneous localization and mapping algorithm (SLAM) which helps in error variation and depth perception.

View: The main purpose of using the view as part of classification is to spotlight how the analyzed data are displayed to the end user through output media. The visually processed data that are obtained from the perception location like patients, real environment, display devices etc. interacts with interaction tools of the view to produce the output in display devices. The display device helps to give output to the end user with a clear view and high-quality images [13]. Monitor, endoscope, monocular and laparoscope are used as 2D display; 3D glasses, augmented microscope and polarized glasses are used as binocular stereoscopic 3D display and as autostereoscopic 3D display; autostereoscopic lenticular LCD, 3D endoscope MATLAB and video display are also used, as shown in Fig. 1 [13].

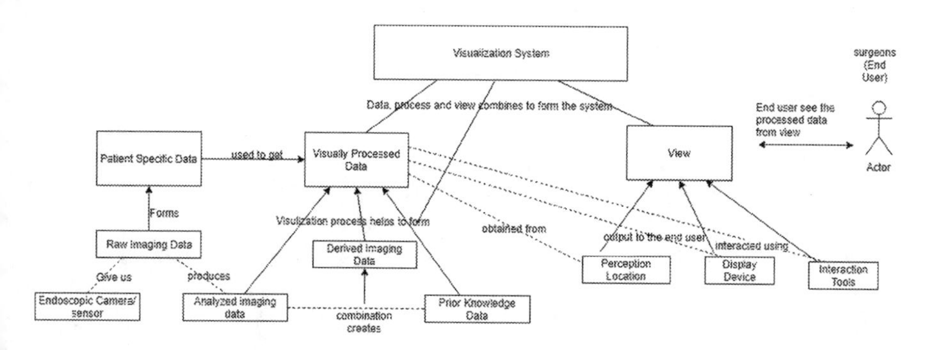

Fig. 1. The DVV classification (Data, visualization process and View), their classes and subclasses (solid-line arrow) [13].

The perception location and display device were specified, whereas the interaction component has less attention from researcher. Kenngott et al. [12], Zou, et al. [17] and Chen, et al. [4] system perception location was patient whereas the remaining 20 paper system perception location was either the patient or a monitor. Bernhardt et al. [2] used an endoscopic camera or digital computer monitor as a display device whereas other paper system consists of a digital computer monitor as a display device. The scope of the interaction tools in the taxonomy is limited to hardware and virtual interaction tools. Some systems didn't specified interaction tool for the view like: Bernhardt, et al. [2], Bourdel et al. [3], Zhao, et al. [15], Cheung et al. [5], Zou, et al. [17], and Kenngott et al. [12] used marker position as interaction tools. However, Chen, et al. [4] used SLAM rendering to dense the surface mesh as the interaction tool.

4 Proposed System Components Evaluation and Validation

The accuracy of the system and depth perception of anatomical organs is proved by the validation and helps to build the right system, while evaluation provides usefulness and value of the system. Table 1 shows these validations and evaluations features.

The accuracy of the system was the focus of validation of most of the papers: Cheung et al. [5], Bourdel, et al. [3], Ganni, et al. [9] and Kenngott et al. [12]. Several papers looked at processing time (speed): Bernhardt et al. [2], Zou, et al. [17]. Few papers focused on the opacity of the system: Rowe, et al. [14] focused on sampling error. Bourdel, et al. [3], and Chen, et al. [4] evaluated and validated their system based upon the component with defined formula and compared those with others. Chen, et al. [4] used the whole system as the component and compared different factors of the output which would affect the accuracy of the system. Bourdel, et al. [3] described the accuracy of the system through segmentation and registration method. Bernhardt et al. [2], Zou, et al.[17], and Rowe, et al. [14] evaluated the system with the theory without any validation using the Vivo model describing the accuracy and processing speed of the system. Bernhardt et al. [2] evaluated all the visualization techniques used but didn't validate his claim in the paper. Another paper analysed the data in vivo model and draw the conclusion without validation. Zhao et al. [15], Ganni, et al. [9], and Kenngott, et al. [12] validated the accuracy of the system with help of phantom and animal models. To get the result as described they used camera movement without proper system evaluation same with the case of Bourdel, et al. [3] where validation of the system using the Vivo model was done in terms of accuracy without evaluation.

Table 1. DVV classification table of augmented reality visualization system

Author	Type of Surgery (Marker base or Marker less)	Domain	Data			Visualization Techniques	View			Component Validated or Evaluated	Study Criteria	Validation/Evaluation method and/or Data Set	Results
			Raw	A	Visually Processed		PL	DD	INT				
Bernhardt, et al. [2]	MB	N/S	MRI CT	S V	A: surface and volume model D: Image intensity, resolution & rigidity PK: Endoscope	Surface rendering & Volume rendering	P/M	EC/M	N/S	Whole system	Anatomical deformation, breathing and heartbeat and processing time.	Direct Measurement	Liver volume variation from 13% to 24%. Liver shift of 28mm whereas kidney shift of 46mm. Discrepancy rise to 44mm. Good frame rate (10fs or 25 for continuous motion perception). latency (up to 300ms or average 250 ms).
Rowe, et al. [14]	MB	Heart	CT	V	A: Volume rendered model D: image intensity PK: N/S	Cinematic rendering using complex lightning model	P/M	M	Transfer function	Image Detection	Opacity	Vivo Model	Clear view of left and right pulmonary arteries, branches of the main coronary artery and aortic arch.
Bourdel et al. [3]	ML	Uterus	MRI	V	A: 2D intraoperative image superimposed on endoscopic image D: recurrence rate PK: monocular laparoscope	AR software using dense structure from motion.	P/M	M	Multiple view using monocular laparoscope	Segmentation and Registration Method	Accuracy	Vivo Model	Laparoscopic myomectomy reaches 50% or more in 5 years. Accuracy is higher in AR group then control group and score difficulty level in between 0 to 4. 2.4 for control group and 0.87 for AR group.
Cheung et al. [5]	N/S	Liver	CT	S	A: monochromatic fluorescence imaging using near infrared light D: operation time PK: near infrared diode, camera and working port	Fluorescence imaging using indocyanine green (ICG)	P/M	M	Move and rotate camera head for multiple view	Image Registration Method	Accuracy	Vivo Model	Less complication rates (15%) and higher survival rates (95%) then open group surgery.
Kenngott et al. [12]	MB	N/S	CT	S	A: 2D CT images are superimposed on video camera images D: N/S PK: N/S	Marker based technique depending on ray casting model	P	M	Markers position determine the view.	Registration method	Accuracy	Phantom model and porcine model	Phantom model: N=10 84% visualization feasibility. 2.8 2.7 mm 95th percentile= 6.7 mm Porcine model: N=5 79% visualization feasibility. 3.5 3.0 mm 95th percentile= 9.5 mm
Zhao, et al. [15]	N/S	N/S	CT	ME	A: 3D mesh patient model D: image quality and effectiveness PK: N/S	3D printing algorithm	P/M	M	N/S	Whole System	Accuracy	Animal model	Root mean square of coordinates defer by 0.598mm. Point cloud coordinates at 60%.
Chen, et al. [4]	ML	N/S	CT	ME	A: 2D intra operative image superimposed on 3D autostereoscopic image D: error variation and depth perception PK: endoscopic camera and endoscope	Simultaneous localization and mapping algorithm using moving least squares	P	M	End user uses SLAM to dense surface mesh	Whole system	Accuracy	Phantom model	Low RMSD value that determines correct visualization of the surfaces.
Ganni, et al. [9]	MB	Gall Bladder	MRI CT	V	A: pre-operative and intra operative image are superimposed in endoscopic images D: scaling and tracking method PK: laparoscopic camera	Motion Tracking	P/M	M	Control view of laparoscopic camera.	Whole system	Accuracy	Phantom model	Clear discrimination between expert and novice performance with no extra instruments.
Zou, et al. [17]	N/S	N/S	CT	PO	A: volume render model. D: operating time PK: computer	Deformable modeling technique	P	M	N/S	Image Detection	Processing time (Speed)	Vivo Model	Less execution and calculation time and low refreshment rate.
Fucentese, et al. [8]	ML	knee	CT	V	A: 2D intra-operative image superimposed on 3D autostereoscopic image D: N/S PK: Computer	Motion Tracking	P/M	M	Move and rotate smart glasses for multiple view	3-dimensional of the ligaments	Accuracy	Direct Measurement	Smart glasses and integrated sensors improves the efficiency of a novel AR-based surgical guidance system
Golse, et al. [10]	ML	Liver	CT	ME	A: 3D mesh patient model D: image quality and effectiveness PK: N/S	green rendered mesh	P/M	M	RGB-D camera	non-rigid registration method	Accuracy	Vivo Model	The vivo AR tests achieved a fast and agile setup installation (<10 min) and ex vivo quantification demonstrated a 7.9 mm root mean square error for the registration of internal landmarks.
Collins, et al. [7]	ML	uterus	MRI CT	V	A: pre-operative and intra operative image are superimposed in endoscopic images D: scaling and tracking method PK: laparoscopic camera	Deformable modeling technique	P/M	EC/M	End user uses SLAM to dense surface mesh and Control view of laparoscopic camera.	Whole system	Accuracy Speed	Vivo Model	3D reconstruction and registration take around 10 min proposed approach for tracking is robust and responsive.
Giselle, et al. [6]	N/S	Myelomeningocele	MRI	S V	A: 3D mesh patient model D: image quality and effectiveness PK: smartphone and tablets	ray casting target object rendering	P	M	Screen capture using smartphone	Whole system	Accuracy Processing time	Direct Measurement	Developing a virtual model for planning fetoscopy repair for myelomeningocele carries out preoperative and postoperative procedures.

PL: Perception location, DD: Display device, INT: Interaction tool, N/S: Not specified, A: Analyzed data, D: Derived data, PK: Prior knowledge, S: Surface(s), V: Volume(s), P: Patient, M: Monitor, EC: Endoscopic camera, PO: Point(s), ME: Mesh(s), ML: Marker less Surgery, MB: MarkerbaseSurgery

System Verification: Evaluation of the framework is the main task in the review report. Chen et al. [4] defined simultaneous localization and mapping (SLAM) algorithm for 3D reconstruction of anatomy structures using both quantitative and qualitative evaluation processes to assess the performance of the SLAM tracking error and quality of the proposed framework. Markerless model helps in increasing the visualization accuracy of abdominal organs. The 3D image construction is built based on the point cloud with the Poisson surface reconstruction algorithm. Bourdel, et al. [3] suggested that the classification can be evaluated and validated using a "system acceptance" measure considering the accuracy of the system in terms of registration and segmentation method.

System Acceptance: To evaluate the DVV classification, We concentrated on the anatomical deformation and sampling error that either boost or reduce the system efficiency. The verification system was not a standard since most of the publications did not consider soft tissue deformation in anatomical deformation during pre-operative and intra-operative data. However, these methods used to find anatomical deformation and sampling error, while checking the accuracy of the system can be an effective way to judge the proposed system. The proposed system's accuracy depends on soft tissue deformation consideration as the registration process may fail due to anatomical deformation. To determine whether this method is acceptable to the user, we thus examined the significance of anatomical deformation and sampling error while making it feasible and reliable in specified publications [13].

System Completeness: For verifying the completeness of the proposed system, we analyzed the existence and non-existence of most fundamental components and subcomponents in state-of-the-art papers. Table 1 summarizes the components to determine the completeness of the system. For completeness of a

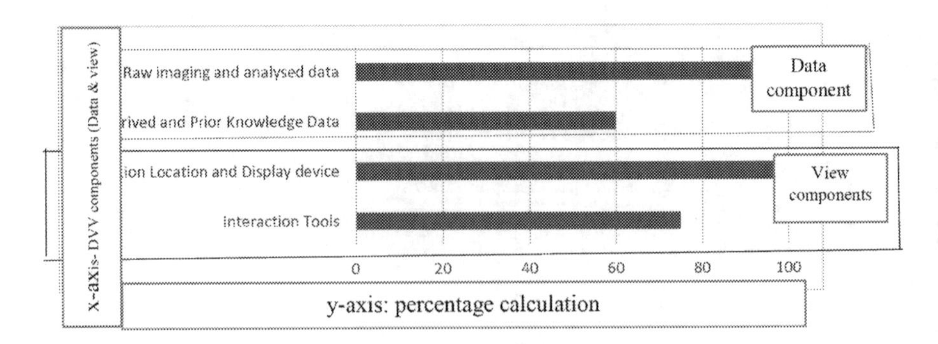

Fig. 2. Represent the percentage of sub factors of main DVV classification that has been described in the selected publications, the bar graph shows 100% and the sub factors which aren't explained in all the papers like derived data, prior knowledge data and interaction tool represents part in the bar graph.

system, all the components and subcomponents of DVV classification must be included that support the objectives of the system as shown in Fig. 2.

System Comparision: To understand the grasp of the proposed system, we analyzed the components by comparing our paper to other works. The proposed classification can be compared with other recent classifications of similar topics, that is anatomical deformation, with proper evaluation and validation. However, the other works classified the system into data types, perception location and display device without interaction tools factors and evaluated the system on basis of anatomical deformation with direct measurement. According to Chen et al. [4], the system would be failed for initialization of the monocular images coordinates. If the surface coordinate datasets are wrongly initialized, then the accuracy of the system will be penalized. As the AR object can be placed anywhere on the patient's surface for correct depth perception, but if the endoscope moves rapidly it may cause a false reading of the analyzed intraoperative data or image. It just reduces the system accuracy and increases the sampling error. If the system fails to address the class or sub-class of the classification, then only the typology should be punished. *So, we believe that these limitations and failing criteria of previous papers must be the focus of current and future research, and these components and subclasses to be integral parts of the classification. Thus, each factor and sub-factors of our proposed system are specified in at least one publication.*

5 Discussion

The discussion is divided into three parts to focus more on each component as follows:

Data: Derived data helps in image intensity in most of the system and sometimes helps in processing time and depth perception. How surgical tools were visualized for navigation purposes is determined by the prior knowledge data. However, in a real surgical environment, sensors are used to track the location of a tool. These tools are visualized as surface and volume models which may be a problem for depth perception or soft tissue deformation cases. Chen, et al. [4] suggested a new algorithm to represent surgical tools which will improve rather than confuse the localization and navigation of the tools. All publications have described only the tools used for navigation but miserly fail to explain the system accuracy and surgery roadmaps on behalf of prior knowledge data. The surgical roadmap isn't explained properly in any of the papers. Chen, et al. [4] explained surgical roadmap as prior knowledge data in the paper describing the soft tissue deformation but couldn't explain clearly and validated their claims. All the common instances of derived data are explained in all the publications, but few works explored the visual representation of derived data [13].

Visualization Techniques: All chosen publications described different visualization techniques used in the AR visualization systems. Most of the papers described the complex light modelling method: Rowe, et al. [14] doesn't have a clear description for that modelling method. The transfer function stated by the author isn't evaluated or validated by other works. Image opacity obtained using the transfer function has a high sampling error which may be problematic, especially in our case where AR is being used.

View: All the publications had perception location and display device, but few only had interaction tools. Without analyzed data being interacted with the interaction tools, the result is obtained based on the theory. How the manipulated tools help to obtain the output is determined by the interaction tool of the view which isn't mentioned in most of the paper. Most of the paper failed to explain the interaction tools as explained in the above sections. Some papers considered hardware interaction tools neglecting virtual interaction tools and vice versa. These results confirmed Kersten-Oertel, et al.[13] study. Chen, et al. [4] considered both interaction tools to produce high accuracy of the system. The lack of prior knowledge and derived data and interaction tools in our classification suggested that shouldn't be considered in this type of data to classify the system. However, we believe that without the prior interaction tools, analyzed data can't be accurately visualized in the display device for the end user and the surgeon's expertise. Therefore, these components need further study for a proper AR visualization system.

6 Conclusion

AR visualization system is a great innovation in the medical field which overcomes the surgeon's limited visual view during surgical procedures. The development of AR visualization systems for incorporating Laparoscopy into Abdominal Surgery helped to reduce surgeons' limited visual field of view with 3D perception. We have described DVV classification based on data type, visualization techniques and view. This visualized data helps to interact with the user in terms of manipulation on screen as well as hardware device interaction. The nomenclature and proposed system in our diagram help to explain the main points of the AR visualization system. The DVV classification shows the classification, evaluation, validation, comparison and verification. The taxonomy was useful for finding the gap between current research and suggesting a new methodology for future study in the field. Our examination showed that few of the components of the system are evaluated, even fewer are validated and least are verified. Therefore, evaluation, validation and verification of the new system must eradicate the absence of such a system in clinical procedures and the operating room. We believed that DVV classification is useful for comparing, analyzing and consistently evaluating the system.

References

1. Barcali, E., Iadanza, E., Manetti, L., Francia, P., Nardi, C., Bocchi, L.: Augmented reality in surgery: a scoping review. Appl. Sci. **12**(14), 6890 (2022)
2. Bernhardt, S., Nicolau, S.A., Soler, L., Doignon, C.: The status of augmented reality in laparoscopic surgery as of 2016. Med. Image Anal. **37**, 66–90 (2017)
3. Bourdel, N., Collins, T., Pizarro, D., Debize, C., Grémeau, A.s., Bartoli, A., Canis, M.: Use of augmented reality in laparoscopic gynecology to visualize myomas. Fertil. Sterili. **107**(3), 737–739 (2017)
4. Chen, L., Tang, W., John, N.W., Wan, T.R., Zhang, J.J.: Slam-based dense surface reconstruction in monocular minimally invasive surgery and its application to augmented reality. Comput. Methods Programs Biomed. **158**, 135–146 (2018)
5. Cheung, T.T., et al.: Pure laparoscopic hepatectomy with augmented reality-assisted indocyanine green fluorescence versus open hepatectomy for hepatocellular carcinoma with liver cirrhosis: A propensity analysis at a single center. Asian J. Endoscopic Surg. **11**(2), 104–111 (2018)
6. Coelho, G.: The potential applications of augmented reality in fetoscopic surgery for antenatal treatment of myelomeningocele. World Neurosurg. **159**, 27–32 (2022)
7. Collins, T., Pizarro, D., Gasparini, S., Bourdel, N., Chauvet, P., Canis, M., Calvet, L., Bartoli, A.: Augmented reality guided laparoscopic surgery of the uterus. IEEE Trans. Med. Imaging **40**(1), 371–380 (2021)
8. Fucentese, S.F., Koch, P.P.: A novel augmented reality-based surgical guidance system for total knee arthroplasty. Arch. Orthop. Trauma Surg. **141**(12), 2227–2233 (2021)
9. Ganni, S., Botden, S.M., Chmarra, M., Goossens, R.H., Jakimowicz, J.J.: A software-based tool for video motion tracking in the surgical skills assessment landscape. Surg. Endosc. **32**(6), 2994–2999 (2018)
10. Golse, N., Petit, A., Lewin, M., Vibert, E., Cotin, S.: Augmented reality during open liver surgery using a markerless non-rigid registration system. J. Gastrointest. Surg. **25**(3), 662–671 (2021)
11. Ivanov, V.M., et al.: Practical application of augmented/mixed reality technologies in surgery of abdominal cancer patients. J. Imaging **8**(7), 183 (2022)
12. Kenngott, H.G., et al.: Mobile, real-time, and point-of-care augmented reality is robust, accurate, and feasible: a prospective pilot study. Surg. Endosc. **32**(6), 2958–2967 (2018)
13. Kersten-Oertel, M., Jannin, P., Collins, D.L.: DVV: a taxonomy for mixed reality visualization in image guided surgery. IEEE Trans. Visual Comput. Graphics **18**(2), 332–352 (2011)
14. Rowe, S.P., Johnson, P.T., Fishman, E.K.: Cinematic rendering of cardiac CT volumetric data: principles and initial observations. J. Cardiovasc. Comput. Tomogr. **12**(1), 56–59 (2018)
15. Zhao, S., Zhang, W., Sheng, W., Zhao, X.: A frame of 3d printing data generation method extracted from CT data. Sens. Imaging **19**(1), 1–13 (2018)
16. Zhao, Z., et al.: Augmented reality technology in image-guided therapy: state-of-the-art review. Proc. Inst. Mech. Engineers Part H: J. Eng. Med. **235**(12), 1386–1398 (2021)
17. Zou, Y., Liu, P.X.: A high-resolution model for soft tissue deformation based on point primitives. Comput. Methods Programs Biomed. **148**, 113–121 (2017)

Cybersecurity Engineering

Open Platform Infrastructure for Industrial Control Systems Security

Guillermo Francia III(✉) and Eman El-Sheikh

Center for Cybersecurity, University of West Florida, Pensacola, FL 32514, USA
{gfranciaiii,eelsheikh}@uwf.edu

Abstract. The introduction of Docker containers ushered the emergence of microservices to facilitate efficient ways to deploy and manage containerized applications. Digital Twins in Industrial Control Systems (ICS) has enabled advances in the test and evaluation of those systems in a low-cost and non-disruptive manner. In this paper, we present our work on advancing the security of Industrial Control Systems through a four-pronged approach: i) provide a safe training infrastructure for ICS security; ii) present an effective avenue for ICS security testing without operational disruption; iii) implement ICS digital twins to enable ICS security training; and iv) facilitate the design, implementation, and evaluation of ICS security tools. To realize these objectives, we propose the utilization of Open Platform Infrastructure (OPI) with Docker technologies to deploy virtualized Programmable Logic Controllers (PLCs), also known as softPLC, and Human Machine Interfaces (HMIs) that can emulate or act as digital twins of ICS. Further, we describe several docker containers instantiated from Dockerfiles to emulate typical Information Technology (IT) and Operation Technology (OT) networks to illustrate the viability and affordability of such implementations for teaching, learning, and testing of ICS security.

Keywords: Docker · Digital Twin · Industrial Control Systems (ICS) Security · Open Platform Infrastructure (OPI) · Virtualization · Programmable Logic Controller (PLC)

1 Introduction

The rapid evolution of technology ushers the proliferation of advanced methodologies of tactics, techniques, and procedures (TTPs) that adversaries employ to carry out unprecedented attacks on Industrial Control Systems (ICS). These ICS are the fundamental drivers of critical infrastructures ranging from power generation to manufacturing. A minor security incident involving these systems can have a devastating effect to society. Thus, it is imperative that these systems be secured and continuously protected. However, there are fundamental challenges that are endemic to these systems that present some hindrance to the implementation of some security measures.

K. Daimi and A. Al Sadoon (Eds.): ACR 2024, LNNS 956, pp. 233–243, 2024.
https://doi.org/10.1007/978-3-031-56950-0_20

1.1 ICS Testbed and Training Workbench

The primary challenge is the scarcity and affordability of testbeds and training workbenches in ICS security. This is widely recognized as a major hurdle by practitioners and trainers because testing and training should never be conducted on live operational systems due to the likelihood of disruptions. Furthermore, the creation of physical twins that can be used to conduct these security activities is prohibitively expensive. For ICS security training purposes, there are two main approaches. One is to put together a portable trainer similar to that described in [1]. This can be built with inexpensive Programmable Logic Controllers (PLCs) running miniature motors and LEDs to mimic an ICS. Another is to use software-based PLCs that are capable of delivering ICS protocols. An open-source system that is readily available for download from the Internet is OpenPLC [2]. It is designed and implemented to emulate a physical PLC and provides several emulated ICS protocols such as Modbus/TCP, Distributed Network Protocol 3 (DNP3) and Ethernet/IP. The Interactive Development Environment of OpenPLC supports ladder logic diagram, structured text, and function block programming for system implementations.

1.2 Contributions to ICS Security Training

The contributions of this work to the advancement of ICS security training include, but are not limited to:

- Presents an affordable infrastructure for an effective ICS security training;
- Provides useful insights into the design and implementation of ICS Open Platform Infrastructure (OPI);
- Facilitates the validation of new ICS vulnerability assessment and security testing tools; and
- Enables the introduction of up-to-date, real-world ICS security scenarios to augment active learning.

To summarize, the topics covered in this paper describe the significance of Open Platform Infrastructure in advancing the state of ICS security training.

The remainder of this paper is organized as follows: Sect. 2 provides some background and related works while Sect. 3 describes our on-going work on ICS Open Platform Infrastructure. Section 4 describes our deployment and dissemination efforts. Finally, Sect. 5 presents our concluding remarks and offers future directions toward enhancing ICS security through OPI technologies.

2 Background and Related Works

2.1 Prior and Similar Works

Virtualization technology is heavily used to implement cyber ranges for cybersecurity education and training. In [3], a virtualization-based infringement incident response tool for cyber security training using Cloud is described. The tool enables scenario-based incident response training, hacking defense practice, and vulnerability measurement exercises.

The issue of resource limitations in training to augment cyber security talent is addressed in [4]. The proposed training platform enables a network information security attack and defense practical training environment on a ThinkPHP framework.

The virtualization of Distributed ICS processes for security research is explored in [5]. The virtualization system, which can be accessed online via the Internet, is built on OpenPLC for the emulation of physical PLCs.

2.2 Digital Twins of Industrial Control Systems

Digital Twins (DTs) are virtual models that emulate their physical counterparts. These vary from one system to another ranging from manufacturing [6], industry [7], power [8], transportation [9], maritime [10], healthcare [11], predictive maintenance [12], and many more.

Dietz and Pernul in [13] present the advantages of enhancing ICS security through DTs. The authors argue for addressing the combination of DT data with known Information Technology (IT) and Operation Technology (OT) system vulnerabilities for the detection of weaknesses. Unlike physical ICS, DTs provide a convenient way of testing for novel ICS vulnerabilities and attack vectors while the system is in operational mode.

An implementation of a DT equipped with an intrusion detection system is described by Akbarian, Fitzgerald and Kihl [14]. The DT facilitates an effective, secure, and safe sandbox for carrying out advanced intrusion detection techniques. In a similar manner, Ekhart, et al. [15] designed DTs to enhance cyber situational awareness. These systems operate in parallel with their cyber-physical counterparts to enable the deep inspection of their behavior without disrupting OT services.

2.3 Open Platform Infrastructure

In [16], Docker is described as

> "... an open platform for developing, shipping, and running applications. Docker enables you to separate your applications from your infrastructure so you can deliver software quickly. With Docker, you can manage your infrastructure in the same ways you manage your applications."

This open platform provides an infrastructure with which lightweight containers can securely run in insolation on a given host. Containers can easily be shared and run on multiple hosts with the assurance that every host gets the identical container that works the same way [16]. We leverage this valuable feature of Docker to create an environment for a practical ICS training platform.

3 ICS Open Platform Infrastructure (ICS-OPI) Development

The development of the ICS Open Platform Infrastructure starts with physical system design requirements and specifications. This is followed by the detailed description of process controls and variables which are mapped to the input/output coils and memory of a PLC. The design is implemented using ladder logic programming and translated to structured text for deployment. The following discussions present the development details and the various scenarios in which the implementation is utilized to its full potential.

The design and implementation of the ICS-OPI system is guided by the following requirements:

- An implementation that works on virtualized PLCs operating on standard ICS protocols;
- An infrastructure that occupies a small footprint and operates in isolation;
- Realization of an IT-OT network infrastructure;
- An infrastructure that facilitates the development of digital twins for ICS security;
- A system that can be interfaced with an external Human Machine Interface (HMI); and
- A system that can be used to simulate ICS attacks and defenses by security purple teams.

3.1 Virtualized PLCs and ICS Protocols

The implementation of virtualized PLCs operating on standard ICS protocols is realized by OpenPLC [2], an open-source software that is designed and implemented to emulate a physical Programmable Logic Controller (PLC). The standard ICS protocols that are emulated by this software are Modbus TCP, Distributed Network Protocol 3 (DNP3) and Ethernet/IP. Modbus TCP, the most widely deployed ICS protocol over TCP/IP, is an application layer messaging protocol [17]. DNP3 is a master/slave control system protocol and is a predominant Supervisory Control and Data Acquisition (SCADA) protocol in the electric, oil & gas, waste/water, and security industries [18]. Ethernet/IP is part of the Common Industrial Protocol (CIP) family of protocols that is in conformance with the Open Systems Interconnection (OSI) model. This protocol enables the deployment of standard Ethernet technology in industrial automation [19]. OpenPLC provides a convenient Integrated Development Environment (IDE) for the implementation of ICS requirements. It supports ladder logic programming for development and structured text for runtime deployment on a web browser using port 8080. A snapshot of the IDE is shown in Fig. 1.

3.2 Small Footprint in Isolation

The requirement for a small footprint in isolation is realized with Docker containers. We started by designing two subnetworks, representing the Information Technology (IT) domain and the Operational Technology (OT) domain connected by a virtual router. The IT subnet is on the 192.168.10.0/24 network and the OT subnet is on the 10.9.0.0/24 network. The network topology is depicted in Fig. 2. Note the port numbers that are being shared by the host and PLC1. A brief description of each port is in order. Port 8080 enables the OpenPLC runtime. Ports 502, 20000, and 44818 are the default ports of the Modbus TCP, the DNP3, and the Ethernet/IP protocols, respectively.

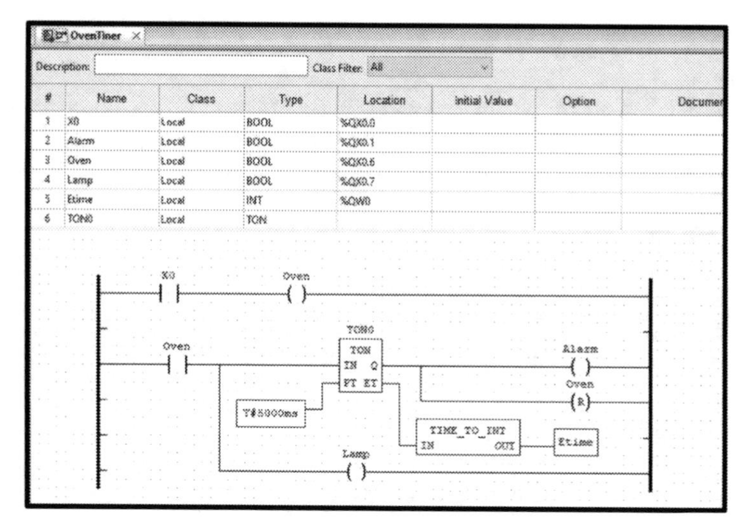

Fig. 1. Integrated Development Environment

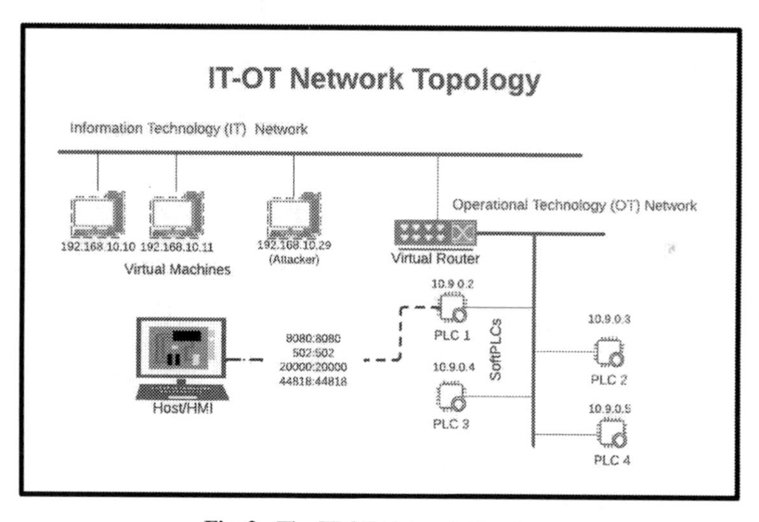

Fig. 2. The IT-OT Network Topology

3.3 Realization of an IT-OT Network Infrastructure

The IT-OT network topology (shown in Fig. 2) is implemented using Docker, an Open Platform Infrastructure. The virtual machines, softPLCs, and virtual router are instantiated as Docker containers. The property of each container is defined in a docker-compose.yml file. Finally, the containers are built using the docker-compose command yielding a realization of the IT-OT network topology as depicted in Fig. 3.

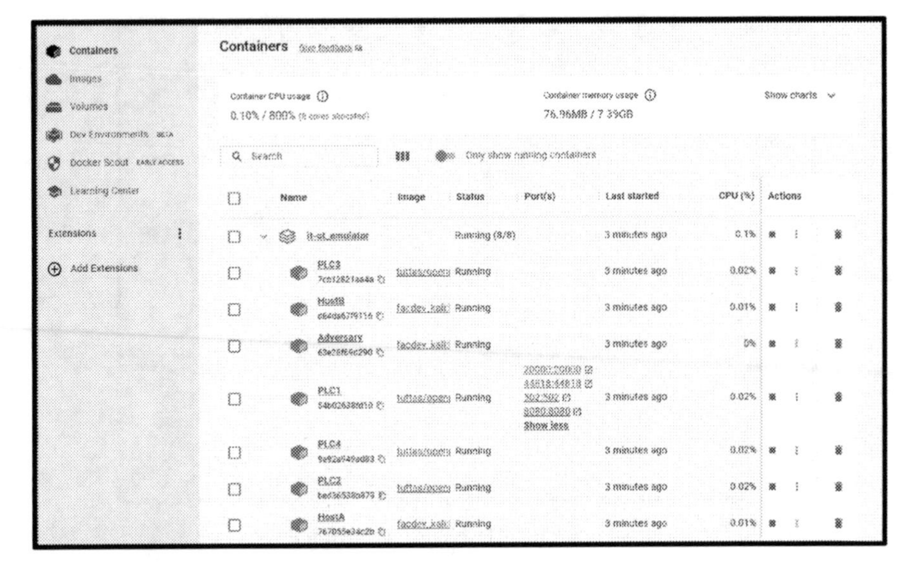

Fig. 3. IT-OT Docker Containers

3.4 Development of ICS Digital Twins

Semenkov, et al. [20] describe a hybrid approach combining virtual machines, emulators, and physical components of a cyber-physical system. In their work, a digital twin of the instrumentation and control components of a nuclear power plant is designed and implemented for testing and verification. In our effort to validate the feasibility of building digital twins using OPI, we designed, implemented, and deployed a similar DT system, which includes an HMI that controls and monitors virtual PLCs created with Docker containers. The HMI of our DT system is depicted in Fig. 4.

3.5 Human Machine Interface for the ICS

A Human Machine Interface (HMI) provides an intuitive interface to facilitate the interaction between the human operator and the control devices. In essence, it enables an effective means of real-time automation and monitoring of process data and system statuses through visualization. By exposing the ICS ports 502, 20000, and 44818 on the virtual PLC to the host machine, an HMI can reach in to emulate process control and monitoring. An example HMI used in the ICS security training is depicted in Fig. 5.

3.6 Simulating ICS Security Attacks and Defense

After creating a sandbox emulation of the IT-OT environment, security red team (attacker) and blue team (defender) activities can commence. Training scenarios focus on both the attacker and the defender viewpoints and include the following:

- Reconnaissance—discovery and probing ICS devices on the network;

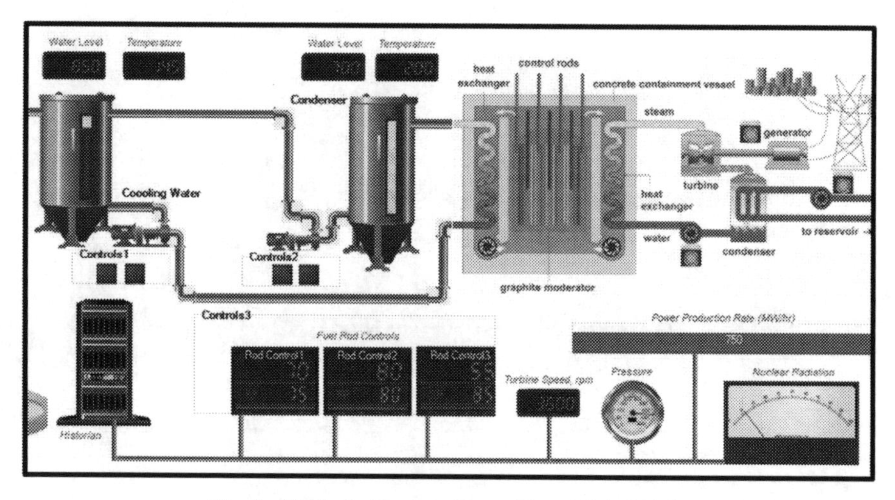

Fig. 4. HMI of a Nuclear Power Plant Digital Twin

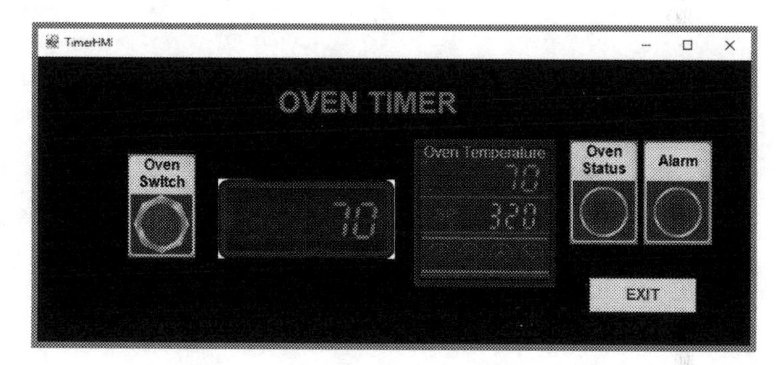

Fig. 5. An Oven Human Machine Interface

- Lateral movement—penetrating adjacent nodes and crossing domain boundaries of IT and OT networks;
- Penetration testing—system intrusion;
- Deep packet inspection—ICS packet capture and analysis;
- ICS packet crafting—creating and injecting malicious ICS network packets that are injected into the OT network;
- Digital forensics—forensic analysis of ICS security artifacts or indicators of compromise;
- Intrusion detection and prevention—crafting Snort [21] rules/filters for intrusion detection of malicious ICS traffic; and
- Threat intelligence and hunting—application of and search for ICS threat intelligence.

To illustrate, we present two red team penetration testing tools in action. The first is an open-source TCP Modbus client tool, Modbus Examiner [22], that can be downloaded from Github. This tool, although functionally limited, can read and write in a Modbus device. Figure 6 depicts an unauthorized writing on a Modbus holding register.

Modbus Examiner

Connection: localhost:502 Slave ID: 1

Register	Alias	Value	Type	Sample rate	
0		0	Holding Registers	3000	Remove
1		595	Holding Registers	3000	Remove
2		0	Holding Registers	3000	Remove
3		0	Holding Registers	3000	Remove
4		0	Holding Registers	3000	Remove

Fig. 6. Modbus Examiner in Action

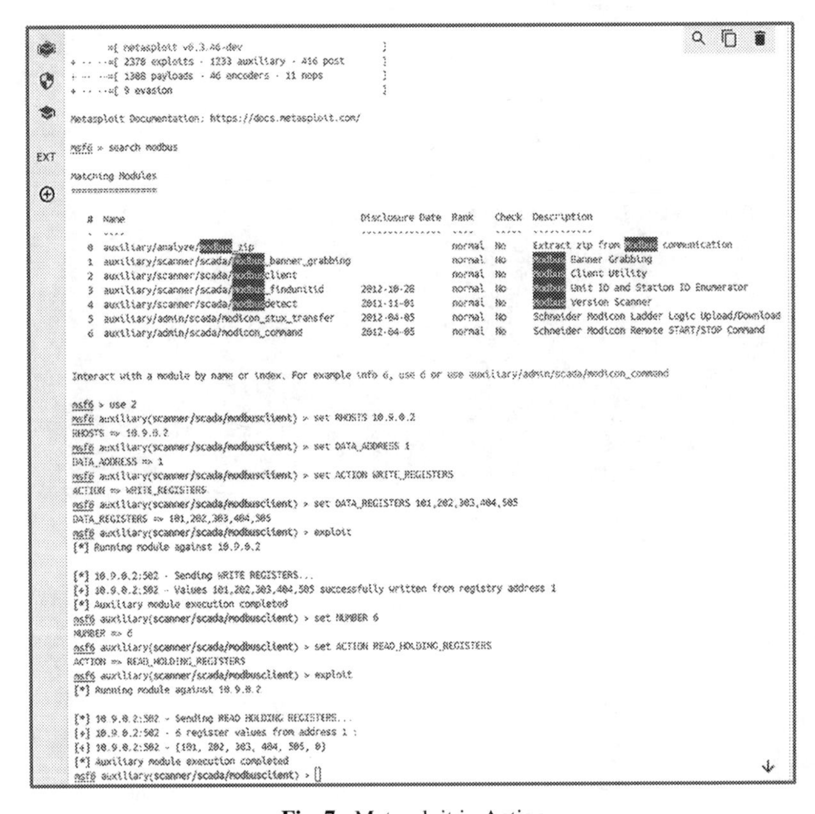

Fig. 7. Metasploit in Action

The second is another open-source tool, the Metasploit Framework [23]. The tool is a de-facto standard in penetration testing and equipped with more than 1,500 exploits. In Fig. 7, we illustrate a penetration testing session performed by a Kali system in the IT network to attack a Modbus device in the OT network. Clearly, this attack scenario illustrates the incursion of an adversary from the IT side into the OT side. The attack consists of writing and reading 5 values in the Modbus registers.

4 Deployment and Dissemination

In order to achieve the full potential of the virtual ICS network on an Open Platform Infrastructure, we designed training exercises that mimic realistic ICS security events. These events are presented as case studies or scenarios to provide an engaging context with which participants can frame their analyses and opinions. These ICS security learning materials were used in the virtual ICS-OPI to train cybersecurity faculty, industry, and government professionals across the United States. The feedback received from these trainees were very positive. Further, the materials were shared in CLARK [24], a public repository of free cybersecurity curriculum.

5 Conclusion and Future Directions

This paper describes an on-going project to enhance the facilitation of ICS security training through virtualization and open platform infrastructure. By leveraging the efficacy and affordability of creating a virtual OPI that can emulate an IT-OT network architecture and the devices contained within, we propose that ICS security training is no longer an arduous and expensive undertaking. The realization of a sand-boxed IT-OT network architecture together with the security purple team exercises illustrate the feasibility of the concepts presented herein. The proposed model facilitates the inclusion of up-to-date, real-world ICS security scenarios to enhance active learning.

As the security of ICS moves to the center stage of cybersecurity, opportunities for future work will abound. Recognizing that state of the technologies and the emerging security issues associated with ICS, we offer the following future directions:

- Expand the collection of ICS security case studies and scenarios to address newly discovered vulnerabilities;
- Create virtual OPIs that incorporate devices found in renewable energy and power grid systems;
- Continue to expand and improve the creation of digital twins as instruments to carry out enhanced ICS security; and
- Automate the process of creating security scenarios for the effective utilization of digital twins in security training and education.

Acknowledgement. This work is partially supported by the University of Colorado at Colorado Springs subaward number 20-144-12 under NSA-NCAE-C grant number H98230-20-1-0385 and the University of West Florida Center for Cybersecurity CyberSkills2Work program funded by the NSA National Centers of Academic Excellence (NCAE) Program under grant number H98230-23-1-0089. The United States Government is authorized to reproduce and distribute reprints notwithstanding any copyright notation herein.

References

1. Francia, G., Bekhouche, N., Marbut, T., Neuman, C.: Portable SCADA security toolkit. Int. J. Inf. Netw. Secur. **1**(4), 265–274 (2012)

2. Alves, T.R., Buratto, M., De Souza, F.M., Rodrigues, T.V.: OpenPLC: an open source alternative to automation. In: IEEE Global Humanitarian Technology Conference (GHTC 2014), pp. 585–589 (2014)
3. Park, Y.S., Choi, C.S., Jang, C., Shin, D.G., Cho, G.C., Kim, H.S.: Development of incident response tool for cyber security training based on virtualization and cloud. In: Proc. of the 2019 International Workshop on Big Data and Information Security (IWBIS), Bali, Indonesia (2019)
4. Ma, S.: Research and design of network information security attack and defense practical training platform based on ThinkPHP framework. In: Proc. of the 2022 2nd Asia-Pacific Conference on Communications Technology and Computer Science (ACCTCS), Shenyang, China (2022)
5. Barinov, A., Beschastnov, S., Boger, A., Kolpakov, A., Ufimtcev, M.: Virtual environment for researching information security of a distributed ICS. In: Proc. of the 2020 Global Smart Industry Conference (GloSIC), Chelyabinsk, Russia (2020)
6. Gericke, G.A., Kuriakose, R.B., Vermaak, H., Mardsen, O.: Design of digital twins for optimization of a water bottling plant. In: IECON 2019-45th Annual Conference of the IEEE Industrial Electronics Society, Lisbon, Portugal (2019)
7. Stein, C., Behr, J.: Industrial use cases: 3D connectivity for digital twins: decoupling 3D data utilization from delivery and file formats on an infrastructure level. In: Proceedings of the 27th International Conference on 3D Web Technology (Web3D 2022), New York, NY (2022)
8. Kummerow, A., Monsalve, C., Rösch, D., Schäfer, K., Nicolai, S.: Cyber-physical data stream assessment incorporating digital twins in future power systems. In: 2020 International Conference on Smart Energy Systems and Technologies (SEST), Istanbul, Turkey (2020)
9. Zhang, Y., Zhang, H.: Urban digital twins: decision-making models for transportation network simulation. In: 2022 International Conference on Computational Infrastructure and Urban Planning (CIUP 2022), New York, NY (2022)
10. Perabo, F., Park, D., Zadeh, K., Smogeli, O., Jamt, L.: Digital twin modelling of ship power and propulsion systems: application of the OpenSimulation platform (OSP). In: 29th International Symposium on Industrial Electronics (ISIE), Delft, Netherlands (2020)
11. Mone, G.: Biomedical digital twins. Commun. ACM **66**(10), 9–11 (2023)
12. Centomo, S., Dall'ora, N., Fummi, F.: The design of a digital twin for predictive maintenance. In: 25th IEEE International Conference on Emerging Technologies and Factory Automation (ETFA), Vienna, Austria (2020)
13. Dietz, M., Pernul, G.: Unleashing the digital twin's potential for ICS security. IEEE Secur. Priv. **18**(4), 20–27 (2020)
14. Akbarian, F., Fitzgerald, E., Kihl, M.: Intrusion detection in digital twins for industrial control systems. In: 2020 International Conference on Software, Telecommunications and Computer Networks (SoftCOM), Split, Croatia (2020)
15. Eckhart, M., Ekelhart, A., Weippl, E.: Enhancing cyber situational awareness for cyber physical systems through digital twins. In: 24th IEEE International Conference on Emerging Technologies and Factory Automation (ETFA), Zaragoza, Spain (2019)
16. Docker, Inc., Docker Overview, Docker, Inc. (2023). https://docs.docker.com/get-started/overview/. Accessed 15 Dec 2023
17. Modbus Organization, MODBUS Messaging on TCP/IP Implementation Guide V1.0b, 24 October 2006. https://modbus.org/docs/Modbus_Messaging_Implementation_Guide_V1_0b.pdf. Accessed 20 Dec 2023
18. Clarke, G., Reynders, D., Wright, E.: Practical modern SCADA protocols: DNP3, IEC 60870.5 and related systems. Burlington, MA: IDC Technologies, Elsevier Ltd. (2004)
19. ODVA, Ethernet/IP, 2023. https://www.odva.org/technology-standards/key-technologies/ethernet-ip/. Accessed 20 Dec 2023

20. Semenkov, K., Promyslov, V., Poletykin, A.: Verification of large scale control systems with hybrid digital models and digital twins. In: 2020 International Russian Automation Conference (RusAutoCon), Sochi, Russia (2020)
21. Cisco, Snort: https://www.snort.org/. Accessed 22 Dec 2023
22. Andrawos, M.: Modbus Examiner, 22 June 2017. https://github.com/minaandrawos/Modbus Examiner. Accessed Dec 2023
23. Rapid7, Rapid7 Metasploit, 2023. https://www.metasploit.com/. Accessed 21 Dec 2023
24. CLARK, Teach Cyber Today...Secure Tomorrow, 2023. https://clark.center/home. Accessed 22 Dec 2023

Towards Hybrid NIDS: Combining Rule-Based SIEM with AI-Based Intrusion Detectors

Federica Uccello[1](✉), Marek Pawlicki[2], Salvatore D'Antonio[1], Rafał Kozik[2], and Michał Choraś[2]

[1] University of Naples 'Parthenope' Centro Direzionale, 80133 Napoli, Isola C4, Italy
federica.uccello@assegnista.uniparthenope.it,
salvatore.dantonio@uniparthenope.it

[2] Bydgoszcz University of Science and Technology, PBS, Bydgoszcz, Poland
{marek.pawlicki,rafal.kozik,chorasm}@pbs.edu.pl

Abstract. The current threat landscape identifies Distributed Denial of Service (DDoS) attacks as one of the most critical hazards for network security. Given the constant variation in attack dynamics, enhancing existing detection techniques has become imperative. Indeed, traditional rule-based Security Information and Event Management (SIEM) systems often fall short in accurately detecting DDoS attacks, due to their evolving nature and complex traffic patterns. To overcome such limitations, Artificial Intelligence (AI) techniques for intrusion detection have garnered increasing attention in the realm of network security. In this paper, we introduce a hybrid approach that amalgamates rule-based SIEM systems with AI-based intrusion detection techniques. Specifically, we present a hybrid Network Intrusion Detection System (NIDS). The proposed approach is aimed at bolstering the security of monitored systems and applications by facilitating a more accurate detection of cyberattacks. We present and test a proof-of-concept architecture against DDoS attacks, yielding promising preliminary results.

Keywords: Denial of Service Attacks · Network Intrusion Detection Systems · Artificial Intelligence · Machine Learning · Rule-Based SIEM

1 Introduction, Problem Statement and Research Questions

1.1 Background and Context

In today's interconnected and data-driven world, network security plays a critical role in safeguarding digital infrastructures from various threats [2,31]. Organizations are becoming more aware of such hazards, fortifying their security measures and adopting proactive defence strategies as a response [1,11]. However, cyberattackers are continuously evolving their tactics and leveraging increasingly

K. Daimi and A. Al Sadoon (Eds.): ACR 2024, LNNS 956, pp. 244–255, 2024.
https://doi.org/10.1007/978-3-031-56950-0_21

sophisticated operations to exploit vulnerabilities in digital systems [30], finding new schemes to avoid classic prevention and detection techniques [12,16,25]. In particular, Distributed Denial of Service (DDoS) attacks pose a significant challenge to network administrators and security professionals [20,32], as they are getting more complex and recurrent [5]. This trend has to be attributed to the geopolitical changes that emerged after the Russian invasion of Ukraine in February 2022 [18].

Traditional rule-based Security Information and Event Management (SIEM) systems have been widely employed for network intrusion detection [15,38,40]. While these systems have shown potential in real-time detection of such attacks, being able to guarantee an accurate discrimination between benign and malicious traffic is not trivial. This limitation arises due to the evolving nature of DDoS attacks, making it challenging to define static rules that can effectively capture their signatures [8,10]. Artificial Intelligence (AI) techniques, specifically AI-based intrusion detectors, can provide a possible solution to overcome the limitations of rule-based SIEM systems. AI-based approaches leverage Machine Learning (ML) algorithms to identify deviations from normal network behaviour, thereby enhancing the detection accuracy of DDoS attacks. However, these techniques alone may suffer from false positives and false negatives due to the lack of contextual information and the complexity of network traffic patterns [13]. In this work, the possibility of combining the two approaches for a comprehensive intrusion detection method is explored.

1.2 Problem Statement

This paper proposes a solution for accurate and efficient detection of DDoS attacks in network traffic, to address the limitations discussed previously. Additionally, the process of gathering and labelling data which enables the use of supervised ML-powered NIDS is a costly and labour-intensive endeavour [27].

Thus, there is a need for an effective, hybrid approach that combines the strengths of rule-based SIEM systems and AI-based intrusion detection techniques to improve the accuracy, timeliness and deployability of DDoS detection.

1.3 Research Questions

To address the problem statement, this paper seeks to answer the following research questions:

RQ1: How can a hybrid approach combining rule-based SIEM systems and AI-based intrusion detectors improve DDoS detection?

RQ2: What is the performance of the proposed hybrid Network Intrusion Detection System (NIDS) compared to traditional rule-based or AI-based approaches?

RQ3: What are the strengths and limitations of the proposed hybrid NIDS?

The paper answers the posed research questions and problem statement by presenting and evaluating a novel approach to leveraging rule-based systems in conjunction with machine-learning-based approaches. The paper is organised as follows: Section 3 describes the materials and methods employed to implement the hybrid approach , with Sect. 3.1 explaining the high-level architecture of the proposed hybrid NIDS. In Sect. 4, the experimental setup and results are presented. Then, the findings are discussed in Sect. 5, including insights of possible further research. Finally, Sect. 6 ends the paper with closing remarks.

2 Related Works

The possibility to enhance classic anomaly detection techniques through ML has gained increasing attention in the literature. To address the limitation of classic SIEM systems against novel and complex attacks, a next-gen SIEM framework leveraging ML is proposed in [6]. The combination of Software-Defined Networking (SDN) and AI is exploited in [33] to create a robust SIEM system, meant to protect Industrial Internet of Things (IIoT) applications.

Other research investigates the application of Deep Reinforcement Learning (DRL) in optimizing post-alert incident responses in SIEM systems [4]. Additionally, the possibility of combining SIEM and Intrusion Detection System (IDS) is explored in [14]. The ML-IDS proposed in [19] aims at detecting Internet of Things (IoT) network attacks. In particular, the paper addresses the privacy and security challenges posed by the proliferation of IoT devices. In the same application domain, [39] proposes an IDS enhanced with a hybrid Convolutional Neural Network (CNN) model. The study [21] proposes a packet-based ML model with deferred decision and a single packet integration classifier for network intrusion detection. The solution proposed in [28] consists of a two-stage hybrid methodology for intrusion detection using ML. A classification-based NIDS using big data analytics tools and deep learning approaches is proposed in [3]. Specifically, a Hybrid Deep Learning (HDL) network consisting of CNN and Long short-term memory (LSTM) is used for better results. The potential of ML-NIDS is also highlighted in [22]. In this work, a robust ML-NIDS is proposed, addressing the limitation of classic hybrid approaches, which are vulnerable to attacks not present in the training set.

In comparison to existing works in the literature, the present paper introduces a novel two-stage hybrid approach that leverages rule-based SIEM and AI-based intrusion detectors for accurate and efficient DDoS attack detection, with no need of a labelled dataset.

3 Proposition of the Combined SIEM-AI Approach

This section overviews the proposed approach, providing details on the architecture, the SIEM system, and the AI-based detectors employed.

3.1 High-Level Architecture of the Proposed Combined SIEM-AI Approach

The proposed approach can be schematised as shown in Fig. 1. Real-time network traffic is simulated by replaying the capture of the original dataset. A network probe ships data to the SIEM through an Apache Kafka producer. A static correlation rule is created to discriminate between regular and anomalous traffic. As a result of the correlation rule, the original samples are labelled as malicious or benign according to the pre-defined criteria. This procedure formulates a novel dataset, which is identical to the original one, with the exception of the labels attributed by the SIEM correlation rule. The SIEM-labelled dataset is used to train the ML models, while the original dataset is used to test them. Subsequently, such analysis is utilised to further improve the detection of anomalous traffic. This turns the SIEM into an effective annotation tool which facilitates the possibility of employing supervised ML algorithms.

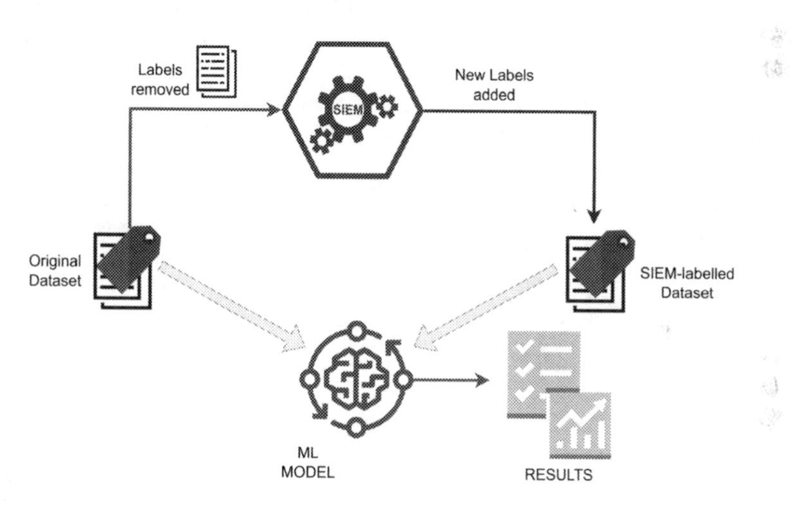

Fig. 1. Architecture of the proposed approach. The correlation logic defined within the SIEM labels the events as benign or anomalies, and the newly labelled dataset is created.

3.2 SIEM Rule-Based Approach

In the proposed approach, a rule-based SIEM has been employed starting from the authors' previous work [9]. The distilled depiction of the architecture of the tool, focusing on the components integral to the research performed in this work, is presented in Fig. 2.

The correlation engine is equipped with a rule designer, which facilitates the formulation of static correlation rules through a user-friendly and intuitive graphical interface. The creation of a rule begins with the definition of a data

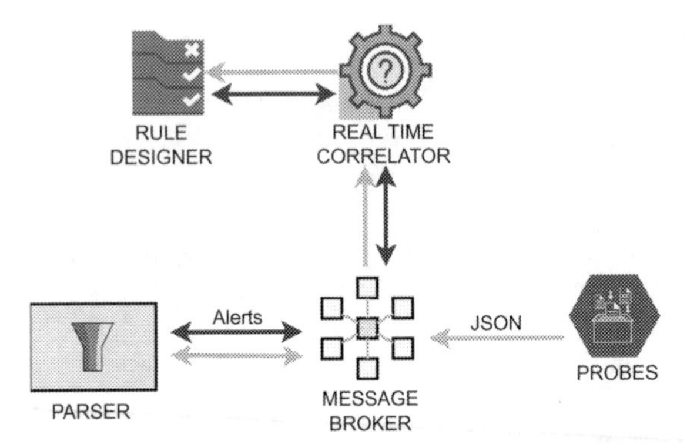

Fig. 2. Streamlined architecture of the SIEM employed in the proposed approach.

source, which is chosen among the available sources on the Kafka broker. In order to design the rules, different building blocks can be used, using all the operations offered by the correlation engine. The building phase of the rule always needs an input block, a set of processing blocks, and an output block. It is possible to perform different operations in the processing blocks, such as: aggregate in the same flow different incoming messages in a defined time window, join different message flows together, filter some events after some parameters exceed a threshold, use the threat intelligence operator to enrich the events and so on. Finally, the result of the correlation is sent to an output topic. In the proposed use case example, the network logs in the original dataset refer to normal traffic, labelled as BENIGN, and intrusion traffic of a DDoS attack. Throughout the experiments conducted, different correlation criteria have been studied to ensure an efficient detection of the anomalous traffic. Hence, the most relevant criteria have been identified, in order to obtain a new labelled dataset.

The logic behind the creation of the SIEM-labelled Dataset can be formalized as follows. Let X represent the set of features in the original dataset D, and let $y = \{DDoS, BENIGN\}$ be the corresponding labels. The aim is to identify x_{rule} and use it as discrimination criteria between DDoS and BENIGN samples. As shown in Eq. 1, to minimize the number of mislabelled samples, the difference between the original set of labels and the SIEM-labelled one must be minimized.

$$x_{rule} \in X : min_{x_{rule}} |y_{siem} \setminus y| \tag{1}$$

In this work, two different SIEM-labelled datasets are considered, corresponding to two different correlation rules.

The SIEM-labelled Dataset D_1 has been created as shown in Eq. 2.

$$y_{D1} = \begin{cases} DDoS & if\ FlowDuration \geq T_{FlowDuration} \\ BENIGN & otherwise \end{cases} \tag{2}$$

where $T_{FlowDuration}$ is the threshold selected for the feature. `Flow Duration` has been selected as the most intuitive criteria to consider for DDoS attacks.

Although the distribution of D_1 was similar to the original dataset, there was still a relevant number of mislabelled samples. As an improvement, a linear correlation analysis has been performed between the dataset features and the DDoS label. Let C be the correlation index and x_i be the ith feature in the dataset. The linear correlation analysis selects the feature x_i with the highest correlation index, as shown in Eq. 3:

$$j = argmax_i(C(f_i, DDoS)) \tag{3}$$

After the analysis, the feature with the highest correlation index (f_j = `Bwd Packet Length Mean`) has been selected for the creation of D_2, following the same logic shown in Eq. 2 for the correlation rule. The thresholds have been set equal to the mean value of the selected feature for the entire dataset,

3.3 AI-Based Intrusion Detectors

The following are the ML algorithms tested with the use of the datasets formulated with the use of SIEM.

Random Forests. The Random Forest classifier is a well-established supervised machine learning technique which leverages the decision trees algorithm improved with bootstrap aggregation (bagging). In principle, the algorithm constructs a multitude of decision trees on random subsamples of the training dataset. This diversity allows the algorithm to capture varied insights about the data. Each individual decision tree becomes a 'weak learner', and their collective input towards the prediction of the entire forest is consolidated via a majority vote [7,17]. The Random Forest algorithm has been found to be very proficient in network intrusion detection [27].

Deep Neural Networks. Artificial Neural Networks (ANNs) use a multitude of neurons and the adjustable weights between those neurons to acquire knowledge from data [34]. In the training phase, the optimisation algorithm uses the discrepancy between the ANN prediction and the factual state to adjust the weights between the nodes and improve the ANNs performance, minimising the error. The neurons can be organised in multiple layers, providing a degree of abstraction, and allowing the network to formulate a more effective set of features from the provided inputs [35,36]. Over the last decade, ANNs and their many flavours have taken the world by storm, starting from the introduction of deep learning [24]. Recently, they have been immensely successful in network intrusion detection as well [29].

To benchmark the algorithms against an approach working in similar conditions, the Isolation Forest is used as an anomaly detector.

Isolation Forest. The 'Isolation Forest' is an unsupervised machine learning algorithm adept at anomaly detection, operating on the principle of isolating anomalies instead of profiling normal data points [26]. The algorithm builds multiple decision trees, much like a Random Forest; however, in each tree, a random feature is selected, and a random split value is defined. This process is repeated until all data points have been isolated or a specified limit on tree depth has been reached. The key intuition is that anomalies are uncommon and different, thus they can be isolated with fewer random partitions than normal points. Consequently, anomalies will tend to have shorter average paths in the isolation trees [26]. The capabilities of Isolation Forest have been effectively utilised in network intrusion detection [23].

4 Experimental Setup and Results

In this section, a detailed description of the experimental setup used to evaluate the proposed hybrid NIDS is presented, starting with the dataset preparation.

In order to train the ML models and generate the events to feed the SIEM system, the CICIDS2017 dataset [37] has been employed.

After the creation of D_1 and D_2, the ML models have been implemented and tested. The first algorithm used for classification is Random Forest. Subsequently, a DNN model has been implemented. The model architecture consisted of an input layer with `ReLU` activation, a hidden layer, and an output layer with `softmax` activation for multi-class classification. The number of units in each layer was determined based on empirical testing to strike a balance between model complexity and performance. The Neural Network model was tuned using a GridSearch to find the optimal combination of hyperparameters. The grid search explored different combinations of hyperparameters, including the choice of optimizer, activation functions, and batch sizes. The best combination of hyperparameters was identified based on cross-validated accuracy scores. In particular, with accuracy score of 0.868696, the following combination has been employed: `GELU` activation, a batch size of 1, and `Nadam optimizer`. The model has been trained for 10 epochs.

Both ML models were evaluated using the testing part of the original dataset as the test set, and the training part of the SIEM-labelled dataset as the train set. Specifically, the efficacy of the Hhybrid NIDS was gauged by employing a variety of evaluation metrics, encompassing Precision (4), Recall (5), F1-Score (6), and Accuracy (7). These metrics provide a holistic overview of the system's performance, each focusing on different aspects of prediction results.

$$\text{Precision} = \frac{\text{True Positive}}{\text{True Positive} + \text{False Positive}} \tag{4}$$

$$\text{Recall} = \frac{\text{True Positive}}{\text{True Positive} + \text{False Negative}} \tag{5}$$

$$\text{F1 Score} = 2 \times \frac{\text{Precision} \times \text{Recall}}{\text{Precision} + \text{Recall}} \tag{6}$$

$$\text{Accuracy} = \frac{\text{Number of Correct Predictions}}{\text{Total Number of Predictions}} \tag{7}$$

The results are summarized in Table 1 for the Random Forest Model and the NN for both SIEM-labelled datasets D_1 and D_2. The benchmark of Isolation Forest is contained in Table 2.

Table 1. Summary of classification reports for different SIEM-labelled dataset implemented using different correlation rules.

Model	Datasets	Precision		Recall		F1-score		Accuracy
		BENIGN	DDoS	BENIGN	DDoS	BENIGN	DDoS	
Random Forest	D_1	0.79	0.62	0.46	0.88	0.58	0.73	0.67
	D_2	0.73	0.96	0.97	0.64	0.83	0.76	0.8
Neural Network	D_1	0.78	0.62	0.45	0.87	0.57	0.72	0.66
	D_2	0.67	0.92	0.96	0.55	0.78	0.67	0.73

Table 2. Classification report using Isolation Forest on the test samples of the original dataset.

Model	Precision		Recall		F1-score		Accuracy
	BENIGN	DDoS	BENIGN	DDoS	BENIGN	DDoS	
Isolation Forest	0.42	0.19	0.67	0.08	0.52	0.11	0.37

The scrutiny of the performance metrics of both the RF and DNN models across datasets D_1 and D_2 highlights that the RF Model consistently exhibits superior performance in terms of Precision, Recall, F1-Score, and Accuracy.

For the RF Model evaluated on dataset D_1, the Precision metric for benign instances (0.79) significantly surpasses that of DDoS instances (0.62). This observation mirrors the performance exhibited by the DNN model. However, the recall for DDoS instances exceeds that of benign instances for both models, thereby suggesting a heightened efficacy of the models in the classification of DDoS instances, at the expense of an increased number of false positives, though. This is in line with the description provided earlier.

Transitioning to the analysis of dataset D_2, the RF Model continues the performance observed in D_1 by exhibiting superior precision for benign instances (0.73) over DDoS instances (0.96). In contrast to D_1, the recall for benign instances (0.97) overwhelmingly outperforms that of DDoS instances (0.64), suggesting a heightened capability of the model to detect benign instances with a lower likelihood of false positives.

In alignment with these observations, the DNN model, when evaluated on D_2, exhibits similar performance characteristics. However, the divergence in precision and recall between benign and DDoS instances is more pronounced in the DNN model than in the RF Model.

Comparing the model performance across the two datasets reveals a clear trend of superior performance on dataset D_2 as opposed to D_1; this observation holds for both models in terms of overall accuracy.

Finally, an evaluation against the benchmark model, namely the Isolation Forest, manifests a substantial performance superiority for both the RF trained with SIEM labelled data and DNN trained with SIEM labelled data across all performance metrics.

These results remain contingent on the specific experimental conditions and dataset characteristics. Consequently, the observed model performance may exhibit variability under different conditions or with diverse datasets. A further exploration of model alternatives or the adoption of ensemble methodologies may present opportunities for additional enhancement in performance.

5 Discussion and Way Forward

In the present section, strengths and limitations of the proposed NIDS are presented, followed by a discussion on threats to validity, and an overview of possible future work.

5.1 Discussion

The hybrid NIDS's major strengths include the ability to adapt to new attack patterns, along with real-time detection capabilities, and improved accuracy compared to individual components. The major benefit of this approach is the ability to employ supervised algorithms with data labelled automatically through the rule-based SIEM. This opens the way to all the benefits of supervised ML, including scalability and efficiency, adaptability to new threats, less human intervention when compared to rule-based SIEMs, and more advanced techniques like the accumulation of knowledge through transfer learning.

The inherent limitations of static correlation logic utilised in the SIEM may hinder the training process of the ML-based detectors. Further advancements in order to optimise the labelling process, reducing the inaccuracies, and improving the quality of data are necessary.

5.2 Threats to Validity

Among the factors that may have influenced the outcomes of the present research study, the dataset selection plays a crucial role. The performance of the hybrid NIDS is dependent on the quality and representativeness of the datasets used for training and testing. While the CICIDS2017 is a well-known and established benchmark, it does not encompass all the possible DDoS attack variants. Additionally, data preprocessing steps such as missing value handling, duplicate removal, dimensionality reduction and data balancing can potentially impact the results, introducing biases or artifacts. A crucial aspect to consider in future work is that the accuracy of the labelled dataset generated by the rule-based SIEM system directly influences the performance of the hybrid NIDS.

5.3 Future Work

The present research provides insights to enhance classic rule-based SIEM and ML detectors. However, further research is required to address the limitations of the preliminary experimental approach. Further improvement could involve a broader dataset collection, more sophisticated data preprocessing techniques, and a thorough investigation of different evaluation metrics. Most importantly, in order to improve the labelling process of the SIEM-labelled dataset, future work will explore advanced correlation techniques and labelling approaches, reducing misclassification and enhancing the quality of the labelled data. As a further advancement, the authors will be using variants of association rule mining to find more advanced criteria for SIEM rules. Finally, while this study focused on combining the rule-based SIEM system with Random Forest and Neural Network classifiers, future research could investigate hybrid approaches with other ML algorithms.

6 Conclusions

The paper presented a novel hybrid approach for improving the accuracy and efficiency of DDoS attack detection in network traffic. By combining a rule-based SIEM system with supervised ML algorithms, the proposed research aims at addressing the limitations of both traditional rule-based approaches and ML techniques. The rule-based SIEM system has been proven as an effective tool to label the data, providing the required labelled dataset for ML. The experimental evaluation has involved RF and DNN classifiers, with the comparison of the performance of the hybrid NIDS against Isolation Forest based anomaly detector. The collaboration between the SIEM and ML models allows to leverage the strengths of each component. Future research will focus on further improving the SIEM-based labelling process, reducing misclassifications, and exploring more advanced correlation techniques. Additionally, investigating hybrid approaches with other AI models may offer further improvements in network intrusion detection.

References

1. Ahmad, A., Desouza, K.C., Maynard, S.B., Naseer, H., Baskerville, R.L.: How integration of cyber security management and incident response enables organizational learning. J. Am. Soc. Inf. Sci. **71**(8), 939–953 (2020)
2. Akter, S., Uddin, M.R., Sajib, S., Lee, W.J.T., Michael, K., Hossain, M.A.: Reconceptualizing cybersecurity awareness capability in the data-driven digital economy. Ann. Oper. Res. **315**, 1–26 (2022). https://doi.org/10.1007/s10479-022-04844-8
3. Al, S., Dener, M.: STL-HDL: a new hybrid network intrusion detection system for imbalanced dataset on big data environment. Comput. Secur. **110**, 102435 (2021). https://doi.org/10.1016/j.cose.2021.102435
4. Alturkistani, H., El-Affendi, M.A.: Optimizing cybersecurity incident response decisions using deep reinforcement learning. Int. J. Electr. Comput. Eng. **12**(6), 6768 (2022)

5. Ardagna, C., Corbiaux, S., Impe, K.V., Sfakianaki, A.: ENISA threat landscape (2022). https://www.enisa.europa.eu/publications/enisa-threat-landscape-2022
6. Ban, T., Takahashi, T., Ndichu, S., Inoue, D.: Breaking alert fatigue: Ai-assisted SIEM framework for effective incident response. Appl. Sci. **13**(11), 6610 (2023)
7. Breiman, L.: Random forests. Mach. Learn. **45**, 5–32 (2001). https://doi.org/10.1023/A:1010933404324
8. Campfield, M.: The problem with (most) network detection and response. Netw. Secur. **2020**(9), 6–9 (2020)
9. Coppolino, L., et al.: Detection of radio frequency interference in satellite ground segments. In: 2023 IEEE International Conference on Cyber Security and Resilience (CSR), pp. 648–653 (2023). https://doi.org/10.1109/CSR57506.2023.10225005
10. Cucu, C., Cazacu, M.: Current technologies and trends in cybersecurity and the impact of artificial intelligence. In: The International Scientific Conference eLearning and Software for Education, vol. 2, pp. 208–214. " Carol I" National Defence University (2019)
11. Dowling, J.F., Sellers, J.E.: Chapter 34 - security awareness. In: Davies, S.J., Fennelly, L.J. (eds.) The Professional Protection Officer (Second Edition), pp. 391–396. Butterworth-Heinemann, Boston, second edn. (2020). https://doi.org/10.1016/B978-0-12-817748-8.00034-1, https://www.sciencedirect.com/science/article/pii/B9780128177488000341
12. Duo, W., Zhou, M., Abusorrah, A.: A survey of cyber attacks on cyber physical systems: recent advances and challenges. IEEE/CAA J. Automatica Sin. **9**(5), 784–800 (2022). https://doi.org/10.1109/JAS.2022.105548
13. Dutta, V., Choras, M., Pawlicki, M., Kozik, R.: Detection of cyberattacks traces in IoT data. J. Univers. Comput. Sci. **26**(11), 1422–1434 (2020)
14. Esseghir, A., Kamoun, F., Hraiech, O.: AKER: an open-source security platform integrating ids and SIEM functions with encrypted traffic analytic capability. J. Cyber Secur. Technol. **6**(1–2), 27–64 (2022)
15. Fakiha, B.S.: Effectiveness of security incident event management (SIEM) system for cyber security situation awareness. Indian J. Forensic Med. Toxicol. **14**(4), 802–808 (2020)
16. Guembe, B., Azeta, A., Misra, S., Osamor, V.C., Fernandez-Sanz, L., Pospelova, V.: The emerging threat of AI-driven cyber attacks: a review. Appl. Artif. Intell. **36**(1), 2037254 (2022)
17. Ho, T.K.: Random decision forests. In: Proceedings of 3rd International Conference on Document Analysis and Recognition, vol. 1, pp. 278–282. IEEE (1995)
18. Jakub, P.: Russia's war on Ukraine: timeline of cyber-attacks (2022)
19. Kayode Saheed, Y., Idris Abiodun, A., Misra, S., Kristiansen Holone, M., Colomo-Palacios, R.: A machine learning-based intrusion detection for detecting internet of things network attacks. Alex. Eng. J. **61**(12), 9395–9409 (2022). https://doi.org/10.1016/j.aej.2022.02.063
20. Khader, R., Eleyan, D.: Survey of DoS/DDoS attacks in IoT. Sustain. Eng. Innov. **3**(1), 23–28 (2021)
21. Kim, T., Pak, W.: Real-time network intrusion detection using deferred decision and hybrid classifier. Futur. Gener. Comput. Syst. **132**, 51–66 (2022). https://doi.org/10.1016/j.future.2022.02.011
22. Kim, T., Pak, W.: Robust network intrusion detection system based on machine-learning with early classification. IEEE Access **10**, 10754–10767 (2022). https://doi.org/10.1109/ACCESS.2022.3145002
23. Laskar, M.T.R., et al.: Extending isolation forest for anomaly detection in big data via k-means. ACM Trans. Cyber-Phys. Syst. (TCPS) **5**(4), 1–26 (2021)

24. LeCun, Y., Bengio, Y., Hinton, G.: Deep learning. Nature **521**(7553), 436–444 (2015)
25. Li, Y., Liu, Q.: A comprehensive review study of cyber-attacks and cyber security; emerging trends and recent developments. Energy Rep. **7**, 8176–8186 (2021). https://doi.org/10.1016/j.egyr.2021.08.126
26. Liu, F.T., Ting, K.M., Zhou, Z.H.: Isolation forest. In: 2008 Eighth IEEE International Conference on Data Mining, pp. 413–422 (2008). https://doi.org/10.1109/ICDM.2008.17
27. Mihailescu, M.E., et al.: The proposition and evaluation of the RoEduNet-SIMARGL2021 network intrusion detection dataset. Sensors **21**(13), 4319 (2021)
28. Narayana Rao, K., Venkata Rao, K., PVGD, P.R.: A hybrid intrusion detection system based on sparse autoencoder and deep neural network. Comput. Commun. **180**, 77–88 (2021). https://doi.org/10.1016/j.comcom.2021.08.026, https://www.sciencedirect.com/science/article/pii/S0140366421003285
29. Pawlicki, M., Kozik, R., Choraś, M.: A survey on neural networks for (cyber-) security and (cyber-) security of neural networks. Neurocomputing **500**, 1075–1087 (2022)
30. Pawlicki, M., Pawlicka, A., Kozik, R., Choraś, M.: The survey and meta-analysis of the attacks, transgressions, countermeasures and security aspects common to the cloud, edge and IoT. Neurocomputing **551**, 126533 (2023)
31. Perwej, Y., Abbas, S.Q., Dixit, J.P., Akhtar, N., Jaiswal, A.K.: A systematic literature review on the cyber security. Int. J. Sci. Res. Manag. **9**(12), 669–710 (2021)
32. Priyanka, S., Vijay Bhanu, S.: A survey on variants of dos attacks: issues and defense mechanisms. J. Appl. Res. Technol. **21**(1), 12–16 (2023)
33. Radoglou-Grammatikis, P.: Securecyber: an SDN-enabled SIEM for enhanced cybersecurity in the industrial internet of things. IEEE COMSOC MMTC Commun. - Front. **18**(2), 16–21 (2023)
34. Rosenblatt, F.: The perceptron: a probabilistic model for information storage and organization in the brain. Psychol. Rev. **65**(6), 386 (1958)
35. Rumelhart, D.E., Hinton, G.E., Williams, R.J.: Learning representations by back-propagating errors. Nature **323**(6088), 533–536 (1986)
36. Rumelhart, D.E., McClelland, J.L., PDP Research Group, C.: Parallel Distributed Processing: Explorations in the Microstructure of Cognition, vol. 1: Foundations. MIT press (1986)
37. Sharafaldin, I., Lashkari, A.H., Ghorbani, A.A.: Toward generating a new intrusion detection dataset and intrusion traffic characterization. ICISSp **1**, 108–116 (2018)
38. Sheeraz, M., et al.: Effective security monitoring using efficient SIEM architecture. Hum. - Centric Comput. Inf. Sci **13**, 1–18 (2023)
39. Smys, S., Basar, A., Wang, H., et al.: Hybrid intrusion detection system for internet of things (IoT). J. ISMAC **2**(04), 190–199 (2020)
40. Tariq, A., Manzoor, J., Aziz, M.A., Tariq, Z.U.A., Masood, A.: Open source SIEM solutions for an enterprise. Inform. Comput. Secur. **31**(1), 88–107 (2022)

Security Challenges and Solutions in Smart Cities

Faisal Alzyoud[1], Ruba Al-Falah[2], Monther Tarawneh[1](✉), and Omar Tarawneh[3]

[1] Computer Science Department, Isra University, Amman, Jordan
{faisal.alzyoud,mtarawneh}@iu.edu.jo
[2] Ministry of Local Administration, Amman, Jordan
ruba.ajarmeh@moma.gov.jo
[3] Software Engineering Department, Amman Arab University, Amman, Jordan
o.husain@aau.edu.jo

Abstract. The increase of smart devices and vast amount of telecommunication growth raise the tendency to convert convolution cities in to emerging smart cities. This paper synthesizes key findings and insights from a comprehensive presentation, addressing critical aspects of smart city security. It underscores the pivotal role of robust security strategies in the development and sustainability of smart urban environments. This paper, encompass three main areas: the integration of Artificial Intelligence (AI) and machine learning for real-time threat detection, the imperative of adopting quantum-safe cryptography, and the evolving nature of security threats in smart cities. These trends and challenges necessitate proactive measures, reinforcing the need for security to be a fundamental component of smart city blueprints. In conclusion, this paper advocates for collaborative efforts and ongoing research in smart city security. It calls upon stakeholders from diverse sectors to join forces, share knowledge, and develop innovative solutions. By doing so, we can navigate the complex security landscape of smart cities and shape a future where technology and security coexist harmoniously, ensuring the well-being and prosperity of urban communities.

Keywords: Artificial Intelligence (AI) · Internet of Things (IoT) · Cyber Security · Smart cities · Threats

1 Introduction

The proliferation of smart devices and the development of communication systems with the rapid global urbanization has concentrated needs to transfer the exist cities to smart ones, since the concept of smart cities has emerged as a focal point for addressing the complex challenges of modern urban life. A smart city represents an innovative and holistic urban ecosystem that harnesses state-of-the-art technologies and data-driven solutions to not only elevate the quality of life for its inhabitants but also to optimize resource utilization, enhance sustainability, and streamline the various intricacies of urban living. At its core, a smart city integrates a sophisticated digital infrastructure, employs advanced data analytics, and fosters seamless connectivity to intelligently manage and

K. Daimi and A. Al Sadoon (Eds.): ACR 2024, LNNS 956, pp. 256–267, 2024.
https://doi.org/10.1007/978-3-031-56950-0_22

distribute resources, boost operational efficiency, and stimulate groundbreaking innovations across key sectors such as transportation, energy management, healthcare, and municipal governance [1]. As urban centers become magnets for population growth and aspirations, the significance of smart cities becomes ever more apparent. The relentless influx of individuals into cities in search of improved opportunities and a higher quality of life amplifies the need for urban spaces to adapt and cater to diverse needs. Smart cities have emerged as a compelling response to these challenges by leveraging technology as a dynamic force to manage resources judiciously, enhance the well-being of residents, and foster an environment that encourages sustainable growth [2]. By intertwining technology and data-driven strategies, smart cities are poised to enhance urban experience, address pressing urban issues, and catalyze advancements that transcend traditional urban planning [3].

In the intricate tapestry of urban existence, smart cities serve as an oasis of innovation amidst challenges posed by congestion, inadequate resource allocation, and environmental degradation. The potential benefits of smart cities are multifaceted and encompass a spectrum of advantages that reverberate throughout urban life [4]. From the efficient management of resources like energy and water to the creation of intelligent transportation systems that mitigate traffic congestion, smart cities hold the promise of a better quality of life for their citizens [5]. Moreover, they champion environmental sustainability through optimized waste management and reduced carbon footprints, thereby contributing to the global fight against climate change. In tandem with technological prowess, smart cities offer economic opportunities by fostering innovation hubs and attracting investments, setting the stage for economic growth that is both inclusive and sustainable [6]. Additionally, these cities amplify citizen participation and engagement, empowering residents to actively contribute to urban development decisions and ensuring a sense of ownership in shaping the city's future. However, the rapid integration of digital systems and the increasing interconnectivity that characterize smart cities also introduce new layers of vulnerability [7]. As the urban landscape becomes more reliant on digital infrastructure, the security and resilience of these systems become paramount. Cybersecurity threats, data breaches, and privacy concerns can undermine the very foundations of a smart city, jeopardizing the benefits they promise. Ensuring the integrity and confidentiality of sensitive data, safeguarding critical infrastructure from cyberattacks, and maintaining the privacy of citizens in a hyper-connected environment are challenges that require immediate attention [8]. The potential consequences of security breaches in a smart city context extend beyond financial losses to encompass compromised citizen safety, loss of public trust, and hindrance to overall urban development progress.

As smart city development surges forward, addressing security issues becomes a critical imperative. The integration of security measures that safeguard data, digital infrastructure, and citizen privacy serves as the cornerstone of sustainable and successful smart city implementation [9]. Only through a comprehensive and proactive approach to security can the potential benefits of smart cities be fully realized, assuring citizens of a safe and resilient urban environment that harmonizes technological innovation with the fundamental principles of security and privacy [10]. As the momentum towards smart cities gains pace, the advantages of harnessing cutting-edge technologies and data-centric solutions to enrich urban living are becoming progressively apparent. Nonetheless, this paradigm shift is accompanied by its own set of hurdles. The fusion of digital systems, in tandem with the proliferation of interconnected devices, gives rise to an intricate security terrain that requires scrupulous consideration. The intricate interplay between technological progress and security susceptibilities underscores the critical need to fully grasp the multifaceted security threat landscape that smart cities traverse.

2 Security Threat Landscape

Smart cities, propelled by advancements in technology and interconnectedness, encounter a wide spectrum of security challenges rooted in their intricate digital ecosystem. The convergence of complex and interdependent digital systems underpins these vulnerabilities. Among the foremost concerns are cybersecurity threats, which encompass hacking, malware, and ransomware attacks that specifically target critical infrastructure, sensitive data, and the network of interconnected devices as it is shown in Fig. 1. The multifaceted physical infrastructure woven throughout smart cities is not immune, facing potential vulnerabilities from physical assaults to tampering with essential components and sensors, which could disrupt crucial services. As the collection of vast volumes of personal and sensitive information accelerates, concerns over data privacy escalate, exposing smart cities to unauthorized access, data breaches, and surveillance risks. The manipulation of human vulnerabilities through social engineering tactics further accentuates the security landscape, coercing individuals into divulging confidential information or granting unauthorized entry. The expansion of the Internet of Things (IoT) ecosystem, while enhancing convenience, introduces novel avenues for exploitation, potentially weaponizing compromised devices to breach digital networks. The threat of insider misuse looms, as authorized personnel might exploit their access privileges to undermine security. Susceptibility to network vulnerabilities, stemming from insecure communication channels or weak points within digital frameworks, provides openings for malicious actors to exploit. The interconnectedness of diverse systems creates a domino effect, enabling threats to spread across sectors, exacerbating the consequences of a breach. External attack vectors, often originating from the broader internet, threaten targeted assaults on smart city infrastructure. Additionally, intercepting data during transmission risks unauthorized access and manipulation of sensitive information. Navigating this intricate security landscape requires a comprehensive understanding to formulate effective strategies that safeguard the intricate components constituting smart cities.

By the overwhelm of modern technology, hacking and data breaches have emerged as critical issues within the context of smart city infrastructure. These external attack vectors, often originating from the broader internet, pose a significant threat to the seamless operation of smart cities. They target vital components such as data centers, communication networks, and IoT devices, aiming to disrupt services and compromise the integrity of data flows. Moreover, intercepting data during transmission poses a substantial risk, potentially leading to unauthorized access and manipulation of sensitive information crucial for efficient urban management. Navigating this intricate security landscape demands a comprehensive understanding of emerging threats and vulnerabilities to formulate effective strategies [11]. It is imperative to implement robust security measures and stay ahead in the constant battle to safeguard the intricate components constituting smart cities, ensuring the resilience and reliability of these innovative urban ecosystems.

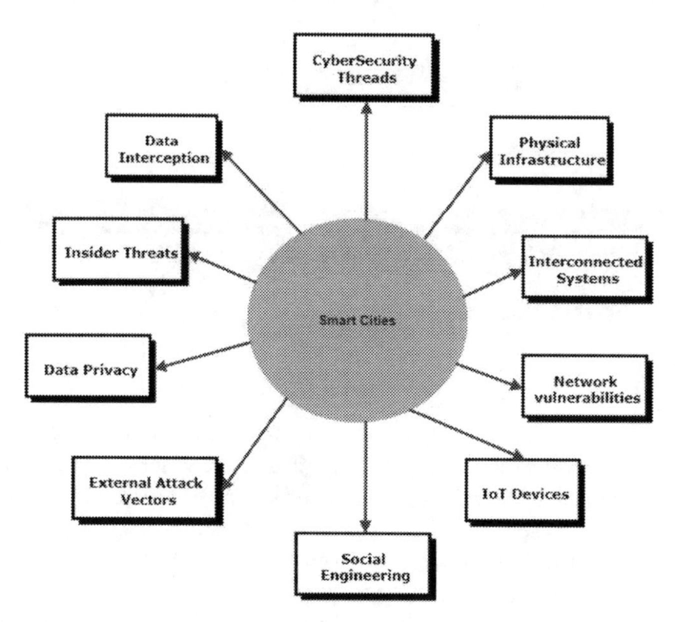

Fig. 1. Smart City Security Threat Landscape

Surveillance and data misuse represent additional layers of concern within the complex security landscape of smart cities. As external attack vectors threaten smart city infrastructure, the extensive surveillance networks deployed within these urban ecosystems are at risk of being exploited for nefarious purposes. Unauthorized access to surveillance feeds or data repositories can compromise citizens' privacy and lead to serious breaches of trust. The potential for data misuse, whether by malicious actors or even well-intentioned authorities, underscores the importance of robust data protection and ethical data handling practices. Safeguarding the integrity of surveillance systems and ensuring responsible data usage is pivotal to maintaining the delicate balance between enhancing urban security and respecting individual privacy in the context of smart cities [12]. Comprehensive strategies must address both external threats and the responsible management of the vast data streams generated by these surveillance networks to preserve the core principles of a truly smart and secure urban environment.

In the intricate realm of smart city security, physical vulnerabilities, such as critical infrastructure attacks and sensor tampering, add yet another layer of complexity to the multifaceted security landscape. External attack vectors and data misuse represent significant threats, but they can be compounded when combined with the potential for direct physical harm to the city's critical infrastructure. Attacks on power grids, transportation networks, or water supply systems can cripple essential services and disrupt urban life [13]. Simultaneously, sensor tampering introduces the risk of false data injection, leading to inaccurate decision-making and potentially dangerous consequences for city operations. The following diagram illustrates the interplay between external attack vectors, data misuse, and physical vulnerabilities, emphasizing the need for a holistic approach to smart city security that addresses both digital and physical threats.

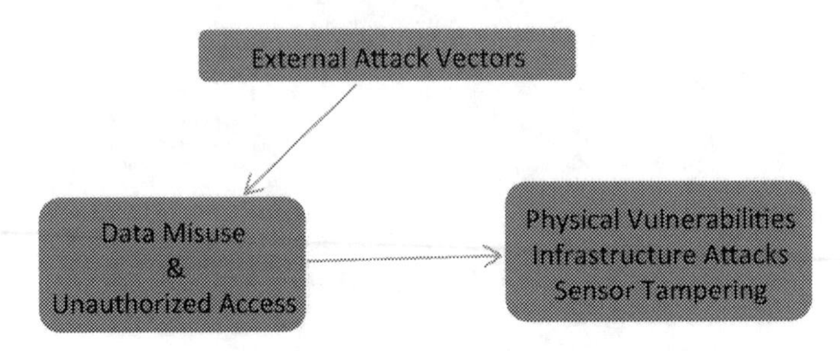

Fig. 2. Interplay of Threat Vectors in Smart Cities.

Figure 2 represents the complex relationship between external attack vectors, data misuse, and physical vulnerabilities, such as infrastructure attacks and sensor tampering, within the context of smart city security. The arrows signify the potential interactions and dependencies among these key security aspects, highlighting the need for a comprehensive security strategy to protect modern urban environments. Within the intricate tapestry sophisticated and web of smart city security considerations, the threat of social engineering, encompassing the manipulation of human behavior, forms yet another critical dimension. Just as external attack vectors, data misuse, and physical vulnerabilities pose tangible risks, human factors can amplify these threats significantly. Social engineering exploits human psychology and trust to deceive individuals into divulging sensitive information or engaging in actions that could compromise the integrity of smart city systems. For example, an attacker might use social engineering techniques to gain access to critical infrastructure control centers or manipulate sensor operators. The potential repercussions of such manipulations on a city's operations are profound, underscoring the importance of holistic security measures that encompass both digital and human centric safeguards. This comprehensive approach aims to protect against not only technical vulnerabilities but also the vulnerabilities inherent in human interactions, creating a robust defense against multifaceted threats [14]. While addressing the multifaceted security challenges in smart cities, it's crucial to recognize the presence of amplifying factors that can exacerbate existing vulnerabilities as shown in the next section which requires proactive measures to enhance security and resilience.

3 Security Amplifying Factors (SAFs) A Subsection Sample

Security Amplifying Factors (SAFs) are crucial elements that enhance the overall security posture of an organization or system. Since, they are used to identify and leverage factors of defenses which are necessary to protect sensitive information. SAFs encompass a wide range of practices, technologies, and strategies, all aimed at minimizing risks and increasing resilience against cyberattacks. Smart cities, which leverage advanced technologies to enhance urban living introduce new challenges and vulnerabilities in security risks [15]. However, this transformation comes with a host of new challenges, especially in the realm of cybersecurity. The security risks in smart cities are amplified by several interconnected factors, which demand careful consideration and proactive measures to mitigate as shown in Fig. 3. These factors include:

- Interconnected Systems that rely on intricate networks of interconnected systems, such as transportation, energy, and public services [16].
- Data Privacy and Surveillance which depends on the collection and analysis of vast amounts of data in smart cities, as this raises the concerns about privacy and surveillance [17].
- IoT Vulnerabilities, this result from the proliferation of Internet of Things (IoT) devices in smart cities which introduces vulnerabilities. Weak device security, unpatched devices, and insecure communications can be exploited to gain unauthorized access [18].
- Vendor Dependencies, smart city projects often rely on various vendors and third-party services, so this will expose cities to several risks such as supply chain attacks, vendor vulnerabilities, and challenges in accountability [19].
- Lack of Awareness, both city officials and residents may lack awareness of the potential security risks associated with smart city technologies. Insufficient training and a lack of security education can result in poor security practice [20].

Complexity and Scale, the sheer complexity and scale of smart city systems can be overwhelming. Managing and securing such vast and intricate networks pose significant challenges, including resource allocation, network architecture, and system overload [21].

Safeguarding smart city infrastructures requires a proactive stance. Leveraging cutting-edge technologies such as advanced encryption, intrusion detection systems, and secure data sharing protocols, combined with comprehensive cybersecurity policies and threat intelligence sharing among cities can help fortify the resilience of smart city ecosystems. Ultimately, addressing these challenges while embracing innovative security solutions is essential to ensuring the safety, privacy, and reliability of our urban environments.

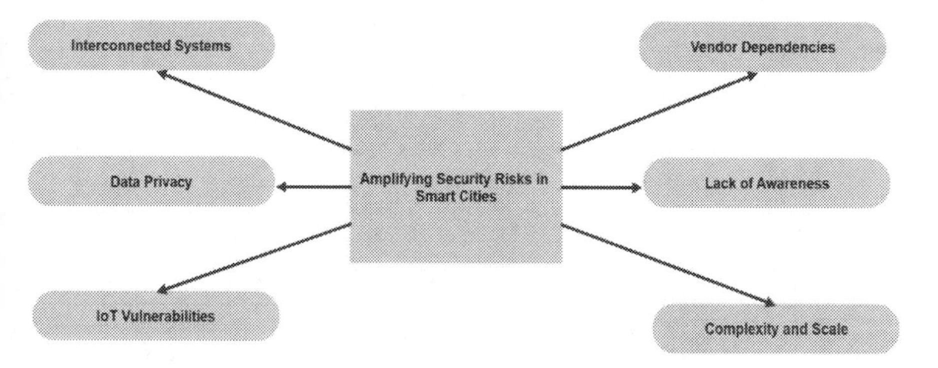

Fig. 3. Cause and Effect Diagram for Security Risks in Smart Cities

4 Security Measures and Solutions

The transformation to smart cities incurs several key security strategies to encompass a multifaceted approach which are essential to protect digital and physical assets. These strategies emphasize the importance of data encryption, stringent access controls, and network security measures to thwart cyber threats. Safeguarding IoT devices, ensuring data privacy, and having a robust incident response plan are vital components. Physical

Table 1. A summarization of Cybersecurity Measures Description and Benefits in Smart Cities

Category	Measure	Description	Benefits
Cybersecurity Measures	Encryption	Data is Protected by converting it into unreadable code, preventing unauthorized access	Protects sensitive data from unauthorized access and ensures data confidentiality
	Intrusion Detection	Monitors network and system activities to detect and respond to unauthorized access or breaches	Detects and mitigates cyber threats in real-time, enhancing overall security
Privacy Techniques	Anonymization	Removes or obscures personally identifiable information from datasets, enhancing privacy	Preserves privacy while allowing data analysis for valuable insights
	Differential Privacy	Adds noise or randomness to data to protect individuals' privacy while still allowing analysis	Balances data utility and privacy, preventing reidentification of individuals
Physical Security Enhancements	Access Controls	Restricts physical access to facilities and systems, limiting unauthorized entry	Prevents unauthorized entry and tampering with sensitive assets
	Surveillance	Uses cameras and sensors to monitor physical spaces and assets, enhancing security	Enhances situational awareness and assists in identifying security threats
User Education	Promoting Responsible Behavior	Educates users about cybersecurity best practices and encourages safe online behaviors	Reduces the risk of social engineering attacks and strengthens overall security

security, public awareness campaigns, and collaboration among stakeholders play pivotal roles in creating a secure urban environment. Compliance with regulations, privacy by design, and continuous monitoring are essential for long-term security, while user education and ethical hacking help fortify defenses. Additionally, implementing secure communication channels, well-defined data retention policies, and exploring emerging technologies like blockchain enhance the overall security posture of smart cities. These strategies underscore the importance of adaptability and vigilance in the face of evolving threats.

Table 1 provides a concise overview of each measure and its role in enhancing cybersecurity, privacy, physical security, and user education within the context of smart cities. As, these measures and techniques work together to create a comprehensive security strategy for safeguarding smart cities and their digital and physical assets while respecting privacy and promoting responsible behavior.

5 Privacy Preservation Techniques and Case Studies

In recent years with the spread of smart devices and developing communication mobile technology, cybersecurity has emerged as a critical concern for organizations worldwide. In this section we are going to highlight the understanding of both the successful security strategies and the lessons derived from security failures.

5.1 Effective Security Strategies Implementation

Effective security strategies are essential factor in developing and safeguarding organizations assets in today's digital landscape. These strategies encompass a multi-faceted approach that includes proactive measures such as robust access control, continuous monitoring, and regular vulnerability assessments. Implementing a zero-trust model, where trust is never assumed by default, has gained prominence. Identity and device verification, coupled with threat intelligence, play a central role in mitigating risks [22]. Furthermore, collaboration and information sharing within the cybersecurity community enhance collective defense against evolving threats. Effective security strategies are necessary for any organization to enhance its defenses by fostering its resilience in the face of dynamic cyber threats, ensuring the confidentiality, integrity, and availability of critical data and systems.

There are several successful examples on the effective security strategies implementation such as:

- Google's BeyondCorp: Google's BeyondCorp security model adopts a zero-trust approach, prioritizing identity, and device security. This proactive strategy has proven its effectiveness on insider threats and external attacks [23].
- Microsoft's Azure Security Center: it implements and adapts comprehensive threat protection and vulnerability identification in Microsoft Azure services. This approach enhances the security posture of cloud users, emphasizing the value of proactive security measures [24].

- Equifax's Post-Breach Transformation: its data breach in 2017 with a significant setback, and the company's post-breach response serves as a valuable case study, highlighting the importance of incident response plans and cybersecurity investments [25].

5.2 Security Failures and Their Implications

Critical cybersecurity failures and their lasting implications have direct impact on smart cities, so there is a growing emphasis on understanding the lessons derived from security failures. By analyzing these failures, we gain invaluable insights into the vulnerabilities and weaknesses that organizations face in an increasingly interconnected world. These case studies serve as powerful cautionary tales, highlighting the potential consequences of inadequate security measures. Understanding the implications of these failures is essential for organizations seeking to bolster their defenses, adapt to evolving threats, and safeguard their digital assets effectively.

Examples on lessons learned from failures that serve as a catalyst for enhanced cybersecurity practices, fostering a more secure digital environment are illustrated below.

- **Target's Data Breach:** its data breach exposed the risks associated with third-party vendor vulnerabilities and the need for continuous monitoring [26]
- **Sony Pictures Entertainment Hack:** it hacks and underscores the importance of protecting intellectual property and implementing robust cybersecurity practices, particularly for entertainment companies [27].
- **WannaCry Ransomware Attack:** it affects the organizations worldwide, emphasizing the critical nature of timely software patch management and cybersecurity hygiene [28].

In conclusion, the dynamic landscape of cybersecurity demands a proactive approach that combines effective security strategies with the wisdom gained from past failures. By embracing these principles, organizations can navigate the ever-evolving threat landscape with confidence, fortifying their defenses, and ultimately, ensuring the integrity, availability, and confidentiality of their vital digital assets. As technology advances and cyber threats evolve, the lessons learned from both successes and setbacks provide a roadmap for continuous improvement, resilience, and a safer digital future.

6 Future Directions and Emerging Trends

The future of smart cities encompasses a multifaceted landscape shaped by technological advancements and evolving threats. Security presents a dynamic landscape characterized by emerging trends and significant challenges. First and foremost, the integration of AI and machine learning stands as a pivotal advancement. These technologies offer enhanced threat detection capabilities, allowing for real-time analysis of vast amounts of data generated within smart cities. However, this integration introduces concerns related to privacy and data protection, necessitating robust regulations and ethical considerations. Another critical aspect is the implementation of quantum-safe cryptography. As quantum computing becomes more potent, traditional encryption methods could become obsolete, posing a substantial security risk. Smart cities must proactively adopt quantum-resistant cryptographic techniques to safeguard sensitive data and communications against future quantum threats. Moreover, the anticipated evolution of security threats is a constant concern. As smart city infrastructures become increasingly interconnected and reliant on IoT devices, the attack surface expands, providing cybercriminals with more entry points. Threats such as ransomware, supply chain attacks, and IoT vulnerabilities are expected to evolve in sophistication, demanding continuous security enhancements. Table 2 highlights the emerging trends and future challenges in smart city security, including the integration of AI and machine learning, quantum-safe cryptography considerations, and the anticipated evolution of security threat.

Table 2. Emerging Trends and Future Challenges in Smart City Security

Trends and Challenges	Description
Integration of AI and Machine Learning	Smart cities leverage AI and machine learning for real-time threat detection and analytics, but face challenges related to algorithm security and data privacy
Quantum-Safe Cryptography Considerations	As quantum computing advances, smart cities must adopt quantum-resistant cryptography to safeguard sensitive data from potential quantum attacks
Anticipated Evolution of Security Threats	Smart cities confront evolving security threats that encompass not only cyber threats but also physical and social engineering attacks, necessitating holistic security strategies

7 Conclusion

In conclusion, this paper has concentrated on the crucial aspects of smart city security, emphasizing the need for forward-thinking strategies to address emerging trends and future challenges. Security undeniably plays a critical role in the development and sustainability of smart cities. Without robust security measures, the very foundations of these technologically advanced urban environments can be compromised, leading to significant risks for both citizens and critical infrastructure. It is imperative that security is not merely an afterthought but an integral part of the smart city blueprint from its inception. As we move forward, we must recognize that the challenges we face in securing smart cities are evolving rapidly. This calls for a collective commitment to collaboration and ongoing research in the field. The proactive sharing of knowledge, best practices, and innovative solutions will be instrumental in bolstering the resilience of smart cities against ever-evolving threats. Let us join forces, across industries and academia, to ensure the safety, security, and prosperity of the smart cities of tomorrow. Together, we can shape a future where technology and security go hand in hand, enriching the lives of citizens and fostering sustainable urban development.

References

1. Gade, D.: Introduction to smart cities and selected literature review. Int. J. Adv. Innov. Res. **6**(2), 7–15 (2019)
2. Bjørner, T.: The advantages of and barriers to being smart in a smart city: the perceptions of project managers within a smart city cluster project in Greater Copenhagen. Cities **114**, 103187 (2021)
3. Farahat, I.S., Tolba, A.S., Elhoseny, M., Eladrosy, W.: Data security and challenges in smart cities. Secur. Smart Cities Models Appl. Challenges 117–142 (2019)
4. Alzyoud, F.Y., Wa'elJum'ah Al_Zyadat, F.H., Shrouf, F.: A proposed hybrid approach combined QoS with CR system in smart city. Eurasian J. Anal. Chem. **13**(6), 178–185 (2018)
5. Alzyoud, F.: Improved model for traffic accident management system using KDD and big data: case study Jordan. Int. J. Comput. Commun. Control **18**(3) (2023)
6. Alzyoud, F., Maqableh, W., Al Shrouf, F.: A semi smart adaptive approach for trash classification. Int. J. Comput. Commun. Control **16**(4) (2021)
7. Nafrees, A.C.M., Sujah, A.M.A., Mansoor, C.: Smart cities: emerging technologies and potential solutions to the cyber security threads. In: 2021 5th International Conference on Electrical, Electronics, Communication, Computer Technologies and Optimization Techniques (ICEECCOT), pp. 220–228. IEEE (2021)
8. Sookhak, M., Tang, H., He, Y., Yu, F.R.: Security and privacy of smart cities: a survey, research issues and challenges. IEEE Commun. Surv. Tutor. **21**(2), 1718–1743 (2018)
9. Xia, L., Semirumi, D.T., Rezaei, R.: A thorough examination of smart city applications: exploring challenges and solutions throughout the life cycle with emphasis on safeguarding citizen privacy. Sustain. Cities Soc. **98**, 104771 (2023)
10. Bianchi, I., Schmidt, L.: The smart city revolution: design principles and best practices for urban transformation. Eigenpub Rev. Sci. Technol. **7**(1), 55–70 (2023)
11. Mughal, A.A.: Cybersecurity hygiene in the era of internet of things (IoT): best practices and challenges. Appl. Res. Artif. Intell. Cloud Comput. **2**(1), 1–31 (2019)
12. Mylonas, G., Kalogeras, A., Kalogeras, G., Anagnostopoulos, C., Alexakos, C., Muñoz, L.: Digital twins from smart manufacturing to smart cities: a survey. IEEE Access **9**, 143222–143249 (2021)
13. Alzyoud, F., Alsharman, N., Almofleh, A.: Best practice fundamentals in smart grids for a modern energy system development in Jordan. In: Proceedings of the 9th International Conference on Advances in Computing, Communication and Information Technology, Rome, pp. 7–8 (2019)
14. Ashraf, I., et al.: A survey on cyber security threats in IoT-enabled maritime industry. IEEE Trans. Intell. Transp. Syst. **24**(2), 2677–2690 (2022)
15. Kitchin, R., Dodge, M.: The (in) security of smart cities: vulnerabilities, risks, mitigation, and prevention. In: Smart Cities and Innovative Urban Technologies, pp. 47–65. Routledge (2020)
16. Gedris, K., et al.: Simulating municipal cybersecurity incidents: recommendations from expert interviews. In: Proceedings of the Annual Hawaii International Conference on System Sciences (2021)
17. Cardullo, P., Kitchin, R.: Being a 'citizen' in the smart city: up and down the scaffold of smart citizen participation in Dublin, Ireland. GeoJ **84**(1), 1–13 (2019)
18. Velazquez-Pupo, R., et al.: Vehicle detection with occlusion handling, tracking, and OC-SVM classification: a high performance vision-based system. Sensors **18**(2), 374 (2018)
19. Ustundag, A., Cevikcan, E.: Industry 4.0: Managing the Digital Transformation. Springer, Cham (2017). https://doi.org/10.1007/978-3-319-57870-5

20. Ghiasi, M., Niknam, T., Wang, Z., Mehrandezh, M., Dehghani, M., Ghadimi, N.: A comprehensive review of cyber-attacks and defense mechanisms for improving security in smart grid energy systems: past, present, and future. Electr. Power Syst. Res. **215**, 108975 (2023)
21. Neirotti, P., De Marco, A., Cagliano, A.C., Mangano, G., Scorrano, F.: Current trends in Smart City initiatives: some stylised facts. Cities **38**, 25–36 (2014)
22. Ray, P.P.: Web3: a comprehensive review on background, technologies, applications, zero-trust architectures, challenges, and future directions. Internet of Things and Cyber-Physical Systems (2023)
23. Buck, C., Olenberger, C., Schweizer, A., Völter, F., Eymann, T.: Never trust, always verify: a multivocal literature review on current knowledge and research gaps of zero-trust. Comput. Sec. **110**, 102436 (2021)
24. Fortino, G., Guerrieri, A., Pace, P., Savaglio, C., Spezzano, G.: IoT platforms and security: an analysis of the leading industrial/commercial solutions. Sensors **22**(6), 2196 (2022)
25. Nield, J., Scanlan, J., Roehrer, E.: Exploring consumer information-security awareness and preparedness of data-breach events. Libr. Trends **68**(4), 611–635 (2020)
26. Shu, X., Tian, K., Ciambrone, A., Yao, D.: Breaking the target: an analysis of target data breach and lessons learned. arXiv preprint arXiv:1701.04940 (2017)
27. Rai, M., Mandoria, H.: A study on cyber-crimes cyber criminals and major security breaches. Int. Res. J. Eng. Technol. **6**(7), 1–8 (2019)
28. Hsiao, S.C., Kao, D.Y.: The static analysis of WannaCry ransomware. In: 2018 20th International Conference on Advanced Communication Technology (ICACT), pp. 153–158. IEEE (2018)

CloudSec: An Extensible Automated Reasoning Framework for Cloud Security Policies

Joe Stubbs(✉), Smruti Padhy, Richard Cardone, and Steve Black

Texas Advanced Computing Center, University of Texas at Austin, Texas, USA
{jstubbs,spadhy,rcardone,scblack}@tacc.utexas.edu

Abstract. Users increasingly create, manage and share digital resources, including sensitive data, via cloud platforms and APIs. Platforms encode the rules governing access to these resources, referred to as *security policies*, using different systems and semantics. As the number of resources and rules grows, the challenge of reasoning about them collectively increases. Formal methods tools, such as Satisfiability Modulo Theories (SMT) libraries, can be used to automate the analysis of security policies, but several challenges, including the highly specialized, technical nature of the libraries as well as their variable performance, prevent their broad adoption in cloud systems. In this paper, we present CloudSec, an extensible framework for reasoning about cloud security policies using SMT. CloudSec provides a high-level API which can be used to encode different types of cloud security policies without knowledge of SMT. Further, it is trivial for applications written with CloudSec to utilize and switch between different SMT libraries. We use CloudSec to analyze security policies in Tapis, a cloud-based API for distributed computational research used by tens of thousands of researchers, and we present a performance case study of using CloudSec with Z3 and cvc5, two popular SMT solvers.

Keywords: Cloud Security Policy · SMT · Extensible Framework · Tapis · Role Based Access Control

1 Introduction

Through the use of cloud-based applications and services, users create valuable digital assets that must be secured. Each cloud platform makes use of a system for managing and enforcing the rules regarding which users have access to which digital assets, and there is little standardization across the vast number of such systems. For example, each of the major cloud computing providers have their own, independent systems for access management: Amazon Web Services makes use of AWS IAM [4], Google Cloud Platform uses Google IAM [14], and Microsoft Azure provides Azure Role Based Access Control (RBAC) [5]. Kubernetes, the popular container orchestration system, has its own RBAC policy system [19].

K. Daimi and A. Al Sadoon (Eds.): ACR 2024, LNNS 956, pp. 268–279, 2024.
https://doi.org/10.1007/978-3-031-56950-0_23

There are also many popular open source projects providing these capabilities, including Casbin [10], KeyCloak [17], Open Policy Agent [22], etc.

The Tapis [24] project represents another such platform. Tapis is an NSF-funded platform providing APIs that enable automated, secure, collaborative research computing to thousands of academic researchers. Using Tapis, researchers store, manage, and share datasets, executable code, execution outputs, project metadata and other resources with individual colleague as well as entire communities of researchers. Tapis stores authorization data in the form of policies describing which users have access to which resources. Tapis policies conform to certain rules governing their format; Table 1 shows an example Tapis policy granting the `jdoe` user `read`, `execute` and `modify` access to all files in her home directory on the Frontera HPC cluster, a world-class supercomputer hosted at the Texas Advanced Computing Center.

Table 1. An Example Tapis Policy

```
username=jdoe,
system=frontera.tacc.utexas.edu,
path=/home/jdoe/*,
action=[READ, EXECUTE, MODIFY],
decision=allow
```

Projects manage thousands of such Tapis policies on behalf of their users, and as these systems evolve, the policies must be updated accordingly. Over time, ensuring that policies are correctly written and match what is being enforced becomes increasingly difficult.

Software based on formal methods such as Satisfiability Modulo Theories (SMT) [9,18] provide techniques for automatically reasoning about entire collections of policies, and to prove or find counter-examples to mathematically precise statements regarding sets of policies. As an example, in the case of Tapis, a project may want to know that all users have modify access to their home directory on all systems but only specific administrative users have access to the root directories. Such statements form the *policy specification* for an application, and the goal is to determine if the actual policies are no more permissive than the policy specification. In general, describing the policy specification is a difficult problem.

While SMT libraries can be used to prove or disprove such statements, the broad adoption of SMT in cloud systems faces the following challenges: 1) the use of these tools requires a sophisticated understanding of the underlying SMT; 2) a significant effort must be made to encode a particular security policy's semantics into an SMT library; and 3) performance on different security policy sets varies across different SMT libraries and even different versions of the same library.

To address these challenges, we built CloudSec [1], an extensible automated reasoning framework for cloud security policies that does not require any SMT knowledge to use or extend to new cloud policy systems. CloudSec provides a core set of data types for defining the semantics of a security policy language, and these data types are linked to SMT solvers through CloudSec's library of `backends`, which implement encodings of the data types as well as proof methods based on the functionality provided by the solver. The initial release of CloudSec includes support for the Z3 [3,21] and CVC5 [2,7] libraries as `backends`. Using CloudSec's building blocks, the policy types for a new system can be defined in just a few lines of Python code without any understanding of SMT. CloudSec's `connectors` abstraction allows policy types to be instantiated with real policies from source systems.

To establish the extensibility of CloudSec, we created basic implementations of policy types for multiple systems, including Tapis and a generic REST API service. For the Tapis platform, we also implement connectors, yielding a tool capable of retrieving and analyzing policies from Tapis's multi-tenant permissions system, which includes hierarchical roles and permission "types" with schemas for many individual services. We automatically establish or find counter-examples to policy requirements across entire sets of Tapis permissions. Finally, we study the scalability of our tool and establish that it performs well when analyzing Tapis policy sets consisting of thousands of policies.

In summary, the main contributions of this paper are:

1. Design and implementation of CloudSec, an extensible Python framework for leveraging SMT for security policy analysis with a user-friendly interface.
2. Description of CloudSec usage in Tapis, a real-world cloud platform used by thousands of researchers.
3. Performance study showing CloudSec scales to thousands of policies.

The rest of the paper is organized as follows: In Sect. 2, we provide background material on Tapis and SMT; in Sect. 3, we describe the CloudSec design, its use in Tapis, and give examples of policy types and encodings; in Sect. 4, we describe our performance study and Sect. 5 compares related work; we conclude in Sect. 6 and outline some areas for future work.

2 Background

In this section, we provide background information on topics used throughout the rest of this paper.

2.1 Tapis

Tapis [24] is a web-friendly, application programming interface (API) for research computing, allowing users to automate their interactions with advanced storage and computing resources in cloud and HPC datacenters. Primary Tapis features include a full-featured data management service, with synchronous endpoints for data ingest and retrieval as well as a reliable asynchronous data transfer facility; workload scheduling and code execution; a highly-scalable document store and metadata API; and support for streaming IoT/sensor data. Tapis supports reproducibility by recording a detailed data provenance and computation history of actions taken in the platform. Additionally, Tapis enables collaboration via a fine-grained permissions model, allowing data, metadata and computations to be kept private, shared with specific individuals or disseminated to entire research communities. Tapis has been used by thousands of researchers across projects funded by a number of government agencies, including CDC, DARPA, NASA, NIH, and NSF.

2.2 Tapis Security Policies

Tapis is organized as a set of 14 independent HTTP web services (sometimes called *microservices*) that coordinate together to accomplish larger tasks. The Tapis Security Kernel (SK) manages all authorization data – information specifying which users have access to which Tapis objects and at what access level. SK stores this authorization data as *permission* objects and provides HTTP endpoints for creating, retrieving, and modifying permissions.

2.3 SMT Solver

CloudSec encodes security access policies into logical formulas represented using Satisfiability Modulo Theories (SMT). Then the satisfiability problem is solved using an SMT solver. An SMT solver is a software that uses decision procedures to report whether a formula is satisfiable in some finite amount of computation and find some counter-example [9,18]. We use two efficient SMT solvers in our backends- Z3 [3] and CVC5 [7].

3 Related Work

There have been several works on cloud-access control policies analysis using SMT [6,11,20,23]. Our work is closely related to the approach used in Zelkova [6], [23]. Zelkova is an AWS policy analysis tool that verifies AWS policies by reasoning if a policy is less or equally permissive than the other. It encodes AWS policies to SMT formulas and uses SMT solvers, Z3, CVC, and Z3AUTOMATA, to verify and prove the properties. Zelkova is not open-source and cannot be extended to other policy languages. CloudSec's approach is similar to Zelkova and other prior works in defining a policy language and translating policies to SMT formulas for reasoning using SMT solvers. The main differences are that 1) CloudSec is an open-source, extensible automated reasoning framework where users or developers can define their policy types not restricted to cloud policies depending on their application, and 2) developers can plug different SMT solvers into CloudSec's extensible backend. Additionally, by defining a policy converter, CloudSec can be easily integrated into existing cloud-hosted services, as demonstrated in Sect. 4.5. In another related work [13], the authors built pySMT, a SMT solver agnostic open-source python library that allows defining, manipulating, and solving SMT formulae. However, to use the pySMT API, one still needs the knowledge of SMT. We envision to support pySMT as one of the backends to Cloudsec.

Eiers et al. [11] proposed a framework to quantify the permissiveness of access policies using model counting constraint solvers and relative permissiveness between the policies. They also built an open-source tool, QUACKY, that analyzes AWS and Azure policies. The CloudSec framework focuses on easy extensibility, defining different policy types, and making the reasoning tool more accessible to users. We envision that QUACKY could potentially be a component in the CloudSec framework to compute relative permissiveness.

Several works have studied the verification of network access control, connectivity, and configuration policies. Jayaraman et al. [15,16] proposed and built a tool called SECGURU that automatically validates network connectivity policies using SMT bit vector theory and the Z3 solver. SECGURU is a closed source tool used in Azure. Fogel et al. [12] proposed and developed an open-source tool, Batfish, that analyzes network configuration and detects errors. Campion [25] is another open-source tool for debugging router configuration and has been implemented as an extension to Batfish. It localizes crucial errors to relevant configuration lines. Beckett et al. [8] proposed a general approach for network configuration that translates both control and data plane behaviors into a logical formula and use SMT solver, Z3, to verify the properties. They have implemented this approach in the tool called Minesweeper. CloudSec could be extended to support network access policies such as Firewall and router policies.

4 Approach

As mentioned in the Introduction, CloudSec provides a toolkit in the form of a Python library for utilizing SMT solvers to analyze security policies in real-world systems such as Tapis. The primary goal of CloudSec is to reduce the expertise needed to apply SMT technology to the study of security policies (Fig. 1).

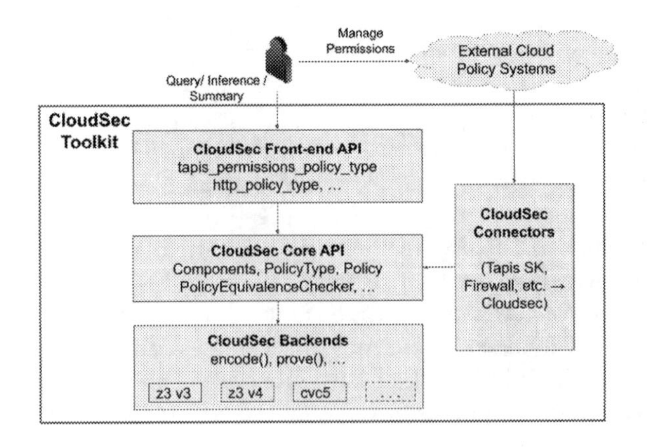

Fig. 1. CloudSec Overview and Usage Model

4.1 CloudSec - Extensible Framework Design

The primary components of the CloudSec framework include (i) the `core` module, with basic data types that can be used to build encodings of real-world security policy systems; (ii) the `backends` library, which provides implementations of encodings of the types provided in the `core` module as well as proof methods for analyzing sets of policies via various solvers, such as Z3 and cvc5; (iii) the `cloud` module, which utilizes the types provided in `core` to define ready-to-use policy types for real systems; and (iv) the `connectors` library, which provides functions for converting security rules in source systems to CloudSec policies.

Central to the design of CloudSec are the concepts of `Component`, `PolicyType`, and `Policy`, provided by the `core` module. Each `Component` type contains a data type, such as a `String`, `Enumeration`, `IP Address` or `Tuple`, the set of allowable values for the data type, and a matching strategy, which defines a "match" relation on two values from the set of allowable values for the data type. Examples of currently supported matching strategies include exact matching and wildcard matching. `PolicyTypes` build on the notion of `Components`, with each `PolicyType` defining a list of `Components` that it is comprised of. Finally, a `Policy` object represents a specific value for a given `PolicyType`.

Using these primary notions, one can create `PolicyTypes` comprised of `Components` for real-world systems in just a few lines of Python without requiring any knowledge of SMT. The `cloud` module provides examples of `PolicyType` objects, including a `tapis_files_policy_type`, used to represent policies related to file objects in Tapis, and an `http_api_policy_type`, which can be used to model policies in an arbitrary HTTP API. Moreover, by decoupling the definitions of `Components` and `PolicyTypes` from their implementations in different backend solvers, CloudSec provides a highly-extensible system in which support for additional solvers can be added independently of defining policy types for new systems.

4.2 An Example Policy Type and Policy Definition

As a first example, we describe the `http_api_policy_type`, available in the CloudSec toolkit. We created this policy type to illustrate what can be achieved with CloudSec. The policy type represents policies governing access to resources defined in a multi-tenant, microservice API platform. The policy type is comprised of three components: *principal*, *resource*, and *action*. A principal is a `Tuple` component type with two fields, `tenant` and `username`, representing a unique user identity in the platform to whom access to some resource is being allowed or denied by the policy. A tenant is a `StringEnum` component with enumerated values representing all possible tenants. We chose a `StringEnum` to model the tenant under the assumption that the number of tenants would be relatively small. On the other hand, the username field is modeled with a `String` component type defined over an alphanumeric set and maximum length.

Similarly, a resource is modeled using a `Tuple` component type with three fields, *tenant, service*, and *path*, that collectively distinguish a specific HTTP endpoint (i.e., HTTP resource) within a service to which access is being allowed or denied in some tenant. A service is a `StringEnum` component with enumerated values representing the names of the APIs in the platform. The path is a String component defined over a path character set with a maximum length. The path represents the URL path corresponding to the resource. Finally, the action is a `StringEnum` that denotes the HTTP method being authorized or not authorized, such as {"GET","POST","PUT","DELETE"}. An example policy definition of `http_api_policy_type` is shown below (Table 2):

Table 2. An Example HTTP Policy

```
p = Policy(policy_type=http_api_policy_type,
    principal=("a2cps","jdoe"),
    resource=("a2cps","files","/ls6/home/jdoe"),
    action="GET",
    decision="allow")
```

Note that all policy types have a special `decision` field which is a `StringEnum` with values "allow" and "deny".

4.3 Tapis Policy Types

The CloudSec toolkit includes policy types representing permissions objects in the Tapis API platform. For example, we provide the `tapis_files_policy_type` for dealing with Tapis permissions related to file objects. The `tapis_file_perm` component is a `Tuple` type representing the Tapis files "perm spec" (see [26]) and includes fields for the tenant, system id, permission level, and file path. Because of the simple and flexible CloudSec core API, the entirety of the Tapis policy type implementations constitutes less than 20 lines of Python code.

4.4 Translating a Policy Set to SMT Formula

A policy set is defined as a set of policies, i.e., $PS = \{P_1, P_2, \cdots, P_i, \cdots, P_{n-1}, P_n\}$ where $1 \leq i \leq n$. Each policy, $P_i = (c_1, c_2, \cdots, c_j, \cdots, c_{m-1}, c_m, Decision)$ where $1 \leq j \leq m$. c_j denotes the value for `Component` C_j of Policy P_i. Note that a policy type determines the number and type of `Components` in a policy. *Decision* is a value from the set $\{``allow", ``deny"\}$ to denote if a policy allows or denies access. A policy is translated to an SMT formula as:

$$\mathcal{P} = \bigwedge_{j=1}^{m} \left(\bigvee_{c \in C_j(P)} C_j = c \right)$$

$C_j(P)$ denotes set of values defined for `Component` C_j in a policy P. If $C_j(P)$ is a `Tuple` component type with k components , let say, $(t_1, t_2, .., t_k)$, then it is further encoded as $\bigwedge_{l=1}^{k} (t_k = v)$ where component t_k takes one of the component allowed values, v.

A policy set can be SMT encoded as:

$$\mathcal{PS} = \left(\bigvee_{AllowSet} \mathcal{P}\right) \bigwedge \neg \left(\bigvee_{DenySet} \mathcal{P}\right)$$

where $AllowSet = \{\forall P \in PS : P.Decision = \text{“}allow\text{”}\}$ and $DenySet = \{\forall P \in PS : P.Decision = \text{“}deny\text{”}\}$.

4.5 Connectors and Converting SK Policies to Cloudsec

Using CloudSec to analyze security rules from a real-world system requires one to generate CloudSec policy objects (of the appropriate type) from authorization data residing in the external system. A CloudSec `connector` can be written for the external system to simplify this effort. The CloudSec toolkit currently includes a connector for Tapis files permissions, allowing CloudSec `tapis_files_policy_type` policies to be generated from Tapis permissions data with a single function call.

Using CloudSec, we developed a program that generates Tapis files policy objects from all Tapis files permissions in the SK for a configurable set of users. The program then uses CloudSec solver backends to prove that the source policies conform to certain rules or find counter examples. For instance, using our program, we analyzed policies for users within a certain project built with Tapis, generating over 3,000 CloudSec policies. We then were able to prove that for this project, no users except for the users in the admin-scientist role had read/write access to files in a protected `data` directory on a specific Tapis system. Similarly, we prove that public access to generated result files is restricted to files with a `.png` extension.

Establishing these kinds of results harnesses the full power of CloudSec – while the Tapis SK is highly efficient at answering the question, “does a given user have access to a specific resource?", it cannot reason about an entire set of permissions at once. Furthermore, our program must use both Z3 and cvc5 to find proofs like the ones above, as some proofs could not be found by one solver or the other.

5 Performance

We did a performance evaluation of the CloudSec toolkit 1) to establish that the CloudSec software was a viable approach (i.e., can be done on commodity hardware in a reasonable amount of time) to analyze policies of the sizes that show up in real systems such as Tapis (i.e., on the order of a few thousand policies) (Sect. 4.5); and 2) to show that CloudSec could be used as a framework for comparing different SMT backends for specific analyses [1]. We also observed that there are scenarios for which either Z3 or CVC5 or both, along with their different versions exhibit performance cliffs. We provide the details of the performance evaluation in subsequent subsections.

We measured the performance to check trivial implications for two policy sets as the number of policies grows. We defined different components (`String` and `StringEnum`) and policy types using those components to create policy sets. Each policy set consists of policies of the same policy type. We repeated the test for both Z3 and cvc5 backends. We ran the tests on a machine with the following configuration: 32 CPUs, Intel(R) Xeon(R) CPU E5-2660 0 @ 2.20 GHz, 128 GB RAM.

5.1 StringEnum Scalability

We defined a policy type containing a `StringEnum` with a variable number, N, allowable values and with wildcard matching. For example, with $N = 5$, the policy type's `StringEnum` will have allowable values { '0', '1','2','3','4'}. We created two policy sets, P and Q. P contained a policy P_i for every allowable value, i.e., $P = \cup_{i=0}^{N-1}\{(P_i, \text{"}allow\text{"})\}$ where $P_i = i$. Q contained a single wildcard policy, $Q = \{(*, \text{"}allow\text{"})\}$. We varied the number of unique elements, N, in the range $10 \leq N \leq 4000$. We measured the time to perform: 1) data load, 2) SMT encoding, 3) $P \implies Q$ and 4) $Q \implies P$ for Z3 as well as for cvc5. In Fig. 2 a, we observed that when using the Z3 backend, the SMT encoding, $P \implies Q$ and $Q \implies P$ took similar amounts of time, while the data load took significantly less time. When we used cvc5, SMT encoding took the most of the computation time while the data load time was more than the implication prove time. For this performance test, cvc5 was roughly 90% faster than Z3 in total time.

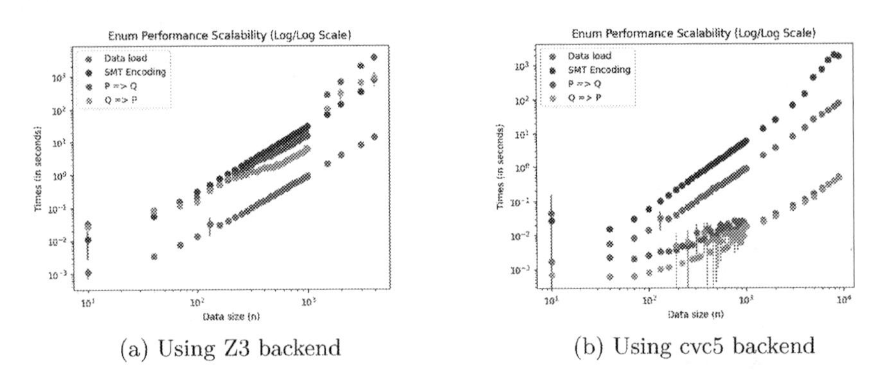

(a) Using Z3 backend

(b) Using cvc5 backend

Fig. 2. Dynamic StringEnum Policy type Scalability

5.2 String with Wildcard Scalability

We defined a policy type with a single `String` component with wildcard matching. The string component was defined over a character set that included alphanumeric characters, '/', and the wildcard character '*'. The maximum length of the string was 100. We created two policy sets, P and Q, for each $10 \leq$

$N \leq 1000$. The policy set $P = \cup_{i=0}^{N-1}\{(P_i, \text{“}allow\text{”})\}$ where each P_i was defined to be the static string “$a1b2c3d4e5/i$”. The policy set $Q = \cup_{i=0}^{N-1}\{(Q_i, \text{“}allow\text{”})\}$ where each Q_i is defined as the string “$a1b2c3d4e5/i*$” ending in the wildcard character. For example, if $N = 2$, $P = \{\text{“}a1b2c3d4e5/1\text{”}, \text{“}a1b2c3d4e5/2\text{”}\}$ and $Q = \{\text{“}a1b2c3d4e5/1*\text{”}, \text{“}a1b2c3d4e5/2*\text{”}\}$. In this case, there are 2 policies in P and two policies in Q.

We varied N and measured the data load, SMT encoding, and $P \implies Q$ times for Z3 as well as for cvc5. Note $Q \implies P$ is not valid. In Fig. 3, we observe that Z3 was faster than cvc5 in total time and, in particular, in proving $P \implies Q$, Z3 was often an order of magnitude or more faster. Both backends follow the same pattern where data load and SMT encoding times are less than implication prove time. Z3 shows good performance even for $N = 1000$, which is 1000 policies in P and in Q.

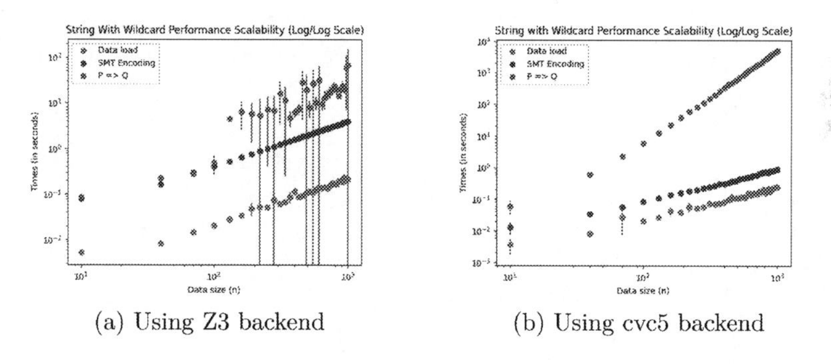

(a) Using Z3 backend

(b) Using cvc5 backend

Fig. 3. String with Wildcard Policy type Scalability

5.3 Performance Cliffs for SMT Solvers

We observed some performance cliffs while using Z3 and cvc5. First, consider two simple policy sets in which the policy type has just one component, *path*, of string type. Let $P = (\text{“}/sys1*\text{”}, \text{“}allow\text{”})$ and $Q = (\text{“}/*\text{”}, \text{“}allow\text{”})$. While trying to prove P is less permissive than Q, the Z3 backend hangs but cvc5 is able to prove it.

Second, consider the policy sets:

$$P = \{(\text{“}jstubbs\text{”}, \text{“}s2/home/jstubbs/*\text{”}, \text{“}*\text{”}, \text{“}allow\text{”}),$$
$$(\text{“}jstubbs\text{”}, \text{“}s2/*\text{”}, \text{“}PUT\text{”}, \text{“}deny\text{”}),$$
$$(\text{“}jstubbs\text{”}, \text{“}s2/*\text{”}, \text{“}POST\text{”}, \text{“}deny\text{”})\}$$

and

$$Q = \{(\text{“}jstubbs\text{”}, \text{“}s2/home/jstubbs/a.out\text{”}, \text{“}GET\text{”}, \text{“}allow\text{”}),$$
$$(\text{“}jstubbs\text{”}, \text{“}s2/home/jstubbs/b.out\text{”}, \text{“}GET\text{”}, \text{“}allow\text{”})\}$$

Z3 was able to to prove $Q \implies P$ but cvc5 hangs.

6 Conclusion and Future Work

In this paper, we presented a description of the CloudSec library, which simplifies the use of SMT in analyzing security policies in real-world systems. We applied CloudSec to the Tapis API platform to analyze thousands of permissions records at once. In the future, we plan to incorporate CloudSec into a public API within Tapis, allowing any user to easily submit security analysis jobs using HTTP requests. Further, we will explore adding support for additional backends to the project and applying CloudSec to additional real-world systems, such as AWS, and Kubernetes.

Acknowledgement. This material is based upon work supported by the NSF OAC Award #1931439.

References

1. CloudSec (December 2023). https://github.com/applyfmsec/cloudsec
2. CVC5: An efficient open-source automatic theorem prover for satisfiability modulo theories (SMT) problems (December 2023). https://cvc5.github.io/
3. Z3 (December 2023). https://github.com/Z3Prover/z3
4. AWS IAM (December 2023). https://docs.aws.amazon.com/IAM/latest/UserGuide/access.html
5. AzureRBAC (December 2023). https://learn.microsoft.com/en-us/azure/role-based-access-control/overview
6. Backes, J., et al.: Semantic-based automated reasoning for AWS access policies using SMT. In: 2018 Formal Methods in Computer Aided Design (FMCAD), pp. 1–9 (2018). https://doi.org/10.23919/FMCAD.2018.8602994
7. Barbosa, H., et al.: cvc5: a versatile and industrial-strength SMT solver. In: TACAS 2022. LNCS, vol. 13243, pp. 415–442. Springer, Cham (2022). https://doi.org/10.1007/978-3-030-99524-9_24
8. Beckett, R., Gupta, A., Mahajan, R., Walker, D.: A general approach to network configuration verification. In: Proceedings of the Conference of the ACM Special Interest Group on Data Communication, pp. 155–168. SIGCOMM 2017 (2017)
9. Bradley, A.R., Manna, Z.: The Calculus of Computation: Decision Procedures with Applications to Verification. Springer, Heidelberg (2007). https://doi.org/10.1007/978-3-540-74113-8
10. Casbin (Dec 2022). https://casbin.org/
11. Eiers, W., Sankaran, G., Li, A., O'Mahony, E., Prince, B., Bultan, T.: Quantifying permissiveness of access control policies. In: Proceedings of the 44th International Conference on Software Engineering, pp. 1805–1817. ICSE 2022 (2022)
12. Fogel, A., et al.: A general approach to network configuration analysis. In: Proceedings of the 12th USENIX Conference on Networked Systems Design and Implementation, p. 469–483. NSDI 2015, USENIX Association, USA (2015)
13. Gario, M., Micheli, A.: PySMT: a solver-agnostic library for fast prototyping of SMT-based algorithms. In: SMT Workshop 2015 (2015)

14. Google IAM (December 2023). https://cloud.google.com/iam/
15. Jayaraman, K., et al.: Validating datacenters at scale. In: Proceedings of the ACM Special Interest Group on Data Communication, pp. 200–213. SIGCOMM 2019 (2019)
16. Jayaraman, K., Bjørner, N., Outhred, G., Kaufman, C.: Automated analysis and debugging of network connectivity policies. Tech. Rep. MSR-TR-2014-102, Microsoft (2014)
17. KeyCloak (December 2023). https://www.keycloak.org/
18. Kroening, D., Strichman, O.: Decision Procedures: An Algorithmic Point of View. In: Juraj, H., Mogens, N. (eds.) Texts in Theoretical Computer Science. An EATCS Series, Springer, Heidelberg (2017). https://doi.org/10.1007/978-3-662-50497-0
19. Kubernetes (December 2023). https://kubernetes.io/docs/reference/access-authn-authz/rbac/
20. Liu, A., Du, X., Wang, N., Wang, X., Wu, X., Zhou, J.: Implement security analysis of access control policy based on constraint by SMT. In: 2022 IEEE 5th International Conference on Electronics Technology (ICET), pp. 1043–1049 (2022). https://doi.org/10.1109/ICET55676.2022.9824517
21. de Moura, L., Bjørner, N.: Z3: an efficient SMT solver. In: Ramakrishnan, C.R., Rehof, J. (eds.) TACAS 2008. LNCS, vol. 4963, pp. 337–340. Springer, Heidelberg (2008). https://doi.org/10.1007/978-3-540-78800-3_24
22. Open Policy Agent (December 2022). https://www.openpolicyagent.org/
23. Rungta, N.: A billion SMT queries aăday (invited paper). In: Shoham, S., Vizel, Y. (eds.) Computer Aided Verification, pp. 3–18. Springer International Publishing, Cham (2022). https://doi.org/10.1007/978-3-031-13185-1_1
24. Stubbs, J., et al.: Tapis: an API platform for reproducible, distributed computational research. In: Arai, K. (ed.) FICC 2021. AISC, vol. 1363, pp. 878–900. Springer, Cham (2021). https://doi.org/10.1007/978-3-030-73100-7_61
25. Tang, A., et al.: Campion: debugging router configuration differences. In: Proceedings of the 2021 ACM SIGCOMM 2021 Conference, pp. 748-761. SIGCOMM 2021 (2021)
26. Tapis: Tapis permissions (2022) (December 2023). https://tapis.readthedocs.io/en/latest/technical/security.html#id3

Optimizing Energy Consumption for IoT Adaptive Security: A Mobility-Based Solution

Asma Arab(✉), Michaël Mahamat, Ghada Jaber, and Abdelmadjid Bouabdallah

Université de Technologie de Compiègne, Heudiasyc (Heuristics and Diagnosis of Complex Systems), CS 60319, 60203 Compiègne Cedex, France
{asma.arab,michael.mahamat,ghada.jaber,madjid.bouabdallah}@hds.utc.fr

Abstract. The Internet of Things (IoT) is transforming communication among devices. The prevalent use of IoT in mobile scenarios introduces vulnerability to attacks, which requires robust security mechanisms. However, the heterogeneity of IoT devices results in diverse security requirements, compounded by varying threat levels across geographical zones. To address this issue, adaptive security solutions that tailor defense mechanisms to the contextual environment (i.e the security requirement of devices and threat level of the environment) are proposed. However, when the threat level increases, the defense mechanism complexity increases. This leads to higher energy consumption and consequently, device failure. To tackle this challenge, we propose in this paper a mobility-based solution to optimize the energy consumption resulting from using adaptive security solutions. Our approach considers the remaining energy of IoT devices, their security requirement and the threat level of the zone in the decision-making process. This task is carried out by an agent trained with Deep Reinforcement Learning. The proposed solution includes Software-Defined Networking and fog computing in order to ensure seamless execution of the security service while the IoT device moves.

Keywords: IoT · Adaptive security · Energy saving · Mobility · Deep Reinforcement Learning

1 Introduction

The rapid expansion of IoT has significantly influenced various industries including healthcare, smart grid, and agriculture [8]. However, IoT encounters challenges arising from the absence of a central controller, device heterogeneity, diverse attacks. Security and energy consumption emerge as pivotal challenges in the IoT domain, particularly in mobile scenarios where devices transition between networks [13]. Furthermore, the heterogeneous nature of IoT networks makes conventional security tools less efficient for addressing these issues. Software-Defined Networking (SDN) and fog computing are two promising technologies to deploy a distributed mobile IoT while ensuring a seamless and continuous execution of security services for mobile IoT devices [12].

K. Daimi and A. Al Sadoon (Eds.): ACR 2024, LNNS 956, pp. 280–291, 2024.
https://doi.org/10.1007/978-3-031-56950-0_24

In the context of a decentralized IoT environment with varying risk levels across geographical zones, designing fixed and static security services becomes challenging due to diverse contextual considerations. Lightweight solutions may render legitimate IoT nodes vulnerable in high-risk areas, while deploying complex solutions could lead to excessive energy consumption, causing IoT nodes to deplete their energy resources even in low-security requirement scenarios. To address this challenge, adaptive security solutions emerge as a viable approach. Adaptive security in the context of the IoT refers to a security approach that can dynamically adjust and modify security measures in response to changing conditions and threats in a system [3]. One of the key benefits is its ability to provide real-time adaptation features for IoT device security [22], ensuring end-to-end security for active IoT devices [21]. Moreover, adaptive security can contribute to the trustworthiness of IoT systems while maintaining their reliability and security [6]. This is crucial for ensuring the overall integrity and resilience of IoT deployments [3].

When the risk level in a geographical zone increases, the automatic response of an adaptive security solution is to employ a complex defense mechanism to secure the IoT environment. This results in higher energy consumption due to the complexity of the security level in the adaptive solution. Therefore, it impacts the network lifetime. To tackle this problem, we propose a mobility-based solution as a preventive measure against device failure resulting from the execution of an adaptive security method. Consequently, our research question is as follows: "Given knowledge of the present energy status of devices, their security requirements, and the threat level in their respective zones, how can we use mobility support for energy consumption optimization during the execution of the adaptive security method for mobile IoT?". In this paper, we present a novel approach that addresses the energy consumption resulting from security defense mechanisms, using mobility support. To the best of our knowledge, we are the first to introduce mobility in this context. The contributions of our work are as follow:

- We firstly present the system model. We detail the role of SDN and fog computing to ensure scalability and the seamless execution of the security service for mobile IoT when moving between zones.
- Then, we provide a comprehensive breakdown of energy consumption for the devices within our system.
- Finally, we formulate our problem as a Markov Decision Process problem and justify the use of Deep Reinforcement Learning (DRL) to determine the actions to be taken for the IoT device whether it should stay, move, or put in sleep mode.

The remainder of the paper is structured as follows: Sect. 2 provides an overview of related works within the adaptive security domain. In Sect. 3, we detail our system model and present our energy-aware and mobility-based adaptive security strategy. The paper is concluded in Sect. 4.

2 Related Works

In mobile IoT with widespread distributed devices, adaptive security solutions play a crucial role in ensuring security while considering the risk level of the device specific zone. Indeed, this approach avoids the use of complex security mechanisms for IoT devices that may necessitate lightweight measures, particularly when these devices do not store sensitive data or operate within safe zones with lower energy levels. There are many research works in this field. For instance, in [2], the authors introduce a risk-based adaptive security solution for smart IoT applications in eHealth. This approach dynamically learns and adjusts to evolving environments.

In [4] an adaptive risk-based access control model is proposed for IoT applications. It dynamically modifies user permissions by incorporating real-time risk assessments and monitoring user activities throughout access sessions. Also, it employs smart contracts to deliver adaptive features. The study outlined in [1] introduces the Adaptive Lightweight Physical Layer Authentication (ALPLA) scheme. This methodology employs a one-class classifier support vector machine (OCC-SVM), using features extracted from the magnitude, real, and imaginary components of the received signal at each antenna. It is specifically crafted for 5G mobile networks in the realm of IoT, with a distinct focus on the physical layer. The survey [16] offers a thorough exploration of adaptive authentication methods harnessing machine learning. Although the survey primarily examines research works focused on web applications and users, it emphasizes that the discussed methods may not be directly applicable to the distinctive context of IoT. The researchers in [19] offer a thorough survey of self-adaptive security mechanisms tailored for IoT-based multimedia services. The paper underscores the lack of a standardized security mechanism for diverse IoT devices and investigates several self-adaptive security approaches, encompassing context-based security, architecture-based self-protection, and self-adaptive authentication.

Other research works have focused on reducing energy consumption in the formulation of their adaptive security solutions. Authors in [17] present a distinctive strategy to tackle the challenges of security in low-power IoT devices. The proposed method advocates for the integration of multiple encryption modes characterized by diverse power consumption and security levels. This is achieved through the Dynamic Partial Reconfiguration (DPR) to dynamically configure the hardware security module, aligning with the available power budget. The article detailed in [10] an adaptive security specification method for 6G IoT networks. The method aims to navigate balance between security and energy consumption. It employs Extended Kalman Filtering (EKF) to predict the harvesting power with high accuracy. Furthermore, it provides joint optimization methods to effectively counter escalating network threats, ensuring both message safety and Quality of Service (QoS).

The research work [7] present an adaptive security framework for 5G-based IoT systems. The proposed approach dynamically adapts security levels in response to changing contextual conditions, aiming to mitigate energy consumption. This departure from a worst-case scenario perspective, known for its energy-intensive nature, marks a noteworthy shift in the quest for enhanced energy efficiency in IoT security. In [18], authors delves into the critical trade-off between security and energy considerations in edge-assisted IoT. It suggests tailoring the complexity of security schemes to specific security levels as a strategy to conserve energy consumption. The paper puts forth an initial solution to navigate the security-energy tradeoff by dynamically adjusting the computational complexity of machine learning-based security schemes through feature selection.

The existing solutions that address energy consumption optimization involves adapting the security method, potentially introducing vulnerabilities and rendering the IoT network susceptible. Instead of modifying or constraining the adaptive security solution, a promising approach is to manipulate the environment to prevent the defense mechanism from depleting the IoT device energy entirely. Thus, we propose an innovative solution based on mobility to optimize the energy consumption of an IoT device during the execution of the adaptive security solution.

3 Our Solution: A Mobility-Based Energy Consumption Optimisation for Adaptive Security in Mobile IoT

In the previous, we outlined that existing works do not consider mobility as a solution to prevent device failure. Indeed, energy consumption resulting from the execution of adaptive security is an issue when complex defense mechanisms are used frequently in zones with a high threat level. A way to counter it, is by my moving the devices to zones with a lower threat level. Therefore, we propose a novel solution to optimize the energy consumption of the execution of security services, using deep reinforcement learning to train an agent for the decision making. It takes into consideration the current threat of the zones, security requirements of the IoT devices, and their energy levels. The learning agent is deployed in a SDN controller that monitors the IoT system with the help of Fog Nodes (FNs). Each fog node will manage the IoT devices of a specific geographical zone (i.e., cluster). This initiative is inspired by the research work presented in [9].

3.1 System Model

We consider an IoT system composed of N clusters $C = \{c_1, c_2, ..., c_N\}$ and a set M of IoT devices $D = \{d_1, d_2, ..., d_M\}$. Each device has a battery with a maximum capacity of R_{max}. Each cluster is a specific geographical zone that has its own FN. Our proposed architecture is tailored for highly distributed mobile IoT environment. The distributed network management for IoT devices is implemented using an SDN controller and FNs in a cluster structure. The proposed architecture is depicted in Fig. 1. This architecture aim to enhance the security of communication between IoT devices, reduce energy consumption, and support the scalability [20]. Indeed, by combining fog computing for local processing and SDN for centralized network management, our architecture aims to create a robust and efficient IoT ecosystem.

To reduce the network delay and overhead in each cluster, the FN acts as a cluster head. The FN is a coordinator and responsible for the management of IoT objects and execution of the adaptive security service. This architecture may also ensure seamless and continuous execution of the security service. Indeed, through the collaboration between FNs and the SDN controller, when a node moves from one cluster to another it will send a request that will be transmitted to the SDN controller. The controller will coordinate with the FN of the destination cluster to enable a seamless handover during the movement of the IoT node. Thanks to the fog computing that is configured at the edge nodes of the network, this architecture avoids frequent handovers. Moreover, the devices in the clusters are SDN enabled, meaning that they are controlled by the SDN controller. This is necessary to make sure that we can make the IoT devices move when needed.

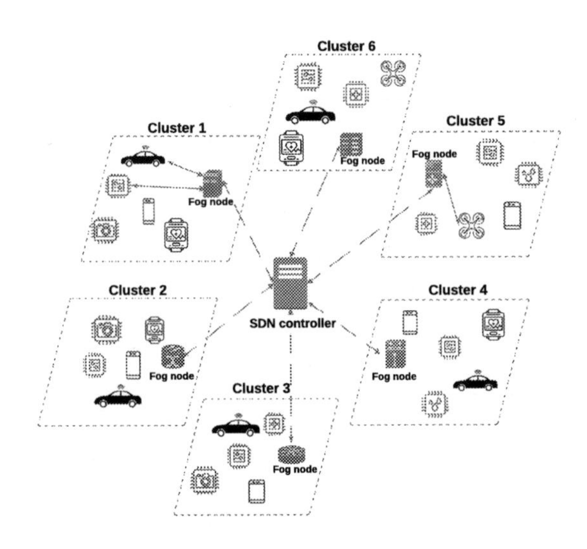

Fig. 1. Architecture of the proposed solution.

3.2 Mobility Support for Adaptive Security

Adaptive security solutions play a vital role in threat mitigation. Nonetheless, the deployment of such solutions introduces variability in energy consumption across IoT devices. Indeed, devices subject to the intricate processes of adaptive security services may deplete their energy reserves at an accelerated rate, which results in device failure. The use of mobility support for an adaptive security solution enables the minimization of energy consumption. Indeed, we can reduce energy consumption IoT device by moving it from a zone with a high threat level that requires complex mechanisms to a less security requiring zone where we can apply a lightweight version of the solution.

Since we focus on the energy consumption optimization through mobility support, in the following, we abstract the threat assessment, the adaptive security solution and the available defense mechanisms. Within our architecture, the threat level assessment module and the adaptive security solution are implemented in each FN. The cluster ($c_j \in C$) threat level is denoted as T_j^t with j and is subject to change at intervals of time. The selection of the defense mechanism of the adaptive security solution is contingent upon both the security requirement of the device and the threat level of the cluster. The set of clusters are under a SDN controller which can control the IoT devices within each cluster.

3.3 Energy Consumption of Adaptive Security Solution for Mobile IoT

In our model, each device $d_i \in D$ is assigned an importance level imp_i, reflecting its significance within the network [9]. Higher values signify critical tasks, where the potential impact on the network is substantial in the event of d_i failure. In this context, we consider $imp_i > 0$ as a fixed parameter that remains constant. Each device possesses a security requirement denoted req_i, which is both task-dependent and constant. When selecting a defense mechanism from the adaptive security solution, the FN considers the device security requirement req_i and the threat level T_j^t within its cluster c_j at a specific time t. This implies that the choice of the defense mechanism in the adaptive security solution for a specific device in a particular cluster can vary over time. Indeed, the threat assessment is continuous in order to ensure that the threat level of each c_j at any moment represent the actual risk in that zone. Furthermore, each defense mechanism sec_k in the adaptive security solution is associated with a known energy consumption rate, denoted as E_{sec_k}. We assume that all E_{sec_k} had already been quantified and are constant.

The energy level of each device is denoted E_i^t, and it can fluctuate over time due to various factors such as task execution, the chosen defense mechanism, and charging activities (which increase the energy level), In our scenario, we posit that the charging activities exhibit a random nature, devoid of any predetermined schedule or dependency on external threats. Additionally, the cluster assignment of d_i may also change as mobile devices move freely between clusters. For simplification, we assume that any changes in the threat level of each cluster and cluster assignment occur at specific times within intervals denoted by Δ_t between s_t and s_{t+1}. Hence, Δ_t remains constant, and every Δ_t the agent determine the action to be taken for each device. E_{rec} signifies the energy acquired during charging, where its value is 0 if no charging occurs during Δ_t. Ep_i corresponds to the energy consumed by task processing in d_i. If d_i stays in the same cluster c_j at t and $t+1$, it remaining energy is:

$$E_i^{t+1} = E_i^t + E_{rec} - (Ep_i + \Delta_t \cdot E_{sec_l}) \tag{1}$$

With E_{sec_l}, the energy consumption resulting from the defense mechanism sec_l used in the c_j. If d_i have been moved (or moved freely) from c_j to $c_{j'}$ where it

Table 1. Notations used in the article.

Notation	Defintions
D	Set of IoT devices
DD	Set of dead devices
SD	Set of sleeping devices
ED	Set of exhausted devices
AD	Set of active devices
ST	set of devices moved between cluster with the same threat level
E_i^t	Remaining energy of device d_i at time t
imp_i	Importance level of device d_i
C	Set of clusters
E_{sec_k}	Energy cost of the k-th defense mechanism
T_j^t	Threat level of cluster c_j at time t

would use $sec_{l'}$, and consumed $E_{mov}(j, j')$ during its transit, then the remaining energy of the device is given by:

$$E_i^{t+1} = E_i^t + E_{rec} - (Ep_i + \Delta_t \cdot E_{sec_{l'}} + E_{mov}(j, j')) \tag{2}$$

Our primary goal is to address the security needs of each device based on its individual requirement and the threat level within its current cluster, all while optimizing the network lifetime by minimizing instances of inactive devices. To realize this objective, we propose to employ a DRL model that trains an agent (the SDN controller) to make decisions based on various parameters (Table 1).

3.4 Optimizing Energy Consumption Through Deep Reinforcement Learning and Mobility-Support

In the envisioned framework, the SDN controller operates as a learning agent, determining the optimal action for each node periodically. This controller integrates a DRL algorithm and interacts with the device layer to perceive the system state space. The reward function assesses the efficacy of the SDN controller actions at a given time step t. At each time step, the agent decides, given the device energy level and its environment, whether the device should remain in its current cluster, relocate to another cluster, or turn to sleep mode to minimize energy consumption.

To address the energy optimization challenge for mobile IoT devices employing adaptive security solutions, we formulate it as a Markov Decision Process (MDP) characterized by the tuple (S, A, R, P). At each time step t, the learning agent observes a state s_t, encompassing the threat levels in each cluster T_j^t, the energy level of each device E_i^t, the cluster assignments for each device $c_{j'}^i$, and the suitable defense mechanism sec_k for each device. The action space A for each device encompasses three options: i) remain in the current cluster, ii) transition to the closest cluster with a lower threat level, iii) enter sleep mode. In this scenario, we contend with a multi-action setting, where the agent must independently make decisions for multiple devices simultaneously, often referred to as a multi-action or multi-dimensional action space [5, 23]. Consequently, at time t, the action is: $a_t = (a_1^t, a_2^t, ..., a_M^t)$, where each $a_i^t = \{stay, move, sleep\}$.

The reward function R, designed to encourage energy-efficient decisions and effective security measures, quantifies the states and actions into numerical values. After executing action a_t, the agent receives a reward $r(s_t, a_t)$ that incorporates the following components:

- A penalty p_{DD} for the failure of a device d_i.
- A penalty p_{SD} for placing a device in sleep mode.
- A penalty p_{ED} for device exhaustion due to relocation.
- A penalty p_{ST} for moving a device to a cluster with an identical threat level.
- Fixed rewards r_{EE} for energy efficiency when energy consumed from moving is less than energy consumption expected when staying and r_{TM} for threat minimization when the decision taken implies using a defense mechanism less consuming.

Penalties are represented as negative values, while rewards are positive. Therefore, the reward $r(s_t, a_t)$ is determined by (3):

$$\begin{aligned} r(s_t, a_t) = \sum_{AD}(r_{EE} + r_{TM}) + \sum_{j \in DD} p_{DD} \cdot imp_j \\ + \sum_{k \in SD} p_{SD} \cdot imp_k + \sum_{l \in ED} p_l \cdot imp_l + \sum_{ST} p_{ST} \end{aligned} \tag{3}$$

Here, DD represents the set of dead devices, SD denotes the set of devices in sleep mode, ED signifies the set of exhausted devices due to relocation, and ST encompasses the devices moved between clusters with identical threat levels. Additionally, future rewards from time step t and onwards are discounted, assigning greater importance to proximate rewards over those in the distant future. To achieve this we introduce a discounting factor γ. This parameter helps the agent to prioritize immediate rewards over delayed ones and encourages it to make decisions more focused on short-term gains. The discounted sum of rewards is calculated as follows:

$$R_t = \sum_{i=t}^{T} \gamma^{(i-t)} \cdot r(s_i, a_i) \tag{4}$$

Ultimately, P denotes the transition probability from state s_t to s_{t+1} when the agent takes action a_t. Given the dynamic nature of the environment and the agent lack of knowledge about the complete model, the transition probability remains unknown. Consequently, we adopt a model-free approach. The agent must acquire knowledge about the most suitable action for each device in every state, necessitating the learning of the policy $\pi(a|s)$ that maps states to actions. To ensure security for all devices and maximize network lifetime, the agent aims to learn the optimal policy π^*. Achieving a balance between exploration and exploitation is facilitated through an ϵ-greedy policy. The term ϵ represents a small positive value, typically between 0 and 1. It works as follows : with probability ϵ, it selects a random action (exploration) and with probability $1 - \epsilon$, it selects the action that maximize the estimated value based on the learned policy (exploitation). The value of ϵ determines the balance between exploration and exploitation. A smaller value encourages more exploitation, while a larger value promotes more exploration.

Due to the considerable size of the state space, that could lead to an excessively memory consumption issue, we chose to consider Deep Reinforcement Learning (DRL) for the resolution of the MDP. DRL is a powerful approach that combines Reinforcement Learning (RL) with deep learning, particularly neural networks, to address complex decision-making problems in high-dimensional action spaces [11,24,25]. Furthermore, DRL has been instrumental in addressing challenges such as the exploration-exploitation trade-off in both episodic and continuous environments, contributing to more effective decision-making processes [15]. These neural networks, commonly referred to as Deep Q-Networks (DQN), inherently learn the unknown transition probabilities implicitly through the Q-network, eliminating the need for explicit knowledge of these probabilities.

When using DQNs, careful consideration is given to a memory pool M that serves to accumulate experiences. At time t, an entry in the memory pool is denoted as $m_t = (s_t, a_t, s_{t+1}, r(s_t, a_t))$. Furthermore, to enhance and stabilize the learning process, the introduction of a target network, denoted as $\tilde{Q}$-network, is necessary [14]. The target network approximates a $\tilde{Q}$-function, referred to as the target function $\tilde{Q}$. Throughout the training process, the parameters of the

Algorithm 1. Pseudo-code of the mobility-support for energy optimization solution

1: **for** each step t **do**
2: Retrieve the current observed threat level of each cluster T_j^t
3: Retrieve the current remaining energy E_t^i of each d_i
4: Retrieve the current cluster assignment energy c_j^i of each d_i
5: Determine the suitable defense mechanism sec_k^i for each device d_i according to T_j^t and req_i
6: Construct the observation of s_t: T_j^t and E_t^i, c_j^i, sec_k^i, for $i = \{1, ..., M\}$ and $j = \{1, ..., N\}$
7: Feed the Q-Network of the agent with the state s_t, the parameters θ
8: Take action a_t according to the ϵ-greedy policy
9: Receive reward $r(s_t, a_t)$ and process to the state s_{t+1}
10: Update the memory pool M with the tuple $m_t = (s_t, a_t, s_{t+1}, r(s_t, a_t))$
11: Use the target Network $\tilde{Q}$ with a sample batch from the memory pool M to minimize a loss function L
12: Update the Q-network thanks to the minimization of L
13: Update the target Network $\tilde{Q}$ every λ steps with the weights of the Q-Network.
14: **end for**

target network undergo updates facilitated by the parameters of the Q-network, θ.

Drawing inspiration from [9], Algorithm 1 outlines the fundamental steps of our mobility-based solution for energy optimization due to the execution of adaptive solutions in mobile IoT. The initial steps (lines 2 to 6) focus on constructing s_t, serving as input to the Q-Network to determine whether each device should stay, move, or enter sleep mode. Subsequently, the reward is obtained (lines 8 to 10). The ensuing steps involve updating the pool, generating a random batch (provided there are sufficient samples in M), and minimizing a loss function, enabling the parameters of the Q-network to be updated (lines 11 to 13). Additionally, at intervals of λ time steps, the parameters of the target network $\tilde{Q}$ are synchronized with the parameters of the Q-network (line 12).

4 Conclusion

Adaptive security solutions are highly effective to address the security needs of distributed IoT systems, considering varying threat levels across different zones. However, such solutions may lead to significant energy consumption due to the execution of complex defense mechanisms. In this paper, we proposed an innovative solution through mobility support to reduce the energy cost of adaptive security mechanisms. By employing deep reinforcement learning, we empower the SDN controller, functioning as a learning agent overseeing clusters in a mobile IoT system, to make decisions for each device. Our proposed approach enables the minimization of energy consumption rates for IoT devices while maintaining the required security level. The ongoing development of this solution is underway. Presently, we are engaged in coding the environment and performing experiments. Therefore, as part of the future work, we aim to finalize the ongoing implementation and explore additional parameters, treating them as variables rather than constants, to account for the dynamic nature of IoT systems. We also plan to evaluate the performance of the proposed solution.

References

1. Abdrabou, M., Gulliver, T.A.: Adaptive physical layer authentication using machine learning with antenna diversity. IEEE Trans. Commun. **70**(10), 6604–6614 (2022)
2. Abie, H., Balasingham, I.: Risk-based adaptive security for smart IoT in ehealth. In: Proceedings of the 7th International Conference on Body Area Networks, pp. 269–275 (2012)
3. Aman, W., Snekkenes, E.: Managing security trade-offs in the internet of things using adaptive security. In: 2015 10th International Conference for Internet Technology and Secured Transactions (ICITST), pp. 362–368. IEEE (2015)
4. Atlam, H.F., Alenezi, A., Walters, R.J., Wills, G.B., Daniel, J.: Developing an adaptive risk-based access control model for the internet of things. In: 2017 IEEE International Conference on Internet of Things (iThings) and IEEE Green Computing and Communications (GreenCom) and IEEE Cyber, Physical and Social

Somputing (CPSCom) and IEEE Smart Data (SmartData), pp. 655–661. IEEE (2017)
5. Chi, C., et al.: Cooperatively improving data center energy efficiency based on multi-agent deep reinforcement learning. Energies **14**(8), 2071 (2021)
6. Ferry, N., et al.: Continuous deployment of trustworthy smart IoT systems. J. Obj. Technol. (2020)
7. Hellaoui, H., Koudil, M., Bouabdallah, A.: Energy efficiency in security of 5g-based IoT: an end-to-end adaptive approach. IEEE Internet Things J. **7**(7), 6589–6602 (2020)
8. Khanna, A., Kaur, S.: Internet of things (IoT), applications and challenges: a comprehensive review. Wirel. Pers. Commun. **114**, 1687–1762 (2020)
9. Mahamat, M., Jaber, G., Bouabdallah, A.: A threat-aware and efficient wireless charging scheme for IoT networks. In: 2023 International Wireless Communications and Mobile Computing (IWCMC), pp. 67–73. IEEE (2023)
10. Mao, B., Kawamoto, Y., Kato, N.: Ai-based joint optimization of QoS and security for 6g energy harvesting internet of things. IEEE Internet Things J. **7**(8), 7032–7042 (2020)
11. Mnih, V., et al.: Human-level control through deep reinforcement learning. Nature **518**(7540), 529–533 (2015)
12. Muthanna, A., et al.: Secure and reliable IoT networks using fog computing with software-defined networking and blockchain. J. Sensor Actu. Netw. **8**(1), 15 (2019)
13. Nahrstedt, K., Li, H., Nguyen, P., Chang, S., Vu, L.: Internet of mobile things: mobility-driven challenges, designs and implementations. In: 2016 IEEE First International Conference on Internet-of-Things Design and Implementation (ioTDI), pp. 25–36. IEEE (2016)
14. Ohnishi, S., Uchibe, E., Yamaguchi, Y., Nakanishi, K., Yasui, Y., Ishii, S.: Constrained deep q-learning gradually approaching ordinary q-learning. Front. Neurorobot. **13**, 103 (2019)
15. Peake, A., McCalmon, J., Zhang, Y., Myers, D., Alqahtani, S., Pauca, P.: Deep reinforcement learning for adaptive exploration of unknown environments. In: 2021 International Conference on Unmanned Aircraft Systems (ICUAS), pp. 265–274. IEEE (2021)
16. Pramila, R., Misbahuddin, M., Shukla, S.: A survey on adaptive authentication using machine learning techniques. In: Shukla, S., Gao, XZ., Kureethara, J.V., Mishra, D. (eds.) Data Science and Security: Proceedings of IDSCS 2022, pp. 317–335. Springer, Heidelberg (2022). https://doi.org/10.1007/978-981-19-2211-4_28
17. Samir, N., et al.: Energy-adaptive lightweight hardware security module using partial dynamic reconfiguration for energy limited internet of things applications. In: 2019 IEEE International Symposium on Circuits and Systems (ISCAS), pp. 1–4. IEEE (2019)
18. Shen, S., Zhang, K., Zhou, Y., Ci, S.: Security in edge-assisted internet of things: challenges and solutions. Sci. China Inf. Sci. **63**, 1–14 (2020)
19. Singh, I., Lee, S.W.: Self-adaptive and secure mechanism for IoT based multimedia services: a survey. Multimedia Tools Appl. **81**(19), 26685–26720 (2022)
20. Sreekanth, G., Ahmed, S.A.N., Sarac, M., Strumberger, I., Bacanin, N., Zivkovic, M.: Mobile fog computing by using SDN/NFV on 5g edge nodes. Comput. Syst. Sci. Eng. **41**(2), 751–765 (2022)
21. Tamizhselvan, C.: A novel communication-aware adaptive key management approach for ensuring security in IoT networks. Trans. Emerg. Telecommun. Technol. **33**(11), e4605 (2022)

22. Tedeschi, S., Emmanouilidis, C., Mehnen, J., Roy, R.: A design approach to IoT endpoint security for production machinery monitoring. Sensors **19**(10), 2355 (2019)
23. Wang, Q., Phillips, C.: Cooperative path-planning for multi-vehicle systems. Electronics **3**(4), 636–660 (2014)
24. Zhang, Q., Lin, J., Sha, Q., He, B., Li, G.: Deep interactive reinforcement learning for path following of autonomous underwater vehicle. IEEE Access **8**, 24258–24268 (2020)
25. Zhang, Y., Cai, P., Pan, C., Zhang, S.: Multi-agent deep reinforcement learning-based cooperative spectrum sensing with upper confidence bound exploration. IEEE Access **7**, 118898–118906 (2019)

Cyber Edge: Mitigating Cyber-Attacks in Edge Computing Using Intrusion Detection System

Waseem AlAqqad[1], Mais Nijim[2(✉)], Ugochukwu Onyeakazi[2], and Hisham Albataineh[3]

[1] Department of Electrical and Computer Engineering, West Virginia University Institute of Technology, Beckley, WV, USA
waseem.alaqqad@mail.wvu.edu
[2] Department of Electrical Engineering and Computer Science, Texas A&M Kingsville, Kingsville, TX, USA
mais.nijim@tamuk.edu
[3] Department of Physics and Geosciences, Texas A&M Kingsville, Kingsville, TX, USA
hisham.albataineh@tamuk.edu

Abstract. Edge computing, an extension of cloud and IoT technologies, introduces unique challenges for intrusion-detection systems (IDS). This study explores IDS architecture in the context of edge computing. We proposed a specialized IDS architecture for edge environments, serving as the foundation for resource allocation strategies. Our chosen allocation model, the single-layer dominant and max-min fair (SDMMF), is theoretically validated to meet hierarchical resource allocation principles. Additionally, we introduce the multilayer dominant and max-min fair (MDMMF) allocation scheme to ensure equitable resource distribution across multiple layers. This research contributes to the enhancement of resource allocation methodologies within IDS, bolstering IoT security in the dynamic edge computing landscape. Given the increasing significance of edge computing, optimizing resource allocation within IDS is crucial for safeguarding critical systems.

Keywords: Edge Computing · Cybersecurity · Machine Learning · Intrusion Detection · IoT

1 Introduction

IoT technology has advanced to the point where many individuals engage with smart devices in their daily lives. [1]. IoT applications typically encompass mobility and latency considerations [2]. To overcome the constraints in the realm of IoT applications, the significance of edge computing has risen substantially as an alternative to traditional cloud computing solutions [3, 4]. By leveraging Edge nodes, positioned in closer proximity to the end-users [5], edge computing enables the delivery provision of services with reduced latency, enhanced access flexibility, and more protected communication for network users [6].

K. Daimi and A. Al Sadoon (Eds.): ACR 2024, LNNS 956, pp. 292–305, 2024.
https://doi.org/10.1007/978-3-031-56950-0_25

In recent years, there has been a notable surge in the proliferation of internet-connected physical devices equipped with sensing and remote communication capabilities. This growth pattern in IoT device internet connectivity is the result of advancements in wireless communications, data analytics, and many other areas [7]. Yet, the proliferation of internet-connected physical devices comes with its share of challenges, particularly in network stability and security [8, 9]. Edge computing networks face a multitude of attacks, and the advantages they offer can be significantly compromised in the absence of robust security and privacy protection mechanisms. To address security threats posed by malicious attackers within the realm of edge computing infrastructure and mitigate potential damages and consequences, our research focuses on evaluating the effectiveness of Intrusion Detection Systems (IDSs).

An Intrusion Detection System (IDS) plays a crucial role as a security barrier by rapidly identifying intrusions and security vulnerabilities within the network [10]. In the context of edge computing, a substantial portion of user service requests are handled by edge nodes. Nevertheless, these edge nodes have limited capacities, making it challenging to conduct comprehensive intrusion detection efficiently [11]. This challenge of resource allocation among edge nodes is focused in our research, for edge computing can be classified into three groups:

1. single-resource allocation,
2. integrated allocation of resources and
3. multi-resource allocation.

The single resource allocation is divided into maximum resource allocation and minimum resource allocation methods and proportional resource allocation techniques [12] [13].

2 Related Work

In this section, we delve into a comprehensive exploration of diverse Deep Learning (DL) techniques employed for the detection of cyberattacks in both conventional and IoT networks. The inherent advantage of DL, which entails automatic feature extraction, has significantly elevated its status in the realm of cybersecurity, particularly within Intrusion Detection Systems (IDS) [14].

In the research documented in [15], S. M. Kasongo and collaborators demonstrated a wireless IDS model's accuracy using the UNSW-NB15 and AWID datasets, while Bae et al. [16] highlighted the effectiveness of an AutoEncoder-based anomaly detection model on the KDD Cup '99 dataset.

Furthermore, [17], authored by M. A. Ferrag and colleagues, revolved around DL models evaluated using the CICIDS2018 and Bot-IoT datasets. These investigations yielded notable accuracy rates, reaching an impressive 97.3%. In [18], Ge, M., Syed, et al. presented an innovative intrusion detection technique rooted in Deep Learning (DL) principles. Their model was thoughtfully constructed with two dense layers, each boasting 512 neurons and employing the ReLU activation function. The final layer, comprising two neurons and utilizing the Softmax function, contributed to the Feedforward Neural Network (FNN) model's remarkable accuracy, which soared to an impressive 99.79%.

Nagisetty et al. [19] provide benchmarks for model accuracy, which we aim to surpass with our proposed schemes. Their findings highlight the importance of high-performance IDS models that are capable of adapting to the dynamic landscape of cyber threats faced by edge networks.

In their work documented in [20], Kasongo, S. M. and colleagues introduced an Intrusion Detection System (IDS) model that relies on Feedforward Neural Networks (FNN). Their approach involved the application of the information gain filter technique for selecting relevant features, and they diligently optimized the model by experimenting with varying numbers of neurons and learning rates. Impressively, when assessed using the NSL-KDD dataset, the model delivered exceptional outcomes. Specifically, for binary classification, the model featured three hidden layers, each with 30 neurons, achieving a remarkable training accuracy of nearly 99.5% and a testing accuracy of 86.19%.

In [21], Fenanir, S., and co-authors presented a lightweight IDS model. They adopted a feature selection strategy that leveraged filter methods and conducted a comprehensive comparative study involving diverse Machine Learning (ML) techniques. Their investigations underscored the superior performance of Decision Trees in classification tasks across multiple datasets. The feature selection process involved the utilization of various filter methods, including correlation filter techniques such as PCC, SCC, and KTC, with different threshold values. Their experiments, conducted on datasets including KDD99, NSL-KDD, and UNSW-NB15, highlighted the Decision Tree classification model's prowess, achieving an impressive accuracy rate of 98%.

In [22], Almaiah et al. conducted a thorough analysis of the Shamoon attack, leveraging Frequency Particle Swarm Optimization (FPSO) to understand its mechanics and propagation through fog nodes. These nodes, pivotal in edge computing, manage diverse and critical data across industrial, medical, and educational sectors—prime targets for the sophisticated Shamoon attacks. The study's focus on the attack vectors and distribution patterns informs our IDS's threat detection capabilities, specifically within edge computing's distributed architecture. By understanding Shamoon's preference for the shortest attack path, we can further refine our SDMMF and MDMMF schemes to proactively anticipate and mitigate such threats. Almaiah et al.'s findings contribute to the threat modeling that underpins our IDS, ensuring it is robust against attacks that exploit the unique topologies of edge computing networks.

In [23], the authors introduced a novel smart health monitoring system within the realm of IoT. This innovative system is designed to monitor critical health parameters, including blood oxygen levels, heart rate, and body temperature, through the utilization of specialized sensors. To bolster data security, the collected information undergoes encryption using the Advanced Encryption Standard (AES) algorithm, providing robust protection against both internal and external threats while the data resides in the cloud. Subsequently, the encrypted data is transmitted to a medical organization, where servers securely receive and decrypt the information. The experimental results strongly support the method's efficacy, with a 95% confidence interval attesting to its reliability. While the smart health monitoring system mentioned in [23] is not directly tied to IDS, it demonstrates DL's role in securing IoT devices—a vital element of edge computing. This reference supports the inclusion of DL in our IDS architecture to ensure comprehensive security in edge computing scenarios.

Kurt et al. introduced a pioneering reinforcement learning-based method for online attack detection, showcasing a notable reduction in false alarms when compared to existing technologies [24]. Despite this success, a current limitation lies in the model's support for only a single agent, prompting the need for expansion to accommodate multiple agents. Transitioning to [25], Morstyn et al. developed an XGboost model adept at predicting global solar radiation (GSR) using climate factors such as temperature and precipitation. Impressively, this model outperformed a support vector machine (SVM)-based counterpart in a case study. In a parallel effort, Cherif et al. [26] proposed an XGboost model for the classification of home network traffic, achieving an impressive accuracy of 99.5% on a dataset with real flows. Despite this success, further enhancements are warranted to fine-tune the model's classification of online traffic. Finally, Camana et al. [27] presented a machine learning-based approach for detecting attacks on smart grids, boasting a quick execution time compared to alternative techniques. It's important to note, however, that this ML-based dimension reduction process may pose a potential risk of data loss.

In their study [28], Su et al. proposed a model designed to identify dynamic load-balancing attacks within smart grid systems, showcasing impressive efficiency with the shortest execution time. However, a notable limitation of this model is the absence of an empirical basis for selecting vulnerable loads or other power system characteristics, suggesting the need for further refinement. In response to this challenge, Patnaik et al. [29] put forth a novel solution employing an XGboost-based classifier. Despite its effectiveness, this approach encounters inefficiencies when dealing with sparse and unstructured data, highlighting potential areas for optimization. Shifting the focus to security concerns, Khamaiseh et al. [30] introduced an innovative adversarial testing strategy tailored for denial-of-service (DoS) attack-detection systems. This strategy adds an extra layer of robustness to the detection mechanisms, showcasing advancements in securing smart grid infrastructures against potential threats. In a separate endeavor [31], Zivkovic et al. employed the firefly algorithm to enhance the effectiveness of the XGBoost classifier for network intrusion detection. This strategy not only minimizes the rates of false positives and false negatives but also demonstrates the potential for combining nature-inspired algorithms with machine learning for improved cybersecurity measures in smart grid systems.

3 III. The Proposed Framework

3.1 A. Architecture

The architecture comprises of Six layers:

User Equipment Layer: It encompasses a diverse range of equipment or devices within the edge computing ecosystem. It includes an array of devices such as private computers, terminals, and various sensors. Those devices can connect to various edge nodes using various protocols tailored to their specific requirements (Fig. 1).

Network Layer: The network layer plays a key role in delivering link services tailored to distinct edge network protocols. Its primary responsibility is to efficiently receive and

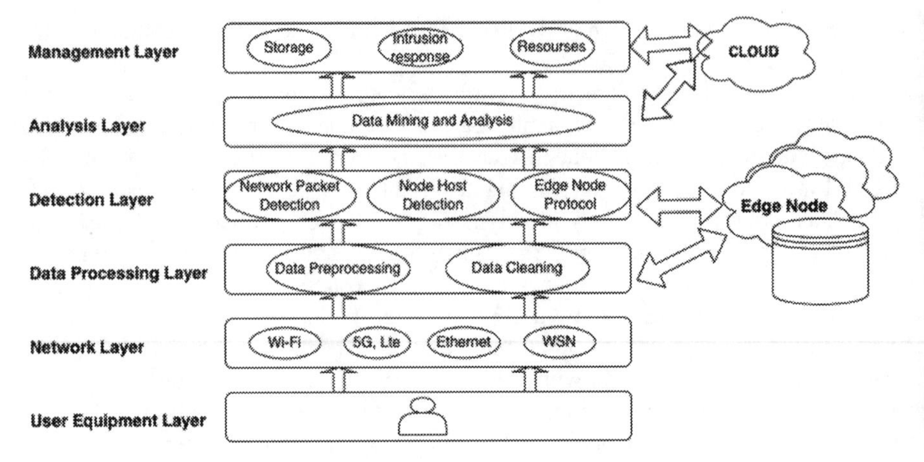

Fig. 1. Architecture of Edge Computing

process data that is transmitted from both the network and the user equipment layer. This layer serves as a crucial intermediary, ensuring seamless communication between the various components of the edge computing system.

Data Processing Layer: At the heart of the edge computing architecture lies the data processing layer. Its primary function revolves around handling network intrusion data originating from user equipment. This intricate task encompasses a spectrum of activities, including packet capture, data cleansing, data filtering, data preprocessing, and other pertinent functions. All these operations are conducted meticulously at the edge nodes, ensuring that the data is prepared and processed effectively to mitigate potential cybersecurity threats.

Detection Layer: Once the intrusion data undergoes preprocessing, this layer comes into play. It serves a crucial role in identifying potential cyberattacks. First, it utilizes a classifier for examining the intrusion data and determining the specific type of attack it corresponds to. This layer incorporates a monitoring system responsible for continuously assessing the state of host devices within the edge nodes. Then, it will actively manage and maintain records of network protocols related to network packets. Once a sufficient volume of data has been collected and stored, the edge node transmits both the test results and relevant logs to the cloud server. Within the domain of intrusion detection systems (IDS) implemented in edge computing, the detection layer holds a central position, and the actual detection procedure occurs within the edge node.

Analysis Layer: The analysis layer plays a vital role. Its main job is to carefully examine the results and logs sent by edge nodes. This thorough analysis is crucial for responding to incidents and conducting digital investigations. Additionally, the analysis layer can turn this information into useful knowledge and provide various services. For instance, it can create reports about the security status of individual edge nodes and store them securely on the cloud server.

Management Layer: Situated within the cloud servers, the management layer takes care of keeping all the edge nodes safe and working properly. It also plays a pivotal role in decision-making and response actions within the IDS. Data and records related to intrusion events on edge nodes are safely maintained, facilitating intrusion forensic investigations. Furthermore, cloud servers are tasked with the strategic distribution of resources among the edge nodes, ensuring efficient and optimized performance.

4 B. Intrusion Detection System of Edge Computing

The figure below illustrates the main role played by an intrusion-detection classifier in processing intrusion data at the detection layer. This classifier has a direct bearing on the subsequent intrusion response activities of a cloud server, ultimately ensuring the overall safety of the system. Consequently, our research focus centers on the development of the intrusion attack detectors. Deploying these detectors on edge nodes harnesses the storing and computational capabilities at their disposal for efficient detection. However, it's important to note that the limited storing and computational capabilities of edge nodes pose constraints on their ability to process and store large-scale data. Furthermore, as previously mentioned, placing detectors exclusively on edge nodes falls short of satisfying the demands of a dynamic network environment (Fig. 2).

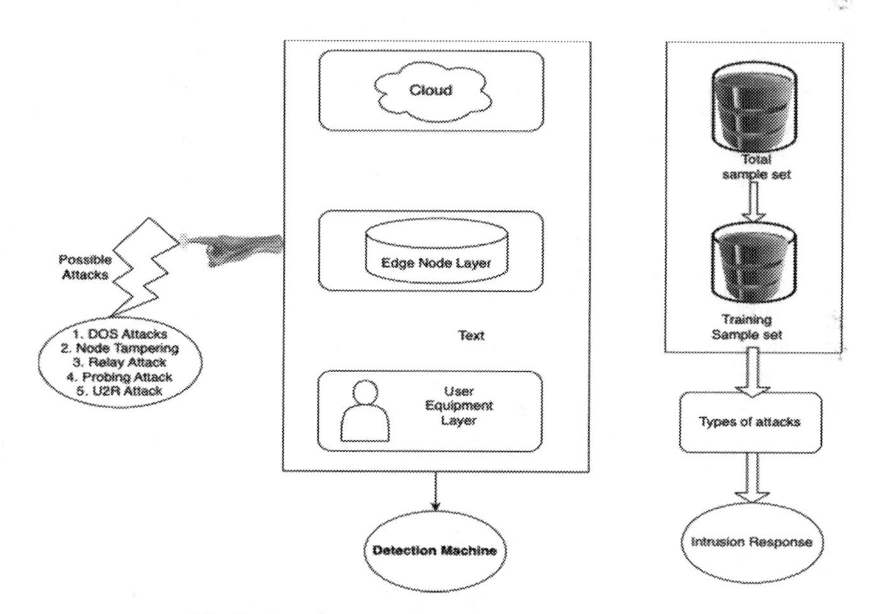

Fig. 2. Intrusion Detection Scheme of Edge Network

In contrast, cloud server possesses significantly larger storage capacity than edge nodes, enabling them to store vast quantities of training sets and associated rules for selecting these sets. Given the diversity of user devices, various edge nodes may introduce substantial variations in the network environment within the edge computing landscape. Additionally, the user population of an edge node experiences dynamic fluctuations, with user devices joining or leaving an edge node at any given time. To address these challenges effectively, a training model generated by the cloud server alone may fall short of meeting the needs of all edge nodes. Moreover, training datasets tend to be large, which could significantly extend training times if conducted solely by central cloud computing, potentially impacting training efficiency.

To overcome these hurdles, a dynamic distribution of training sets to edge nodes for localized training can be implemented. This approach ensures that each edge node is tailored to its specific and ever-changing environment. The workflow for this scheme unfolds as follows:

1. User equipment creates a connection by accessing the edge node.
2. The cloud server will store the entire training dataset and samples are selected based on predefined rules.
3. The chosen training set will be sent to the edge node with the help of a cloud server.
4. The edge node completes its training activity
5. The interaction between the edge node and user equipment results in the generation of a data stream, with intrusion detection conducted locally on the edge node.

At the edge node layer, ensuring the safety and reliability of edge nodes requires a dual focus on intrusion detection and rapid response. In cases where external intruders target edge nodes, the node must possess the capability to promptly detect the intrusion type and trigger a notification as a preemptive security measure. Leveraging their compute and store data locally, enabling low-latency operations, efficiently perform local computations to ensure minimal latency. To achieve this, Efficient and lightweight algorithms with minimal energy consumption specifically designed for intrusion detection can be deployed on edge nodes, optimizing their performance in this critical security domain.

4.1 Resource Allocation Process

For edge nodes, the job of figuring out how to use the resources is done on the cloud server. To distribute resources to edge nodes fairly, we use important settings. These resources include the CPU, storage space, memory for running programs, and other things on the cloud server. Each edge node requires different resources to do the job of detecting intrusions. A big challenge in making the best use of resources is deciding how to share them between the cloud server and edge nodes. We have two resource-sharing plans that are suitable for the setup we're suggesting: SDMMF allocation and MDMMF allocation [24].

Our proposed IDS framework introduces two tailored resource allocation schemes to address the unique demands of edge computing environments. The Single-layer Dominant and Max-Min Fair (SDMMF) scheme is designed specifically for simpler, single-layer network architectures prevalent in smaller-scale edge setups. It efficiently balances resource allocation to optimize the detection and response capabilities of the IDS without overburdening the network. This scheme operates on a two-step allocation process: firstly, it employs the Dominant Resource Fairness (DRF) method [25] to allocate available resources equitably among all requesting nodes. Subsequently, any surplus resources are distributed using the Max-Min Fairness (MMF) method [25] to ensure that the least served nodes are prioritized, thereby maximizing overall network service quality.

In contrast, the Multilayer Dominant and Max-Min Fair (MDMMF) scheme is crafted for more complex, multilayered network infrastructures that are characteristic of large-scale edge computing systems. This scheme not only recognizes but also strategically manages the varying resource demands across different network layers. For instance, it coordinates resource distribution between high-priority edge nodes and subserves, ensuring that each layer receives an appropriate share of resources, such as CPU cycles, storage space, and process memory. The MDMMF builds upon the SDMMF foundation but adds a layer-specific allocation strategy that adapts to the hierarchical nature of resources in multilayer networks. This additional layer of resource management ensures that our IDS can function at scale, accommodating a more diverse set of edge computing scenarios. By establishing these two distinct allocation strategies, our framework is equipped to cater to a wide range of edge computing architectures, from the simplest to the most complex, with precision and adaptability.

5 Simulation and Results

5.1 Simulation Environment: NS3

In our study, we have employed the Network Simulator (NS3) as the primary tool for simulating the proposed Intrusion Detection System (IDS) in edge computing scenarios. NS3 is renowned for its robustness and flexibility, making it an ideal choice for simulating complex network architectures and protocols. Its ability to accurately model both wired and wireless networks allows us to closely emulate the real-world conditions of edge computing environments.

5.2 Simulation Parameters and Key Performance Metrics

Our simulation focuses on four crucial metrics: detection rate, false positive rate, latency, and resource utilization.

- **Detection Rate:** This metric measures the IDS's ability to correctly identify malicious activities. In edge computing, where security threats are diverse and evolving, a high detection rate is crucial for protecting sensitive data and maintaining system integrity.
- **False Positive Rate:** An equally important measure, the false positive rate, indicates the frequency of benign activities being wrongly classified as threats. Minimizing false positives is essential to avoid unnecessary disruptions in edge computing operations.
- **Latency:** In the context of IDS, latency refers to the time taken to detect and respond to a threat. Low latency is vital in edge computing, given the need for real-time or near-real-time data processing and decision-making.
- **Resource Utilization:** This metric assesses how efficiently the IDS utilizes computational and network resources. Efficient resource utilization is a key concern in edge computing due to the limited resources available at the edge of the network.

5.3 Attack Simulation and Dataset Utilization

To create a realistic simulation environment, we incorporated a variety of attack scenarios. These include common threats in edge computing such as DDoS attacks, malware injections, and unauthorized access attempts. In our simulation, we used publicly available datasets like NSL-KDD and UNSW-NB15 which are commonly used in cybersecurity research, particularly for training and testing Intrusion Detection Systems (IDS).

5.4 Simulation Goals

The primary aim of our simulation is to validate the efficacy of our IDS framework in accurately detecting and responding to cyber threats in edge computing environments, while efficiently utilizing available resources. By analyzing the results against the key performance metrics, we aim to demonstrate the advantages of our proposed SDMMF and MDMMF allocation schemes over traditional IDS approaches.

5.5 Baseline Models for Comparison Comparative Analysis and Established Models

In our methodology, we conduct a comparative analysis with established models in the field of Intrusion Detection Systems (IDS), specifically focusing on models that are pertinent to both traditional and IoT-focused network security. Our comparison includes various baseline models as outlined in academic papers [15–24]. However, to maintain a focused and relevant comparison, we have primarily concentrated on models that closely align with the operational context and objectives of our proposed IDS framework, particularly in the edge computing environment.

Our selected baseline models, derived from papers [17, 19, 20], and [22], represent the current state-of-the-art in IDS. These studies were chosen for their direct relevance to the aspects of IDS that our SDMMF and MDMMF schemes aim to enhance, such as detection accuracy, resource allocation efficiency, and adaptability to edge computing dynamics. While references [15, 16, 18, 21, 23], and [24] provide valuable insights into the broader domain of cybersecurity and IDS, our analysis specifically targets those models that offer the most direct comparison and benchmarking for our proposed framework in the context of edge computing.

5.6 Proposed Framework Specifics SDMMF and MDMMF Schemes

Both SDMMF and MDMMF schemes introduced by our framework are expected to enhance the performance of IDS in edge computing by optimizing resource distribution, thus improving detection rates and reducing latency without sacrificing network stability.

5.7 Simulation Results

In the simulated environment, our proposed SDMMF and MDMMF models exhibited significant improvements over the baseline models in all key performance metrics.

Specifically, the detection rate was enhanced by approximately 5%, and the false positive rate was reduced by 3%. Importantly, our models demonstrated a notable reduction in latency, a critical factor in edge computing. Furthermore, both SDMMF and MDMMF schemes showed superior resource utilization, essential for the resource-constrained environments of edge computing.

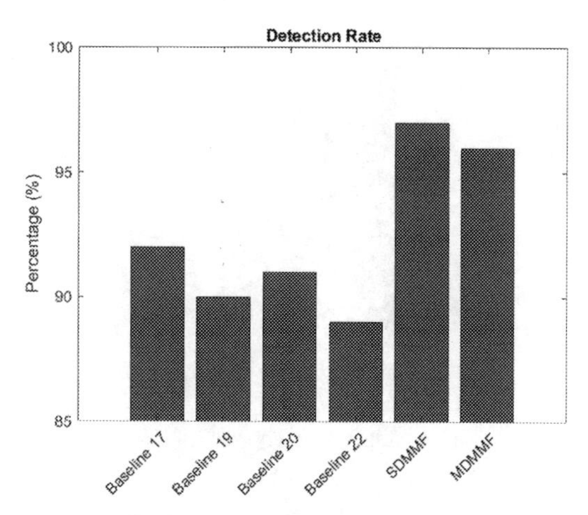

Fig. 3. Detection Rate Comparison

Figure 3 demonstrates that the proposed SDMMF and MDMMF models significantly outperform the baseline models concerning detection rate, which is a testament to their ability to accurately identify cyber threats within an edge computing environment.

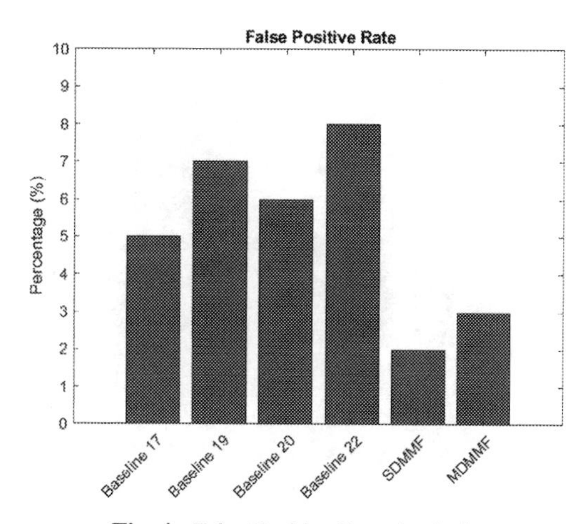

Fig. 4. False Positive Rate Analysis

Figure 4 presents the false positive rates across the baseline models and our frameworks. Notably, the SDMMF and MDMMF models exhibit a significant reduction in false positives, underscoring their precision and reducing the likelihood of benign activities being misclassified as threats.

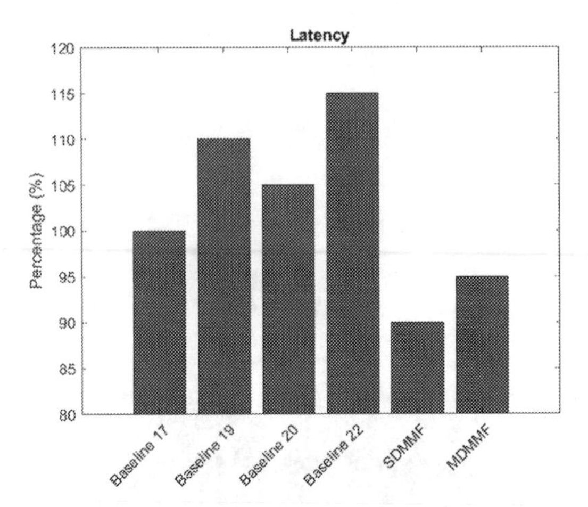

Fig. 5. Latency in Threat Detection

Figure 5 presents a latency comparison, where both SDMMF and MDMMF models outperform the baseline models. This improvement is critical in edge computing environments where reduced latency is imperative for timely threat detection and response.

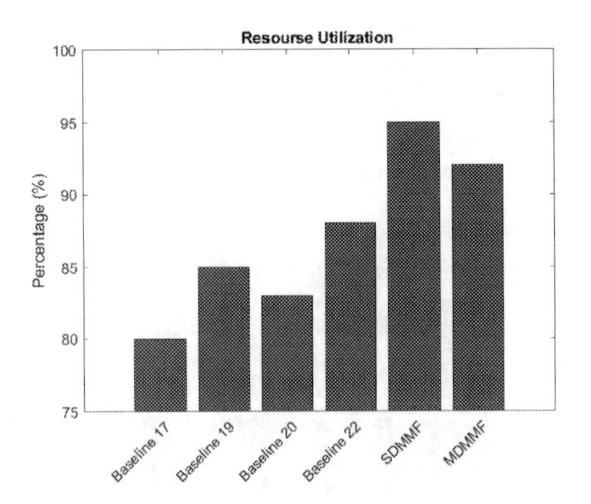

Fig. 6. Resource Utilization Efficiency

Figure 6 compares the efficiency of resource utilization between the baseline models and our proposed schemes. The SDMMF and MDMMF schemes demonstrate enhanced resource management, which is vital in the resource-limited context of edge computing.

5.8 Analysis and Interpretation of Results

The simulation results affirm that the specialized design of the SDMMF and MDMMF models is highly effective in the context of edge computing. The improved detection rate and reduced false positives contribute to more reliable and trustworthy IDS functionalities. The low latency and efficient resource utilization further underscore the suitability of these models for the unique demands of edge computing, where swift response times and judicious resource management are paramount. The empirical evidence provided by Figs. 3, 4, 5 and 6 validates the performance superiority of the proposed SDMMF and MDMMF models over the baseline models. The quantitative advancements illustrated in Fig. 3 for detection rates and Fig. 4 for false positive rates not only reflect the models' accuracy but also their operational efficiency as seen in Figs. 5 and 6 for latency and resource utilization, respectively. These enhancements are pivotal for edge computing environments where the balance between performance and resource management is critical.

6 Conclusion and Future Work

In conclusion, our research introduces innovative approaches within Intrusion Detection Systems (IDS) for edge computing, focusing on the pivotal challenges of resource allocation and threat detection efficiency. The simulations conducted using Network Simulator 3 (NS3), as demonstrated in Figs. 3, 4, 5 and 6, clearly indicate that our proposed Single-layer Dominant and Max-Min Fair (SDMMF) and Multilayer Dominant and Max-Min Fair (MDMMF) schemes significantly enhance the security posture of edge computing environments. These figures highlight the tangible improvements in detection rates, false positive rates, latency, and resource utilization, underscoring the practical impact of our findings.

As we look toward future work, we plan to transition from simulated models to real-world implementation and testing. This transition includes exploring adaptive learning mechanisms for IDS and conducting a thorough analysis of the scalability and robustness of our models across various edge computing scenarios. Despite the promising results achieved in simulated environments, we recognize that applying these findings in actual deployments entails confronting a series of challenges and potential limitations:

1. **Scalability in Diverse Environments:** The effectiveness of the SDMMF and MDMMF schemes in simulated edge computing scenarios is established, but their scalability in heterogeneous real-world environments, characterized by varying network sizes and loads, demands extensive testing.
2. **Integration with Existing Infrastructure:** Implementing our proposed IDS models in existing network infrastructures, especially within legacy systems, requires careful consideration of compatibility and integration challenges.
3. **Resource Constraints:** Practical deployments might encounter more severe resource constraints than our simulations, which could influence the performance efficacy of the IDS.
4. **Operational Overheads:** The deployment of these IDS schemes might introduce additional operational costs, including maintenance, monitoring, and management.

These overheads need to be carefully weighed against the security benefits they provide.

Moving forward, our goal is to prototype and rigorously evaluate these IDS approaches through collaborations with real-world organizations. This step is crucial to verify the practicality and effectiveness of our models in actual edge computing deployments, thereby translating theoretical advancements into tangible cybersecurity improvements.

References

1. Maddikunta, P.K.R., Gadekallu, T.R., Kaluri, R., Srivastava, G., Parizi, R.M., Khan, M.S.: Green communication in IoT networks using a hybrid optimization algorithm. Comput. Commun. **159**, 97–107 (2020). https://doi.org/10.1016/j.comcom.2020.05.020
2. Chang, C., Narayana Srirama, S., Buyya, R.: Indie fog: an efficient fog-computing infrastructure for the Internet of Things. Computer **50**(9), 92–98 (2017)
3. Sabella, D., Vaillant, A., Kuure, P., Rauschenbach, U., Giust, F.: Mobile-edge computing architecture: the role of MEC in the Internet of Things. IEEE Consum. Electron. Mag. **5**(4), 84–91 (2016)
4. Corcoran, P., Datta, S.K.: Mobile-edge computing and the Internet of Things for consumers: extending cloud computing and services to the edge of the network. IEEE Consum. Electron. Mag. **5**(4), 73–74 (2016)
5. Masip-Bruin, X., Marín-Tordera, E., Tashakor, G., Jukan, A., Ren, G.J.: Foggy clouds and cloudy fogs: a real need for coordinated management of fog-to-cloud computing systems. IEEE Wirel. Commun. **23**(5), 120–128 (2016)
6. Roman, R., Lopez, J., Mambo, M.: Mobile edge computing, Fog et al.: a survey and analysis of security threats and challenges. arXiv (2016)
7. Lee, I., Lee, K.: The Internet of Things (IoT): applications, investments, and challenges for enterprises. Bus. Horizons **58**, 431–440 (2015). https://doi.org/10.1016/j.bushor.2015.03.008
8. Esposito, C., Castiglione, A., Pop, F., Choo, K.R.: Challenges of connecting edge and cloud computing: a security and forensic perspective. IEEE Cloud Comput. **4**(2), 13–17 (2017)
9. Osanaiye, O.A., Chen, S., Yan, Z., Lu, R.X., Choo, K.R., Dlodlo, M.E.: From cloud to fog computing: a review and a conceptual live VM migration framework. IEEE Access **5**, 8284–8300 (2017)
10. Peng, J., Choo, K.R., Ashman, H.: User profiling in intrusion detection: a review. J. Netw. Comput. Appl. **72**, 14–27 (2016)
11. Iqbal, S., et al.: On cloud security attacks: a taxonomy and intrusion detection and prevention as a service. J. Netw. Comput. Appl. **74**, 98–120 (2016)
12. Amaldi, E., Capone, A., Coniglio, S., Luca, G.: Network optimization problems subject to max–min fair flow allocation. IEEE Commun. Lett. **17**(7), 1463–1466 (2013)
13. Mankar, P.D., Das, G., Pathak, S.S.: A novel proportionally fair spectrum allocation in two-tiered cellular networks. IEEE Commun. Lett. **19**(4), 629–632 (2015)
14. Ma, W.: Analysis of anomaly detection method for Internet of things based on deep learning. Trans. Emerg. Telecommun. Technol. **31**(12), e3893 (2020)
15. Kasongo, S.M., Sun, Y.: A deep learning method with wrapper-based feature extraction for wireless intrusion detection system. Comput. Secur. **92**, 101752 (2020)
16. Bae, G., Jang, S., Kim, M., Joe, I.: Autoencoder-based on anomaly detection with intrusion scoring for smart factory environments. In: Park, J.H., Shen, H., Sung, Y., Tian, H. (eds.) PDCAT 2018. CCIS, vol. 931, pp. 414–423. Springer, Singapore (2019). https://doi.org/10.1007/978-981-13-5907-1_44

17. Ferrag, M.A., Maglaras, L., Moschoyiannis, S., Janicke, H.: Deep learning for cyber security intrusion detection: approaches, datasets, and comparative study. J. Inf. Secur. Appl. **50**, 102419 (2020)
18. Ge, M., Syed, N.F., Fu, X., Baig, Z., Robles-Kelly, A.: Towards a deep learning-driven intrusion detection approach for the Internet of Things. Comput. Netw. **186**, 107784 (2021)
19. Nagisetty, A., Gupta, G.P.: Framework for detection of malicious activities in IoT networks using Keras deep learning library. In: 2019 3rd International Conference on Computing methodologies and Communication (ICCMC), pp. 633–637. IEEE (2019)
20. Kasongo, S.M., Sun, Y.: A deep learning method with filter-based feature engineering for wireless intrusion detection system. IEEE Access **7**, 38597–38607 (2019)
21. Fenanir, S., Semchedine, F., Baadache, A.: A machine learning-based lightweight intrusion detection system for the Internet of Things. Revue d'Intelligence Artif. **33**(3) (2019)
22. Almaiah, A., Almomani, O.: An investigation of digital forensics for Shamoon attack behavior in FOG computing and threat intelligence for incident response. J. Theor. Appl. Inf. Technol. **15**, 98 (2020)
23. Siam, A.I., et al.: Secure health monitoring communication systems based on IoT and cloud computing for medical emergency applications. Comput. Intell. Neurosci. **2021** (2021)
24. Kurt, M.N., Ogundijo, O., Li, C., Wang, X.: Online cyber-attack detection in smart grid: a reinforcement learning approach. **10**, 5174–5185 (2019). https://doi.org/10.48550/arXiv.1809.05258
25. Fan, J., et al.: Comparison of support vector machine and extreme gradient boosting for predicting daily global solar radiation using temperature and precipitation in humid subtropical climates: a case study in China. **164**, 102–111 (2018). https://doi.org/10.1016/j.enconman.2018.02.087
26. Cherif, I.L., Kortebi, A.: On using eXtreme gradient boosting (XGBoost) machine learning algorithm for home network traffic classification, pp. 1–6. https://doi.org/10.1109/WD.2019.8734193
27. Camana Acosta, M.R., Ahmed, S., Garcia, C.E., Koo, I.: Extremely randomized trees-based scheme for stealthy cyber-attack detection in smart grid networks **8**, 19921–19933 (2020). https://doi.org/10.1109/ACCESS.2020.2968934
28. Qingyu, S., Li, S., Gao, Y., Huang, X., Li, J.: Observer-based detection and reconstruction of dynamic load altering attack in smart grid. J. Franklin Inst. **358**(7), 4013–4027 (2021). https://doi.org/10.1016/j.jfranklin.2021.02.008
29. Patnaik, B., Mishra, M., Bansal, R.C., Jena, R.K.: MODWT-XGBoost based smart energy solution for fault detection and classification in a smart microgrid **285**, 116457 (2021). https://doi.org/10.1016/j.apenergy.2021.116457
30. Khamaiseh, S.Y., Alsmadi, I., Al-Alaj, A.: Deceiving machine learning-based saturation attack detection systems in SDN. In: 2020 IEEE Conference on Network Function Virtualization and Software Defined Networks (NFV-SDN), Leganes, Spain, pp. 44–50 (2020). https://doi.org/10.1109/NFV-SDN50289.2020.9289908
31. Zivkovic, M., Tair, M., Venkatachalam, K., Bacanin, N., Hubálovský, Š., Trojovský, P.: Novel hybrid firefly algorithm: an application to enhance XGBoost tuning for intrusion detection classification. PeerJ Comput. Sci. **8**, e956 (2022).https://doi.org/10.7717/peerj-cs.956
32. Lin, F.H., Su, J.T.: Multi-layer resources fair allocation in big data with heterogeneous demands. Wirel. Personal Commun. **98**(7), 1–16 (2017)
33. Ghodsi, A., Zaharia, M., Shenker, S., Stoica, I.: Choosy, max–min fair sharing for data center jobs with constraints. In: Proceedings of the 8th ACM European Conference on Computer Systems, Prague (2013)

A New Security Mechanism for IoT Devices: Electroencephalogram (EEG) Signals

Ahmet Furkan Aydogan[1], Cihan Varol[1](✉), Aysenur Vanli[1], and Hacer Varol[2]

[1] Sam Houston State University, Huntsville, TX 77384, USA
{axa184,cxv007,axv176}@shsu.edu

[2] Stephen F. Austin State University, Nacogdoches, TX 75962, USA
varolh@sfasu.edu

Abstract. The variety and high usage rate of Internet of Things (IoT) devices make them a prime target for cyber-attacks. Unfortunately, the limited physical size of IoT devices prevents the use of powerful computing components to secure these devices with sophisticated encryption methods. Hence, typically, symmetric-asymmetric, lightweight, and hybrid methods are used to secure IoT devices. However, each of these approaches has its disadvantages; thus, none of them is considered successful in preventing cyber-attacks on IoT devices. On the other hand, security procedures based on biological uniqueness can be effective in solving this predicament of IoT devices. While biological singularity methods such as fingerprint and facial recognition systems are also utilized to secure IoT devices, technological innovations such as artificial intelligence and deepfake still lead to vulnerabilities in IoT. Nonetheless, because of the uniqueness of the biological singularity, here, we present a mechanism to secure such devices that combines the encryption and the human factor while minimizing the possible attack surface to the system. Specifically, in this paper, we propose the use of users' brain frequencies as a security mechanism in IoT devices. The work showed that obtained data from AF3-Pz-T8-AF4 electrodes can be used to secure IoT devices.

Keywords: Brain Frequencies · Cyberwarfare · Human-Machine-Encryption Integration · IoT Security · Social Engineering

1 Introduction

Human vulnerability is one of the main effective weapons used in cyber warfare. Attacks carried out mainly with the effective use of social engineering methods reach a level that can cause a high level of vulnerability. Moreover, the incomplete encryption of the data obtained in PlugX attacks or the lack of FTP server encryption in the 2020 United States federal government data breach are signs of how vital encryption methods are [1].

IoT devices are increasingly used in many areas, such as police departments, power generation plants, education, finance, living spaces, and armies which is becoming the core of cyber warfare. Their encryption mechanisms' success rates determine the fate of IoT devices in cyberattacks. Encryption methods that provide high security require

K. Daimi and A. Al Sadoon (Eds.): ACR 2024, LNNS 956, pp. 306–317, 2024.
https://doi.org/10.1007/978-3-031-56950-0_26

high processing capacities, while encryption methods that require low processing are insufficient to provide complete protection. Unfortunately, the physical size of IoT is an obstacle to the use of powerful hardware components to secure these devices.

The use of passwords with encryption methods is a well-known technique to mitigate security risks on IoT devices. However, the generated passwords' security (considering the vulnerability of the human factor), naturally negatively impacts the security procedures established for the devices. Although creating a security procedure that is both personalized and unaffected by manipulations may seem complicated, it may also make the system more secure.

To eliminate the vulnerability of the human factor to manipulation, there are efforts to introduce a method of encryption based on biological singularity. Some of them aim to ensure system security with facial recognition and fingerprinting. In attacks where almost all social engineering strategies are carried out remotely, no matter how much the human factor is manipulated, the fact that security is provided by biological singularity naturally limits the impact of attacks. However, with the development of artificial intelligence, the ability to imitate the human face with so-called deepfake methods [2] or to use fingerprints after converting them into numerical values so that systems can comprehend them has led to the re-emergence of vulnerabilities [3]. Therefore, we argue that combining the concepts of humans, IoT devices, and encryption in a single framework can address this problem. Therefore, this paper introduces a security mechanism utilizing Electroencephalogram (EEG) signals to secure IoT devices. Specifically, brain signals obtained from humans are used as an encryption method. The benefit of our proposal is that it enables a new encryption method based on biological singularity for which even low-performance components in IoT devices will suffice. In addition, brain signals are resistant to imitation and remote access.

2 Literature Work

Various encryption methods have been used to increase the security of IoT devices. Encryption methods for IoT devices include symmetric-asymmetric, lightweight, hybrid, and biological singularity. One of the most significant factors that cause variations is because of IoT devices' processing capacity. Encryption methods that provide high security require high processing capacities, while encryption methods that require low processing are insufficient to provide complete protection [4].

Symmetric encryption is based on determining a sequence of randomly generated letters or numbers (secret key). Two different approaches can be used in symmetric encryption, block cipher and stream cipher. The main difference between the two methods is that the block cipher stores the data to be encrypted in memory, while the stream cipher stores the data integrated into the algorithm [5].

The study conducted by Fischer et al. [6] uses a symmetric encryption method to ensure IoT devices' security contains the steps to modify the CP-ABE process. During the development phase of the new method, the key revocation problem in the ABE method was taken as the primary objective. Key revocation consists of revoking the privileges of users who have public keys. According to the article, the ABE method allocates too much time to the key revocation part, which increases production costs.

The method presented as a solution is to remove the ABE method's key revocation and process it in a different section called proxy. ABE will see the key revocation values as a constant with the specified method before processing the text to be encrypted. At the same time, key revocation values will be created in the Proxy section. Besides, the values in the proxy content will not be enough to decrypt. The methodology performed better than the total ABE conversion and encryption phases [6].

In asymmetric encryption, a pair of keys called public and private keys are used. The public key can be shared with anyone and does not create a security vulnerability. However, the private key is the only way to make encrypted data readable, so it should only be shared with those who have permission to access it [7]. Diffie–Hellman key exchange, one of the earliest known studies of asymmetric encryption, was announced in 1976. The advantage of the Diffie–Hellman key exchange method is that the text encrypted by the public key can be read with many private keys. It should be noted that Diffie–Hellman is a key exchange method, not an encryption method [8]. The Rivest–Shamir–Adleman (RSA) encryption method was announced in 1977. Although public and private keys are produced in RSA encryption, there is a mathematical connection between the two keys. With this mathematical connection, the data is encrypted by the keys and becomes readable only by people with the private key. The benefit of this strategy is that even if the public key is transferred insecurely, it makes the system secure against attacks since the private key is not owned [9].

Hussain et al. [10] created a new encryption method inspired by asymmetric encryption to secure IoT devices' communication. The generated encryption method aims to obtain security by processing the user's data, along with a unique key code received from the user. The user can select a number between 0 and 255, and then transfer the unencrypted data. Pure data received from the user is converted to ASCII codes. The cipher from 0 to 255 previously supplied by the user is inserted into the XOR process with plaintext and converted to ASCII. Then, the results are converted to decimal values using the n-bit & n/2-bit sequence path. The encryption becomes decrypted when both data are retrieved from the user [10].

Lightweight Encryption Algorithms (LEAs) developed by Hong et al. [11] emerged in 2013. Hong et al. proposed software-based encryption with key sizes of 128, 192, or 256 bits and named LEA-128, LEA-192, and LEA-256. LEA focuses on modular addition, bit rotation, and XOR operations (ARX) as its operating principle. Another specific aspect of LEA is that the first and last loop functions are the same. This way, unlike other encryption methods, it focuses on performance by not using more processing capacity. Hong et al. argue that encryption is used more than decryption in IoT devices and has provided 1.5 to 2.0 times better performance than the frequently used Advanced Encryption Standard (AES) [11]. As a result of all these developments, LEA has become a phenomenon and opened the door to different studies to create the security of IoT devices in the academic field.

Understandably, lightweight encryption methods follow different strategies to reduce processing power. One of these strategies is the lightweight encryption methods integrated with cloud systems. The technique developed by Belguith et al. [12] is the attribute-based encryption (ABE) method. Changes to the policies of the ABE method provided different advantages, and the technique was named PU-ABE. PU-ABE has three distinct advantages. First, it created data that can be easily re-encrypted with cloud technology. Second, the public key can be shared with specific accounts or completely hidden. Third, the data shared with the end user is of fixed size and low cost.

Hybrid encryption combines the strengths of symmetric and asymmetric encryptions. However, in general, the bit lengths used by the encryption have been reduced. Jian et al. [13] aimed to provide security on IoT devices by hybridizing asymmetric and symmetric encryption methods. During data transfer between IoT and other devices, it is first suggested that the IoT device control the network to coordinate which and how many devices are connected. In the first step, called the self-identification procedure, the MAC addresses of each device connected to the network are recorded by IoT modules. In short, each device connected to the network shares its MAC addresses for later use in encryption and storing valuable data such as manufacturer information. Then those devices will register with the database. In the second step, public keys can be shared between the predefined devices. When transferring the data, IP addresses and MAC addresses are controlled via the server, and if the match is achieved, the data process is performed. Finally, 751 bytes of a private key and 498 bytes of a public key were obtained. This way, the authors achieved data security since the private key size starts with 256 bytes [13].

Chandu et al. [14] aimed to secure IoT devices in a hybrid way using RSA, AES, and e-mail verification methods. The changes on the Field Programmable Gate Array (FPGA) of the devices were applied using Xilinx SPARTAN-6, and the results were analyzed with the synthesis tool of Xilinx ISE-Design 14.5 software. Finally, methods such as brute force attacks on IoT devices have been experimented with using cloud technology to point out vulnerabilities [14].

Biological singularity is effectively used in system security procedures. The idea of using security applications created with various biological characteristics of users, such as fingerprints and face recognition, in IoT devices has created a harmonious process. Considering the capacity of the sensors in IoT devices to recognize these biological characteristics, it is possible to develop security procedures [15]. Hossain et al.'s work using biological singularity for IoT devices focuses on face recognition. The face image obtained from the user, after being subjected to orientation, is transformed into a histogram of differential excitation and Weber local descriptor (WLD). Simultaneously, the outputs of the two histograms, combined with the Local Binary Pattern Histogram (LBP), were compared against a database of 1204 images, with a maximum success rate of 99.5 percent, depending on the alpha values [16]. Sarika et al. present an implementation of a door lock sensor created by interacting the RS03 fingerprint module with the Arduino Uno microcontroller [17]. However, the uses of fingerprint data do not have to be directly IoT embedded. As an example, Golec et al. presented a scheme called BioSec, in which the data obtained from the fingerprint sensor on a Raspberry Pi 4 device was successful in identifying the user. However, since the data belonging to the singularity still needs to be secured in the proposed systems, the user data is subjected to relatively low 128-bit encryption in both the transfer and read-back phases using the DES method [18].

Different approaches have been developed to secure IoT devices. Symmetric and asymmetric methods are strong in terms of protection but costly. Lightweight methods are much less costly but can be weak in terms of protection. Hybrid methods are based on modifications of symmetric and asymmetric encryption but are not as strong and still costly. Finally, security procedures based on biological uniqueness have weaknesses due to the risk of being imitated by technological innovations such as deepfake and artificial intelligence. This paper proposes a new mechanism to go beyond general IoT security methods. It presents EEG signals as a security method to overcome the problems encountered in biological singularity.

3 Experimental Setup and Test Case

The experimental scenario aims to find the possibility of establishing secure communication with IoT devices by collecting/analyzing the frequencies produced by the human brain. Brain frequencies have a unique production sequence for each individual. Brain signals repeat a particular frequency generation sequence when considering a specific subject. This way, secure communication aims to obtain the brain frequency, a unique production of the person with a special remembrance. Specifically, the user of the IoT device will be able to generate a unique brain frequency by thinking of remembrance, and the obtained frequency will be used in replacement of the classical username/password type of authentication mechanisms. An electroencephalogram (EEG) device, which resembles a computer headset, was used to acquire brain frequencies. While creating the test case, the effect of the ability to make decisions quickly on brain frequencies and the elimination of stress-related artifacts that ambient factors may cause were aimed. This ensures that fast decision-making is possible even under a cyber-attack, which could be encountered in real life, and the system can function correctly even under stress.

In the scenario created to identify the evidential features of matching memories, photographs from four different locations are included. As can be seen in Fig. 1, photo "A" contains a dresser with an antique telephone on it and a chair. The second photo "B" is a library. The third photo "C" contains an old television and a cabinet. The fourth photo is the workspace with many drawers and cabinets. Notice that each photo contains a drawer or cabinet. The benefits of this feature in the photographs will be revealed in free choices.

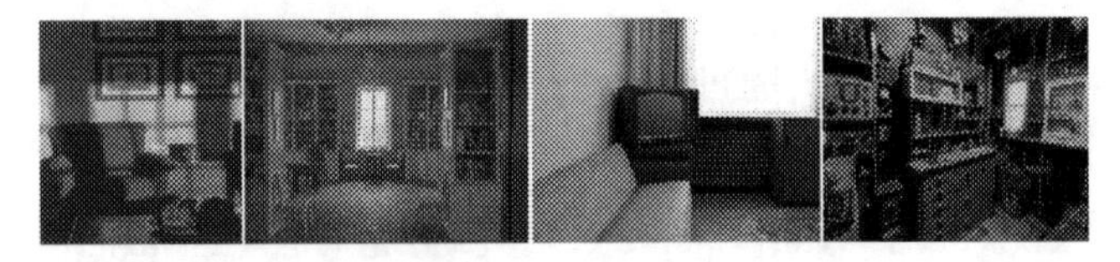

Fig. 1. Used pictures for the scenario.

At the beginning of the experiment of the scenario, the subjects were expected to take a position in front of the computer screen. When the EEG data started to be acquired, each subject looked at a blank screen for the first 10 s. The purpose of showing the blank screen is to reduce the stress level of the subjects and to allow time for noises to be avoided during the correction of their posture. Then, a photograph is shown on the screen for 50 s. In this way, a total of 1 min of EEG data is obtained from each subject, with 10 s of blank screen and the remaining 50 s of content. After the subjects have seen three photographs, before they see the last photograph, a recall is imposed as "The next picture requires your focus. Imagine that you have an imaginary wallet and hide it in a suitable spot you see in the picture." However, the recall was imposed on different photographs for each subject. So, if subject 001 sees photo "D" in the 4th column, subject 002 sees photo "C" in the 4th column. That is, each subject is exposed to the recall imposed by the photo shifted one backward from the previous subject. In this case, subjects are specified as the images to focus on, but the place to hide the imaginary wallet is left to their free will. To determine whether the memory imposed here would cause a match in the future, some changes were made in the next stage. Namely, in the second stage, the pictures were shown to the subjects again, but no comment was made. In addition, while the blank screen duration was kept constant at 10 s, the total duration was reduced to 40 s (30 s of it for the content), in order to control the rapid response process in a short time.

In the experimental scenario, the main expectation is that the density and distribution of subject frequencies shaped by the imposed recall would match. As an example, from the scenario, subject 001 chooses "A" as the main photo. In this case, the 1-min recording of subject 001 should match the 30-s recording. However, this match should only be on photo "A" because the thought constrained and induced by the imposed recall will be similar in the main pictures. Other combinations such as A-B, A-C, and A-D are less likely to match. Table 1 shows the expected responses when these combinations occur. Combination A-A is expected to produce more similar values, while combinations A-B, A-C, and A-D are expected to produce less similar values. In addition, it should be noted that the combinations are always based on 1-min recordings. The reason for this is the relationship between door keys and padlock. The 1-min recordings are used to create the padlock. Whereas 30-s recordings are only useful if they produce a key that matches the padlock.

Table 1. Combinations of 1-min and 30-s EEG data from subject 001.

Subject 001 Padlock Photo A 1 Minute Rec.	→	Subject 001 Key Photo A 30 Sec. Rec.	→	More Similar
Subject 001 Padlock Photo A 1 Minute Rec.	→	Subject 001 Key Photo B 30 Sec. Rec.	→	Less Similar
Subject 001 Padlock Photo A 1 Minute Rec.	→	Subject 001 Key Photo C 30 Sec. Rec.	→	Less Similar
Subject 001 Padlock Photo A 1 Minute Rec.	→	Subject 001 Key Photo D 30 Sec. Rec.	→	Less Similar

Unsupervised machine learning methods allow inferences to be made based on the structural relationships of data. Clustering, an unsupervised method, aims to ensure that data with the same characteristics are placed in the same clusters, even if the data has not been processed before. Applying the clustering method to perform data synchronization and density measurements in the scenario can provide a general solution. For example, let's take subject 001 for the scenario. Subject 001 used picture C as a padlock. Subject 001 will provide the key to open the padlock only with the frequencies he/she will produce in a 30-s recording after seeing the same picture. Now, let us assume that the combinations C-A, C-B, C-C, and C-D are processed by the clustering method. If the clustering method is applied to the aforementioned 1-min and 30-s data, the combinations that should provide the most matches are expected to be C-C, as stated in the hypothesis.

4 Results and Discussion

The first method to be used in the observation phase of the data is the extraction of normal (Gaussian) distributions. The data are distributed on an electrode-based basis. It has already been mentioned that the recordings had a blank screen time of 10 s in all scenarios. The main purpose of these recordings was to eliminate movement, stress, and excitement-induced contractions that may occur in the subjects during the initial stages of data recording. While blinking, heartbeat, and other muscle-related noises may occur as the data recording continues, they will be much less than during the first 10 s of the experiments. The data were simply reformatted to detect changes due to the effects of noises that occurred in the first 10 s of the experiments. Since EEG data produces 128 data samples per second and the total artifact avoidance time is 10 s, deleting the first 1280 data lines of each electrode will eliminate noises. Let's take subject 001 as an example. 001 selected "C" as a padlock photograph. When subject 001's 1-min and 30-s recordings of the photograph "C" are distributed, the electrodes AF3 (frontal cortex), AF4 (frontal cortex), Pz (side of the skull), T7 (center of the skull) and T8 (center of the skull) can be observed side by side. Figure 2 shows the density of the data on the y-axis, while the x-axis shows the single measured value of each feature (EEG.AF3, EEG.AF4, EEG.Pz, EEG.T7, and EEG.T8). The electrodes AF4, Pz, T7, and T8 in the figure have great similarities. There are small differences between the data obtained from the AF3 electrode.

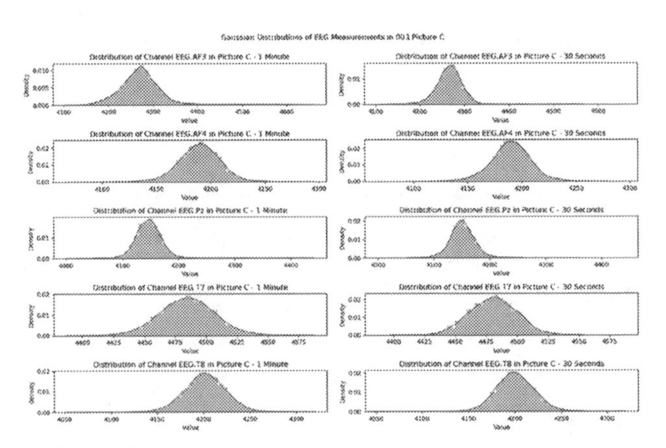

Fig. 2. Gaussian distribution of 1-min padlock (left) and 30-s key (right) picture C records of Subject 007 by electrode basis.

This time the data of subject 001 was analyzed with the C-A combination. Recall that 001 chose "C" as the padlock photo. It is expected that there will be differences between the data when a different key, the 30-s photo "A", is used. As can be seen in

Fig. 3, there are differences in the data obtained from AF4, Pz and T8 electrodes, the electrode where this is most easily observable is AF4. The data obtained from electrode AF4 for the 1-min "C" photograph shows that the EEG measurements obtained from subject 001 never produced a signal corresponding to the 4250 value that appeared in the previous recording and was caused by a momentary high concentration. However, subject 001 produces brain signals corresponding to 4275 in the 30-s photo "A".

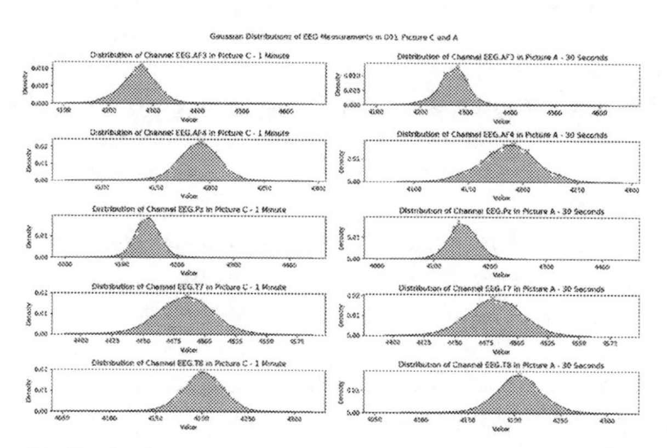

Fig. 3. Gaussian distribution of 1-min padlock picture C (left) and 30-s key picture A (right) records of Subject 001 by electrode basis.

In order to better perceive the differences or similarities between the 1-min and 30-s recordings in the scenario, it may be necessary to display the frequency distributions of the subjects on the same axis. In Fig. 4, the 1-min padlock and 30-s key data of subject 001 photograph "C" are shown on the same axis with respect to the electrodes. In particular, it is observed that the intensity measurements of the 30-s recordings are larger for each electrode in the matched images.

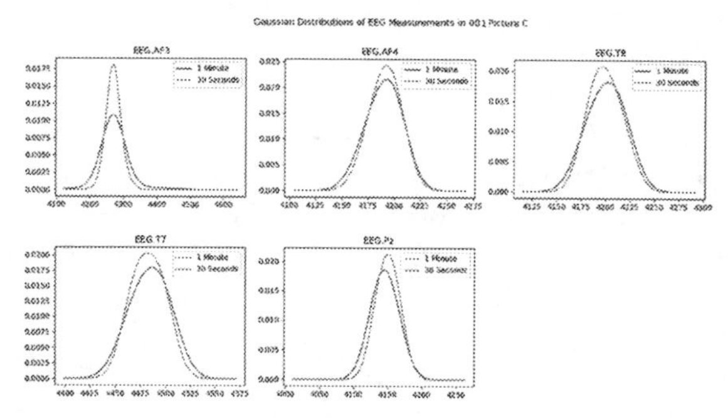

Fig. 4. Gaussian distribution in same axis of 1-min padlock and 30-s key picture C records of Subject 001 by electrode basis.

However, for subject 001, when the 1-min recording remained the padlock photograph "C" and the 30-s key recording belonged to another photograph, the above-mentioned situation remained only for limited electrodes. Figure 5 shows the distributions of the 1-min padlock photograph "C" and the key 30-s photograph "D" for subject 001 on the same axis. As can be seen, the 30-s intensities were higher than the 1-min recording only at electrode AF3.

Recall that the assumption was made that the correct padlock-key combinations would result in a proportionally larger cluster of data points. Simpson's Rule was used to make a comparison of overlap rates between combinations. Simpson's Rule is used to calculate the fractional integral of a function. This approach divides the interval into subregions to calculate the area under the curve and approximates the curve in each subregion as a quadratic function. Initially, the main objective is to approximate the curve with a series of parabolic arcs and find the area of each parabolic segment. Applying Simpson's Rule, the intersection points in experimental data points were first identified. Then, the area shared by the slopes between the detected points is calculated. As a result of the calculations, the combination of subject 001 "padlock C - key C" in Fig. 5 has 7.69% more overlap than subject 001 "padlock C - key B".

In order to further investigate the amount of matching suggested by Simpson's Rule, it is essential to combine the possible output of each subject. In addition, different electrode combinations were created, considering that the use of more limited electrodes would also reduce the power consumption of the IoT device. For example, each padlock and key output from each subject were combined and then processed with all possible electrode combinations, such as only AF3 and Pz or AF3, T8, and AF4. Finally, the z-score is obtained by subtracting each value in the data set from the mean and dividing it by its standard deviation. The z-score normalization helps to reveal relationships between data more easily. The output data is clustered using the Expectation Maximization (EM) algorithm to reveal hidden connections between the data distributed in Gaussian Mixture Modeling (GMM). EM adopts the Mahalanobis Distance method. Mahalanobis Distance takes into account data distributions to find data similarities, which is exactly what is desired. Logarithmic likelihood is used to measure the performance of the resulting clusters. EM data is repeated three times with K-fold cross-validation to get a better clustering performance.

There are several aspects that are included in the GMM algorithm when obtaining the results. The first one is the number of components. This value represents the clustering boundary, which is set as two. Another variable is the covariance matrix, which helps to make sense of the relationship between variables. Covariance matrix types that can be used in GMM include full, tied, diag, and spherical. When the covariance matrix is selected as full type, it ensures that each electrode in a combination has a unique covariance matrix. If the bound type is selected, each element of the electrode combination will share the same covariance matrix values. In the Diag selection, the covariance matrix values will be unique for each combination element, but the covariance values will be shaped diagonally. In global selection, although each component has a unique variance, the main element of the variance consists of the scalar product of the covariance matrix.

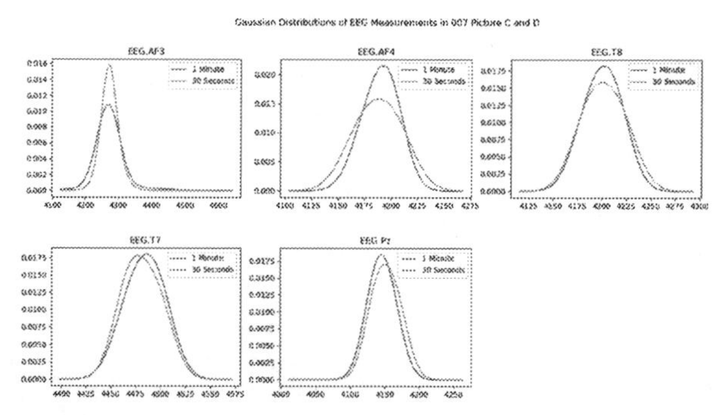

Fig. 5. Gaussian distribution in same axis of 1-min padlock picture C and 30-s key picture D records of Subject 001 by electrode basis.

After the GMM settings, the number of iterations in the EM algorithm was set to 500. While the default iteration value was 100, this number was increased to avoid ignoring data points that were not previously represented. The initialization parameter is used to obtain the initial reference points of the clustering. Kmeans measures the proximity of other data to a randomly selected point and then continues clustering by finding the main cluster center with the data obtained.

Another parameter in the EM algorithm, splitting, is used to determine how many subsets the data will be divided into when analyzing. In the experiments, the splitting parameter was given as three. The last EM parameter, randomness, is intended to prevent the EM algorithm from having random initial values each time it is run. Fixing the randomness to a value will result in the same initial selection values for each subject.

In the light of the data obtained from all tables, the most repeated combinations were AF3-Pz-T8-AF4 and AF3-Pz-AF4 with 5 repeats each. These combinations are followed by AF3-T7-AF4, AF3-T8, and Pz-T8 with 3 repeats each. At this stage, all experiments based on the two combinations with the most repetitions are repeated. However, the number of iterations was increased to 1000 to obtain more accurate results during the repetitions. The results showed that the EM algorithms, where the covariance matrix was set to diag and the initialize parameter was set to k-means, detected successful matches for each subject. In addition, when the settings were set to spherical and random from data, matches were also found for each subject.

5 Conclusion

This work is based on the idea that the human factor can be integrated with device and encryption concepts using brain frequencies. The main reason for choosing brain frequencies is their unobservability and dynamic nature, unlike other biologically based security procedures such as fingerprint and face recognition systems. Experiments prove that human factors can be digitized and make IoT systems more secure. Specifically, AF3-Pz-T8-AF4 combinations can be chosen to create a successful security mechanism for IoT Devices. In the future, we intend to increase the test case numbers and utilize deep-learning methods to increase the success rate of the correct prediction.

References

1. Fruhlinger, J.: The OPM hack explained: Bad security practices meet China's Captain America. CSO Online (2018)
2. Hussain, S., et al.: Exposing vulnerabilities of deepfake detection systems with robust attacks. Digit. Threats Res. Pract. (DTRAP) **3**(3), 1–23 (2022)
3. Hamilton-Nyu, K.: Artificial Intelligence Fools Fingerprint Security Systems. Futurity (2018)
4. Lata, N., Kumar, R.: Analysis of lightweight cryptography algorithms for IoT communication. In: Sharma, H., Saraswat, M., Yadav, A., Kim, J.H., Bansal, J.C. (eds.) Congress on Intelligent Systems, CIS 2020. Advances in Intelligent Systems and Computing, vol. 1335, pp. 397–406. Springer, Singapore (2021). https://doi.org/10.1007/978-981-33-6984-9_32
5. Crane, C.: Block Cipher Vs Stream Cipher: What They Are and How They Work. Hashed Out by the SSL Store, 30 November 2021
6. Fischer, M., Scheerhorn, A., Tonjes, R.: Using attribute-based encryption on IoT devices with instant key revocation. In: 2019 IEEE International Conference on Pervasive Computing and Communications Workshops (PerCom Workshops). IEEE (2019)
7. Stallings, W: Cryptography and Network Security: Principles and Practice, 7th ed. Pearson (2016)
8. Diffie, W., Hellman, M.E.: New directions in cryptography. In: IEEE Transactions on Information Theory, vol. 22(6), pp. 644–54. Institute of Electrical and Electronics Engineers (IEEE) (1976)
9. Rivest, R.L., Shamir, A., Adleman, L.: A method for obtaining digital signatures and public-key cryptosystems. Commun. ACM, **21**(2), 120–126 (1978). Association for Computing Machinery (ACM)
10. Hussain, I., Negi, M.C., Pandey, N.: Proposing an encryption/ decryption scheme for IoT communications using binary-bit sequence and multistage encryption. In: 2018 7th International Conference on Reliability, Infocom Technologies and Optimization (Trends and Future Directions) (ICRITO). IEEE (2018)
11. Hong, D., Lee, J.K., Kim, D.C., Kwon, D., Ryu, K.H., Lee, D.G.: LEA: A 128-Bit block cipher for fast encryption on common processors. In: Kim, Y., Lee, H., Perrig, A. (eds.) Information Security Applications, WISA 2013. Lecture Notes in Computer Science, vol. 8267, pp. 3–27. Springer, Cham (2014). https://doi.org/10.1007/978-3-319-05149-9_1
12. Belguith, S., Kaaniche, N., Russello, G.: PU-ABE: lightweight attribute-based encryption supporting access policy update for cloud assisted IoT. In: 2018 IEEE 11th International Conference on Cloud Computing (CLOUD). IEEE (2018)
13. Jian, M.S., Cheng, Y.E., Shen, C.H.: Internet of Things (IoT) cybersecurity based on the hybrid cryptosystem. In: 2019 21st International Conference on Advanced Communication Technology (ICACT). IEEE (2019)
14. Chandu, Y., Kumar, K.S.R., Prabhukhanolkar, N.V., Anish, A.N., Rawal, S.: Design and implementation of hybrid encryption for security of IOT data. In: 2017 International Conference on Smart Technologies for Smart Nation (SmartTechCon). IEEE (2017)
15. Yang, W., Wang, S., Sahri, N.M., Karie, N.M., Ahmed, M., Valli, C.: Biometrics for internet-of-things security: a review. Sensors **21**(18), 6163 (2021)
16. Hossain, M.S., Muhammad, G., Rahman, S.M.M., Abdul, W., Alelaiwi, A., Alamri, A.: Toward end-to-end biometrics-based security for IoT infrastructure. IEEE Wirel. Commun. **23**(5), 44–51 (2016)

17. Sarika, C.G., Bharathi, M.A., Harinath, H.N.: IoT-based smart login using biometrics. In: Smys, S., Bestak, R., Chen, J.Z., Kotuliak, I. (eds.) International Conference on Computer Networks and Communication Technologies. Lecture Notes on Data Engineering and Communications Technologies, vol. 15, pp. 589–597. Springer, Singapore (2019). https://doi.org/10.1007/978-981-10-8681-6_54
18. Golec, M., Gill, S.S., Bahsoon, R., Rana, O.: BioSec: a biometric authentication framework for secure and private communication among edge devices in IoT and industry 4.0. IEEE Consum. Electron. Magaz. **11**(2), 51–56 (2020)

An Assessment of the Cyber Security Challenges and Issues Associated with Cyber-Physical Power Systems

Abubakar Bello[1], Farnaz Farid[1](✉), and Fahima Hossain[2]

[1] Western Sydney University, Penrith, Australia
{A.bello,Farnaz.farid}@westernsydney.edu.au
[2] Hamdard University, Dhaka, Bangladesh

Abstract. Cyber-Physical Power Systems (CPPS) are innovative technologies that combine physical systems with control, computing, and communication technology. Its significance has grown because of improved efficiency and safety in various applications such as smart grids, smart cities, CNC matching monitoring systems, intelligent manufacturing systems, smart transportation, smart government, smart healthcare, smart environments, smart homes, and so on. These smart applications not only cause accidental failure and errors but also pose numerous security and privacy issues, such as cyber-attacks that cause physical harm to the system and its environment. Due to the heterogeneity, scalability, and dynamic nature of these intelligent applications, existing security solutions cannot be directly applied to them; therefore, when developing and implementing new mechanisms or systems, it is essential to be aware of security and privacy risks. This paper examines the security challenges and issues associated with CPPS in response to this concern. The review gives a general overview of the CPPS interdependence framework and numerous CPPS applications. The security challenges and solutions are then evaluated, followed by describing the cyber threats that can exploit CPPS using an analysis, defense, and protection model. Other critical CPPS issues, which include the development of secure and sustainable power systems, are summarized along with current research challenges and suggestions for future work.

Keywords: CPS · CPPS · CPPS Design · CPPS Framework · CPPS Modeling · CPPS Applications · CPPS Security Issues · Critical Issues

1 Introduction

ICT technologies in the electric power system have become the norm in every aspect to meet the increasing demand for the power system. [1]. A heterogeneous multi-dimensional system with integrated cyber components (control, computation, and communication) is referred to as a Cyber-Physical System (CPS) to achieve stability, robustness, efficiency, and reliability in applications involving physical systems. To complete the shared objectives, the physical system receives a control signal from the cyber system, which in the CPS collects data from the physical system via sensors [2]. CPSs are

K. Daimi and A. Al Sadoon (Eds.): ACR 2024, LNNS 956, pp. 318–333, 2024.
https://doi.org/10.1007/978-3-031-56950-0_27

tightly coupled cyber and physical systems with integrated intelligence. Such systems' computational and physical processes are tightly interconnected and coordinated to work effectively together, often with humans in the loop. The growing coupling and dynamic interactions between cyber and physical systems have transformed the modern power system into the Cyber-Physical Power System (CPPS) [3]. It is comprised of a large number of computing devices (such as servers, computers, and embedded computing equipment), data acquisition equipment (such as sensors, phasor measurement units, and embedded data acquisition equipment), and peripherals (such as generator sets, various distributed generations, microgrids, and loads) [3]. Usage of CPPS is growing because of its promising potentials, such as robustness, autonomy, self-organization, self-maintenance, self-repair, transparency, predictability, efficiency, interoperability, global tracking and tracing and so on. CPPSs encompass all the critical domains in power systems, including electricity generation, transmission, transformation, distribution, consumption, and sale [4]. These complex systems typically operate in a dynamic and uncertain environment due to various factors such as time-varying utilization, hardware and software component failures, physical degradation and malfunction, and an incomplete understanding of the system's operating state [5]. The CPPS's reliability and resilience depend on properly operating related subsystems such as computing, communications, and control, as illustrated in Fig. 1.

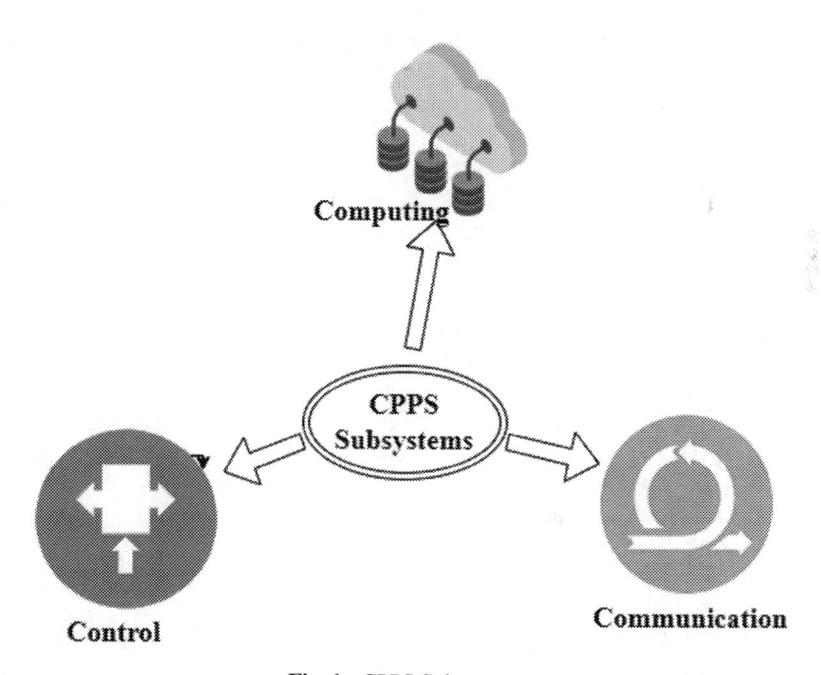

Fig. 1. CPPS Subsystems.

The dynamic physical system consists of a generator, transformer, transmission line, load, and other components physically connected to energy flow. In contrast, a cyber system is a static system comprising cyber components linked together via an information-flowing communication network [2]. Due to its complex coupling relationship, the power network is more vulnerable to natural disasters and malicious attacks [3].

A stable and secure power supply is a crucial foundation for national and social development, so the CPPS is one of the country's most critical infrastructure systems. Thus, the security of the energy system must be considered for the proper functioning of a society. Technological advancements in the power sector determine cyber security vulnerabilities [6]. The power system increasingly relies on secondary information systems for measurement, sensing, and control. As a result, it is critical to assess power systems from a CPSstandpoint. Privacy protection is a type of cyber security issue that focuses on the confidentiality of information during transmission and decision-making [6]. Malfunctions on the cyber side, such as large-scale cascading failure, may reduce the reliability of power system operating conditions and jeopardize the CPPS's safe and stable operation state [3]. A major cyber incident in the power system could have severe consequences for the operation of the CPPS in terms of socioeconomic impacts, market impacts, equipment damage, and large-scale blackouts [6]. Cyber-attacks on power systems may attempt to disrupt communication to impede monitoring and control via denial of service attacks [1]. Insiders, amateur hackers, political activists, criminal organizations, governments, and terrorists may all launch attacks on the power system. The communication infrastructure and protocols for monitoring power system states introduce many cyber security issues. Because of the vast geographical and cyberspace distribution and the deep integration of the cyber and physical sides, it is challenging to protect CPPS from cyber-attacks. A CPPS's main application is to make the most of solid computing ability and a wide range of information to promote optimal decision-making. As a result, the power system's safety, reliability, and efficiency are enhanced [7]. A critical understanding of CPPS complexity and interdependence, as well as analysis of both qualitative and quantitative approaches between physical and cyber systems, will aid in preventing catastrophic cascading failure events in a networked CPPS [2]. Resilience has emerged as a critical topic in avoiding and mitigating the risks posed by large-scale CPPS blackouts [3]. Indeed, continuous assessment of the power system should be expanded to include intentional incidents such as cyber-attacks [8].

This paper aims to assess the issues and challenges associated with power systems, specifically in the context of a Cyber-Physical Power System (CPPS). The purpose of this paper is to answer the following three research questions:

1. What are the available interdependence frameworks for applications in CPPS?
2. What are the critical cyber security vulnerabilities on CPPS?
3. What are the existing solutions to address the vulnerabilities associated with CPPS?

The first question focuses on comprehending the CPPS's complex cyber and physical components interdependence. The paper will most likely investigate various models and frameworks that demonstrate how these components interact and affect one another. The second question seeks to identify and analyze potential vulnerabilities within the CPPS, particularly regarding cyber security. The paper will most likely discuss the challenges and threats CPPS faces due to its integration of cyber components. The third question seeks information about strategies and mechanisms for mitigating CPPS vulnerabilities. The paper may look into existing solutions, technologies, and best practices for improving the security and resilience of the CPPS.

The paper is organized as follows to address these research questions. Section II describes the detailed interdependence modelling of CPPS and its various applications, focusing on how cyber and physical systems are interconnected and coordinated. Section III presents existing CPPS security assessment challenges and solutions. This section will almost certainly delve into the cybersecurity aspects of CPPS. Section IV describes cyber-attacks that exploit CPPS vulnerabilities, detection methods, and protection mechanisms. It focuses on identifying potential threats and determining how to counteract them. Section V describes other critical CPPS issues. Beyond security vulnerabilities, this section may discuss additional challenges or considerations. Section VI discusses potential future directions and advancements in the field of CPPS, emphasizing the importance of ongoing research and development. Section VII draws conclusions based on the paper's findings and discussions.

2 Interdependence Framework of CPPS

The CPPS comprises many physical and cyber devices that work together to form a large-scale, interdependent, complex system. The integration relationship between the cyber and physical devices is modeled as interdependent modeling of CPPS, which evolves, as illustrated in Fig. 2.

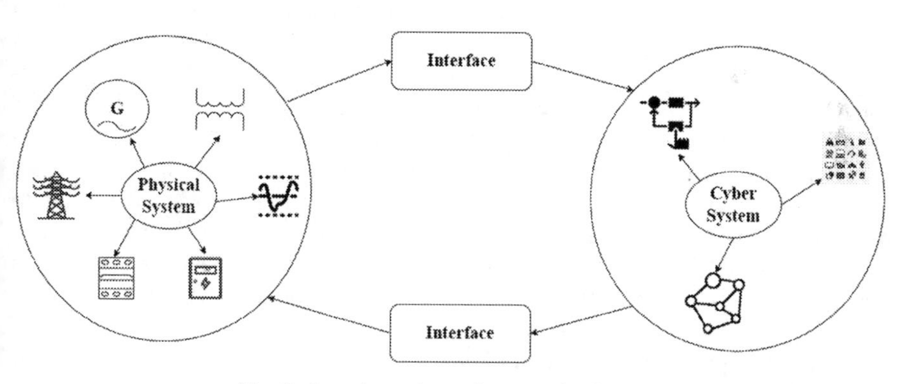

Fig. 2. Interdependence framework of CPPS.

The CPPS is modeled as an interdependent complex network-based model that includes power flow analysis at the physical layer, cyber layer information, edge capacity checks, delay analysis, transmission analysis, and an indirect interaction mechanism between the two layers. The interdependent CPPS is divided into the physical, cyber, and interface-mapping layers. The physical layer node represents the generator, transformer, substation, and so on, and the physical layer edge represents the transmission lines in the electric power grid network. The cyber layer nodes are comprised of computational systems, communication equipment, and control algorithms, with the primary function of monitoring and controlling CPPS. The network edges represent the cyber nodes' communication links. Typically, the physical and cyber layers operate independently of one another. Because the topology and operational relationships of the two layers differ, it is necessary to consider the interdependency effect and apply mitigation strategies in both layers simultaneously. Based on cyber layer nodes, there are two types of interdependencies in CPPS: one-to-one and one-to-multiple interdependency. The single cyber node monitors (detecting the status of the physical node) and controls (issuing control commands) each physical node in the one-to-one interdependency. The control center then collects the information from the distributed cyber nodes. Each physical node in the one-to-multiple interdependencies is monitored by more than one cyber node, which is extremely useful for securing data against cyber-attacks [2]. When the physical outage remedial control fails due to a concurrent cyber-side failure, the cyber-physical coupling failure in the strong interdependent CPPS increases the risk of power systems. To improve the robustness of power systems in the face of possible cyber-physical coupling failures, critical information about the CPPS should be transmitted via a reliable path to ensure its accessibility [2].

CPPS is applied in a variety of applications such as smart grids, smart cities, Computer numerical control (CNC) matching monitoring systems, intelligent manufacturing systems, smart transportation, smart government, smart healthcare, smart environments, smart homes, and so on, as shown in Fig. 3 due to its improved efficiency and safety.

Using the smart grid, smart transportation systems, smart manufacturing, and smart building infrastructure, CPSs are essential to national initiatives to improve performance, reliability, productivity, and energy efficiency across economic sectors [9]. Increasing demand for reliable energy and numerous technological advancements have motivated the development of a smart electric grid for rising control and advancing sensing technologies to make it dynamically available at various locations [10]. The future requirements for smart grids are attack resistance, self-healing, consumer motivation, power quality, generation and storage accommodation, enabling markets, and asset optimization [10]. The smart grid operates without human intervention, which induces more security concerns that target individual entities' availability, integrity and confidentiality. Different kinds of attacks, such as Denial of Service (DoS), false data injection, and Man in the Middle (MiTM), can disrupt the network services, cause significant damages such as a power outage, modify the data of smart meters, violate the privacy, and so on [11].

Smart city deployments of Cyber-Physical Power Systems (CPSSs) are poised to significantly improve healthcare, transportation, utilities, safety, and environmental health [11]. Unexpected and large-scale DDoS attacks and ransomware threats, such as cryptowall and Wannacry, hampered security and privacy in smart city systems. Televisions, refrigerators, video cameras, routers, and other smart devices are used by attackers as attack vectors or resources for malicious activity.

Electric vehicles have several environmental and economic advantages. Electric vehicles (EVs) can reduce reliance on fossil fuels, lower operating costs compared to combustion engine vehicles, and lower emissions [12]. Cyber-attacks launched from the EVI can spread quickly due to the ubiquity of communications and the mobility of EVs

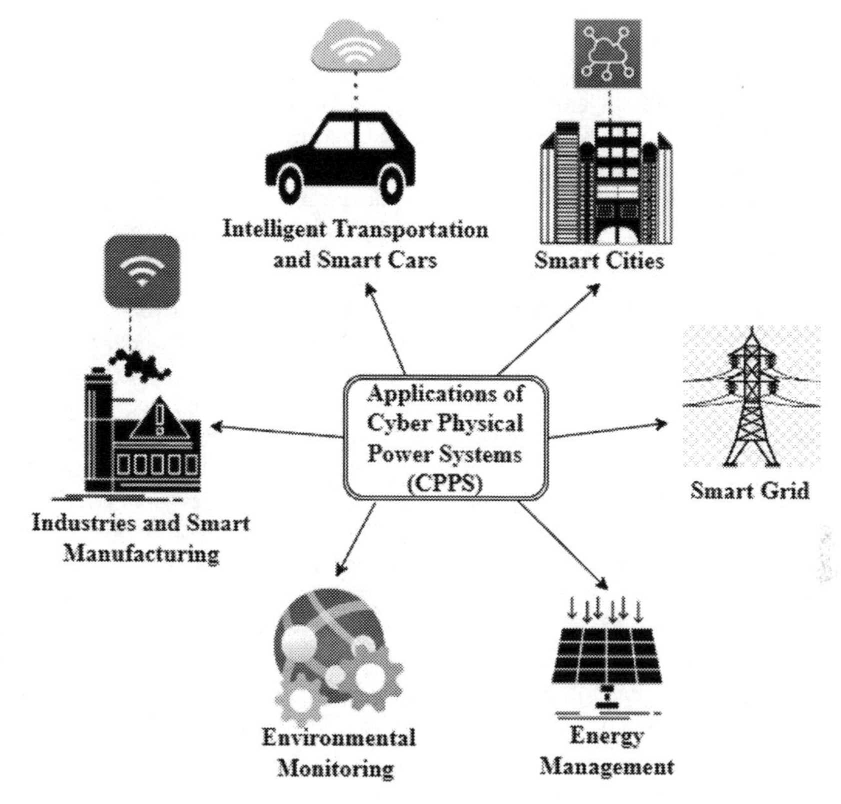

Fig. 3. Various applications of CPPS.

[13]. Customers and power system installations can benefit from intelligent control and management of EV charging operations.

The introduction of the Internet of Things (IoT) and the Internet of Services (IoS) in manufacturing has transformed today's factories into smart ones, thanks to advances in information and communication technology (ICT). IoT and CPPS technologies and sensor networks now provide advanced monitoring and control of real-world processes on a previously unheard-of scale [14].

Using a CPPS in conjunction with Building Information Modeling (BIM) presents a powerful paradigm for effectively monitoring and utilizing existing energy use for optimization, analysis, and calculation to minimize environmental impact [15]. To develop resilient and sustainable design, operations, and management strategies, domain knowledge for each infrastructure and its organizational characteristics must be integrated with those of other infrastructures [13].

3 Existing Security Assessment Challenges and Solutions on CPPS

Researchers use CPPS modeling as the foundation for vulnerability assessment, simulation, and optimization in CPPSs. CPPS modeling typically begins with analyzing the mutual coupling effects between power and cyber networks [16]. This modeling investigates the impact of invalid control commands on power systems. Three techniques are used to model the effects of outsider attack and defender strategy in CPPSs: monitoring, contingency, and preventive control actions.

- **Monitoring:** CPPS has connected numerous devices, causing network anomalies to emerge. The analysis of anomaly monitoring aids in determining whether or not the system is abnormal, allowing the system to avoid anomalies and recover as quickly as possible [17]. Most anomaly monitoring employs data mining and other technologies to achieve the best monitoring possible by learning from log data.
- **Contingency analysis:** The interaction of power physical and cyber systems in CPPS is a crucial problem in CPPS vulnerability analysis. A contingency is the loss or failure of a small part of the power system (e.g. a transmission line) or the loss/failure of individual equipment such as a generator or transformer. Contingency analysis is performed to evaluate the effects and calculate any overloads resulting from each outage event. It simulates and quantifies the results of problems that could occur in the power system in the immediate future. Problems and unstable situations can be identified, critical configurations can be recognized, operating constraints and limits can be applied, and corrective actions can be planned by analyzing the effects of contingency events in advance.
- **Preventive control actions:** To enhance the safety of the power system, effective preventive control strategies must ensure stable grid operation and regular power supply in the event of a typical single fault. When multiple serious accidents damage the power system, these devices can be urgently started for emergency control to prevent the expansion of accidents and large-scale power outages [18]. This technique rapidly recovers the service path by network self-healing protection functions, analogous to the power system's emergency control strategy, to quickly remove failures.

4 Cyber Attacks Exploiting CPPS Vulnerabilities

Cyber-attacks on CPPS refer to the attack behavior of tracking the communication network or control commands without permission and exploiting the system's vulnerability for system destruction or function reduction [3]. The CPPS requires cyber security on multiple levels, including information, ICT infrastructure, and application-level security. Cyber-attacks pose a substantial security threat to Cyber-Physical Power Systems (CPPS), with increasing frequency and diverse impacts. These include cascading failures that can lead to system-wide collapse and blackouts, disruptions to stable power system operations by injecting false or misleading data, and economic consequences that can disrupt the economic development of nations. Cyber-attacks are a significant security risk to CPPS, occurring more frequently and having more varied effects. These include cascading failures that can cause systemic failures and blackouts, interference with the stable power system's ability to function due to the introduction of false or misleading data, and economic consequences that can impede the growth of nations' economies [27]. Various attack detection methods have been proposed to address these challenges and mitigate the negative effects of cyber-attacks. To assess the security of CPPS, four steps are followed: categorization of cyber-attacks, attack types, evaluation of attacks, defense mechanisms of attacks, and mitigation and protection from attacks.

4.1 Classification of Attacks on CPPS

1. Attacks targeting the cyber domain

   Attackers target communications and protocols, asset control commands, and data storage in cyber domains [19]. Attackers attempt to gain unauthorized access through communication and protocols by exchanging remote access credentials, measurements, system reports and warnings, and so on, or by inserting malicious modifications (data alteration). Attackers target the CPPS data integrity by using asset control commands to mask counterfeit system data. Attackers target the accuracy and non-repudiation of CPPS data through data storage, such as asset setpoint modifications, user sign-ins and action histories, inbound/outbound connections and traffic, and so on.
2. Attacks targeting the physical domain

   Physical domain attacks can be invasive, non-invasive, or semi-invasive [19]. To manipulate it, physical access to the CPPS asset is required for invasive attacks. Non-invasive attacks that do not necessitate physical tampering with the ICs on the CPS assets. Because no traces are left after the attack, they are the most challenging type of attack to detect. Power analysis attacks, timing attacks, electromagnetic emission attacks, brute force attacks using physical means, hall sensor spoofing, and other non-invasive attacks are common examples. Semi-invasive attacks are a compromise between invasive and non-invasive attacks in that they are not as difficult to execute as invasive attacks and can be repeated as quickly as non-invasive attacks. Semi-invasive attacks commonly include fault injection, laser scanning, ultraviolet radiation, and control process tampering.

4.2 Attack Types

Attackers employ carefully designed and diverse attack methods, beginning attacks in the information domain and focusing specifically on the physical domain to maximize power system loss [20]. Attacks that are sophisticated, well-crafted, and coordinated may have cascading effects and affect a large portion of the power system across a large geographical area [21]. Table 1 provides a summary of attacks and scenarios concerning CPPS.

4.3 Evaluation of Attacks on CPPS

CPPS security has gained more importance in terms of cyber security and control security in light of emerging cyber threats [3]. The vulnerability assessment process typically consists of identifying vulnerable points and conducting quantitative assessments. To begin

Table 1. CPPS Attack Types and Scenarios

Attack Method	Scenario
Data Tampering Attack	A data tampering attack is a network cooperative attack that can result in large-scale power outages, casualties, and other major power outages. The purpose of the power CPS data tampering attack is to illegally tamper with the measurement data of physical nodes by invading the information system. It invariably leaves traces on the information and physical systems' data levels [21]
Man-in-the-Middle Attack (MITM)	In a MiTM attack, the intruder can perform false data injection (FDI) and false command injection (FCI) attacks that can compromise power system operations, such as state estimation, economic dispatch, and automatic generation control (AGC) [22]
Aurora attack	An Aurora attack is a malicious command injection attack in which critical circuit breakers are opened and closed without authorization. The attacker continuously sends trip and reclose commands to a vulnerable breaker, causing the generator to lose synchronization with the transmission grid. This type of attack can be launched both locally and remotely. This condition can lead to severe system instability and cascading failures [21]
False data injection	False data injection attacks change the results of power system state estimation [21]
Switching attack	A switching attack uses a state-dependent controlled switching sequence to destabilize the power system by targeting relays and breakers [21]
Reconnaissance attacks	Reconnaissance attacks seek out vulnerable systems and devices in a network to support future attacks. Many industrial network protocols lack features for authenticating the provenance or originality of network packets. As a result, industrial systems are vulnerable to injection, modification, and replay attacks. Injection attacks deliver malicious network packets to targets [21]
Alteration attack	Alteration attacks, such as via a man-in-the-middle attack, change network packet contents before delivery [21]
Replay attack	Replay attacks resend packets from earlier periods. The attacks can target operator commands, control signals, and sensor measurements [21]
DoS and DDoS attack	Denial of service attacks on a power system can prevent system state monitoring and operators and automated algorithms from delivering commands to control the system [21]

(*continued*)

Table 1. (*continued*)

Attack Method	Scenario
Eavesdropping attack	The system intercepts all data sent by it. Transferring control information from sensor networks to CPPS applications for monitoring purposes could be vulnerable to eavesdropping. Additionally, user privacy may be jeopardized because the system is being monitored [23]
Data Diddling	Data Diddling Attacks involve unauthorized changes to a database, including altering file statuses and making improper modifications that undermine data integrity [28]
Salami Attacks	Salami Attacks discreetly target a network data system, allowing attackers to extract sensitive information without detection gradually. These small-scale attacks can accumulate and substantially damage a company [28]
Spoofing attack	Spoofing occurs when an attacker gains access to information and can change, delete, or insert data [23]
Resonance Attack	Resonance Attack causes compromised sensors or controllers to operate at a different resonance frequency [23]
Integrity Attack	The Integrity Attack tries to destabilize the system by injecting external control inputs and falsifying sensor data [23]
Jamming	Jamming occurs when noise or a signal with the same frequency is introduced into the wireless channel between sensor nodes and the remote base station. This attack could cause DoS by introducing deliberate network interference [23]
Buffer Overflow	Buffer overflow attacks take advantage of any vulnerabilities that result in buffer overflow vulnerabilities [23]
Malicious Code	Attacks the user application by launching malicious code, such as viruses and worms, causing the network to slow down or malfunction [23]
Social Engineering	Social engineering cyberattacks use persuasion strategies to trick victims into disclosing private information. Criminals frequently use publicly available personal information from social media sites to profile victims for attacks using techniques like phone calls, emails, or social media interactions. Social engineering attacks can take many forms, such as phishing, grooming, and pretexting [28]
Traffic Analysis Attack	This attack examines communication traffic between a sender and receiver to gather sensitive data and spot network flaws. Although it is a passive attack that compromises the confidentiality and privacy of user data, this analysis helps plan theft [28]

modeling and quantitative analysis of cyber-attacks, vulnerable points must be identified, and quantitative evaluation is accomplished through empirical weights methods or modeling calculation methods.

There are numerous manifestations of cyber-attacks that have an impact on CPPS functions, such as safety, stability, and economy. To evaluate the consequences of attacks, assessments should develop quantitative evaluation standards based on specific scenarios and attack models [3]. The standards should focus on the economic consequences and stability consequences. In terms of the economy, cyber-attacks may cause changes in real-time electricity prices and regional marginal electricity prices, so the income of the attacker can be used as a criterion. In terms of stability, cyber-attacks may cause tripping of breakers, load imbalance and ultimately reflect on the frequency of instability or load loss [3].

4.4 Defense Mechanisms for Attacks on CPPS

Detecting an attack aims to determine whether an abnormal event occurs in the system. According to the specific identification basis, existing anomaly detection methods can be divided into deviation-based and feature-based detection [3]. Deviation-based detection methods typically monitor one or more variables related to attacks strongly related to defense targets and determine an attack when the value of the variables deviates from the normal range to a certain threshold. The most commonly used deviations are statistical distribution deviation, control effect deviation, and prediction deviation [3]. Feature-based detection methods use physical mechanism analysis or artificial intelligence to extract features in regular operation and attacked scenarios and detect cyber-attack occurrence through feature comparison. There are two standard methods for extracting features: the physical model of the system and the artificial intelligence method [3]. In order to achieve the goal of attack detection, model-based methods aim to quantify the changes in the system's internal state under cyber-attacks. For the latter, a classifier for attack detection is trained using an artificial intelligence-based method [27].

4.5 Mitigations/Protection of Attacks on CPPS

The security of CPPS includes both the cyber environment security and the physical environment stability. Protection can be achieved through collaboration between the cyber and physical environments, which can aid in maintaining the security of coupling and association properties [3].

Protection Means of Cyber Environment
Cybersecurity techniques are divided into two categories: prevention and recovery. Standard preventative measures include certification checks, encryption, network isolation, and access management. Post-event cyber measurements include damaged equipment isolation and control strategy adjustment. Countermeasures for a DDoS attack, for example, include traceability, network reconfiguration and redirection, filtering, speed limitation, legality detection, and attack resource exhaustion [3].

Protection Means of Physical Environment
Physical protection methods include resource preparation methods and information interaction-based correction methods. Resource-preparing methods deploy redundant resources in advance and allocate them in an emergency to provide backup for CPPS and maintain the system's stable operation state after attacks. The information interaction-based correction methods use knowledge of attack vectors and the system to correct tampered signals or data and achieve the desired control effects [3].

5 Other Critical issues of CPPSs

The following sections examine significant problems and difficulties relating to Cyber-Physical Power Systems (CPPSs). These discussions highlighted the need for thorough analysis and protection by illuminating contemporary power systems' complex interdependencies and vulnerabilities.

A. **Cyber-Physical Modeling and Interdependent Analysis**
The power system depends on a communication network to transmit data and control information due to the interdependence of the two heterogeneous networks [24]. A cascading failure in a system can occur in many different types of systems, including physical resource and computational-resource networks like power grids, the Internet, and traffic networks. The interdependence of physical-resource and computational-resource networks in cyber-physical systems complicates the analysis of system cascading failure. As a result, understanding the underlying cascading failure patterns is essential for protecting such interdependent cyber-physical systems [25]. The integrated cyber-physical model facilitates the interdependent security analysis of CPPS.

B. **Cyber Security and Privacy-Persevering**
A plethora of scenarios characterized by collaborative operation among multiple entities have emerged for cyber security and privacy protection. Coordination between various parties exposes the power system to potential privacy and cyber security risks while also providing more flexibility to support their operation and help with the best use of resources on a larger scale. Although the power system is regulated in relatively isolated and secure cyberspace, the cyber systems of these third-party resources make it more vulnerable to malicious cyber-attacks, ultimately jeopardizing power grid operation. Besides cyber security concerns, privacy concerns have grown in importance. Data exchange between entities is required to enable collaborative operation [26].

C. **Co-Optimization and Market Design**
Regulating information flow for co-optimization and market design will also affect energy flow for CPPSs [26]. There is significant potential to significantly impact CPPS interdependence and analyze the interconnections of cyber-physical flexibility. Additionally, the cyber and physical sides of the market mechanisms for CPPS should be fully considered. Data sources can benefit entities in overcoming inconvenience and diseconomy caused by information asymmetry or incompleteness.

D. **Resilience of Cyber-Physical Power Systems**

With the exception of traditional power system resilience analysis, resilience assessment and enhancement strategies for CPPSs should account for the interdependent characteristics of cyber-physics, primarily due to cyber-physical coupling failures caused by extreme hazards and cyber-physical attacks [19].

E. **Time-Delay Effects on Cyber-Physical Power Systems**

The coupling of time delays in information systems and physical power system dynamics will exacerbate problems with CPPS dynamic performance and stability concerning time-delay effects on CPPS stability [26]. The hindrance to developing wide-area control systems (WACS) for large-scale power systems and fast-response massively scalable control for power systems is time delay on the cyber side.

F. **Digital Twin and Co-Simulation for Cyber-Physical Power Systems**

Digital Twin (DT) technology is an integrated multi-physics, multi-scale, probabilistic simulation of a system that uses high-precision physical models, real-time data, and so on. The use of DT in the simulation of CPPSs is also beneficial in identifying CPPS weaknesses in the context of various types of cyber threats or cyber-physical coupling abnormalities [2]. This Working Group should consider DT toward CPPS- for precise large-scale real-time simulation and pre-decision-making of complex CPPS.

Table 2. Summary of Critical Issues in Cyber-Physical Power Systems (CPPS).

Section	Key Issues Discussed
A. Cyber-Physical Modeling and Interdependent Analysis	The interdependence of physical and computational networks in CPPS makes analyzing cascading failures crucial. An integrated cyber-physical model facilitates security analysis
B. Cyber Security and Privacy-Preserving	Collaboration in power systems introduces privacy and cyber security risks. The power system becomes more vulnerable to malicious cyber-attacks. Privacy concerns are also growing
C. Co-Optimization and Market Design	Regulating information flow for co-optimization and market design affects energy flow in CPPS. Market mechanisms should consider both cyber and physical aspects
D. Resilience of Cyber-Physical Power Systems	Resilience strategies for CPPS must consider interdependence due to cyber-physical coupling failures caused by extreme hazards and attacks
E. Time-Delay Effects on Cyber-Physical Power Systems	Time delays in information and physical power systems impact CPPS stability and control systems
F. Digital Twin and Co-Simulation for Cyber-Physical Power Systems	Digital Twin technology is helpful in simulating and identifying weaknesses in CPPS, especially in the context of cyber threats and coupling abnormalities

We summarise the main ideas from each section in Table 2 to provide a brief summary and enable quick access to the major issues covered in the paper.

6 Discussion and Future Directions

Integrating information and communication technology with power systems has transformed a power system into a CPPS that significantly improves the system's efficiency and overall reliability while conveying potential failure risks. Failures negatively impact the overall reliability of the power system. The CPPS will enable effective management of the complexity of power systems with enhanced operational capabilities. CPPS reliability and resilience depend on properly operating related subsystems such as computing, communications, and control. Due to the interdependent framework, the power system is more vulnerable to natural disasters and malicious attacks. To address the research questions in this paper, a detailed overview of the interdependence framework and different application areas of CPPS are covered. Moreover, security issues such as cyber-attacks, their detection, defense and mitigation approaches, which may lead to large-scale failures of power systems, are discussed. Other issues cause damage to the working of CPPS that have been examined. The recommendations are as follows:

- To overcome failures in cyber environments of CPPS, cyber-physical coupling failure, and to mitigate risks in power systems as CPPS works independently in its three layers, security must be designed in each layer of CPPS.
- A dynamic and interactive infrastructure should be established with new energy management capabilities to protect CPPS from security threats.
- A comprehensive protection strategy is required for CPPS to mitigate the impact of cyber-attacks, such as load loss, stability issues, economic loss, or equipment damage. CPPS requires cyber security on multiple levels, including information security, ICT infrastructure security, and application-level security.

7 Conclusion

This study examined the security issues and challenges associated with CPPS. It analyzed the CPPS interdependent framework, the launching of cyber-attacks within this framework, various CPPS applications, their working procedures, and vulnerability assessment. The review also evaluated existing security assessment challenges and solutions, such as monitoring, contingency analysis, and preventive control actions. Better architectural security solutions can be implemented by understanding the security issues in the power system, how they can be exploited, and the outcomes of such actions. Furthermore, by researching the potential effects of malicious attacks on the power system, including cyber-attacks targeting different layers of the CPPS, attack types, cyber-attack defense mechanisms, and attack prevention, an efficient strategy for securing the power system and mitigating existing and emerging risks can be proposed. Overall, this review is intended to assist researchers in identifying security issues and challenges associated with various CPPS applications, building models that take these considerations into account, and overcoming these issues. It also provides information on the CPPS's defense and prevention mechanisms against cyber-attacks.

References

1. Jimada-Ojuolape, B., Teh, J.: Impact of the integration of information and communication technology on power system reliability: a review. IEEE Access **8**, 24600–24615 (2020). https://doi.org/10.1109/access.2020.2970598
2. Yohanandhan, R.V., Elavarasan, R.M., Manoharan, P., Mihet-Popa, L.: Cyber-physical power system (CPPS): a review on modeling, simulation, and analysis with cyber security applications. IEEE Access **8**, 151019–151064 (2020). https://doi.org/10.1109/access.2020.3016826
3. Cai, X., Wang, Q., Tang, Y., Zhu, L.: Review of cyber-attacks and defense research on cyber physical power system. In: 2019 IEEE Sustainable Power and Energy Conference (ISPEC) (2019). https://doi.org/10.1109/ispec48194.2019.8975131
4. Shi, L., Dai, Q., Ni, Y.: Cyber-physical interactions in power systems: a review of models, methods, and applications. Electr. Power Syst. Res. **163**, 396–412 (2018). https://doi.org/10.1016/j.epsr.2018.07.015
5. Morris, T.H., et al.: Engineering future cyber-physical energy systems: challenges, research needs, and roadmap. In: 41st North American Power Symposium (2009). https://doi.org/10.1109/naps.2009.5484019
6. Dogaru, D.I., Dumitrache, I.: Robustness of power systems in the context of cyber attacks. In: 2017 21st International Conference on Control Systems and Computer Science (CSCS) (2017). https://doi.org/10.1109/cscs.2017.78
7. Tang, Y., et al.: A hardware-in-the-loop based co-simulation platform of cyber-physical power systems for Wide Area Protection Applications. Appl. Sci. **7**(12), 1279 (2017). https://doi.org/10.3390/app7121279
8. Zonouz, S., Davis, C.M., Davis, K.R., Berthier, R., Bobba, R.B., Sanders, W.H.: Socca: a security-oriented cyber-physical contingency analysis in power infrastructures. IEEE Trans. Smart Grid **5**(1), 3–13 (2014). https://doi.org/10.1109/tsg.2013.2280399
9. Carreras Guzman, N.H., Wied, M., Kozine, I., Lundteigen, M.A.: Conceptualizing the key features of cyber-physical systems in a multi-layered representation for safety and security analysis. Syst. Eng. **23**(2), 189–210 (2019). https://doi.org/10.1002/sys.21509
10. Sridhar, S., Hahn, A., Govindarasu, M.: Cyber–physical system security for the Electric Power Grid. Proc. IEEE **100**(1), 210–224 (2012). https://doi.org/10.1109/jproc.2011.2165269
11. Radoglou-Grammatikis, P.I., Sarigiannidis, P.G.: Securing the smart grid: a comprehensive compilation of intrusion detection and prevention systems. IEEE Access **7**, 46595–46620 (2019). https://doi.org/10.1109/access.2019.2909807
12. Mohandes, B., Hammadi, R.A., Sanusi, W., Mezher, T., Khatib, S.E.: Advancing cyber–physical sustainability through integrated analysis of smart power systems: a case study on electric vehicles. Int. J. Crit. Infrastruct. Prot. **23**, 33–48 (2018). https://doi.org/10.1016/j.ijcip.2018.10.002
13. Franco, P., Martínez, J.M., Kim, Y.-C., Ahmed, M.A.: A cyber-physical approach for residential energy management: current state and future directions. Sustainability **14**(8), 4639 (2022). https://doi.org/10.3390/su14084639
14. Yao, X., Zhou, J., Lin, Y., Li, Y., Yu, H., Liu, Y.: Smart manufacturing based on cyber-physical systems and beyond. J. Intell. Manuf. **30**(8), 2805–2817 (2017). https://doi.org/10.1007/s10845-017-1384-5
15. Zhang, Y., Beetz, J.: Building-CPS: cyber-physical system for building environment monitoring. In: CIB W78, vol. 2021, pp. 11–15. New Zealand (n.d.)
16. Chen, K., Wen, F., Palu, I.: Cyber contingencies impacts analysis in cyber physical power system. In: 2019 IEEE International Conference on Energy Internet (ICEI) (2019). https://doi.org/10.1109/icei.2019.00013

17. Li, Q., et al.: Safety risk monitoring of cyber-physical power systems based on ensemble learning algorithm. IEEE Access **7**, 24788–24805 (2019). https://doi.org/10.1109/access.2019.2896129
18. Yang, T., Liu, Y., Li, W.: Attack and defence methods in cyber-physical power system. IET Energy Syst. Integr. **4**(2), 159–170 (2022). https://doi.org/10.1049/esi2.12068
19. Zografopoulos, I., Ospina, J., Liu, X., Konstantinou, C.: Cyber-physical energy systems security: threat modeling, risk assessment, resources, metrics, and case studies. IEEE Access **9**, 29775–29818 (2021). https://doi.org/10.1109/access.2021.3058403
20. Ping, G.: Detection of power data tampering attack based on gradient boosting decision tree. J. Phys: Conf. Ser. **1846**(1), 012057 (2021). https://doi.org/10.1088/1742-6596/1846/1/012057
21. Adhikari, U., Morris, T., Pan, S.: WAMS cyber-physical test bed for power system, cybersecurity study, and data mining. IEEE Trans. Smart Grid **8**(6), 2744–2753 (2017). https://doi.org/10.1109/tsg.2016.2537210
22. Wlazlo, P., et al.: Man-in-the-middle attacks and defence in a power system cyber-physical testbed. IET Cyber-Phys. Syst. Theory Appl. **6**(3), 164–177 (2021). https://doi.org/10.1049/cps2.12014
23. Dixit, M.K.: Attack taxonomy for cyber-physical system. Int. J. Res. Appl. Sci. Eng. Technol. **10**(1), 194–200 (2022). https://doi.org/10.22214/ijraset.2022.39734
24. Zhang, H., Peng, M., Guerrero, J.M., Gao, X., Liu, Y.: Modelling and vulnerability analysis of cyber-physical power systems based on interdependent networks. Energies **12**(18), 3439 (2019). https://doi.org/10.3390/en12183439
25. Huang, Z., Wang, C., Stojmenovic, M., Nayak, A.: Characterization of cascading failures in interdependent cyber-physical systems. IEEE Trans. Comput. **64**(8), 2158–2168 (2015). https://doi.org/10.1109/tc.2014.2360537
26. Guo, Q.: Interdependence and security of cyber-physical power system. CIGRE (n.d.). https://www.cigre.org/article/GB/news/the_latest_news/interdependence-and-security-of-cyber-physical-power-system. Accessed 26 Oct 2022
27. Du, D., et al.: A review on cybersecurity analysis, attack detection, and attack defense methods in cyber-physical power systems. J. Mod. Power Syst. Clean Energy **11**(3), 727–743 (2023). https://doi.org/10.35833/mpce.2021.000604
28. Ribas Monteiro, L.F., Rodrigues, Y.R., Zambroni de Souza, A.C.: Cybersecurity in cyber–physical power systems. Energies **16**(12), 4556 (2023). https://doi.org/10.3390/en16124556

Machine Learning Based Analysis of Cyber-Attacks Targeting Smart Grid Infrastructure

Mais Nijim[1(✉)], Viswas Kanumuri[1], Waseem Al Aqqad[2], and Hisham Albataineh[3]

[1] Department of Electrical Engineering and Computer Science, Texas A&M University-Kingsville, Kingsville, TX, USA
mais.nijim@tamuk.edu,
satya_viswas_varma.kanumuri@students.tamuk.edu

[2] Department of Electrical and Computer Engineering, West Virginia Tech, Beckley, WV, USA
waseem.alaqqad@mail.wvu.edu

[3] Department of Physics and Geosciences, Texas A&M University-Kingsville, Kingsville, TX, USA
hisham.albataineh@tamuk.edu

Abstract. The transformation of traditional electric power systems into smart grids has allowed for improved monitoring and control capabilities. However, this evolution has also brought about new challenges in the form of malware and vulnerabilities, creating significant security concerns. To address this issue, sensors are being deployed to the grid, leading to a large influx of data that needs to be analyzed for accurate results. Machine learning algorithms are being utilized to process this data and extract important information. This paper explores the application of various machine learning algorithms in smart grids, with a specific focus on their use in cybersecurity. We identify different types of cyber threats affecting smart grids and examine defense strategies to counter these threats. Through this study, we provide insights into the potential of machine learning in addressing the cybersecurity challenges in smart grids.

Keywords: Smart grid · Cybersecurity · Machine learning · Attack detection · False data injection

1 Introduction

The smart grid serves as energy efficient than the old traditional grids, but it has a high chance of cyber threats in the physical layer as well as the logical layer. Issues regarding the physical layers are Energy theft, load forecast due to theft, stability, etc. Whereas in the logical layer the biggest threat is data confidentiality or data privacy [1]. Many smart grids are designed and developed in a way to withstand high energy generation and energy transmission to the consumers is done in a Bi-directional flow. It also contains renewable energy resources on large scale along with traditional energy generation. Renewable energy resources are highly scalable and can produce energy without any interception compared to traditional power grids [2].

K. Daimi and A. Al Sadoon (Eds.): ACR 2024, LNNS 956, pp. 334–349, 2024.
https://doi.org/10.1007/978-3-031-56950-0_28

In Smart grid technology, the mechanical meters which are used in past are converted into electric meters which are also known as smart meter, which helps to share real-time data with the central servers of the smart grid. Smart meters consist of sensors, communication controllers, metering Ic(which converts analog signals into Digital signals), communication modules, power management, and Digital Display [3]. In a smart grid, the smart meters are key changing tools for the operation of the energy grids, these can be used to find fault data that is used for wrong approaches, by using this data it can perform tasks much more efficiently like (response, operations, and planning) and will increase the reliability of the smart meter [4]. Every smart grid runs on a communication link which is known as a network. Advance Metering Infrastructure is a communication link connected to the smart grid network, it involves the bi-directional flow of data among consumers and utilities. For better quality of power, it contains 3 phases: Smart meters at the consumer end, the bi-directional flow communication path between consumer and utilities, and lastly central server unit of the smart grid controlled for better data processing, these all help in maintaining the grid powerful [5].The grids mainly work on two types of networks, 1. HAN (Home Area Network) is pre-installed in all houses and all the smart devices like home appliances, electric charging devices, etc. are connected to the smart meter. The devices in the house and the smart meter will communicate with each other and exchange data using a network or Bluetooth. Whereas 2. WAN (Wide Area Network) is connected to wide range of devices. It acts as a communication bridge between the smart meter and the server, it frequently communicates through the network [6].

2 Literature Survey

The In a smart grid, there are different types of computational equipment one of such systems is a Cyber-Physical Systems (CPS) that contains embedded machines which will monitor and suggest the physical processes through assessment connections that will keep us in the loop. The Smart grid System (SGS) is one example that integrates both the power sources of the grid and the devices and sensors, which serve as an advantage to the grid through better Communication, Supervision, and Analysis [7]. With the help of cyber systems, we can have many advantages such as optimal and accurate pricing, Bi-directional flow of power with optimal utilization, theft detection, Stability of the power grid, lower voltage losses etc. Along with the increase in technology the challenges to secure it have increased in the form of cyber threats. So, the security of the smart grid has become a big challenge. Cyber attackers may attack the grid and can access all the sensitive information of the customers which makes us to consider cyber infrastructure seriously [8] which makes us consider cyber infrastructure seriously. We were in a situation where electric utilities aimed at installing around 90 million smart meters by 2020, thus increasing the need for security manifold.

Recently, a lot of cyber-attacks took place across the world in recent years and it has rapidly increased in the past decade. For instance, if you consider the year 2016 alone, there had been more than 50 cyber-attacks reported in the energy sector [9]. Among them, the cyber attackers mostly targeted the software devices and sensors for the customer's data. If you consider the real-life figures in the cyber-attack that happened in Ukraine in December 2016, more than 2,25000 consumers had been affected for many hours [10].For e.g., the cyber-attacks in Ukraine were the most prolific attacks involving the energy sector. The attacks launched on 3 different energy distribution firms in Ukraine clearly show the necessity for securing the Power infrastructure against cyber-attacks. Not only Ukraine, many other developed and powerful countries like USA and Israel are attacked in the years 2018 and 2016 respectively [11].

A study on cyber security attacks reveals that the Stuxnet - style attack that happened in the USA on the smart grid could be the worst, which costs nearly an estimation of 1 trillion US dollars. By considering many incidents along with this, it became very essential to predict such cyber-attacks that can happen in the future. The defense mechanisms which we use in the smart grid are becoming outdated as the technology advances at a high rate. Y. wang discussed methods to secure power grids in detail [12]. To counter all the cyber-attacks, there is a need to develop an Intrusion Detection System (IDS). That helps to prevent cyber-attacks, IDS is a proven technology that is used to monitor and find the intrusions of devices aiming to keep its security. An intrusion Detection System (IDS) could be either a hardware or can be software component within the system [13]. we can separate the attacks into two types, one is based on the Signature (SIDS) and the second is on the Anomaly (AIDS). Also adds one more class known as Stateful Protocol Analysis. In the Signature-based IDS (SIDS), it matches the patterns in the data with the preserved values to identify an attack that is already known. But this won't work in the case of a new type of attack being attempted because such type of attack never happened, and it can't predict the signature of the attack. Whereas in Anomaly-based IDS these kinds of attacks can be interpreted as an intrusion. In AIDS they are classified into three types: 1. Statistics Approach, 2. Knowledge approach, 3. Machine learning based [14].

The Statistics-based model will collect each data point in the record and with the help of the data, it will analyze it and from that, it will build a model which will help to track consumer behavior [15]. Based on the data the anomaly count will be noted and tested to describe the degree of intrusion but predicting the threshold value is very hard for such models.

Secondly, The Knowledge-based model, which is also called an expert system, will try to build in a way that reflects the general functioning of the system. Developing such big knowledge data needs resources and updating all time [15]. The previous Statistics model and Knowledge model comes under the same class called a programmed-based class. ML models themselves understand the complex data and do the pattern matching technique for huge data and that data is used for IDS. It has the capability of changing the processing technique when it is executing in a real-time environment. Machine learning models are one of the best choices used to detect the outliers in the system [16]. These techniques are mainly implemented in the Anomaly Intrusion Detection system of the grid. Here we need Machine Learning models for smart grid security.

In this paper, we are more focused on reviewing the Machine learning Algorithms used in smart grids. This paper focuses on Sect. 3 Machine learning Algorithms applied to smart grid, Sect. 4 Infrastructure of smart gird, Sect. 5 Treats to smart grid, and Sect. 6 Analysis of various Machine learning techniques applied to the security of the smart grid.

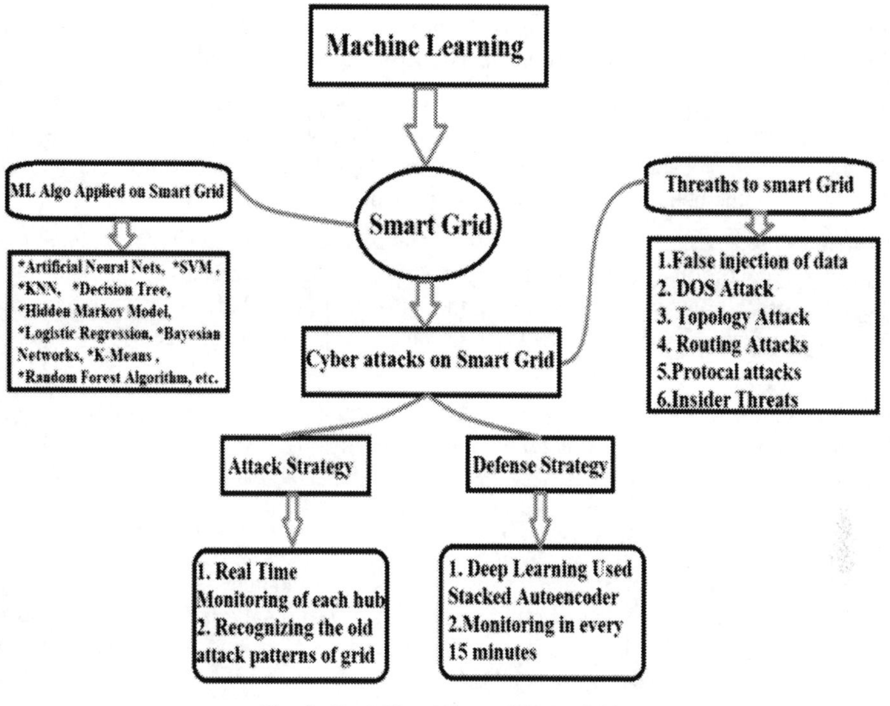

Fig. 1. Real-Time Flow of Smart Grid.

Section 7, Case Study on Detection of cyber-attacks using deep learning in smart grid. Lastly, in Sect. 8, all the results. The plan is as per focused in Fig. 1.

3 Machine Learning Algorithms Applied on Smart Grid

The ML models like Linear regression, logistic regression, ANN, K-means, Hidden Markov model, and many others are applied for the betterment of smart gird. Now let's see in detail which model is applied to which area. Figure 1: Real-Time Flow of Smart Grid.

Artificial Neural Nets: ANN can be useful as a classification system to identify the quality of the power because it has the ability to think itself and it can make independent decisions for tough decision-making problems. This is the reason why it is mostly used for error detection. Whenever the grid fails to deliver the energy, it can automatically switch to another grid to send the interfered electricity. ANN has three layers, 1. An input layer, 2. Hidden layer and 3. Output layer, different Machine Learning models are used in the hidden layer to train the data and to get better results. Finally, the output layer gives us 2 values 0 or 1 [17].

SVM: In SG, the Support vector Machine model is mostly used in the areas like Load Forecasting, which helps in predicting the generation of a correct number of power units utilized by the consumer and balancing the needs according to the demand and supply. To figure out the correct output, it draws a hyperplane to predict [18].

KNN: K-Nearest Neighbors model is used to find the alternate way of power supply, if some microgrid or grid has a difficulty in power supply, it automatically connects the alternate power grid source with it and helps in establishing the connection efficiently, it can identify the behavior of each node for providing the better results [18].

Decision Tree: It is mostly used to know the status of the grid because it is a combination of different conditions. It helps to identify the FDIA attack that creates a disturbance in the smart grid. It also helps in certifying the individual grid whether it's working well or not in the case of an FDIA Attack. The accuracy of the Decision tree Model is very high in detecting these attacks.[19].

Hidden Markov model (HMM): It mainly helps in solving the Islanding Issues, because to predict something it relays on probability. By using the smart grid Phasor measurements, it can predict the hidden state's probability, it basically performs statistical analysis [20], which is not useful in the case of a new attack. This algorithm can identify the existing malware well.

Logistic Regression: For optimal results, this model is used in cyber-physical systems, where it can provide a stable and efficient power grid. Anomaly detection is very easy using logistic regression because it uses the binary classifier, and it can also identify whether the grid is healthy or not [21].

Bayesian Networks: Bayesian Networks are used in diversified services of smart grids, and this has existed for a long back. On a Bayesian Network basis, we can predict the required resource allocation and also transportation in a smart grid. It can also identify the voltage loss and will suggest the load forecast if any additional supplies are needed in the smart grid [22].

K-means: In Machine Learning k-means comes under an unsupervised clustering technique which is useful for unlabeled data, it is mainly used in an environment like smart buildings which reflect like a cluster in the real world, it can automatically find the neighboring nodes themselves. It can also note the power consumption of each microgrid. The author worked on the real-time data of Singapore smart homes and showed the best results using Kmeans [23].

Random Forest: RF model is used when we have a huge inflow of data from the devices and sensors in the smart grid. For optimal results, we should never provide raw data to this algorithm instead need to filter the data and need to provide the data having the correct feature selection dataset. Accordingly, to Jian Zhou [24] the random forest model is best used for detecting the false record in a smart grid [24]. A random forest Algorithm can help in maintaining smart grids like Smart cities.

4 Infrastructure of Smart Grid

The infrastructure of a smart grid comprises a sophisticated network of devices, sensors, and communication systems that work together to enhance the efficiency, reliability, and sustainability of electricity distribution. The smart grid is an advanced power grid

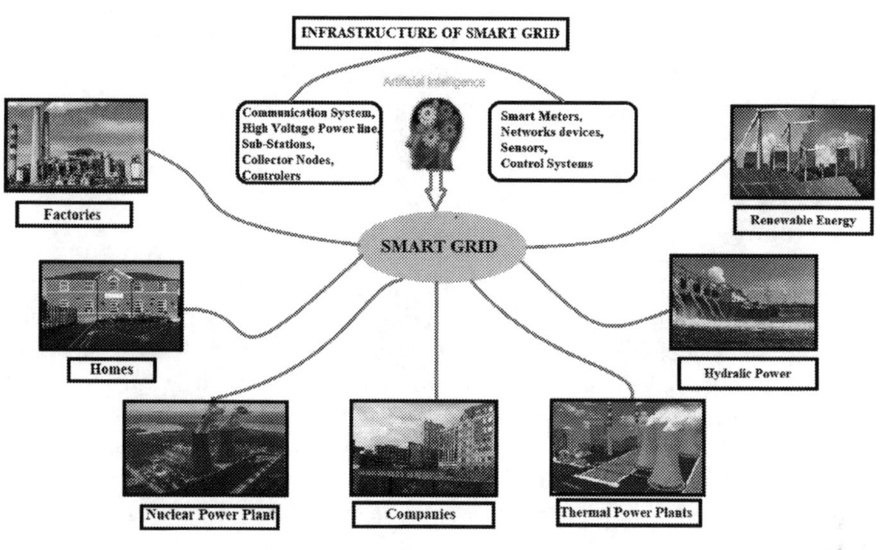

Fig. 2. Infrastructure of the smart grid with AI

that uses digital technology to monitor and manage the flow of electricity, infrastructure includes various components such as power generation sources such as power plants, solar panels, and wind turbines. High-voltage power lines are used to transmit electricity over long distances, while medium- and low-voltage power lines deliver electricity to homes and businesses. Substations are responsible for regulating and controlling the flow of electricity between the transmission and distribution networks. Smart meters are used to track energy consumption in real-time, and the data is transmitted to utility companies for billing purposes. The infrastructure also includes communication networks such as wired and wireless networks, satellite, and cellular communication systems. Control systems are software applications that monitor and manage the flow of electricity on the grid, using data from sensors and other devices to optimize the grid's performance and prevent outages. By using these infrastructures, we can collect the data from the devices and will feed that data as input to the ML algorithms for optimal results as shown in Fig. 2. Overall, the smart grid infrastructure utilizes digital technology to monitor and manage the flow of electricity in real-time, improving the efficiency, reliability, and sustainability of the power grid.

5 Threats to Smart Grid

The major threat to the smart grid comes from the Unauthorized devices and applications used by consumers, these all need to be analyzed correctly to prevent cyber-attacks [25]. Also, there are a lot of issues with the communication networks within the smart grid which is used as a loophole by cyber attackers [26]. Different kinds of threats are possible.

False Injection of Data: In the smart grid, the false injection of data is one kind of attack which is very complex to detect and is highly impressive. For this Y.Liu proposed two distributed detection models to find the false injection of data. First is DOID (Distributed Observable Island Detection algorithm), which is completely based on the observable islands model. it says that, if a connection is established between two nodes, then it should pass with various observable islands, and we can identify the false injection of data in this line. The Second approach is DTAD, which stands for Distributed Time Approaching Detection algorithm. Here for every measuring point, if the estimated value is always differing, then we can detect the attack, this can find the threats efficiently with a minimum budget [27].

The false injection of data attacks can be considered for unstructured data as well, the main aim is to find the false data injection using Distributed way, based on distributed state estimation model. In this model, the connection between the different computation nodes should be defined. The divergent way is used as a cooperation between the computing units, which needs each individual node to interchange the data with its neighboring nodes. There will be a huge flow of data, but the expected results will be good. In Fig. 3, H, R, and z are designated according to the following representation, where H is a matrix with dimensions m x n, R is the covariance matrix of the measurement error "e" in the system. And it is assumed to have the properties of a normal distribution. R represents the statistical relationships between different components of the measurement errors in the system and z represents the measurement values in the system (Fig. 3).

$$H = \begin{bmatrix} H_1 \\ H_2 \\ \vdots \\ H_p \end{bmatrix}, R = \begin{bmatrix} R_1 \\ R_2 \\ \vdots \\ R_p \end{bmatrix}, z = \begin{bmatrix} z_1 \\ z_2 \\ \vdots \\ z_p \end{bmatrix},$$

Fig. 3. False Data Impact: Analyzing H, R, and z in Power System Estimation

In the event of false data injection with in the DC model, a visual representation of this injection is provided in Fig. 4. The model incorporates essential components: the attack vector a = (a1,a2,…,ap)T and the measurement error vector e = (e1,e2,…,ep)T. These vectors are meticulously partitioned into distinct elements, denoted as a1,a2,…,ap and e1,e2,…,ep respectively. This partitioning delineates the various aspects and individual elements linked to both the attack vector and the measurement error vector, contributing to a comprehensive understanding of the injection model [27, 28].

$$\begin{bmatrix} z_1 \\ z_2 \\ \vdots \\ z_p \end{bmatrix} = \begin{bmatrix} H_1 \\ H_2 \\ \vdots \\ H_p \end{bmatrix} x + \begin{bmatrix} a_1 \\ a_2 \\ \vdots \\ a_p \end{bmatrix} + \begin{bmatrix} e_1 \\ e_2 \\ \vdots \\ e_p \end{bmatrix}$$

Fig. 4. False data injection in Direct Current(DC) Model

Topology attacks: In the smart grid, the topology attack will be done on the network of the grid, and a middleman will alter the measurements. By altering the measurements of the grid, from then the grid is made to accept that, the power grid topology has been modified. In these modern days, it is difficult to launch such topology attacks, because technology has increased and it can easily detect these attacks[29]. To start this kind of attack, we need to alter two things simultaneously, one is network data and the other is meter data, then only it can be consistent along with the data. we can denote the topology attack as shown below.

$z = H^\wedge \theta + e.$
$H^\wedge = H + a.$
Here, the variables are defined as follows [23]:

- z represents the measurement vector.
- H is a matrix.
- θ is a vector.
- e is an error term.
- a represents a certain term.

Denial of Service Attack: This attacks on load frequency control (LFC) of smart grids, which is different from the topology, here in the control center, only some measurements are available. The DoS attack causes distributed denial of service, which is intended to utilize various gadgets to focus on a server by overpowering the organization with various requests. Basically, this attack is simplest to execute and hard to find. A DoS attack on the smart grid can decrease the health of the grid, as a portion of these frameworks is not intended to endure this kind of attack. At times, it may cause energy interference, and the controls must be reestablished physically by the administrator. The serious issue with DoS identification is that it is hard to recognize genuine and DoS traffic. To identify and recognize the sorts of such goes after on the power foundation, the SG network should be fit for observing the marks of give and take (IOCs) to make the location signal reliable. [30]. Table 1. mentioned several types of attacks.

Table 1. Different Kind of Attacks

Type Of Attack	Affected Properties	Victims
False Data Injection Attacks	Data Integrity DoS Confindentiality	Neighbourhood-House, PowerSupplying Unit
Network-Based Attacks	Availability Confidentiality Devices with Personal Information	WANs, Household, PowerSupplying Unit
Smart Meter Attack	Integrity Non-repudiation Confidentiality	Networks, Neighbourhood area, House
Scada	Integrity Confidentiality	LANS

6 Analysis of Various Machine Learning Techniques Applied on Security of Smart Grid

Various Machine learning models have been tried in the domain of smart grids in the field of security. Different Machine Learning designs for recognizing the attacks on the smart grid are utilized in [31] like KNN, SVM, ANN, CNN, Logistic regression, XGBoost e.t.c. The design will be having four sections as follows. In finding the feature's importance, the creators built 16 new Attributes or features to improve the accuracy. They divided the data in a ratio of 9:1 for finding the accuracy and the cross-validation. Various classifiers were trained and the majority voting will be applied to it to get more accuracy The Article closes with the comment that information handling strategies alongside AI are a decent choice to further develop the discovery precision of the models. Moreover, [32] likewise utilizes three unique Machine Learning models to find the more important features.

In [33] and [34], For the different types of objectives, reinforcement learning is used to identify the attack sequence by using the Q-learning approach, it can easily find the attacks. In a proper OS, the attack sequence will be started, and with the initial attack, the stability mode will be activated in the system. If it tackled the attack, then system starts the second attack, in this way the attack goes on. If the agent fails, then it results in power outages. Here the attacks are continuous and help the agent to learn by himself and rewards and depreciations are given accordingly to make the agent learn. This goes on until the complete blackout happens. The author discussed the trade-off related to power loss. In Reference [33], in two-man collaboration. The primary individual can be considered a cyber attacker and the other as a safeguard. The author has proposed a game with 2 persons and with a zero-sum game In this multistage game, the attacker finds the best attack succession, to apply on the lines of transmission, and the protector safeguards a bunch of lines. In the wake of learning, the activities will be utilized as a security setting in the safeguard. This recommends that learning reproduced attackers assists in protecting with getting ready for better safeguard systems [35].

Repetitive Artificial Neural nets are a kind of Neural network, that extracts the transient relationship between the data elements which are close in order. The result of a Repetitive Neural Network relies upon the given inputs, and also past inputs and results. Reference [36] outlines the undertaking of recognizing FDI attacks as an order issue utilizing RNN. They utilize the power estimations, as a contribution to RNN. The attack vector presence in order will be noted as a positive instance and negative instances will be taken when we have normal measurements. A LSTM design of RNN for Interruption, Identification, and through execution test is utilized in [37], Here the Deep learning Technique ended up being better for detecting Intrusions. Numerous other AI has additionally been tried in the domain of Smart Grid. To distinguish data integrity attacks on smart grid communications, [38] utilizes the Isolation forest technique which is the unsupervised machine learning technique used on unlabeled data. Reference [39] worked on detecting the DOS attacks, they also used the same unsupervised methods as auto-encoders, and multi-level features from various kernel algorithms for building a final detection model.

7 Discussion and Analysis of Cyber Attacks in Smart Grid Using Machine Learning

To tell the utilization of ML strategies in improving the SG network protection, and to acquire knowledge about the advantages these techniques offer, a current IDS based on machine Learning as proposed in [40] is carried out as a contextual analysis, as made sense of straightaway. The strategy comprises 2 sections, which are 1) carrying out the going after techniques with complete organization data wherein a given electrical cable is over-burden by changing minimum meters in the grid, and 2) executing the shielding model for a similar utilizing DL.

1) Attack strategy on Smart Grid: The methodology is planned in 2 phases. Coming to the main stage, the optimal flow program runs, which yields power streaming among every hub. The subsequent stage is figured out as an improvement that is not direct and expects to limit the extent of non-zero components in the attack vector. Thus, is displayed as the L0 standard of (zt − h(xt)), dependent upon the different power framework working requirements. Likewise, it is guaranteed that the power coursing through the line to be gone after is more prominent than its most extreme indicated esteem.
2) Defense Strategy on Smart Grid: The safeguard system is likewise inherent in 2 sections. First is the disconnected part where a model is prepared to conjecture the electric burden. The engineering utilized for determining is a stacked autoencoder that uses deep learning, where initially, every layer is independently prepared, and next kept on one another. The loads were calibrated by utilizing an essential layer toward the last.

In the web-based stage, the heap will be gauged like clockwork for 15 min, the middle-of-state factors are acquired by carrying OPF on the estimated values. Generally, some mistakes exist in the gauge information and the gauging blunder is displayed with Gaussian appropriation. To do an information commotion examination, the blunder dataset DSdn will be produced as:

$$DSdn = ((rl - y^\wedge(\chi 1)), ...(rNs - y^\wedge(\chi Ns)))$$

For a set of Ns instances, DSdn represents the vector of differences between the actual response values (r) and the corresponding predicted values (y^). These differences are pivotal in quantifying the model's predictive accuracy. The expression DSdn = ((rl − y^(χ1)),…,(rNs − y^(χNs))) signifies Ns as the number of samples or data points in the dataset. Each term in the tuple (ri − y^(χi)) corresponds to the difference between the observed value ri and the predicted or estimated value (y^(χi) for the i-th sample. These differences play a crucial role in assessing the model's accuracy. The term (rNs − y^(χNs)) represents the difference between the observed value rNs and the predicted or estimated value (y^(χNs) for the Ns-th sample or data point in the dataset. This difference, often referred to as the residual or error, quantifies how much the prediction (y^(χNs)) deviates from the actual observed value (rNs) for the Ns-th instance. In simpler terms, it measures the accuracy of the model for the specific data point indexed by Ns. If the model is accurate, this difference should ideally be close to zero, indicating a minimal deviation between the predicted and observed values. The vector DSdn contains similar differences for all Ns samples in the dataset, providing an overall assessment of the model's predictive performance. Furthermore, Gaussian Model computations are employed on the dataset to determine mean and variance for load values. The assessment of timespan state factors involves solving a nonlinear optimization problem to limit the power balancing interval at each node rationally. Additionally, the evaluations include the incorporation of dynamic and responsive electricity in the gauge assessments.

$$[\Delta x\gamma t, \Delta x\gamma t] = [\min^{\rightarrow} eT\gamma t\Delta^{\rightarrow} xt, -\min^{\rightarrow} eT\gamma t\Delta^{\rightarrow} xt]$$

This expression defines a vector interval, denoted by $[\Delta x\gamma t, \Delta x\gamma t]$. This interval is determined by evaluating the minimum and maximum values of the expression $^{\rightarrow}eT\gamma t\Delta^{\rightarrow}xt$ across different instances or scenarios.

- $^{\rightarrow}eT$ represents the transpose of the error vector.
- γt is a parameter associated with the model.
- $\Delta^{\rightarrow}xt$ is a vector representing changes in input variables.

The minimum value in the interval is obtained by evaluating "$^{\rightarrow}eT\gamma t\Delta^{\rightarrow}xt$", and the maximum value is the negation of this minimum value," – min $^{\rightarrow}eT\gamma t\Delta^{\rightarrow}xt$". This interval essentially captures the range of values that the expression "$^{\rightarrow}eT\gamma t\Delta^{\rightarrow}xt$" can take across different scenarios. Analyzing this interval provides insights into how sensitive the model is to variations in the input variables $\Delta^{\rightarrow}xt$ and the impact of the error term $^{\rightarrow}e$. The minimum and maximum values help understand the potential variability in the outcome of the expression under different conditions.

8 Results

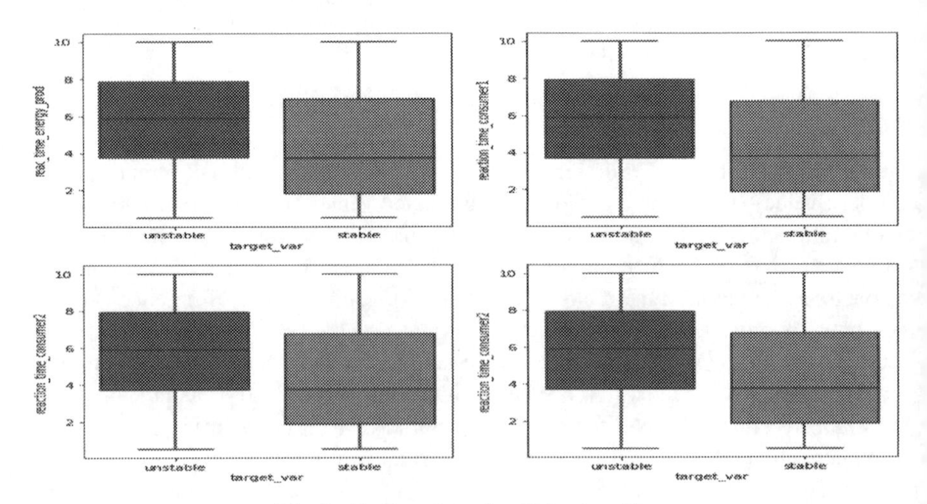

Fig. 5. Outliers detection Using box Plot

In Fig. 5, we present the results of our outliers detection analysis on Mississippi State University and Oak Ridge National Laboratory dataset, a crucial aspect of our research. It is essential to clarify that outliers, in this context, refer to data points that deviate significantly from the expected patterns in the household power consumption dataset. To elaborate on the dataset used, our analysis is conducted on the Household Power Consumption dataset, encompassing comprehensive data from consumers recorded at frequent time intervals. This dataset serves as the foundation for our experiments, executed in Python and Google Colab using various machine learning algorithms and Python libraries. To ensure the integrity of our analysis, we performed outlier detection on this dataset. Specifically, we used Python and leveraged outlier analysis techniques to identify and handle unwanted data points, including null values. The preprocessing steps involved data cleaning, where null values were either deleted or replaced with appropriate measures such as the mean, mode, or median, depending on the nature of the data. The outcomes of this process are depicted in Fig. 5, showcasing the effectiveness of our approach in enhancing the dataset's quality and reliability.

The python code is performed to calculate the flow of electricity among each node, by this we can find the attack that occurred. Many machine learning algorithms are performed to find the best results. When we plot the results in a graph then we can identify the results as shown in Fig. 6.

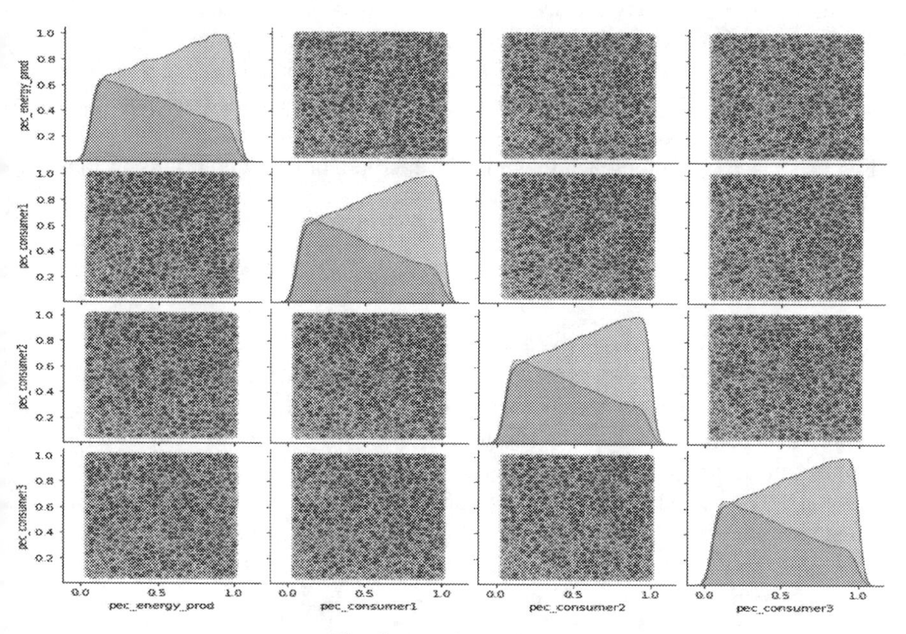

Fig. 6. Attack Possibility

Among all the algorithms, in our analysis Random Forest Algorithm gave us the better results with high accuracy. Anyways, in the occasion of attack, the values of the nodes which are attacked have flown outside of the expected interval, different experiments uncovered that the proposed Analysis strategies have an extremely good accuracy in this

Table 2. Outcome of various Algorithms

Algorithm	Precision	Recall	F1-score	Accuracy
Random Forest	0.953945	0.955	0.953945	0.959457
Ensemble	0.930326	0.939826	0.929913	0.939889
Logistic Regression	0.929304	0.929826	0.929565	0.925444
Decision Tree	0.915406	0.915343	0.915454	0.915787
Multinomial	0.638000	0.777438	0.778999	0.638000

analysis. In extension to this research, In our next research paper, we provided better results for the same dataset collected by Mississippi State University and Oak Ridge National Laboratory, which amalgamates three distinct datasets, comprising a total of 37 power system event scenarios. The decision to use this specific dataset was motivated by its unique attributes that align with the objectives of our research. Each component of the dataset contributes valuable insights into diverse attack scenarios on smart grids, and the collaboration between Mississippi State University and Oak Ridge National Laboratory ensures the dataset's credibility and relevance to real-world power system security challenges. To provide transparency in our methodology, we offer a detailed breakdown of dataset utilization. The scenarios were divided into training, validation, and testing sets, with an 80–10-10 split to balance model performance and generalization. While acknowledging the dataset's comprehensiveness, we also recognize potential biases in representing specific attack vectors. In our analysis, we conscientiously consider these biases and discuss their implications on the interpretation of our results in our next research paper (Table 2).

9 Conclusion

This work presents an analysis of various machine learning that helps in detecting cyber-attacks on smart grids. In the case study, we focused on showing, how autoencoders are used to find a cyber-attack. Many Authors used machine learning, deep learning, and reinforcement learning to detect cyber-attacks on smart grids. Here we did an analysis of some of the techniques and a lot needs to be done in the future to identify other cyber-attacks on the smart grid. Machine Learning models are applied to create an attack vector, that can overcome the existing cyber-attack detectors. This will help us to build a more robust model in the future. In our next paper, we will perform based on Deep learning to detect the cyber-attack on the smart grid.

References

1. Yadav, S.A., Kumar, S.R., Sharma, S., Singh, A.: A review of possibilities and solutions of cyber attacks in smart grids. In: 2016 International Conference on Innovation and Challenges in Cyber Security (ICICCS-INBUSH), pp. 60–63 (2016). https://doi.org/10.1109/ICICCS.2016.7542359

2. Zahran, M.: Smart Grid Technology, Vision Management and Control. Wseas Trans. Syst. **12**(1) (2013)
3. Sreedevi, S.V., Prasannan, P., Jiju, K., Indu Lekshmi, I.I.J.: Development of indigenous smart energy meter adhering indian standards for smart grid. In: 2020 IEEE International Conference on Power Electronics, Smart Grid and Renewable Energy (PESGRE2020), pp. 1–5 (2020). https://doi.org/10.1109/PESGRE45664.2020.9070245
4. Barai, G.R., Krishnan, S., Venkatesh, B.: Smart metering and functionalities of smart meters in smart grid - a review. IEEE Electr. Power Energy Conf. (EPEC) **2015**, 138–145 (2015). https://doi.org/10.1109/EPEC.2015.7379940
5. National Energy Technology Laboratory (NETL), Advanced metering infrastructure, NETL Modern Grid Strategy Powering our 21st-Century Economy, Report prepared for the U.S. Department of Energy Office of Electricity Delivery and Energy Reliability (2008)
6. Alohali, B., Kifayat, K., Shi, Q., Hurst, W.: Group authentication scheme for neighbourhood area networks (NANs) in smart grids. J. Sens. Actuator Netw. **5**(2). 9 (2016). https://doi.org/10.3390/jsan5020009
7. Arnold, G.W.: Challenges and opportunities in smart grid: a position article. Proc. IEEE **99**(6), 922–927 (2011)
8. Sun, C.-C., Hahn, A., Liu, C.-C.: Cyber security of a power grid: state-of-the-art. Int. J. Electr. Power Energy Syst. **99**, 45–56 (2018)
9. Team, I., et al.: Ics-cert year in review (2016)
10. Rao, P.U., Sodhi, B., Sodhi, R.: Cyber Security Enhancement of Smart Grids Via Machine (2020)
11. Khandelwal, S.: Israeli electrical power grid suffers massive cyber attack (2016)
12. Wang, Y., et al.: Analysis of smart grid security standards. In: 2011 IEEE International Conference on Computer Science and Automation Engineering, vol. 4, pp. 697–701 (2011)
13. Liao, H.-J., Lin, C.-H.R., Lin, Y.-C., Tung, K.-Y.: Intrusion detection system: a comprehensive review. J. Netw. Comput. Appl. **36**(1), 16–24 (2013)
14. Khraisat, A., Gondal, I., Vamplew, P., Kamruzzaman, J.: Survey of intrusion detection systems: techniques, datasets and challenges. Cybersecurity **2**(1), 20 (2019)
15. Hodo, E., Bellekens, X., Hamilton, A., Tachtatzis, C., Atkinson, R.: Shallow and deep networks intrusion detection system: a taxonomy and survey. arXiv preprint arXiv:1701.02145 (2017)
16. Amin, B.M.R., Taghizadeh, S., Maric, S., Hossain, M.J., Abbas, R.: Smart grid security enhancement by using belief propagation. IEEE Syst. J., 1–12 (2020). (Many References should come for ml algo in smart grid)
17. Alshahrani, S., Abbod, M., Alamri, B.: Detection and classification of power quality events based on wavelet transform and artificial neural networks for smart grids. In: 2015 Saudi Arabia Smart Grid (SASG), pp. 1–6 (2015).https://doi.org/10.1109/SASG.2015.7449296
18. Ali, M., Khan, Z.A., Mujeeb, S., Abbas, S., Javaid, N.: Short-term electricity price and load forecasting using enhanced support vector machine and k-nearest neighbour. In: 2019 Sixth HCT Information Technology Trends (ITT), pp. 79–83 (2019).https://doi.org/10.1109/ITT48889.2019.9075063
19. Lu, X., Jing, J., Wu, Y.: False data injection attack location detection based on classification method in smart grid. In: 2020 2nd International Conference on Artificial Intelligence and Advanced Manufacture (AIAM), pp. 133–136 (2020). https://doi.org/10.1109/AIAM50918.2020.00033
20. Kumar, D., Bhowmik, P.S.: Hidden markov model based islanding prediction in smart grids. IEEE Syst. J. **13**(4), 4181–4189 (2019). https://doi.org/10.1109/JSYST.2019.2911055
21. Noureen, S.S., Bayne, S.B., Shaffer, E., Porschet, D., Berman, M.: Anomaly detection in cyber-physical system using logistic regression analysis. In: 2019 IEEE Texas Power and Energy Conference (TPEC), pp. 1–6 (2019).https://doi.org/10.1109/TPEC.2019.8662186

22. Yang, J., Song, Y.: Bayesian model based services awareness of power line communications for smart power grid. In: 2018 2nd IEEE Advanced Information Management,Communicates,Electronic and Automation Control Conference (IMCEC), pp. 871–874 (2018).https://doi.org/10.1109/IMCEC.2018.8469494
23. Li, W., Logenthiran, T., Phan, V.-T., Woo, W.L.: Power alert system using K-means for smart home. IEEE Innov. Smart Grid Technol. Asia (ISGT Asia) **2018**, 722–727 (2018). https://doi.org/10.1109/ISGT-Asia.2018.8467949
24. Zhou, J.,Ge, Z., Gao, S., Yanli, X.: Fault record detection with random forests in data center of large power grid. In: 2016 IEEE PES Asia-Pacific Power and Energy Engineering Conference (APPEEC), pp. 1641–1645 (2016).https://doi.org/10.1109/APPEEC.2016.7779771
25. Stoyaov, I.S., Iliev, T.B., Mihaylov, G.Y., Evstatiev, B.I., Sokolov, S.A.: Analysis of the cybersecurity threats in smart grid university of telecommunications and post, Sofia, Bulgaria. In: 2018 IEEE 24th International Symposium for Design and Technology in Electronic Packaging (SIITME), pp. 90–93 (2018). https://doi.org/10.1109/SIITME.2018.8599261.n
26. Marah, R., Gabassi, I.E., Larioui, S., Yatimi, H.: Security of smart grid management of smart meter protection. In: 2020 1st International Conference on Innovative Research in Applied Science, Engineering and Technology (IRASET), pp. 1–5 (2020). https://doi.org/10.1109/IRASET48871.2020.9092048
27. Liu, Y., Yan, L., Ren, J.-W., Su, D.: Research on efficient detection methods for false data injection in smart grid. Int. Conf. Wirel. Commun. Sens. Netw. **2014**, 188–192 (2014). https://doi.org/10.1109/WCSN.2014.45
28. Junwei, C., et al.: Information system architecture for smart grid. Chin. J. Comput. **36**(1), 143–167 (2013)
29. Kim, J., Tong, L.: On topology attack of a smart grid: undetectable attacks and countermeasures. IEEE J. Sel. Areas Commun. **31**(7), 1294–1305 (2013)
30. Merlino, J.C., Asiri, M., Saxena, N.: DDoS cyber-incident detection in smart grids. School of Computer Science & Informatics, Cardiff University, Cardiff CF10 3AT, UK
31. Wang, D., Wang, X., Zhang, Y., Jin, L.: Detection of power grid disturbances and cyber-attacks based on machine learning. J. Inf. Secur. Appl. **46**, 42–52 (2019)
32. Sakhnini, J., Karimipour, H., Dehghantanha, A.: Smart grid cyber attacks detection using supervised learning and heuristic feature selection. In: 2019 IEEE 7th International Conference on Smart Energy Grid Engineering (SEGE), pp. 108–112 (2019)
33. Ni, Z., Paul, S.: A multistage game in smart grid security: a reinforcement learning solution. IEEE Trans. Neural Netw. Learn. Syst. **30**(9), 2684–2695 (2019)
34. Ni, Z., Paul, S., Zhong, X., Wei, Q.: A reinforcement learning approach for sequential decision-making process of attacks in smart grid. In: 2017 IEEE Systems Series of Information computing(SSIC) (2017)
35. Rao, P.U., Sodhi, B., Sodhi, R.: Cyber security enhancement of smart grids via machine learning - a review. In: 2020 21st National Power Systems Conference (NPSC), pp. 1–6 (2020). https://doi.org/10.1109/NPSC49263.2020.9331859
36. Ayad, A., Farag, H.E.Z., Youssef, A., El-Saadany, E. F.: Detection of false data injection attacks in smart grids using recurrent neural networks. In: 2018 IEEE Power Energy Society Innovative Smart Grid Technologies Conference (ISGT), pp. 1–5 (2018)
37. Kim, J., Thi Thu, H.L., Kim, H.: Long short term memory recurrent neural network classifier for intrusion detection. In: 2016 International Conference on Platform Technology and Service (PlatCon), pp. 1–5 (2016)
38. Ahmed, S., Lee, Y., Hyun, S., Koo, I.: Unsupervised machine learning-based detection of covert data integrity assault in smart grid networks utilizing isolation forest. IEEE Trans. Inf. Forensics Secur. **14**(10), 2765–2777 (2019)

39. Ali, S., Li, Y.: Learning multilevel auto-encoders for ddos attack detection in smart grid network. IEEE Access **7**, 108647–108659 (2019)
40. Wang, H., et al.: Deep learning-based interval state estimation of ac smart grids against sparse cyber attacks. IEEE Trans. Ind. Inform. **14**(11), 4766–4778 (2018)

Cyber Attack Detection on IoT Using Machine Learning

Mohamed Haddadi[1(✉)], Eralda Caushaj[2], Ala Eddine Bouladour[3], and Adbeldjabar Nedjai Dhirar[3]

[1] Université de M'hamed Bougara de Boumerdes, Boumerdès 35000, Algérie
m.haddadi@univ-boumerdes.dz
[2] Oakland University, Rochester Hills, MI 48309, USA
ecaushaj@oakland.edu
[3] Université de Ferhat Abbess Sétif1, Setif, Algérie

Abstract. In recent years, there has been a rapid increase in the adoption of Internet of Things (IoT) devices due to their significant advantages in modern society. However, this surge has created a substantial opportunity for hackers to carry out malicious attacks. Detecting and mitigating these attacks necessitates the use of innovative techniques, given their severity. Machine learning, a subfield of Artificial Intelligence (AI, is a vital tool in addressing this issue. Techniques such as random forest, decision tree, k-nearest neighbors, support vector machine, logistic regression, extreme Gradient Boosting, Adaptive Boosting, and Gradient Boosting must be employed to effectively classify IoT attacks using two types of classification: binary and multiple classes. To evaluate the detection accuracy of various ML techniques, the IoTID20 dataset was created. We conducted a comparative analysis between our results and those obtained by others using similar ML techniques. The findings demonstrate that our models outperform others in terms of detection accuracy, both in binary and multiclass classifications.

Keywords: Internet of Things · Machine Learning · IoT Network · Cyber-attacks · IoTID20 dataset

1 Introduction

Globally, the Internet of Things (IoT) plays a crucial role in our daily lives due to its numerous benefits, notably its ability to collect and transfer data without human intervention. These data originate from a wide range of sources, including self-driving cars, sensors, and more. However, this IoT network is susceptible to various attacks, which can be categorized as cyberattacks and physical attacks. Cyberattacks can be either active or passive. Active attacks involve manipulating system configurations and disrupting services, while passive attacks focus on manipulating and decrypting confidential information [1].

K. Daimi and A. Al Sadoon (Eds.): ACR 2024, LNNS 956, pp. 350–358, 2024.
https://doi.org/10.1007/978-3-031-56950-0_29

In general, the detection of these attack types is of utmost importance, as there are inherent limitations in various fields. To address these limitations, the vast majority of the research community has turned to a new concept known as Artificial Intelligence (AI). In today's world, AI is being widely employed in a multitude of fields, including economics, military, scientific research, and more.

Finally, within the realm of AI, a novel branch known as Machine Learning (ML) has emerged. ML involves learning from training datasets to develop the capacity to make new decisions based on new data. However, these datasets often contain missing values, errors, outliers, and noisy data. It is essential to filter out these unwanted or incomplete data before initiating any ML training process. As a result, data preprocessing in Machine Learning (ML) is a pivotal step that can enhance data quality, leading to more consistent datasets. Currently, it plays a crucial role in achieving high-performance metrics when employing ML techniques. These techniques can be broadly categorized into two main groups. The first category comprises supervised learning techniques such as K-Nearest Neighbors (KNN), Random Forest (RF), Support Vector Machine (SVM), and Naïve Bayes (NB), which rely on labeled data. In contrast, the second category encompasses unsupervised learning techniques, which can work with unlabeled data, including algorithms like K-means and Principal Component Analysis (PCA).

Numerous researchers have utilized various IoT datasets to assess the effectiveness of their proposals. One of the most commonly employed IoT datasets is IoTID20, which was recently released for the purpose of detecting intrusions in IoT networks [2]. In our study, we applied certain preprocessing techniques, including under-sampling, to the IoTID20 dataset with the aim of improving the accuracy of IoT attack detection using ML techniques.

The rest of this paper is organized into the following sections. Section 2 provides an overview of related work, while Sect. 3 details the IoTID20 dataset. Our proposed model is presented in Sect. 4, and the results are discussed in Sect. 5. Finally, Sect. 6 concludes the paper.

2 Related Work

In this section, we will reference recent literature in the field of cyber-attack detection on IoT using ML techniques. We start with the work of Vikas et al. [3], who introduced an ensemble approach involving various ML techniques to detect attacks in IoT networks. The primary objective of their study was to identify the most effective technique for real-time IoT attack detection. The results indicate that K-Nearest Neighbors (KNN), Naïve Bayes (NB), and Decision Trees (DT) exhibit strong performance.

Another framework was devised by Pokhrel et al. [4], who presented an innovative approach employing an ML model to identify and counter Distributed Denial of Service (DDoS) attacks within an IoT network. The findings of their study demonstrate that K-Nearest Neighbors (KNN) outperforms Naïve Bayes (NB) and Multi-Layer Perceptron Artificial Neural Network (MLP ANN) in terms of accuracy. Hussain et al. [5] introduced an innovative two-fold ML approach designed to prevent and detect botnet attacks in IoT networks, achieving an impressive accuracy of 98.89%. In another study, Htwe et al. [6] developed an architecture utilizing ML techniques, including Classification and Regression Trees (CART) and Naïve Bayes (NB). They conducted an evaluation using N-BaIoT and found that CART outperformed NB, boasting an accuracy of 99%. Chesney et al. [7] presented an approach aimed at assessing the effectiveness of ML algorithms in countering IoT-related cyber-attacks. They utilized the Logistic Regression (LR) technique with the CICDDoS2019 dataset and achieved an impressive prediction accuracy of 99.7%.

Kumar et al. [8] introduced a framework that establishes an intelligent cyber-attack detection system for IoT networks, employing a novel hybrid feature-reduction technique. They conducted evaluations using the Bot-IoT dataset to calculate the accuracy of various ML techniques. The results indicate that XGBoost and Random Forest (RF) achieved a remarkable accuracy of 99.99%, while K-Nearest Neighbors (KNN) reached an accuracy of 85.92%. Mandal et al. [1] proposed the utilization of machine learning to enhance security in an IoT intrusion detection system. The results demonstrate that the highest accuracy achieved is 94.57%.

3 IOTID20 Dataset

IoT instruction dataset, known as IoTID20, was introduced by I. Ullah et al. [9]. This dataset comprises 83 features and includes 3 labels: 'Label,' 'Category,' and 'Subcategory,' as outlined in Table 1. Out of a total of 625,783 records, 40,073 records are designated as part of the normal class, while the remaining 585,710 records are categorized as anomalies. Furthermore, the dataset encompasses various types of IoT attacks, such as scanning, Denial of Service (DoS), Mirai, and Man-in-the-Middle (MITM) attacks.

Table 1. Two different instances extracted from IoTID20 dataset.

Instances	Label
192.168.0.13–222.61.154.61–554-5346–6,222.61.154.61,5346, 92.168.0.13,554,6,26/05/2019 10:11:16 PM,2228,0,2,0.0, 0.0,0.0,0.0,0.0,0.0,0.0,0.0,0.0,0.0,0.0,897.6660682226213,2228.0 ,0.0, 2228.0,2228.0, 0.0,0.0,0.0,0.0,0.0,2228.0,2228.0,0.0,2228.0,2228.0,0,0,0,0,0,44,0.0 ,897.6660682226213,0.0,0.0,0.0,0.0,0.0,0,1,0,0,0,0,0,0.0,0.0,0.0,0.0,0,0,0,0,0,0,0,2,0, –1,14600, 0,0,0.0,0.0,0.0,0.0,2228.0,0.0,2228.0,2228.0, Anomaly, DoS, DoS-Synflooding	DOS
192.168.0.13–192.168.0.16–9020-49784–6,192.168.0.13,9020,192.168.0.16,49784,6,20/05/2019 04:57:57 AM,73,0,2,0.0,0.0,0.0,0.0,0.0,0.0,0.0,0.0,0.0,0.0,0.0,27397.260273972603,73.0,0.0,73.0,73.0,0.0,0.0,0.0,0.0,0.0,73.0,73.0,0.0,73.0,73.0,0,0,0,0,0, 0,64,0.0,27397.260273972603,0.0,0.0,0.0,0.0,0.0,0,0,0,1,0,0,0,0.0,0.0,0.0,0.0,0,0,0,0,0,0,0,0,2,0, –1,32683,0, 0,0.0,0.0,0.0,0.0,73.0,0.0,73.0,73.0, Normal, Normal, Normal	Normal

4 Proposed Model

In this section, we have developed our proposed model based on ML techniques to detect IoT attacks. For our study, we employed nine classifiers: Decision Tree (DT), Logistic Regression (LR), Random Forest (RF), Naïve Bayes (NB), K-Nearest Neighbors (KNN), Support Vector Machine (SVM), Adaptive Boosting (AdaBoost), Extreme Gradient Boosting (XGBoost), and Gradient Boosting (GB) to assess the effectiveness of these techniques. The implementation of this proposed model involves a series of steps, as illustrated in Fig. 1.

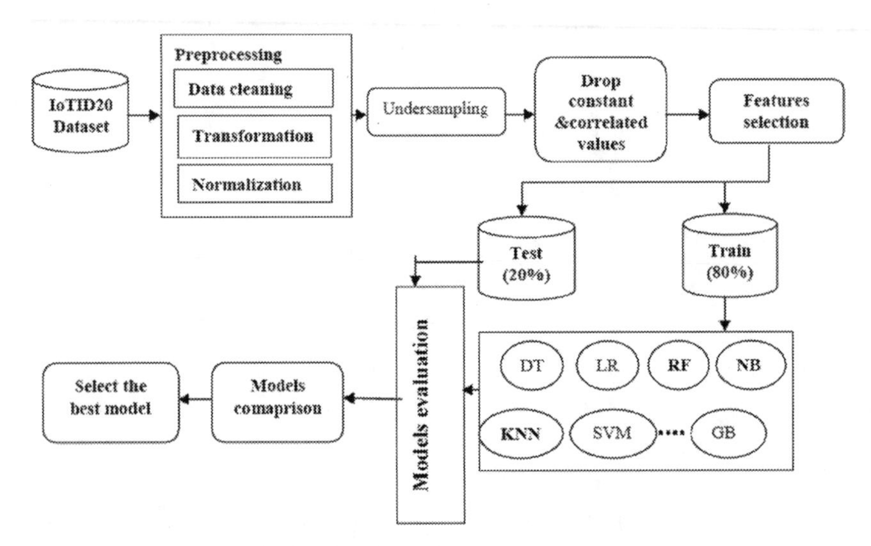

Fig. 1. Flowchart of our proposed model.

In Fig. 1, we commence with the preprocessing stage, which is a critical step in the development of an ML model. This stage encompasses the following operations:

- Data Cleaning: Our first task is to eliminate missing values and duplicated rows. To achieve this, we utilize the drop_duplicates() method in the Python programming language.
- Categorical to Numerical Transformation: Next, we convert categorical values into numerical values. This transformation is carried out using the Python method LabelEncoder(), where 'Normal' is encoded as 1 and 'Anomaly' as 0.
- Normalization: The final step in this phase involves data normalization. This process scales the data to a fixed range of [0, 1]. To do this, we apply the following Python statement:

$$Y_{norm} = (Y - Y_{\min})/(Y_{\max} - Y_{\min}) \tag{1}$$

Following that, we perform an under-sampling operation to achieve a balanced dataset, with the aim of preventing overfitting. The next crucial step is feature selection, which involves choosing the most relevant features from the IoTID20 dataset to enhance the accuracy and efficiency of our ML models. To accomplish this, we employ Recursive Feature Elimination (RFE) with the use of Python. Finally, we partition our refined IoTID20 dataset into two distinct sets: a training set consisting of 80% of the data and a testing set containing the remaining 20%.

5 Results and Discussions

In this section, we will evaluate the performance of several well-known ML techniques using confusion matrices. This will allow us to assess their effectiveness through a commonly used metric, accuracy, in two classification scenarios: binary classification and multi-class classification. Accuracy is defined as follows:

$$Accuracy = (TP + TN)/(TP + FP + FN + TN) \tag{2}$$

5.1 Binary Classification

We employ binary classification to compare our models with those presented in reference [10]. This comparison is conducted using the widely-used programming language Python to calculate the accuracy of each model. In this comparative study, we use the IoTID20 dataset to determine accuracy, as depicted in Fig. 2. This dataset is well-recognized for its application in training and testing models for the detection of cyber-attacks in IoT networks. Table 2 provides a comparison of accuracy between our results and those mentioned in [10] using binary classification.

Table 2. Comparison of the accuracy between our results and others [10] using binary classification.

Models	Our results	others of [10]
DT	99.6%	98.56%
RF	99.50%	98.62%
XGBoost	99.74%	98.64%
Adaboost	99.57%	98.02%
KNN	99.16%	98.43%
SVM	90.88%	87.22%
NB	70.68%	18.79%
GB	99.41%	98.34%
LR	91.59%	93.27%

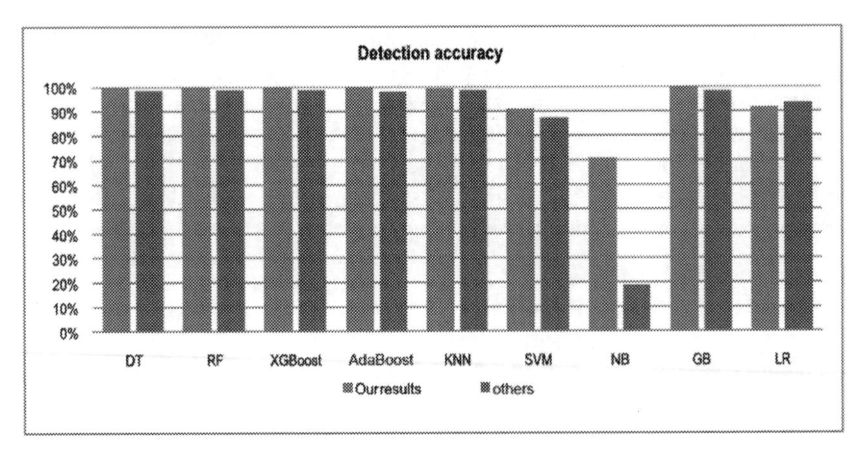

Fig. 2. Accuracy comparison between our results and others [10] using binary classification.

According to Fig. 2, the algorithms we utilized, such as XGBoost, RF, AdaBoost, KNN, SVM, and GB, demonstrate the highest accuracy in comparison to other algorithms mentioned in [10]. Notably, LR achieves a competitive accuracy of 91.59% in contrast to the LR accuracy reported in [10], which is 93.27%. On the other hand, our results indicate that NB has the lowest accuracy at 70.68%, while the accuracy mentioned in [10] is 18.79%. It's important to note that this comparison is conducted using a similar IoTID20 dataset.

5.2 Multi-classification

In the following sections, we employ multi-classification to compare our models with others as mentioned in [10]. This comparison is conducted using the widely-used programming language Python to calculate the accuracy of each model. In this comparative study, we utilize the IoTID20 dataset to determine accuracy, as illustrated in Fig. 3. This dataset is well-recognized for its application in training and testing models for detecting cyber-attacks in IoT networks. Table 3 provides a comparison of accuracy between our results and those mentioned in [10] using multi-classification.

Based on the observations from Fig. 3, our employed algorithms, including XGBoost, RF, AdaBoost, KNN, SVM, and GB, exhibit higher accuracy compared to the existing algorithms mentioned in [10]. Notably, in our results, LR demonstrates competitive detection accuracy at 75.30%, whereas in [10], the result is slightly higher at 75.86%. It's essential to highlight that this comparison is conducted using a similar IoTID20 dataset.

Table 3. Compares the accuracy between our results and others [10] using multi-classification.

Models	Our results	others [10]
DT	98.84%	83.41%
RF	97.91%	83.55%
XGBoost	99.21%	83.71%
Adaboost	98.42%	57.91%
KNN	96.98%	81.29%
SVM	76.56%	68.23%
NB	63.27%	57.38%
GB	97.12%	83.09%
LR	75.30%	75.86%

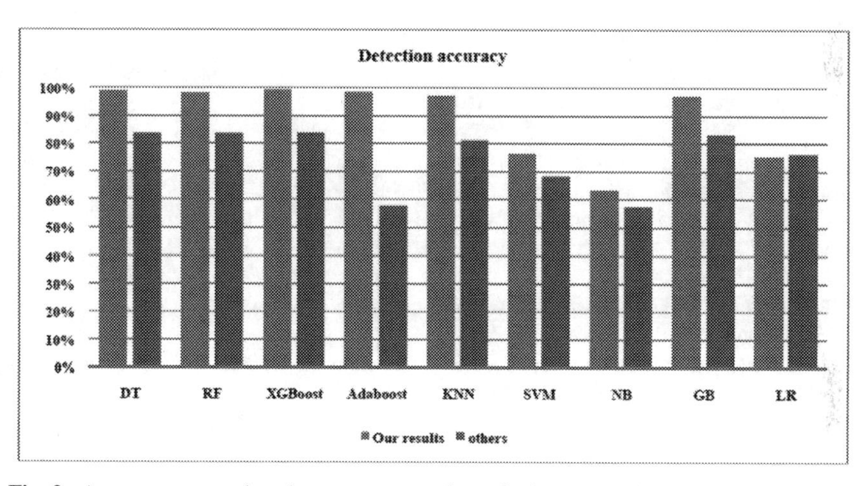

Fig. 3. Accuracy comparison between our results and others [10] using multi-classification.

6 Conclusion

In our study, we improved several algorithms, specifically DT, LR, RF, NB, KNN, SVM, AdaBoost, XGBoost, and GB. We employed the IoTID20 dataset to detect attacks on IoT networks using these nine enhanced ML techniques. Our enhancements were based on various data preprocessing operations, including data cleaning, undersampling, removing constant and correlated values, and feature selection using Recursive Feature Elimination (RFE). These operations were conducted to ensure the dataset's consistency, as an inconsistent dataset can potentially lead to issues in the accuracy of IoT attack detection.

The results demonstrate that the XGBoost classifier outperforms all other models in both binary and multi-class classifications. It achieves an accuracy of 99.74 in binary classification and an accuracy of 99.21 in multi-class classification. On the other hand, the

NB model shows lower efficiency in both binary and multi-class classification tasks. A comparison reveals that our proposed model attains the highest accuracy when compared to the work mentioned in [10]. Notably, our results using AdaBoost, XGBoost, RF, and DT outperform other approaches, underscoring their effectiveness and the capability of our proposed model for accurate classification.

References

1. Ullah, I., Mahmoud, Q.H.: A Scheme for generating a dataset for anomalous activity detection in IoT networks. In: Goutte, C., Zhu, X. (eds.) Canadian AI 2020. LNCS (LNAI), vol. 12109, pp. 508–520. Springer, Cham (2020). https://doi.org/10.1007/978-3-030-47358-7_52
2. Tomer, V., Sharma, S.: Detecting IoT attacks using an ensemble machine learning model. Future Internet **14**(4), (2022)
3. Pokhrel, S., Abbas, R., Aryal, B.: IoT security: botnet detection in IoT using machine learning. arXiv preprint arXiv:2104.02231 (2021)
4. Hussain, F., et al.: A two-fold machine learning approach to prevent and detect IoT botnet attacks. IEEE Access **9**, 163412–163430 (2021)
5. Htwe, C.S., Thant, Y.M., Thwin, M.M.S.: Botnets attack detection using machine learning approach for IoT environment. J. Phys. **1646**(1), 1–7 (2020)
6. Chesney, S., Roy, K., Khorsandroo, S.: Machine learning algorithms for preventing IoT cybersecurity attacks. In: Intelligent Systems and Applications: Proceedings of the 2020 Intelligent Systems Conference (IntelliSys), vol. 3, pp. 679–686 (2021)
7. Kumar, P., Gupta, G.P., Tripathi, R.: Toward the design of an intelligent cyber-attack detection system using hybrid feature reduced approach for IoT networks. Arab. J. Sci. Eng. **46**, 3749–3778 2021)
8. IoT Intrusion Dataset. https://sites.google.com/view/iot-network-intrusion-dataset/home. Accessed 06 Nov 2023
9. Bajpai, S., Kapil, S.: A Framework for Intrusion Detection Models for IoT Networks using Deep Learning (2022)

Using Multivariate Heuristic Analysis for Detecting Attacks in Website Log Files: A Formulaic Approach

Peter Smith(✉), John Robson, and Nick Dalton

Department of Computer Science, Northumbria University, Newcastle, UK
{peter.t.smith,john.c.robson,nick.dalton}@northumbria.ac.uk

Abstract. As cyberattacks on websites evolve and become more sophisticated, there is a pressing need for detection methodologies that can adapt to this ever-changing landscape. This pilot study evaluates current methodologies in order to identify gaps in current literature and assesses their ability to be deployed in a real-world scenario. In order to do this, we propose a shift towards a multivariate framework, which measures the influence of several key factors. It was hypothesised that historic data is useful in predicting attacks. The study was given access to real website data in order to verify the efficacy of a multivariate approach on finding a variety of attacks. Results indicated a significant improvement in accuracy, specificity and sensitivity in attack detection in comparison to previous methods. This empirical evidence highlights the importance of using real-world data in cyber security and takes an essential preliminary step to be expanded by future research.

Keywords: Cyber Security · Multivariate Analysis · Network Traffic Analysis · Pattern Recognition · Heuristic Algorithms

1 Introduction

1.1 Background

The dependency on websites in daily life is trending upwards [1]. Increasingly, people use websites for activities such as; e-commerce, socialising, medical care, particularly post-Covid [2]. Thus, sensitive information is stored online at higher frequencies [3]. Consequently, becoming a more coveted target for hackers, who employ novel techniques to circumvent existing security measures. Moreover, they are trying to disrupt websites functionality, while causing reputational and monetary harm through volumetric Denial of Service attacks. High-rate attacks have for a long time been mitigated against, so they no longer pose a significant risk [4]. On the other hand, previous research may be unable to detect low-rate attacks [5]. Generally, these can look like legitimate traffic but on a slow connection, highlighting the need for an effective way to distinguish attack and non-attack traffic, without this it is unclear how widespread attacks are.

K. Daimi and A. Al Sadoon (Eds.): ACR 2024, LNNS 956, pp. 359–370, 2024.
https://doi.org/10.1007/978-3-031-56950-0_30

1.2 Review of Current Website Protection

Given that 92% of websites have vulnerabilities that could be exploited at any one time [6]; most websites use a Web Application Firewall (WAF). These use pre-defined rules to inspect traffic and block malicious requests, reducing the risk of hackers exploiting these weaknesses. The importance of a WAF was highlighted by the mitigation of the log4j vulnerability. Cloudflare, one of the biggest WAF providers, saw an average of 27,000 blocked requests per minute on December 12th, 2021 for this vulnerability [7]. However, a WAF rule can only be implemented after a vulnerabilities' attack signature has been discovered. Consequently, unascertained attacks expose a weakness; WAFs are not an effective precautionary security measure, diminishing their utility [8].

While there are indications of individuals searching for vulnerabilities, they may go unnoticed for extended periods if not actively monitored. Evidenced in the Log4J vulnerability which went undetected from 2013–2021 [9,10]. Additionally, WAFs must strike a balance between detecting potential threats and avoiding false positives, potentially resulting in a high false negative rate. For instance, a common tactic may be repeatedly attempt to access login pages using POST requests, but at a low rate that may evade the WAF as login attempts can be legitimate user behaviour. This indicates a need for assessments of threats over an increased time-frame, requiring large amounts of data to be collected which can be classified [11]. However, this volume of data may be hard to store [12]; web-servers already generate a large volume of data, negating the need for additional data collection if this data can be analysed. This data quantity is necessary due to the ability of low-rate attacks to pose as legitimate user activity, when looked at over short time periods they are difficult to detect. Furthermore, there is a lack of research into low-rate attacks and none of this uses real world data.

1.3 Proposed Approaches to Detect Low Rate Attacks

Systems have been proposed to alert when the CPU was depleted which should theoretically detect low rate attacks [13]. However, there are two issues with the methodology, other confounding variables can cause high CPU depletion such as writing to disc. Furthermore, Adi states that "auxiliary mechanisms ought to be deployed for identifying the volumes and patterns of network traffic" [13], which shows his methodology needs backup detection. Given current methodology's software only alerted to CPU depletion, leading to the conclusion that attack traffic may have different characteristics. These methodologies only inform if there is an attack, without providing sufficient information on the cause of the attack and, thus, how to mitigate them.

A technique for measuring the Chi Squared differential between sets of simulated data depicting normal and attack traffic has been proposed. High accuracy and a zero false positive rate was claimed [14]. While the use of simulated data may be useful for preliminary model verification, it can be argued that it is a sub-optimal benchmark for hypothesis testing. In the mentioned study the lack of external data also suggests little attempt to disprove the hypothesis. Real world data may have additional background noise, that may increase false positive rates, opposed to the predetermined attack intervals utilised in the study. This assumption of linearity contradicts the typical non-linear nature of website traffic, this is a contributing factor in their detection difficulty [15]. This provides a rationale for cyber security researchers to advocate for the increased use of real world data [16].

The User Agent (UA) String contains discernable information that can be used for identification [17]. Including the type of browser and device in use and can thus, be used to detect suspicious traffic. As UAs can have different combinations of the same words, using a bag-of-words approach can be useful for classifying each part of the UA independently. However, UA's can also be falsified to evade detection [18], this invalidates using them as a univariate analysis. UAs can be used as part of a multivariate analysis in a bag-of-words format in order to classify how likely it is that a request is automated. For example, if a UA contains 'python', it is likely automated, increasing the likelihood of an attack.

AI systems have been proposed to detect cyberattacks and may achieve satisfactory results [19]. There is a danger that, because of the way that AI works, it classifies data incorrectly and a human interpreter does not know why. While AI may be able to detect known attacks, in a similar way to WAF, it may lack vital context. When looking at cyberattacks, F-Secure Global suggest that 'context is everything' [20] It has been argued that a human may be a better judge of context compared to AI [21]. Despite this, the current paper doesn't discount AI being beneficial to cyber security, such that it may be used in a learning capacity, however the internal workings of cyber security software should be clear and easy to follow.

1.4 Aims and Hypothesis

The main hypothesis is automatically collected data, specifically log files, provides adequate information to detect attacks and that a multivariate approach to website attacks can improve the accuracy of detection.

It has been highlighted that low-rate DDoS attacks and their defence mechanisms are not well addressed in existing literature [22], showing the need for a novel detection system that can be used in a real-world environment. This paper proposes a multivariate approach to low-rate DDoS attack detection, that could be used to enhance protection.

The main aims of this pilot study are:

1. To use authentic website data for training and verifying security models, as advocated by Rajbahadur et al.
2. To assess if combining UA with other methods is better than UA alone
3. To use large amounts of historical data to aid in the detection of attacks.

2 Methods

The present methodology aimed to facilitate the identification of risk within log files. This was done by submitting log file data for analysis through the proposed detection system, as outlined in subsections A, B and C, using a multivariate, comprehensive model with variables weighed according to their respective designated confidence of reliability. For example, the country that an IP belongs to was given a relatively high weighting in comparison to the other variables, as this can strongly predict risk. The present paper describes risk as the likelihood that an IP is attacking a website. This was translated onto a scale from 0–100, where 0 denotes an absence of risk and 100 implies a high likelihood of an attack. The model was refined such that, it is uncommon to get a score, of 0 or near to 100 and values are carefully calibrated to achieve this. The IP addresses and log files were anonymised using a one way hash function. The log files were submitted for analysis in a raw form with the IP, however the output used the same hash so that they could be matched with the raw log file (Fig. 1).

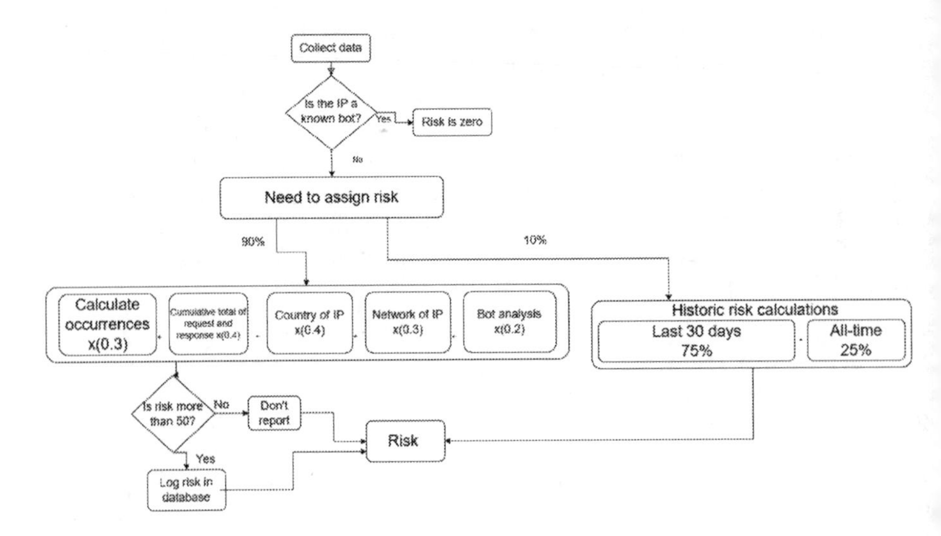

Fig. 1. Risk flow

2.1 Analysis of Traffic Features

A key variable in the proposed detection system is the number of occurrences of an IP in the submitted data. The occurrences can be any real number, therefore it was important to establish a reliable method for determining the risk of occurrences. This was achieved by using a sigmoid function as can be seen in Eq. 1, in order to transform a high variance of numbers into a range.

$$\frac{10}{5 + (e^{-0.1 * occurences})} \tag{1}$$

In order to differentiate between trustworthy and suspicious UAs, a bag of words was generated based on the data. Researchers assigned the words to one of two conditions; Good or bad. For example, Yandex was classified as bad, due to the fact that it is a browser primarily used in Russia, a country which a large number of cyber attacks come from. The bag of words was a list of words that should be in the UAs string of text, these were cut into individual words and then analysed, as can be seen in Fig. 2. The analysis was completed in three stages; first, the UAs string was split into words, a word is defined in this context as anything with a space either side. Second, the number of words were multiplied by a constant (x). Lastly, for every bad UA, x was added to this total; then, for every good word found, x was subtracted.

Initial State
Mozilla/5.0 (Macintosh; Intel Mac OS X 12_5) AppleWebKit/537.36 (KHTML, like Gecko) Chrome/103.0.0.0 YaBrowser/22.7.0 Yowser/2.5 Safari/537.36

Good	Bad
Mozilla/5.0	YaBrowser/22.7.0
(Macintosh;	Yowser/2.5
Intel	
Mac	
OS	
X	
12_5)	
AppleWebKit/537.36	
(KHTML,	
like	
Gecko)	
Chrome/103.0.0.0	
Safari/537.36	

Fig. 2. UA classification

2.2 User Behaviour

Another variable is the resources that an attacker is attempting to access. In order to measure this, a blacklist of known URL patterns were used to identify potential malicious requests similar to the way a WAF works. This list was generated using known attack vectors that are commonly exploited, such as attempting to access config files. Unlike a WAF, this blacklist can be highly sensitive as it was used to determine risk, flagging the suspicious requests that, after being considered in the context of other factors, may not be harmful. It should be noted that some URL patterns are given a higher risk as their presence in normal traffic should be minimal; the greater the risk the more confidence there is in them being an attack and the likely severity of it.

In order to determine the legitimacy of a request, the HTTP response codes were analysed; allowing the formula to assign a risk level to the request. As the codes are standard, confidence in a meaning is high. For example, if the request is processed without issue, the server returns a 200 code; whereas a 401 error indicates a user is not authorised to view the requested item.

These URL patterns were based upon known, currently exploited attacks. For example, one attack that is commonly exploited is the Wordpress login attack. So one of the URL patterns was WP-login.

2.3 Context

The formula's accuracy increases with context. The country that the IP belongs to is given a value to quantify risk. Due to a lack of publicly available data on attacks by country, the risks were derived from experience of looking at prior attacks. A similar methodology was applied to network risk as another variable. For example, many attacks come from public cloud servers which are low cost and easy to set up, so these networks are given a higher risk value compared to home broadband providers. These variables add crucial context to the IP and requests, which makes it easier to reliably judge behaviour, thus, making the formula more accurate.

If an IP scores a significant risk, it's recorded in the database. So that it can be taken into account if an occurrence of this IP is seen again. Additionally, having a record of high-risk IPs can aid in identifying patterns or trends in cyber attacks, which can inform more effective security measures.

2.4 Formulating Risk

The extracted features from the log files provide insight into the IP behaviour on a website, therefore, this makes up the majority of the resulting risk analysis. Comparatively, a lower proportion of the risk comes from the historic risk calculation. Of this, a higher weighting is given to the last 30 days, and a lower weighting is given to the all time activity, as IPs can change locations and users, making it a less valid determinant of risk. However, the all time activity still provides useful context.

2.5 Procedure for Analysis

In order to analyse the accuracy of the proposed formula, two scenarios were performed. One looking at just the UA, resembling the research conducted by TANAKA et al. (2020) and the second looking at the multivariate analysis, as proposed by the present paper as being more effective in detecting attacks. After running each scenario, genuine bots were excluded from the sample. This was done by comparing the IP addresses in the logfiles to a list in the database to remove these from the sample. Additionally, we could guarantee that these were legitimate traffic however the detector a have misidentified them. The data was then compared with the raw log data and an expert classified the results for each procedure into four categories: True Positive (TP), True Negative (TN), False Positive (FP) or False Negative (FN). The expert looked at similar variables to the multivariate approach assessing an IP's occurrences, pages accessed and UAs, to determine risk. If there were any that the expert was unsure about, AbuseIPDB was used to see if that website had flagged the IP as malicious.

Using machine learning techniques, the data was measured by four performance metrics. These included Accuracy. This is the key metric as it measures how many times an attack is correctly identified, and was defined as:

$$\frac{TP + TN}{TP + TN + FP + FN} \tag{2}$$

Sensitivity (Se) is designed to measure what proportion of actual positives were identified correctly and was measured using the formula:

$$\frac{TP}{TP + FN} \tag{3}$$

Another key metric measured was Specificity (Sp), which checked how many of the items labelled as 'positive' were actually considered a threat by the expert. as calculated by:

$$\frac{TP}{TP + FP} \tag{4}$$

The F1 score was measured to asses how many classifications were correct. This score indicates the harmonics between Specificity and Sensitivity and is calculated using:

$$2 \times \frac{Sp \times Se}{Sp + Se} \tag{5}$$

The results of each of these variables will be discussed in the results section.

3 Results

This pilot study had three key aims; to use authentic website data for training and verifying security models, to analyse multiple data points within the data set and to use large amounts of historical data to aid in the detection of attacks. To assess the first aim, random samples from multiple websites were collected in Apache extended format, which is automatically collected by servers. The study sought permission from the owners of live websites to analyse its data. One website was that of a researcher from a different institution, who's website was in information wiki and this website was known to be under attack, therefore provided a higher density of attacks in comparison to other data sets used. The second websites used provided a normal distribution of attack traffic, more representative of regular website traffic. We used 148 data points in total, which was comprised of a 50/50 split between both data sets. After analysis, the software was able to identify a high number of attacks. The second research aim was accomplished by conducting an analysis of various data points within the data set, consisting of country, network, occurrences, requests, responses and the UA. By amalgamating the analysis of these data points, our employed formula yielded greater accuracy in comparison to the univariate approach. Comparatively, an anomalous data set would only be assigned a high risk if it was apparent amongst all more than one variable. Thirdly, by utilising log files, this study was able to collect a large amount of data from a website without the need for sophisticated materials to fulfil the use of large amounts of historical data. The use of this data allowed for reliable analysis overall.

Table 1 shows how each methodology performed in comparison to the expert assessment. The multivariate approach had significantly increased the true predictions, particularly when it comes to TPs. However, the number of FNs is still significantly high, despite being lower than the univariate.

Table 1. A table showing the difference in classification for each methodology

	TP	TN	FP	FN
Univariate	36	16	12	84
Multivariate	45	18	9	76

Table 2. A table showing percentage differences in Univariate and multivariate approaches across different attack surfaces, as measured by real website data

	Accuracy	Sensitivity	Specifcity	F1 score
Univariate	35.14%	30.00 %	57.14%	42.86%
Multivariate	42.57%	37.19%	66.67%	51.43%
Change	+7.43%	+7.19%	+9.52%	+8.57%

Data analysis revealed that the multivariate approach proved to be more precise than a univariate approach, with a 7.43% increase in accuracy, as depicted in Table 2. While sensitivity is low the multivariate performance is in line with the univariate approach, however does still show an improvement. Additionally, the multivariate methodology yielded a greater degree of specificity. These findings suggest a higher detection rate and legitimate traffic to a website is not adversely impacted by the multivariate approach. Furthermore the higher F1 score shows that, the multivariate analysis has a greater harmony between sensitivity and specificity.

The present study hypothesised that automatically collected data, specifically log files, provide adequate information to detect attacks. Also, a multivariate approach to the detection of website attacks may improve the accuracy without affecting false classification. The findings suggest that this hypothesis can be accepted under the present conditions, such that the multivariate approach significantly improved the accuracy of detection in the sample.

4 Discussion

The results of this pilot study indicate that there is sufficient data in website log files to detect a variety of attacks that may be missed by previous methodologies. In order to give a comparison point Tanaka's methodology, looking at UAs only in a univariate context [23]. This univariate approach is aligned with other contemporary research [13,14], that may have a blind spot to some attack traffic. After applying the work done by Tanaka to the data set used in this study, the achieved accuracy was 35.14% which is lower than the 90.2% reported by Tanaka, demonstrating a potential weakness with Tanaka's methodology.

The present methodology provides several strengths that greatly expand on the current literature. The main strength is the use of real-world data, which allows researchers to validate the present study and demonstrate its applicability to real websites. Previous studies in this field used artificial data to identify malicious traffic and thus did not obtain representative samples [13,14]. By using real-world data, this study was able to fine-tune the proposed model to consider a wider range of factors that successfully determine risk, such as the country and network posing a more significant threat, as well as how much of a risk they represent, as demonstrated by a numerical scaling framework of 0–100. This process enabled researchers to build a more reliable model that effectively responds to real-world data. The current model used data that had already been collected by websites, resulting in easy and accurate data from web servers. This made it easy to implement on a larger scale and clarified the scope of the research as replicable.

The data from the present study came from a variety of websites. Random sampling of data ensured an equal balance between attack and non-attack traffic, allowing for increased differential opportunities between the two in order to effectively test the performance of the methodology in both conditions.

The higher accuracy observed within the results section shows that increasing the number of variables assessed, results in better determination of risk. However, due to the complex nature of the data and subsequent calculations, it necessitates a greater allocation of computational resources over a sustained period of time. This calls for a balance between accuracy and resource management in future methodologies. The resources required could be lessened making the process faster but, this comes at the detriment of accuracy. This highlights the need for a human moderator, who would be required to do more detailed analysis. Which is why a human should be kept "in the loop" [21].

4.1 Limitations

Classification of the data was conducted in order to ascertain an expert's assignment of risk to assess the effectiveness of both approaches. This classification was conducted by only one researcher. Consequently, the methodology may yield low inter-rater reliability and have a moderate margin of error when assigning levels of risk. Low levels of reliability can negatively affect the findings, such that it may elicit a Type 1 error, which may result in an increase in FP ratings. This effect could also be attributed to researcher bias. Therefore, in elaborative studies, it's incumbent that researchers employ more concrete classification techniques to ensure high reliability.

Selection of the appropriate data set was conducted with great care, this contained a random sample from multiple websites. However, this sample was relatively small and may not necessarily represent traffic on a global scale. This was primarily due to the manual classification technique undertaken by the researcher so, given time constraints, a smaller data set needed to be analysed. Future studies that expand on this premise may utilise more researchers to categorise greater data sets with a more representative sample.

5 Conclusion

This paper aimed to assess the use of a multivariate approach in the detection of website attacks, while assessing the merits in using real world data when verifying security models. Utilising a multivariate approach results in more accurate classification of website traffic and the risks associated with an IP address, this is due to the added context that additional variables provide. The use of simulated data in cyber security should be questioned, as this work has shown that when methods are applied in a real world environment, the accuracy may fluctuate.

This work has shown a way to collect large amounts of data about website traffic, without the need for additional software that can be used to detect attacks using a multivariate framework. The high accuracy of the multivariate methodology also demonstrates its ability to detect different attacks. Therefore, providing an all-encompassing solution to website protection that opens up new avenues for future evaluation, focusing on the exploration of log file data to detect potential attacks. Furthermore, it implores the use of real world data by demonstrating responsible, ethical handling of IP addresses and log files that includes standardised protocols to anonymise IP addresses.

5.1 Future Work

Future work should be carried out to refine the calibration of the multivariate analysis. This research may include the employment of AI for the classification of data, as well as improvements in the speed of model training. Future work should also look at methodologies that use a multivariate approach in real time to detect low rate attacks. This work can also be further developed by comparing the multivariate analysis to traditional WAF rules to see if this system is more effective than a WAF, using a range of dimensional feedback measures, such as the likes of efficiency and ease of use by users.

In order to advance the field of cyber security, it is imperative that all future work be conducted using authentic, real-world data. This would enable researchers to develop methodologies that can be readily implemented in practical settings. Additionally, we implore researchers to prioritise a thorough understanding of the ecosystems and technologies that encapsulate websites and website owners. We advocate for researchers to involve website owners in the development of methodologies to protect websites. Only when this has been achieved, can we be confident that researchers understand the challenges of cyber security.

References

1. Diomidous, M., et al.: Social and psychological effects of the internet use. Acta Informatica Medica **24**(1), 66 (2016)
2. Arzhanova, K.A., Beregovskaya, T.A., Silina, S.A.: The impact of the Covid-19 pandemic on consumer behavior and companies' internet communication strategies. In: Research Technologies of Pandemic Coronavirus Impact (RTCOV 2020), pp. 50–57. Atlantis Press (2020)
3. Young, S.D., Schneider, J.: Clinical care, research, and telehealth services in the era of social distancing to mitigate COVID-19. AIDS Behav. **24**, 2000–2002 (2020)
4. Bawany, N.Z., Shamsi, J.A., Salah, K.: DDoS attack detection and mitigation using SDN: methods, practices, and solutions. Arab. J. Sci. Eng. **42**, 425–441 (2017)
5. Zhou, L., Liao, M., Yuan, C., Zhang, H.: Low-rate DDos attack detection using expectation of packet size. Secur. Commun. Netw. **2017** (2017)
6. Razzaq, A., Hur, A., Shahbaz, S., Masood, M., Ahmad, H.F.: Critical analysis on web application firewall solutions. In: 2013 IEEE Eleventh International Symposium on Autonomous Decentralized Systems (ISADS), pp. 1–6 (2013). https://doi.org/10.1109/ISADS.2013.6513431
7. Graham-Cumming, J., Martinho, C.: Exploitation of Log4j CVE-2021-44228 before public disclosure and evolution of evasion and exfiltration (2021). https://blog.cloudflare.com/exploitation-of-cve-2021-44228-before-public-disclosure-and-evolution-of-waf-evasion-patterns//. Accessed 06 Nov 2022
8. Kozik, R., Choraś, M., Renk, R., Hołubowicz, W.: A proposal of algorithm for web applications cyber attack detection. In: Saeed, K., Snášel, V. (eds.) CISIM 2015. LNCS, vol. 8838, pp. 680–687. Springer, Heidelberg (2014). https://doi.org/10.1007/978-3-662-45237-0_61
9. Ko, W.: Jndi lookup plugin support (2013). https://issues.apache.org/jira/browse/LOG4J2-313
10. Gabor, G.: CVE-2021-44228 - log4j RCE 0-day mitigation (2022). https://blog.cloudflare.com/cve-2021-44228-log4j-rce-0-day-mitigation/
11. Zhijun, W., Wenjing, L., Liang, L., Meng, Y.: Low-rate dos attacks, detection, defense, and challenges: a survey. IEEE Access **8**, 43920–43943 (2020). https://doi.org/10.1109/ACCESS.2020.2976609
12. Staniford, S., Hoagland, J.A., McAlerney, J.M.: Practical automated detection of stealthy portscans. J. Comput. Secur. **10**(1–2), 105–136 (2002)
13. Adi, E., Baig, Z.A., Hingston, P., Lam, C.P.: Distributed denial-of-service attacks against http/2 services. Cluster Comput. **19**, 79–86 (2016)
14. Tripathi, N., Hubballi, N.: Slow rate denial of service attacks against http/2 and detection. Comput. Secur. **72**, 255–272 (2018)
15. Fang, X., Maochao, X., Shouhuai, X., Zhao, P.: A deep learning framework for predicting cyber attacks rates. EURASIP J. Inf. Secur. **1–11**, 2019 (2019)
16. Rajbahadur, G.K., Malton, A.J., Walenstein, A., Hassan, A.E.: A survey of anomaly detection for connected vehicle cybersecurity and safety. In: 2018 IEEE Intelligent Vehicles Symposium (IV), pp. 421–426 (2018). https://doi.org/10.1109/IVS.2018.8500383
17. Zhang, Y., et al.: Detecting malicious activities with user-agent-based profiles. Int. J. Netw. Manage **25**(5), 306–319 (2015)
18. Grill, M., Rehak, M.: Malware detection using http user-agent discrepancy identification. In: 2014 IEEE International Workshop on Information Forensics and Security (WIFS), pp. 221–226 (2014). https://doi.org/10.1109/WIFS.2014.7084331

19. Taddeo, M., McCutcheon, T., Floridi, L.: Trusting artificial intelligence in cybersecurity is a double-edged sword. Nat. Mach. Intell. **1**(12), 557–560 (2019)
20. F-Secure Global. How to detect targeted cyber attacks: The importance of context (2018). https://blog.f-secure.com/detect-targeted-cyber-attacks-importance-context/. Accessed 02 Mar 2023
21. Cranor, L.F.: A framework for reasoning about the human in the loop (2008)
22. Agrawal, N., Tapaswi, S.: Defense mechanisms against DDoS attacks in a cloud computing environment: state-of-the-art and research challenges. IEEE Commun. Surv. Tutorials **21**(4), 3769–3795 (2019)
23. Tanaka, T., Niibori, H., Shiyingxue, L.I., Nomura, S., Kawashima, H., Tsuda, K.: Bot detection model using user agent and user behavior for web log analysis. Proc. Comput. Sci. **176**, 1621–1625 (2020). ISSN 1877-0509. https://doi.org/10.1016/j.procs.2020.09.185. URL https://www.sciencedirect.com/science/article/pii/S1877050920320871. Knowledge-Based and Intelligent Information & Engineering Systems: Proceedings of the 24th International Conference KES2020

Computational Intelligence

Integrating Lean Healthcare and Machine Learning for Cancer Risk Prediction

Mohammad Shahin, Mazdak Maghanaki, F. Frank Chen, and Ali Hosseinzadeh(✉)

The University of Texas at San Antonio, San Antonio, TX 78249, USA
{Mohammad.Shahin,Mazdak.mohammadimaghanaki,ff.chen,
ali.hosseinzadehghobadlou}@utsa.edu

Abstract. The rising global threat of cancer has gained significant attention within the scientific community. The integration of Lean Healthcare principles with cutting-edge Machine Learning (ML) techniques has emerged as a promising approach to transform healthcare systems and enhance patient care. One of the most critical areas where this integration is making significant strides is in predicting the risk of developing cancer. This article explores the synergy between Lean Healthcare and ML in the context of cancer risk prediction, highlighting its potential to revolutionize early detection and personalized preventive care. Utilizing five distinct Machine Learning models, the analysis leveraged the Cancer Patients dataset, a publicly accessible resource containing 1000 patient profiles with diverse information related to the risk of cancer development in the human body. The study assessed various ML algorithms in cancer detection and also underscored the potential of Industry 4.0 technologies in improving patient outcomes. Assessment using performance metrics like accuracy, sensitivity, and F-score demonstrated AI's potential in improving detection accuracy. The results have shown that Multilayer Perceptron (MLP), Random Forest (RF) with Principal Component Analysis (PCA), and Logistic Regression (LR) with PCA exhibit significant efficacy in cancer detection. Consequently, the integration of supervised machine learning methods is poised to offer substantial assistance in the early diagnosis and prognosis of cancer.

Keywords: Lean Healthcare · Artificial Intelligence · Machine Learning · Industry 4.0 · early diagnosis

1 Introduction

Cancer is a complex disease involving uncontrolled cell growth that varies by gender and age. Early cancer detection is vital for better treatment outcomes. It allows for less invasive interventions and improves the chances of successful recovery [1]. Machine learning models show great promise in improving cancer detection by quickly identifying patterns in medical imaging and genetic data, leading to better treatment outcomes and increased survival rates. They also help healthcare professionals make informed decisions and create personalized treatment plans, enhancing patient care [2, 3]. Figure 1 outlines the block diagram of a basic cancer detection model.

K. Daimi and A. Al Sadoon (Eds.): ACR 2024, LNNS 956, pp. 373–381, 2024.
https://doi.org/10.1007/978-3-031-56950-0_31

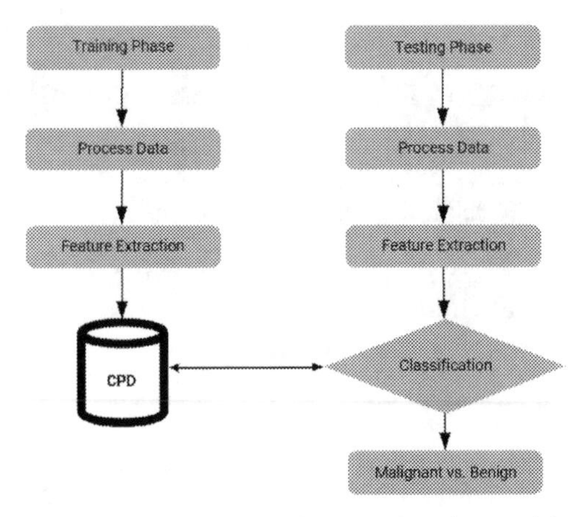

Fig. 1. Block diagram of cancer detection model

1.1 Integration of Lean Healthcare with AI

While the potential of ML models in cancer detection is promising, their successful integration into clinical practice demands meticulous validation, precise result interpretation, and continual enhancements. It becomes imperative to establish a robust system that encourages perpetual progress in cancer detection through ML models. This system should enable seamless data validation, seamless integration of feedback, and iterative optimization of models, thereby creating a dynamic feedback loop involving clinicians, data scientists, and industry experts. Lean Healthcare is a methodology derived from Lean Manufacturing principles, initially developed by Toyota. It focuses on eliminating waste, optimizing processes, and improving efficiency in healthcare delivery. Key components of Lean Healthcare include continuous improvement (Kaizen), reducing non-value-added activities, enhancing patient-centric care, and streamlining workflows [4]. In the context of Industry 4.0 and lean principles, the integration of ML models for cancer detection can be further enhanced through continuous improvement initiatives. Leveraging Industry 4.0 technologies such as IoT (Internet of Things) and advanced data analytics can facilitate the collection of real-time patient data, enabling more comprehensive and dynamic training of ML algorithms. Concurrently, adopting lean methodologies can streamline the validation and interpretation processes, optimizing the integration of ML models into clinical workflows. This collaborative approach fosters a dynamic environment for ongoing refinement, ensuring that ML models for cancer detection are constantly updated and improved to achieve higher efficacy and reliability in clinical practice [5]. Figure 2 illustrates AI's role in the medical industry, while Fig. 3 depicts the utilization of AI, ML, and DL in Digital Healthcare.

This study highlights how integrating Lean Healthcare with advanced Machine Learning techniques can significantly improve cancer risk prediction and early detection. Using five Machine Learning models, including MLP, RF with PCA, and LR with PCA, the study underscores their efficacy in detecting cancer. This integration has the potential to revolutionize healthcare, offering more personalized care and improved patient outcomes.

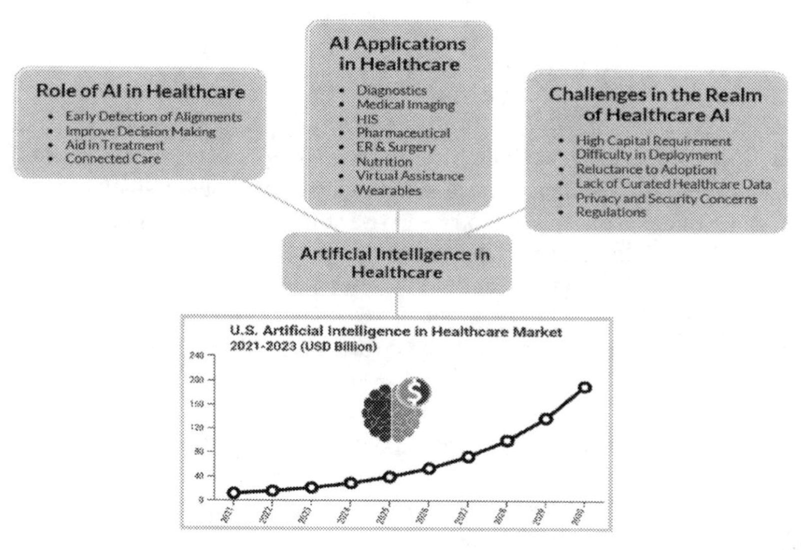

Fig. 2. AI's role in the medical industry

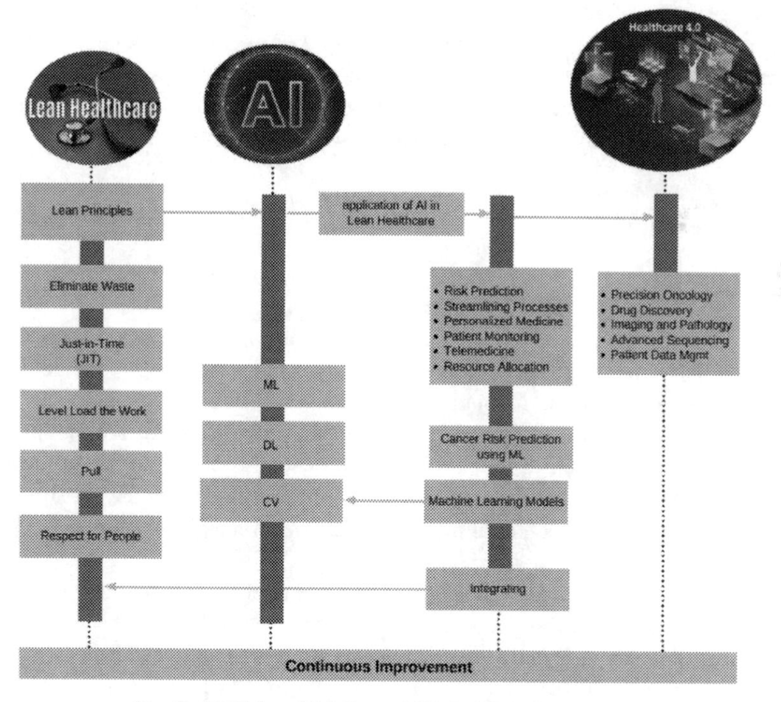

Fig. 3. Utilizing AI, ML, and DL in Digital Healthcare

1.2 Predicting Cancer Risk

Predicting the risk of developing cancer is a complex and multifaceted challenge. It involves analyzing various factors, including genetic predisposition, lifestyle choices, environmental exposures, and health history. ML algorithms excel at processing and interpreting these diverse data sources, making them invaluable tools for cancer risk assessment. Lean Healthcare principles encourage the consolidation of data silos and the efficient flow of information [4]. ML algorithms can ingest data from electronic health records, genetic profiles, and patient surveys, offering a holistic view of an individual's health history.

This integrated data enhances the accuracy of cancer risk predictions. Lean's Kaizen philosophy aligns with ML's iterative model refinement. ML models can continuously learn and adapt to new data, ensuring that predictions remain up-to-date and accurate. Regular model updates based on real-world outcomes contribute to ongoing improvements in cancer risk assessment [6]. ML algorithms excel at tailoring predictions to individual patients. By considering a person's unique genetic makeup, lifestyle choices, and environmental exposures, ML models can provide personalized risk assessments. This enables healthcare providers to offer targeted interventions and preventive measures. The integration of Lean Healthcare and ML supports early cancer detection [2].

ML algorithms can identify subtle biomarkers and early signs of cancer, allowing for timely intervention and improved patient outcomes. Lean principles emphasize efficient resource allocation. ML-based risk prediction can help healthcare organizations allocate resources, such as screening tests and preventive programs, to those individuals at the highest risk of developing cancer, optimizing resource utilization [7].

2 Methodology

2.1 Dataset

The Cancer Patients Dataset [8], a key element of this paper, underwent advanced ML algorithm processing. To ensure model robustness and generalizability, the dataset was split into 75% for model training and 25% for testing, following best practices in data science and machine learning. This study evaluates various ML algorithms in cancer detection and also underscores the potential of Industry 4.0 technologies in improving patient outcomes. Assessment using performance metrics like accuracy, sensitivity, and F-score demonstrates AI's potential in enhancing detection accuracy. Table 1 describes each of the variables found in this dataset.

A confusion matrix evaluates machine-learning models by summarizing correct and incorrect predictions on a test dataset. Performance, especially for ML and computer-based vision, relies heavily on this matrix's elements: True Positive (TP), False Positive (FP), False Negative (FN), and True Negative (TN). From the confusion matrix, metrics like accuracy, precision, recall, and F1 score can be derived, offering insights into model strengths and weaknesses. In medical testing, various metrics assess model performance. Accuracy measures overall correctness, precision evaluates the accuracy of positive predictions, sensitivity assesses the ability to identify positive cases, and the F1 Score strikes a balance between precision and recall. Specificity gauges the ability to identify

Table 1. Overview of Variables in the Cancer Patients Dataset

Age	Dust allergy	Balanced diet	Chest pain	Obesity	Frequent cold
Air pollution	Occupational hazards	Shortness of breath	Coughing of blood	Wheezing	Dry cough
Gender	Genetic risk	Smoking	Fatigue	Weight loss	Snoring
Alcohol use	Chronic lung disease	Passive smoking	Clubbing of fingernails	Swallowing difficulty	Tendency to develop cancer

negative cases, while the G-mean1 Score evaluates performance in imbalanced datasets. These metrics ensure a comprehensive evaluation of a model's performance in medical testing, considering the risks of both false positives and false negatives.

Accuracy is a key metric in machine learning (ML) used to assess a model's performance. It measures the number of correct predictions divided by the total predictions, which is crucial in medical applications like disease diagnosis, prognosis, and treatment planning. However, relying solely on accuracy may not suffice, especially in medical scenarios where false positives and false negatives can have severe consequences.

Precision evaluates a model's ability to correctly identify positive cases. It's calculated as the number of true positive cases divided by the total predicted positive cases. In medical applications, precision is vital to minimize false positives, which can lead to unnecessary treatments and procedures.

Sensitivity gauges a model's ability to correctly identify actual positive cases. It's computed as the number of true positive cases divided by the total actual positive cases. A high sensitivity value is crucial, especially in disease diagnosis or screening tests, to ensure early detection and treatment.

The F1 score is a metric that balances precision and sensitivity, providing a comprehensive measure of a binary classification model's performance. It is especially valuable in medical testing, ensuring accurate diagnoses while minimizing false positives and negatives.

Specificity is essential in assessing a model's performance in correctly identifying negative cases. It measures the proportion of true negative cases among all actual negative cases, crucial in tests where false positives can have serious consequences.

The G-mean, or geometric mean, is instrumental in evaluating a model's performance in imbalanced classes, particularly in medical applications where the cost of misclassification can be high. It provides a balanced measure of the model's performance across positive and negative classes.

2.2 Machine Learning Algorithms Used on Cancer Prediction Dataset

Principal Component Analysis (PCA) is a method in machine learning that reduces dataset dimensionality while retaining crucial information by identifying high-variance directions. It transforms data into a lower-dimensional space, creating new features that capture the data's variability. Logistic Regression (LR) is a binary classification algorithm that predicts outcomes by transforming input features into probabilities using a logistic function. It is simple and interpretable, suitable for linear relationships, but may not handle complex, nonlinear data well. Random Forest (RF) is an ensemble learning algorithm that combines multiple Decision Trees (DT) to predict outcomes. It reduces overfitting risk and efficiently handles high-dimensional data. Extreme Gradient Boosting (XGBoost) is a powerful gradient boosting algorithm that uses parallel tree construction, regularization, and a customized loss function to prevent overfitting. It is fast, scalable, and widely used for various tasks in real-world applications. Multilayer Perceptron (MLP) is a neural network in machine learning that processes input through interconnected nodes, adjusting weights to minimize a loss function. It excels in complex tasks where traditional methods are insufficient. Figure 4 depicts MLP training loss without PCA.

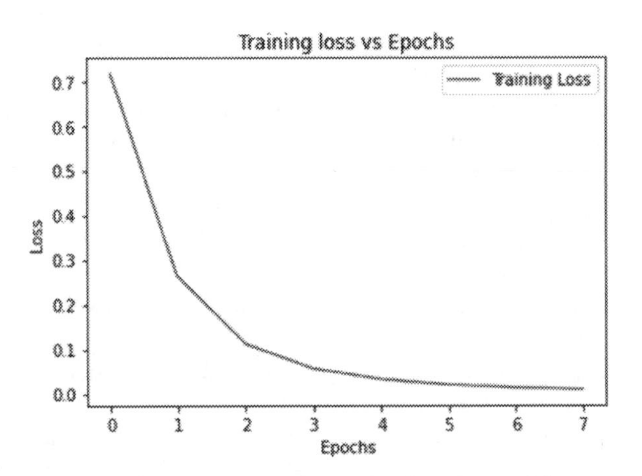

Fig. 4. The loss per epoch value for MLP model

Convolutional Neural Network (CNN) is a versatile neural network known for image processing, but it's also valuable for structured numerical data. In numerical analysis, CNNs handle one-dimensional arrays representing sequences. They use convolutional layers to extract local patterns [9], followed by activation functions like ReLU. Pooling layers down sample, and fully connected layers make predictions [10]. Training optimizes weights via backpropagation. CNNs excel in tasks like time series prediction, anomaly detection, and signal processing across industries. Figure 5 shows CNN training loss without PCA.

Certain ML models demands numeric features. To tackle categorical data, we employ one hot encoding. Here, each category becomes a binary vector with a length matching category count. A 1 goes where the category matches, and 0 fills other slots. ML, especially DL, often uses this before processing. It's vital because many algorithms can't handle categories directly, needing numeric data. One hot encoding transforms categorical data into numeric form while preserving category details.

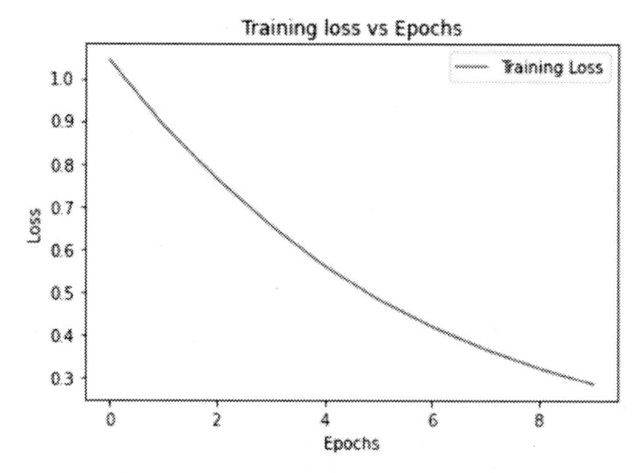

Fig. 5. The proposed architecture of the CNN model

3 Results and Discussion

In this study, five distinct Machine Learning models analyze the Cancer Patients Dataset, a publicly accessible resource containing 1000 patient profiles with diverse information related to the risk of cancer development in the human body [8]. To enhance the model's strength and optimize its performance across different situations, the dataset was divided, with 75% designated for model training and the remaining 25% reserved for testing purposes. This division aligns with the recognized standards and conventions in the domains of data science and machine learning. Performance metrics for the five mentioned algorithms are shown in Table 2.

Table 2. TP, FP, TN, and FN results for all algorithms

Custom Built Ml Model	Class Risk Level	TP	TN	FP	FN
RF with PCA	Low	73	177	0	0
	Medium	84	166	0	0
	High	93	157	0	0
XGBoost with PCA	Low	83	167	0	0
	Medium	83	167	0	0
	High	84	166	0	0
CNN	Low	74	164	2	10
	Medium	69	169	12	0
	High	93	153	0	4

(continued)

Table 2. (*continued*)

Custom Built Ml Model	Class Risk Level	TP	TN	FP	FN
LR with PCA	Low	71	175	3	1
	Medium	82	164	1	3
	High	93	157	0	0
MLP	Low	84	166	0	0
	Medium	71	179	0	0
	High	95	155	0	0

Table 3 shows a summary of the average values of performance measurements for all models. The accuracies of MLP, RF with PCA, and LR with PCA were found to be 100%, while the CNN algorithm exhibited an accuracy of 96.27%. This indicates that the CNN model demonstrates relatively lower performance when applied to tabular datasets, particularly when the dataset is relatively small.

Table 3. Average values of performance measurements for all models

Prediction Models	Accuracy	Precision	Sensitivity	F1 score	Specificity	G-meanl
RF with PCA	100.00%	100.00%	100.00%	100.00%	100.00%	100.00%
XGBoost with PCA	100.00%	100.00%	100.00%	100.00%	100.00%	100.00%
CNN	96.27%	94.18%	94.66%	94.13%	97.39%	95.95%
LR with PCA	98.93%	98.25%	98.36%	98.29%	99.24%	98.79%
MLP	100.00%	100.00%	100.00%	100.00%	100.00%	100.00%

4 Conclusions

The fusion of Lean Healthcare principles with advanced Machine Learning techniques holds great promise for reshaping cancer risk prediction and prevention. This synergy can optimize healthcare processes, integrate data seamlessly, and provide personalized risk assessments, potentially redefining early cancer detection and patient-centered care. As technology advances and healthcare organizations adopt these strategies, cancer risk prediction could become more precise, accessible, and globally impactful. This article explores how this partnership can revolutionize early detection and personalized prevention, emphasizing its potential to enhance patient care. The proposed model in this paper presents a comparative study of the largely popular machine learning algorithms and techniques commonly used for cancer prediction, namely MLP, RF with PCA, LR with PCA, XGBoost and CNN. The Cancer Patients Dataset served as the training set for evaluating the performance of different machine learning techniques, focusing on key parameters like accuracy and precision. Notably, each algorithm exhibited an accuracy exceeding 96% in distinguishing between benign and malignant tumors. Analysis from Table 3 highlights the superior effectiveness of MLP, RF with PCA, and LR with PCA in cancer detection. Consequently, supervised machine learning methods are poised to play a crucial role in enabling early diagnosis and prognosis of cancer. Further exploration in future research could delve into the utilization of advanced models such as MosaicML and Google's ViT-22B.

References

1. Hanahan, D.: Hallmarks of cancer: new dimensions. Cancer Discov. **12**(1), 31–46 (2022)
2. Shahin, M., Chen, F.F., Hosseinzadeh, A., Koodiani, H.K., Shahin, A., Nafi, O.A.: A smartphone-based application for an early skin disease prognosis: towards a lean healthcare system via computer-based vision. Adv. Eng. Inform. **57**, 102036 (2023). https://doi.org/10.1016/j.aei.2023.102036
3. Shahin, M., Chen, F.F., Hosseinzadeh, A., Bouzary, H., Rashidifar, R.: A deep hybrid learning model for detection of cyber attacks in industrial IoT devices. Int. J. Adv. Manuf. Technol. **123**(5), 1973–1983 (2022). https://doi.org/10.1007/s00170-022-10329-6
4. Shahin, M., Chen, F.F., Bouzary, H., Krishnaiyer, K.: Integration of Lean practices and Industry 4.0 technologies: smart manufacturing for next-generation enterprises. Int. J. Adv. Manuf. Technol. **107**, 2927–2936 (2020)
5. Shaheen, M.Y.: Applications of Artificial Intelligence (AI) in healthcare: a review. Sci. Prepr. (2021)
6. Kilic, A.: Artificial intelligence and machine learning in cardiovascular health care. Ann. Thorac. Surg. **109**(5), 1323–1329 (2020)
7. Yang, C., Zhang, Y.: Delta machine learning to improve scoring-ranking-screening performances of protein-ligand scoring functions. J. Chem. Inf. Model. **62**(11), 2696–2712 (2022)
8. "Cancer Patients Data. https://www.kaggle.com/datasets/rishidamarla/cancer-patients-data. Accessed 12 Mar 2023
9. Shahin, M., Chen, F.F., Hosseinzadeh, A., Khodadadi Koodiani, H., Bouzary, H., Shahin, A.: Enhanced safety implementation in 5S + 1 via object detection algorithms. Int. J. Adv. Manuf. Technol. **125**(7), 3701–3721 (2023). https://doi.org/10.1007/s00170-023-10970-9
10. Shahin, M., Chen, F.F., Bouzary, H., Hosseinzadeh, A.: Deploying convolutional neural network to reduce waste in production system. In: 51st SME North American Manufacturing Research Conference (NAMRC 51), vol. 35, pp. 1187–1195, August 2023. https://doi.org/10.1016/j.mfglet.2023.08.127

Innovating Project Management: AI Applications for Success Prediction and Resource Optimization

Monther Tarawneh[3](✉), Huda AbdAlwahed[2], and Faisal AlZyoud[1]

[1] Computer Science Department, Isra University, Amman, Jordan
faisal.alzyoud@iu.edu.jo
[2] Software Engineering Department, Isra University, Amman, Jordan
ae2110@iu.edu.jo
[3] Information Technology Department, Tafilah Technical University, Tafila, Jordan
mtarawneh@ttu.edu.jo

Abstract. The revolution of Artificial Intelligence (AI) has made transformative changes in all industries. The field of software engineering has great benefit from AI by Automat all process. Applying Artificial intelligence (AI) technologies, particularly Deep Neural Network (DNN) models, to project management will transform traditional methodologies to new ways. This work investigates how AI can be used within project management to better allocate resources, estimate time, and predict costs. Data from many recourses used to improve accuracy in project planning, refine how risks are managed, and develop new methods. Data includes real projects portfolio, open-source data, and simulated data. The integration of AI in project management examines project success and client satisfaction. This work shows 99% accuracy for learning and 78% for testing of predicting project success and highlights the need to constantly update methods to effectively use the big potential changes AI can bring to project management.

Keywords: Artificial Intelligence · Deep Neural Networks · Project Management · Predictive Modeling · Data-driven Decision-making · Optimization Techniques

1 Introduction

In this advanced world, the success of an organization's depends on its ability to manage projects, guarantee quality of outcomes within planned budgets and schedules [1]. Traditional methods of project management have been in place for a long time, and advanced technology offers innovative paths to improve the efficiency of project management practices. Artificial Intelligence (AI) is one of the advanced technologies that has emerged as a powerful tool with great power to redesign the project management landscape.

Artificial Intelligence, represents an innovative model that fills many aspects of human activities. As a field in computer science, AI simulates human intelligence using

K. Daimi and A. Al Sadoon (Eds.): ACR 2024, LNNS 956, pp. 382–391, 2024.
https://doi.org/10.1007/978-3-031-56950-0_32

machines [2]. The fast development of AI is making it more effective across a many areas [3]. AI's abilities is beyond human expectations, it moves us virtual assistants, data analytics and optimization. Therefore, the combination of AI and project management is a great transformation.

AI's ability to automat data analysis, resource allocation, real-time communication, and risk mitigation can improve the practice of project management. The integration of AI technologies has the benefit of rearrangement project activities, planning, speed up processes, and improve the accuracy of decision-making [4]. These improvements has great outcomes compared to traditional approaches. By coupling AI tools and algorithms, the classical patterns of project management can define how projects are abstracted, executed, and monitored [5].

Project management, as a multifaceted discipline, entails planning, organizing and controlling resources to achieve specific objectives within pre-determined time frames. AI enhances project management practices such as data-driven efficiency and increased responsiveness. The main goal of this project is to demonstrate the integration of AI within a project management framework, with the main goal of increasing project success rates and overall productivity.

In this project, the power of artificial intelligence employed in project management. The main objectives are to improve project planning, resource management, risk assessment and decision-making by exploiting artificial intelligence technologies. The aims to improve project efficiency, output, and success rates, and finally reach project outcomes.

2 Background

Recently, the world witnessed many crises. These crises served as an incentive to reconsider the traditional way of working, as weaknesses emerged in various industries [1]. This was an incentive to search for innovative ways to face the challenges and activate the role of the sectors in all situations. The most active and innovative way that can be used to shift whole sectors is artificial intelligence. Artificial intelligence technologies have evolved to become more powerful and easy to use, which has led to them being increasingly used as vital components of new software systems. This new application can allow for new functionality and often allows for better adaptation to user needs. Artificial Intelligence (AI) is a subfield Computer Science. That creates smart machines and computer programs to perform several tasks that need human intelligence. It can considered as a system that simulates many functions a person can perform [2]. Deep learning (DL) is a branch of Machine Learning that relies on Deep Neural Network (DNN) models. DNN models, like other machine learning models, require identifying the inputs from the dataset, and the output to be predicted. In addition, the model needs to be built, the data needs to be pre-processed for training, and performance measures are needed too [3, 4].

The great progress that the field of artificial intelligence has witnessed in recent years is that it can be used in a variety of software engineering applications. Intelligent technologies are being used as key elements in modern software systems, and these technologies allow the development of new functions and better adaptation to user needs [5]. The relationship between software engineering and AI can be classified into three main aspects: first Point of Application (PA) where AI technology is applied, with three main levels being process level, product level, and operation level. Second: Type of AI applied (TAI): define the approaches to implement AI. This includes the symbolic approach, the connectionist approach, and others. Third: Level of Automation (LA): This aspect denotes the degree of self-application of AI technology, ranging from low levels where AI provides data to high levels where AI autonomously makes and implements decisions without human intervention [6]. This classification will give more understanding on the best way to apply AI in SE.

The great progress that the field of artificial intelligence has witnessed in recent years is that it can be used in a variety of software engineering applications. Intelligent technologies are being used as key elements in modern software systems, and these technologies allow the development of new functions and better adaptation to user needs [5].

Where the stages of development and application of artificial intelligence in the project life cycle discussed from the stage of idea and conceptualization until reaching the production stage, the stages reviewed as follows:

1. The Idea and Planning Phase: This phase focuses on defining the main idea of the AI project and developing a detailed plan for its implementation. Applying smart tools must help to identify correct project objectives, needed resources, and economic feasibility.
2. Design and development phase: This stage includes translating the idea of the smart system to be developed into a practical design.
3. Experiment and Test Phase: The developed model will be tested to evaluate its performance and see if it requires modification or not.
4. Improvement and modification stage: After the testing phase, necessary adjustments should be made to improve performance.
5. Production and application phase: This is the final phase where the smart system is implemented in the real environment and used on a large scale. All optimizations should have been applied and the system should be production ready.

The phase of artificial intelligence includes critical steps to achieve success and effectiveness in applying smart technologies in projects. Planning, design, testing, and optimization aspects must be considered to ensure AI's successful development and effective use [7].

Project managers is important guiding the project team, coordinating efforts, and fostering collaboration among stakeholders to achieve project success. A project is the method of change that an organization or an individual has something new which they do not have, and which in some respects can be guaranteed to work within the system in society, in the marketplace, etc. Usually, organizations use different tools and techniques in implementing projects to help manage them. Accordingly [8], Armenia and others dealt with this in their research on the challenges facing companies in achieving sustainability of their business activities by integrating social, economic, and environmental perspectives. The study also reviews how project management can be integrated with sustainability concepts. The results concluded that the academic literature on this topic is still in its infancy, but the interest of researchers is increasing, which opens up new research directions. Based on the literature review findings, a new conceptual framework is proposed linking five key dimensions of sustainable project management:

corporate policies and practices, resource management, life-cycle orientation, stakeholder engagement, and organizational learning. On this front, Müller et al. [9]. Discuss Organizational Project Management (OPM) and how to complement project, program, and portfolio management with emerging elements such as governance, project implementation, project management office (PMO), and organization design. Hence, these topics require an integrated model that defines the content and roles in managing organizational projects. This paper addresses this issue by developing a seven-layer model that organizes 22 elements of organizational project management.

Hence, Ika et al. [10] dealt with the issue of project management and international development as two fields of knowledge and practice that grew in the twentieth century. Both areas share a central concern with organizing action and achieving change. Although international development had a role in defining the field of project management in the 1950s and 1960s, there has been little exchange between them in recent decades. Projects are important to international development efforts and the need to help project management address global challenges that overlap with international development, such as climate change and the COVID-19 pandemic. Accordingly, this research addresses, for exchange and integration, what links and distinguishes the two fields, project management, and international development, whether in terms of concepts or through the nature of their service delivery. The research highlights an agenda for research at the intersection between project management and international development.

The PMO has been considered in previous studies as a knowledge broker that can improve the communication between these levels. However, these studies were considered a one-sided perspective that lacked defining the specific roles of PMO and provided fragmentary evidence for cofactors associated with it. To bridge this gap, Ali et al. [11]. Used mediation theory to develop a comprehensive theoretical framework that identifies the specific roles of the knowledge mediator (PMO) and articulates the enablers to facilitate multidirectional knowledge transactions. Three groups of knowledge mediation roles described, each corresponding to one of three classes of knowledge transactions. Our model demonstrates how PMO can facilitate the mediation of knowledge confined in organizational cages by striking a balance between experiential learning from below and informed learning from above while maintaining horizontal knowledge synchronization. In this paper, Magano et al. [12]. Dealt with project management education strategies for engineering students and how to attract the interest of millennials (Generation Z) in this field. The article points out that engineering students although they gain remarkable theoretical knowledge during their studies, lack transferable competitiveness such as soft skills, which are rarely given attention in project management education. Also, a correlational analysis was used to link the personality traits of Generation Z with the soft skills of project management. These findings reveal interesting personality traits of Generation Z engineering students in project management. However, this sample showed a low recognition of individuality and a lack of interpersonal relationships and did not place value on their creative potential.

A model B proposed where projects can be effectively managed in small and medium enterprises (SMEs) [13], i.e. in areas where the available international methodologies for project management have not generally been adopted. The proposed model has been verified on projects in various SMEs in Slovakia. The mathematical assessment, knowledge and experience from this verification were summarized, and the proposed in a model called SMEPM (Small and Medium Enterprises Project Management), which was modified so that it could be used in the implementation of other projects in the conditions of small and medium enterprises. The concept of a sustainable approach to managing IT projects through the participation of the client in the stage of selecting the project management methodology explored by [14]. The study focuses on IT projects that aim to develop software commissioned by organizations. The study aims to assess how the internal perspective of sustainability in information technology projects, which is represented by the conformity of the project management methodology with the needs of the client, affects the overall customer satisfaction with the technology project, its products, and its results.

The latest developments in project management education identified and examined by evaluating improvements made by blended learning models, curricula, and play [11]. It mainly aims to summarize these aspects' impact on project management education by evaluating empirically confirmed research. The main findings indicate that most of the studies used the blended learning model, which combines advanced e-learning with traditional face-to-face educational practices. They proposed a class system aimed at summarizing the essential components of blended learning and its benefits. Challenges, gaps, and open issues in project management education are presented. Accordingly, a project-centered model was also proposed to support learning outcomes in project management provide guidance to teachers, and improve their performance through integrated educational experiences in this domain. The importance of project management principles studied in promoting competitive business strategies, indicating that success in projects may be achieved by following the principles of project management and the project's success. Research has been conducted to identify best methods to manage projects and define its success factors. Information can explain project success factors by applying research methodologies and integrating findings into a conceptual framework.

The integration between artificial intelligence (AI) and project management aim to improve many aspects of project management:

- Improving Project Planning and Scheduling Accuracy: The main goal is to use AI algorithms to increase the accuracy of project planning and scheduling. Projects can be more accurately planned and schedules by testing AI's on large datasets and identifying complex patterns.
- Optimizing Risk Assessment and Mitigation Plans: sing AI to analyze historical data and suggest risk mitigation strategies AI enables the project manager to identify potential risks with high accuracy.
- Automating Repetitive Tasks: The main goal is to automate routine tasks that consume significant time and resources. The use of artificial intelligence shifts guidance and focuses it on other value-added activities, which ultimately enhances productivity.
- Real-Time Monitoring: Artificial intelligence helps monitor the progress of the project in real time by collecting and analyzing data. Its main benefit is that it allows appropriate decisions to be made more quickly.
- Facilitating Data-Driven Decision-Making: Using AI's predictive capabilities, which are based on data analysis, provides project stakeholders with a clear picture that helps them make decisions based on accurate analyses.

To achieve the previous goals, artificial intelligence must be integrated into project management to increase efficiency and use available resources well in order to achieve better results. Achieving these goals works to redefine traditional project management practices and transfer them within an environment full of data and supported by artificial intelligence.

3 Methodology

Deep learning models have shown great potential in handling complex and large-scale data, which is often the case in project management scenarios. The primary objective of this research is to leverage the capabilities of deep learning models to forecast critical project parameters, facilitating more accurate project planning and decision-making. By binding the ability of neural networks and innovative data processing techniques, this methodology aims to improve the accuracy and resource allocation, time estimation, and cost prediction, eventually contributing to enhanced project outcomes. The main stages of the model are illustrated in Fig. 1.

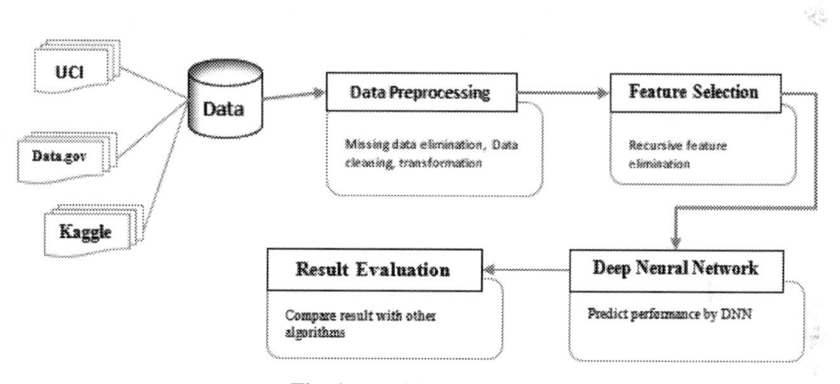

Fig. 1. Model architecture

3.1 Data Collection and Pre Processing

Data collected from various sources to facilitate the development and validation of the deep learning-based predictive models for project management parameters. These sources include publicly available datasets from repositories such as Kaggle [15], UCI [16] Machine Learning Repository, and Data.gov [17], as well as project management tools, academic research databases, industry associations, and potentially company-specific data, subject to permissions and ethical considerations. The following data collected:

- Real projects: The dataset comprises completed real projects managed within a portfolio over an extended duration it encompasses a cohesive collection of resources, both consumable and non-consumable, interconnected in a complex, multi-dimensional manner, with significant correlations among quantity, productivity rates of key resources, and cost rates for materials, labor, equipment, and subcontract resources. The data is publicly available for download, hosted in a repository.

- Data. World: The dataset for projects collected from Data.gov, a publicly accessible repository known for hosting diverse datasets. Specifically focusing on projects, the data extracted from Data.gov encompasses a comprehensive collection of project-related information. It contains project details such as attributes, resources, schedules, costs and other important features relevant for project management analysis.
- Kaggle repository: Projects portfolios obtained from Kaggle. The portfolio stored as excel file contains all necessary detail about the project.
- Simulated data: In addition to the data retrieved from Data.gov and Kaggle, a simulated dataset containing 1000 project records was generated attributes specifically for this research project

Data collected from various sources was converted into an XML (Extensible Markup Language) file to organize project characteristics, such as project duration, budget, team size, complexity, risk factors, and success indicators, uniformly. This facilitates data processing and analysis because it is comprehensive for different projects from different sources. The data contains information about a set of simulated projects, each of which has specific characteristics that reflect different aspects of complexity. A sample of the XML is shown in Fig. 2.

```
<project>
    <pname>Regional Airport Car Park</pname>
    <pid>1</pid>
     <complexity>
        <scope>
        <objectives>
        <deliverables>
        <resources>
            <labours>
            <MATERIAL RESOURCES>
            <PLANT RESOURCES>
            <SUBCONTRACT RESOURCES>
        </resources>
        <risk factors>
 </complexity>
    <team>
       <size> 12</size>
        <stackhoders> 62 </stackhoders>
     </team>
     <time>
        <start>5/05/11</start>
        <end>6/11/11</end>
        <duration>185</duration>
     </<Time>>
    <budget>
            <BAC>1965174</BAC>
            <AC>1,898,995</AC>
            <value>1,902,511</value>
            <final_value>2,280,303</final_value>
    </budget>
    <risk_level>
        <level>Medium</level>
    </risk_level>
</project>
```

Fig. 2. XML format for the data

The score is calculated for each feature in the XML file using multiple classifiers. The analysis includes an evaluation of all factors related to the project, which include duration, budget, number of team members, risk level, project complexity, and project number. This approach aims to know all possible influences on predicting project outcomes.

It allows for a comprehensive understanding of the factors that contribute to project success. Extracted project attributes are summarized in Table 1.

Table 1. Project attributes

ATTRIBUTE	DESCRIPTION
PROJECT ID	An identifier uniquely assigned to each project for reference.
DURATION	Represents the projected duration of the project in months, ranging from 1 to 12 months.
BUDGET	Indicates the estimated budget allocated for the project
TEAM SIZE	Denotes the estimated number of team members assigned to work on the project.
COMPLEXITY	An attribute that represents the complexity level of the project. It includes various project features such as technical challenges, scope, required resources, stakeholder contribution, regulatory compliance, risks, and other aspects.
RISK LEVEL	Categorizes the perceived risk level associated with the project, indicating 'Low', 'Medium', or 'High' risk factors.
SUCCESS	Represent project success, where '1' indicates a successful project, and '0' represents a failed project that did not meet the success measures

4 Experiment Result

The model was developed and tested using the Python programming language in the COLAB environment. Deep neural network with 3 hidden layers is implemented and the number of neurons are 5, 10, and 20 respectively for layer 1, 2, and 3. The input layers are six and the output is one. The output is one layer because the output can be inferred as zero or one. The deep neural network (DNN) runs for 10 epochs on the dataset. The accuracy of the training data started from 48.86% and then gradually increased to 62.29% at the end of training. After training, the model reached 66% accuracy on the test dataset.

The model's accuracy improved pointedly after increasing the number of epochs from 10 to 20. The accuracy on the training data increased from 68.6% to 99.5%, which indicate that the model is learning data patterns efficiently. This increased learning is also reflected in the test accuracy, rising from 66% to 99%, demonstrating that the model's generalization to unseen data has improved remarkably. The model's performance seems promising, achieving a high accuracy rate and suggesting it effectively captures the underlying patterns in the dataset.

Figure 3 illustrate the Accuracy regarding the number of epochs during training and testing. Initially, the model's accuracy, both in training and testing, increases rapidly with each epoch, indicating the learning process effectively captures patterns in the data. However, after several periods, the testing accuracy level stabilizes while the training accuracy continues to increase. This difference can be explained by model fit, as the model has learned too much from the training data, making it less able to recognize unseen data. The figure illustrates the need for good techniques such as modifications in model structure to mitigate overfitting and improve generalization to enhance performance on new data. Table 2 shows a comparison between models accuracy.

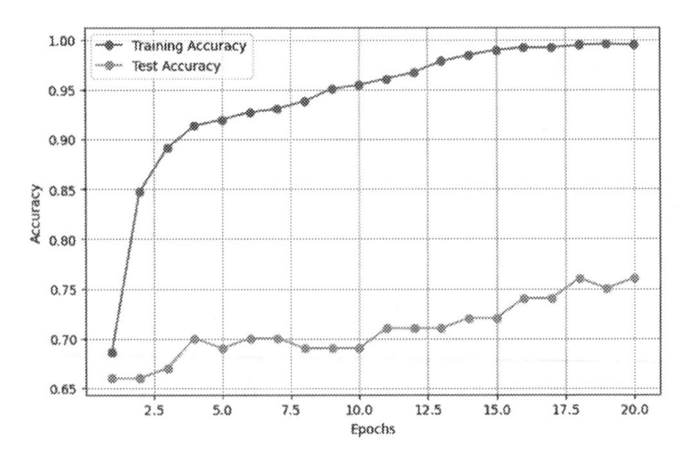

Fig. 3. Model accuracy over epochs

Table 2. Comparison between Models Accuracy

Model	Accuracy
Neural Network (MLP)	0.65
Logistic Regression	0.74
Support Vector Machine	0.725
DNN	0.77

5 Conclusion

The combination of artificial intelligence and project management has transformed traditional methods into automation. In this research, the impact of applying artificial intelligence techniques using a deep neural network (DNN) was studied. The results were excellent, as the accuracy rate in predicting the project's success reached 99%. Although it requires continuous preparation and training for optimal performance. Data was collected from various sources and then converted into XML format. Then, it went through a pre-processing phase that included feature selection. Visual illustrations of the model performance show the need to balance learning from training data and simplify new data to mitigate overfitting. This study visualizes AI's role in project management, from refining planning accuracy to facilitating real-time monitoring and data-driven decision-making. Also, it prove the importance of integration between AI, Software Engineering, and Project Management.

References

1. Taboada, I., Daneshpajouh, A., Toledo, N., de Vass, T.: Artificial intelligence enabled project management: a systematic literature review. Appl. Sci. **13**, 5014 (2023)

2. Fathima Anjila, P.: What is artificial intelligence? Success is no accident. It is hard work, perseverance, learning, studying, sacrifice and most of all, love of what you are doing or learning to do, p. 65 (1984)
3. Sharrab, Y.O., Alsmirat, M., Hawashin, B., Sarhan, N.: Machine learning-based energy consumption modeling and comparing of H. 264 and Google VP8 encoders. Int. J. Electr. Comput. Eng. (IJECE) **11**, 1303–1310 (2021)
4. Tarawneh, M., Al Zyoud, F., Sharrab, Y.: Artificial intelligence traffic analysis framework for smart cities. In: Arai, K. (eds.) Intelligent Computing. SAI 2023. LNNS, vol. 711, pp. 699–711. Springer, Cham (2023). https://doi.org/10.1007/978-3-031-37717-4_45
5. Meziane, F., Vadera, S.: Artificial intelligence applications for improved software engineering development: New prospects: New Prospects: IGI Global, 2009
6. Feldt, R., de Oliveira Neto, F.G., Torkar, R.: Ways of applying artificial intelligence in software engineering. In: Proceedings of the 6th International Workshop on Realizing Artificial Intelligence Synergies in Software Engineering, pp. 35–41 (2018)
7. De Silva, D., Alahakoon, D.: An artificial intelligence life cycle: from conception to production. Patterns **3** (2022)
8. Armenia, S., Dangelico, R.M., Nonino, F., Pompei, A.: Sustainable project management: a conceptualization-oriented review and a framework proposal for future studies. Sustainability **11**, 2664 (2019)
9. Müller, R., Drouin, N., Sankaran, S.: Modeling organizational project management. Proj. Manag. J. **50**, 499–513 (2019)
10. Ika, L.A., Söderlund, J., Munro, L.T., Landoni, P.: Cross-learning between project management and international development: analysis and research agenda. Int. J. Proj. Manag. **38**, 548–558 (2020)
11. Hadi, A., Liu, Y., Li, S.: Transcending the silos through project management office: knowledge transactions, brokerage roles, and enabling factors. Int. J. Proj. Manag. **40**, 142–154 (2022)
12. Magano, J., Silva, C.S., Figueiredo, C., Vitória, A., Nogueira, T.: Project management in engineering education: providing generation Z with transferable skills. Ieee Revista Iberoamericana De Tecnologias Del Aprendizaje **16**, 45–57 (2021)
13. Nagyová, A., Pačaiová, H., Markulik, Š, Turisová, R., Kozel, R., Džugan, J.: Design of a model for risk reduction in project management in small and medium-sized enterprises. Symmetry **13**, 763 (2021)
14. Woźniak, M.: Sustainable approach in it project management—methodology choice vs. Client satisfaction. Sustainability **13**, 1466 (2021)
15. Kaggle. https://www.kaggle.com/datasets/
16. D. a. G. Dua, C.: UCI Machine Learning Repository. http://archive.ics.uci.edu/ml
17. Projects datasets. https://www.data.gov/dataset/

Optimizing Feature Selection for Binary Classification with Noisy Labels: A Genetic Algorithm Approach

Vandad Imani[1](✉), Elaheh Moradi[1], Carlos Sevilla-Salcedo[2], Vittorio Fortino[3], and Jussi Tohka[1]

[1] A. I. Virtanen Institute for Molecular Sciences, University of Eastern Finland, Kuopio, Finland
{vandad.imani,elaheh.moradi,jussi.tohka}@uef.fi

[2] Department of Computer Science, Aalto University, Espoo, Finland
carlos.sevillasalcedo@aalto.fi

[3] Institute of Biomedicine, University of Eastern Finland, Kuopio, Finland
vittorio.fortino@uef.fi

Abstract. Feature selection in noisy label scenarios remains an understudied topic. We propose a novel genetic algorithm-based approach, the Noise-Aware Multi-Objective Feature Selection Genetic Algorithm (NMFS-GA), for selecting optimal feature subsets in binary classification with noisy labels. NMFS-GA offers a unified framework for selecting feature subsets that are both accurate and interpretable. We evaluate NMFS-GA on synthetic datasets with label noise, a Breast Cancer dataset enriched with noisy features, and a real-world ADNI dataset for dementia conversion prediction. Our results indicate that NMFS-GA can effectively select feature subsets that improve the accuracy and interpretability of binary classifiers in scenarios with noisy labels.

Keywords: Genetic algorithm · Feature selection · Noisy labels · Classification · Mild cognitive impairment · Magnetic resonance imaging · ADNI · Converter dementia · Alzheimer's disease

1 Introduction

In the era of big data, machine learning (ML) algorithms are increasingly facing the challenges of high data dimensionality and redundant features. This can make it difficult to extract valuable knowledge from the massive feature space, and can lead to overfitting and poor generalization performance, known as the "curse of dimensionality" [1]. This makes it hard for conventional ML methods to find valuable information from an expansive feature space laden with irrelevant and redundant features present in data [2]. Feature selection (FS) algorithms can be used to address these challenges by identifying a subset of features that are most relevant to the classification task [3]. These algorithms consider the

J. Tohka—For the Alzheimer's Disease Neuroimaging Initiative.

K. Daimi and A. Al Sadoon (Eds.): ACR 2024, LNNS 956, pp. 392–403, 2024.
https://doi.org/10.1007/978-3-031-56950-0_33

relationship between features and labels, and depending on this relationship, they can help improve the accuracy and interpretability of ML models.

There are three main types of FS algorithms: filter-based, wrapper-based, and embedded. The filter-based algorithms assess features using an evaluation index that is independent of the learning algorithm [4–6]. Embedded algorithms perform FS as part of the classification algorithm by simultaneously learning the classifier, either within the algorithm or as an added functionality [7–9]. Wrapper-based algorithms search for the optimal subset of features by evaluating their performance on the classification algorithm [10,11].

Traditionally, FS algorithms have been tailored for clean datasets, where all the labels in the training set are correct. However, in many practical situations, obtaining a training set with correct labels is difficult, but the labels must be assumed to contain noise. This can be caused by a variety of factors, such as human error, data collection imperfections, or ambiguities in labeling criteria. The presence of noisy labels can severely impact the accuracy and generalization of ML models.

There are a number of methods for addressing noisy labels. One approach is to identify and eliminate samples with noisy labels from the training dataset [12]. Another approach is to design loss functions that are less sensitive to label noise [13]. These loss functions can be categorized into two main types: symmetric and asymmetric. Symmetric loss functions [13] penalize errors equally, regardless of whether the error is an underprediction or an overprediction, making them less sensitive to label noise when compared to their asymmetric counterparts. In contrast, asymmetric loss functions [14] may penalize false positives and false negatives differently, potentially leading to higher sensitivity to label noise. A third approach is to correct the loss function based on the estimated label flip rates [15,16]. The label flip rate is the probability that a label is incorrect. By estimating the label flip rate, we can adjust the loss function to be more robust to noise. The work in [16] proposed a simple loss function that combines a symmetric loss function and an asymmetric loss function, and the weights of the two loss functions are determined by the estimated label flip rate.

However, FS with noisy labels remains an understudied topic. Addressing this gap, our primary aim in this paper is to introduce and validate a novel approach to FS in noisy label scenarios. Specifically, we propose a novel FS approach, called Noise-Aware Multi-objective Feature Selection with Genetic Algorithm (NMFS-GA), based on our recently presented MMFS-GA framework [10] for FS with noisy labels. The algorithm can effectively select informative feature subsets that enhance the accuracy and interpretability of binary classifiers in the presence of noisy labels. The proposed method is evaluated on different datasets to assess its performance. We conducted experiments on synthetic datasets, and applied NMFS-GA to a real-world Breast Cancer dataset that has been enriched with noisy features to simulate challenging conditions. In both synthetic and Breast Cancer datasets, we explored varying degrees of label noise, including 5%, 10%, 15%, and 20% noise levels, capturing different levels of noise severity. Furthermore, NMFS-GA is evaluated on another real-world ADNI dataset, where we focused on the classification task of stable MCI (sMCI) versus progressive MCI (pMCI). This dataset presents a scenario of asymmetric label noise, which adds to the complexity of the classification problem.

2 Proposed Method

In this section, we present the proposed Genetic Algorithm (GA) designed for FS in the context of binary classification with noisy labels (NMFS-GA). We define $\mathbf{D}$ as the underlying joint distribution of a pair of random variables $\{(\mathbf{x}, y)|\mathbf{x} \in \mathbf{X} \text{ and } \mathbf{y} \in \mathbf{Y}\} = \mathbf{X} \times \mathbf{Y}$. Here, $\mathbf{X} \subset \mathbb{R}^d$ represents the feature space from which the samples are drawn, and $\mathbf{Y} = \{0, 1\}$ denotes the output label space. In the ideal noise-free classification scenario, we consider that a training set $S = \{(\mathbf{x}_1, y_1), \ldots, (\mathbf{x}_N, y_N)\}$ of N samples are drawn independently and identically from $\mathbf{D}$. In this case, all labels $\{y_i\}_{i=1}^N$ are correct. However, in real-world classification tasks, noisy labels often exist, leading us to work with a noisy training set $\tilde{S} = (\mathbf{x}_i, \tilde{y}_i)_{i=1}^N$ obtained from a noisy distribution $\tilde{\mathbf{D}}$. Here $\tilde{y}$ is a contaminated version of y:

$$\tilde{y}_i = \begin{cases} 1 - y_i & \text{with probability } \rho_{\text{noise}} \\ y_i & \text{with probability } (1 - \rho_{\text{noise}}) \end{cases}. \tag{1}$$

Our objective is to use a GA to identify important features in the input data and address the challenges posed by noisy labels to develop effective strategies to learn from the noisy training set, $\tilde{S}$. Specifically, our objective is to identify relevant features in the input data while minimizing the estimated generalization error of the model. To achieve this, we introduce a set of membership indicators, $\mathbf{c} \in \{0, 1\}^{1 \times d}$, where $c_j = 1$ indicates the presence of feature x_j in the optimum set of features, while $c_j = 0$ indicates its absence. We define the loss function $\ell : \mathbb{R} \times \mathbf{Y} \to \mathbb{R}$ to penalize the difference between the model output $h(\mathbf{x})$ and the noisy ground truth label $\tilde{\mathbf{y}}$. The empirical risk of h in the noisy training set $\tilde{\mathbf{S}}$ is represented as:

$$\hat{\mathbf{R}}(h, \tilde{\mathbf{S}}) = \frac{1}{N} \sum_{i=1}^{N} \ell(h(\mathbf{x}_i), \tilde{y}_i) \tag{2}$$

Ideally, we hope to find an unbiased estimator $\hat{\mathbf{R}}(h, \tilde{\mathbf{S}})$ for $\hat{\mathbf{R}}(h, \mathbf{S})$ given $\tilde{\mathbf{S}}$ so that the adverse impact caused by noisy labels can be removed. In this work, we consider linear h implemented through linear discriminant analysis (LDA).

2.1 NMFS-GA Framework

In this section, we describe a GA-based framework, called NMFS-GA (Noise-Aware Multi-objective Feature Selection Genetic Algorithm), designed to address the FS problem using multiniche techniques. We formulate FS as a multiobjective optimization problem [17], with the following objective functions:

$$f_1(\mathbf{c}) = \mathcal{E}(\tilde{y}, h(\mathbf{x}; \mathbf{c})); f_2(\mathbf{c}) = \sum_{j=1}^{d} c_j \tag{3}$$

Here, $f_1(\mathbf{c})$ measures the classification performance though a specific loss function ℓ when only specific features ($c_j = 1$) are considered useful and $f_2(\mathbf{c})$ calculates the total number of selected features. The objective is to simultaneously minimize the classification error while selecting the most informative features. To avoid premature convergence and enhance the identification of important features, NMFS-GA employs multiple niches, each independently evolving its populations through GA operators.

The proposed algorithm consists of the following steps, repeating steps from 2 to 5 until convergence:

1. **Initialization**: The algorithm randomly generates a population of C chromosomes, each of which represents a potential solution in the form of a feature subset.
2. **Fitness evaluation**: The fitness of each chromosome is evaluated using objective functions in Eq. (3) calculated through 10-fold cross-validation using LDA as the classifier.
3. **Crossover and Mutation**: The variation operator produces new offspring through crossover or mutation to develop better solutions that will emerge in the population during evolution. In the case of the crossover process, the elements of two solutions of the parental population mate to produce a single offspring. The algorithm uses binomial crossover to generate the offspring since this method is less dependent on the size of the population. In the event of mutation, an element of one solution from the parental population is selected at random and mutated according to the probability rate of mutation to produce a single offspring.
4. **Selection**: The tournament selection operator, adopted by the Nondominated Sorting Genetic Algorithm II [17] as the selection operator, works by randomly selecting two solutions from the population, comparing the solutions with respect to their front ranks and their crowding distance, and selecting the best one.
5. **Migration**: Niches independently evolve their populations through crossover and mutation; nevertheless, niches interact with each other every 5% of the total generations through a genetic operator termed migration, which swaps the top 25% of their populations.
6. **Termination**: The algorithm terminates after 1000 generations.

2.2 Loss Functions: Theoretical Analysis

We can approximate $\mathcal{E}(\tilde{y}, h(\mathbf{x};\mathbf{c})) \approx \frac{1}{N}\sum_{i=1}^{N} \ell(h(\mathbf{x}_i;\mathbf{c}), \tilde{y}_i)$ through various loss functions, summarized in Table 1, which have been proposed to deal with noisy labels. Note that, when needed, LDA outputs classification probabilities, $h(\mathbf{x};\mathbf{c})$ presenting the probability of the class 1. **Cross-entropy** loss (ℓ_{CE}) [18], known as log loss, is a commonly used loss function for classification tasks, including those with noisy labels [19]. It measures the dissimilarity between the predicted probability distribution of the model and the true distribution of the target variables. **Symmetric cross-entropy** loss (ℓ_{SCE}) [13], is a modified version of CE loss function that addresses the issue of imbalanced class distributions. It assigns different weights to positive and negative samples, allowing for more balanced training. **Generalized cross-entropy** loss (ℓ_{GCE}) [20] loss function is a flexible variant of the CE loss that encompasses multiple loss functions by introducing a parameter, q. It generalizes the standard cross-entropy loss and allows for various levels of optimization. **Joint optimization** loss (ℓ_{JOL}) [21], is designed to streamline model training by optimizing multiple objectives simultaneously. It consists of three key components: ℓ_c measures the Kullback-Leibler divergence loss, assessing the difference between predicted probabilities and noisy labels; ℓ_p acts as a penalty to encourage accurate probability predictions; and ℓ_e penalizes significant deviations in model parameters to prevent overfitting. **Peer loss function** (ℓ_{PL}) [22] is a robust loss function that can be used to learn from noisy labels without knowing the noise rate. The peer loss function penalizes the model for making different predictions for two similar examples. **Class-Wise denoising loss function** (ℓ_{CWD}) [15] is a robust loss function that can be used to learn from noisy labels in a class-wise manner. The CWD loss function first estimates the centroid of each class in the training set. Then, it penalizes the model for making predictions that are far from the centroid of the class. In addition, we use **balanced accuracy** (ℓ_{BA}) as our baseline metric to evaluate loss function performance with noisy labels.

Table 1. Summary of Loss Functions, we define $\tilde{\iota} = 1-\tilde{y}$, $\psi = 1-h(\mathbf{x};\mathbf{c})$ and $a = 1-\alpha$.

Loss Function	Formula	Description
Cross-entropy	$-[\tilde{y}\log(h(\mathbf{x};\mathbf{c})) + \tilde{\iota}\log(\psi)]$	Measures the dissimilarity between the predicted and true probability distributions
Symmetric cross-entropy	$-(\alpha\tilde{y}\log(h(\mathbf{x};\mathbf{c})) + a(\tilde{\iota})\log(\psi))$	α is a balancing parameter between positive and negative samples
Generalizedcross-entropy	$\tilde{y}\frac{1-h(\mathbf{x};\mathbf{c})^q}{q} + \tilde{\iota}\frac{(1-\psi^q)}{q}$	$q > 0.5$ more noise tolerance, slower convergence; $q < 0.5$ Faster convergence, less noise tolerance
Joint optimization	$\ell_c(h(\mathbf{x}_i;\mathbf{c}), \tilde{y}_i) + \alpha\ell_p(h(\mathbf{x};\mathbf{c})) + \beta\ell_e(h(\mathbf{x};\mathbf{c}))$	α balances loss and prediction penalty; β balances between predicted probabilities and model parameters
Peer loss	$\ell(f(x_n), \tilde{y}_n) - \ell(f(x_{n1}), \tilde{y}_{n2})$	$\ell(.)$ is 0-1 loss; Two randomly sampled peer samples are $(x_n, \tilde{y}_n)$ and $(x_{n1}, \tilde{y}_{n2})$
Class-Wisedenoising	$h(\mathbf{x};\mathbf{c})^2 + 1 + Q\langle\tilde{\mu}, \mathbf{w}\rangle$	For squared loss, Q is a constant value, and $\tilde{\mu}$ is a dataset centroid estimate, $\mathbf{w}$ are LDA coefficients

3 Experimental Results

We evaluated the proposed NMFS-GA algorithm on four different datasets, two synthetic and two real world data sets.

3.1 Synthetic Data

We constructed two synthetic 500-dimensional datasets (A and B) similar to that of [23] with three simulated label noise rates by flipping the true label with a probability of 0.05, 0.1, or 0.15. The data is structured in a way that it is challenging for feature-ranking or greedy FS methods to find an optimal feature subset. Specifically, in dataset A, only 6 features exhibit discriminative power, while the other 494 features are non-informative. Moreover, dataset B is designed with 7 discriminative features and 493 non-informative features. The informative features of the samples in each dataset have the same covariance matrix but with different means, and the classes are normally distributed. For dataset A, LDA achieved an accuracy of 72% for dataset A and 69% for dataset B without label noise. The Bayes error rates for datasets A and B obtaining values of 0.046 and 0.141, respectively. We evaluate the actual probability of correct classification (PCC) under the assumption of an infinite number of (noiseless) test samples by using conditional PCC as a performance measure. The conditional PCC was computed with the Monte Carlo integration with 10 million simulated test samples.

Comparison of Loss Functions. Table 2 presents the performance comparison of various loss functions under different label noise rates. The results with the dataset A indicate that all loss functions can achieve PCCs that are close to the optimal (1 - Bayes error rate) when 5% of the labels are noisy. However, PCCs decrease as the noise ratio increases, which is expected. The CWD and BA losses prove the most robust, consistently achieving the highest PCCs. The other loss functions are less noise-resistant, with mean PCCs ranging from 0.84 to 0.87 at 5% noise. At 10% noise, CWD, BA, and GCE maintain their PCC at 0.79, while others drop to 0.70–0.75. Notably, as the noise ratio escalated to 15%, the BA achieved a mean a PCC of 0.70, closely followed by CWD and GCE loss functions.

The comparison of results with the dataset B across different noise levels reveals insights into loss function performance. At 5% noise, most loss functions perform similarly, the CWD achieved an average PCC of 78%. At this level, the choice of loss function has minimal impact. At 10% noise, CWD maintains its competitiveness (PCC 72%), followed by BA (PCC 71%), with others showing little difference. As noise rises to 15%, the impact of label noise on accuracy becomes clear. The CWD remains robust with PCC of 61%, but all loss functions suffer reduced PCC, indicating the challenge posed by substantial label noise.

Across all noise levels (5%, 10%, and 15%), mean PCC differences between loss functions are not substantial. BA, CWD, and GCE consistently demonstrate similar performance, suggesting that the choice of loss function may have limited impact on classification accuracy when using the NMFS-GA algorithm in scenarios with varying label noise. Given this consistent performance, these three loss functions-BA, CWD, and GCE-were selected for the subsequent experiments.

Table 2. Comparison of different loss functions used in NMFS-GA algorithm with synthetic data. The table displays the average PCC and its standard deviation across 10 experiments for each loss function under three different label noise rates. There were 100 training samples per class.

Experiments	Noise rate	Accuracy					
	ρ_{noise}	BA	CWD	SCE	GCE	JOL	PL
Dataset A	0.05	0.87 ± 0.039	$\mathbf{0.88 \pm 0.039}$	0.85 ± 0.031	0.87 ± 0.040	0.84 ± 0.032	0.86 ± 0.026
	0.1	$\mathbf{0.79 \pm 0.063}$	$\mathbf{0.79 \pm 0.049}$	0.73 ± 0.075	$\mathbf{0.79 \pm 0.085}$	0.75 ± 0.070	0.70 ± 0.068
	0.15	$\mathbf{0.70 \pm 0.060}$	0.65 ± 0.064	0.61 ± 0.038	0.65 ± 0.096	0.62 ± 0.089	0.60 ± 0.063
Dataset B	0.05	0.77 ± 0.028	$\mathbf{0.78 \pm 0.044}$	0.77 ± 0.045	0.77 ± 0.033	0.73 ± 0.026	0.73 ± 0.047
	0.1	0.71 ± 0.034	$\mathbf{0.72 \pm 0.048}$	0.68 ± 0.061	0.70 ± 0.034	0.63 ± 0.082	0.68 ± 0.048
	0.15	0.58 ± 0.074	$\mathbf{0.61 \pm 0.055}$	0.56 ± 0.040	0.58 ± 0.052	0.59 ± 0.032	0.58 ± 0.050

Effect of Sample Size on Algorithm Robustness. Table 3 explores the robustness of NMFS-GA algorithms with reduced dataset sizes (25 and 50 instances per class). As sample size decreases, the PCC of all loss functions tends to decline. Despite smaller datasets of type A, our NMFS-GA algorithm, utilizing GCE loss, maintains competitiveness with an average PCC of 64%, closely followed by CWD (PCC 63%) at a 10% noise ratio. Experiments with type B dataset (Bayes error rate of 0.141) also show CWD achieving 62% accuracy. At a 15% noise ratio with a dataset size of 50 samples per class, Table 3 reveals a drop in classification accuracy, reflecting the challenges posed by substantial label noise. CWD achieved a mean accuracy of 52% and 57%, while GCE reaches 58% and 57% for higher and lower discriminative power datasets, respectively.

Increasing the sample size to 50 instances per class yields substantial accuracy improvements across all methods. In Table 3, for experiments with 50 samples per class, GCE loss function achieves an average accuracy of 73% for higher discriminative power, closely followed by CWD at 72% at 10% noise. In the lower discriminative power dataset, CWD loss function reaches 70% PCC, with GCE at 69%.

Turning to the 15% noise ratio results, a consistent decline in PCC is observed for all loss functions due to the increased noise levels. In the dataset with higher discriminative power, the average PCC for GCE loss function is 65%, while CWD achieved PCC of 59%. In the dataset with lower discriminative power, CWD loss function achieved average accuracy of 63%, followed by GCE at 62%.

Table 3. Comparison of loss functions with 25 and 50 samples per class. The table displays the average PCC and its standard deviation across 10 experiments for each loss function.

Experiment	Noise rate	BA		CWD		GCE	
	ρ_{noise}	50	100	50	100	50	100
Dataset A	0.1	0.57 ± 0.080	0.64 ± 0.084	0.63 ± 0.108	0.72 ± 0.022	$\mathbf{0.64 \pm 0.096}$	$\mathbf{0.73 \pm 0.052}$
	0.15	0.50 ± 0.000	0.60 ± 0.070	0.52 ± 0.070	0.59 ± 0.094	$\mathbf{0.58 \pm 0.089}$	$\mathbf{0.65 \pm 0.103}$
Dataset B	0.1	0.56 ± 0.079	0.64 ± 0.031	$\mathbf{0.62 \pm 0.102}$	$\mathbf{0.70 \pm 0.032}$	0.58 ± 0.089	0.69 ± 0.039
	0.15	0.51 ± 0.043	0.58 ± 0.071	$\mathbf{0.57 \pm 0.084}$	$\mathbf{0.63 \pm 0.110}$	$\mathbf{0.57 \pm 0.095}$	0.62 ± 0.083

3.2 Breast Cancer Dataset

The publicly available breast cancer dataset [24] comprises 569 samples of which 212 represent malignant and 357 benign cases. Each sample has 30 features, and we further added 300 noise features, drawn from the Gaussian distribution. The features were randomly permuted to prevent any FS algorithm from learning the feature order. To assess the impact of label noise on the performance of our model, we employed 10-fold cross-validation and experiments with two simulated noise rates adding label noise to the training set, flipping the true label with a probability of 0.1 or 0.2.

In Table 4, we compare the classification performance of various loss functions in the NMFS-GA algorithm at noise levels of 10% and 20%. At 10% noise, all three loss functions achieve similar balanced accuracy values, approximately ranging from 0.85 to 0.88. Even at 20% noise, they perform well, with balanced accuracy values of 0.72 to 0.77. CWD consistently outperforms others, followed by BA, and GCE performs slightly worse but still reasonably well. These findings underline the effectiveness of the NMFS-GA algorithm in handling noisy data using various loss functions.

Table 4. Performance comparison of the NMFS-GA Algorithm using different Loss Functions, across two distinct noise rates (10% and 20%). The evaluated metrics were balanced accuracy, sensitivity (SEN), specificity (SPE), and area under the curve (AUC), each represented as the mean value across the folds of 10-fold cross-validation ± standard deviation.

Method/	Balanced Accuracy		SEN		SPE		AUC	
ρ_{noise}	0.1	0.2	0.1	0.2	0.1	0.2	0.1	0.2
BA	0.87 ± 0.061	0.76 ± 0.074	0.75 ± 0.113	0.55 ± 0.129	0.99 ± 0.028	0.96 ± 0.043	**0.98 ± 0.025**	**0.90 ± 0.063**
CWD	**0.88 ± 0.044**	**0.77 ± 0.039**	0.75 ± 0.088	0.58 ± 0.087	1.00 ± 0.000	0.97 ± 0.030	**0.98 ± 0.017**	0.89 ± 0.058
GCE	0.85 ± 0.056	0.72 ± 0.044	0.73 ± 0.115	0.53 ± 0.076	0.97 ± 0.022	0.90 ± 0.045	0.95 ± 0.025	0.82 ± 0.046

3.3 ADNI Data

We used ADNI data (http://adni.loni.usc.edu) to predict future dementia in participants experiencing Mild Cognitive Impairment (MCI) [25] as a real-world test-bed for our algorithm. The ADNI was launched in 2003 as a public-private partnership, led by Principal Investigator Michael W. Weiner, MD. For up-to-date information, see (www.adni-info.org).

We used volumes of specific brain structures, extracted from magnetic resonance images (MRI,) as features. MRIs were processed through the CAT12 pipeline [26]. Processed MRIs were averaged into regional volumes according to the neuromorphometrics atlas, which is based on MR images from 30 subjects from the OASIS database with 138 manually annotated structures provided by Neuromorphometrics, Inc. (http://neuromorphometrics.com) [27]. The MCI participants were categorized into two groups according to their follow-up diagnosis: stable MCI (sMCI) and progressive MCI (pMCI). The sMCI group consisted of 191 participants with consistent MCI diagnosis and available follow-up diagnosis at least for 5 years. To introduce label noise we also included 189 participants in sMCI group with available follow-up diagnoses for only 3 years. For the pMCI group, we included all MCI participants who converted to dementia during the available follow-up period. Within this category, we identified a consistent pMCI subgroup consisting of 261 participants who consistently received a dementia diagnosis in their last two available follow-up diagnoses. Additionally, there was a noisy pMCI group consisting of 112 pMCI participants who received a dementia diagnosis only in their last available follow-up diagnosis.

According to Table 5, all four loss functions performed well on the ADNI dataset, with balanced accuracy values ranging from 0.76 to 0.80. This suggests that the NMFS-GA algorithm, regardless of the specific loss function used, is effective in achieving a reasonable balance between sensitivity and specificity. The sensitivity and specificity metrics, which quantify the ability to correctly identify true positive and true negative cases, respectively, range from 0.73 to 0.77 and 0.78 to 0.84 across different loss functions. This indicates that the algorithm performs consistently well in predicting future dementia in MCI patients by classification of pMCI vs. sMCI groups. The GCE achieved the highest Balanced Accuracy value, followed by the CWD.

Table 5. Performance comparison of the NMFS-GA algorithm using different loss functions for sMCI vs. pMCI on the ADNI dataset. The evaluated metrics include balanced accuracy, sensitivity (SEN), specificity (SPE), and area under the curve (AUC), each represented as the mean value across the folds of 10-fold cross-validation ± standard deviation.

sMCI vs pMCI				
Method	Balanced Accuracy	SEN	SPE	AUC
BA	0.77 ± 0.045	0.73 ± 0.063	0.81 ± 0.097	0.84 ± 0.047
CWD	0.78 ± 0.036	0.74 ± 0.042	0.82 ± 0.045	0.85 ± 0.036
GCE	0.80 ± 0.052	0.77 ± 0.085	0.84 ± 0.077	0.86 ± 0.050

4 Conclusion

We investigated the efficacy of the Feature Selection Genetic Algorithm (NMFS-GA) for binary classification tasks with noisy labels, employing various loss functions. Our experiments consisted of synthetic datasets with varying levels of label noise, the Breast Cancer dataset augmented with noise features, and a real-world

ADNI dataset for the classification of stable Mild Cognitive Impairment (MCI) versus converter Dementia (CDE). NMFS-GA, equipped with multiple loss functions, demonstrated notable robustness to label noise. It consistently outperformed across different noise ratios, underscoring its reliability in handling noisy data. Across all datasets and noise conditions, NMFS-GA consistently achieved competitive classification accuracy. Variations in the choice of loss function did not lead to drastic differences in performance, indicating the algorithm's versatility and effectiveness. Our experiments revealed that as sample sizes decreased, classification accuracy naturally decreased. However, NMFS-GA remained effective even with limited training data, highlighting its adaptability and potential for various applications.

Acknowledgments. Supported by grants 346934, 332510 from the Academy of Finland; grant 351849 from the Academy of Finland under the frame of ERA PerMed ("Pattern-Cog"); Sigrid Juselius Foundation; grant 220104 from Jenny ja Antti Wihurin; grant 65221647 from Pohjois-Savon Rahasto; and the Doctoral Program in Molecular Medicine (DPMM) from the University of Eastern Finland. The computational analyses were performed on servers provided by UEF Bioinformatics Center, University of Eastern Finland, Finland.

Data collection and sharing regarding ADNI data was funded by the Alzheimer's Disease Neuroimaging Initiative (ADNI) (National Institutes of Health Grant U01 AG024904) and DOD ADNI (Department of Defense award number W81XWH-12-2-0012). ADNI is funded by the National Institute on Aging, the National Institute of Biomedical Imaging and Bioengineering, and through generous contributions from the following: AbbVie, Alzheimer's Association; Alzheimer's Drug Discovery Foundation; Araclon Biotech; BioClinica, Inc.; Biogen; Bristol-Myers Squibb Company; CereSpir, Inc.; Cogstate; Eisai Inc.; Elan Pharmaceuticals, Inc.; Eli Lilly and Company; EuroImmun; F. Hoffmann-La Roche Ltd and its affiliated company Genentech, Inc.; Fujirebio; GE Healthcare; IXICO Ltd.; Janssen Alzheimer Immunotherapy Research & Development, LLC.; Johnson & Johnson Pharmaceutical Research & Development LLC.; Lumosity; Lundbeck; Merck & Co., Inc.; Meso Scale Diagnostics, LLC.; NeuroRx Research; Neurotrack Technologies; Novartis Pharmaceuticals Corporation; Pfizer Inc.; Piramal Imaging; Servier; Takeda Pharmaceutical Company; and Transition Therapeutics. The Canadian Institutes of Health Research is providing funds to support ADNI clinical sites in Canada. Private sector contributions are facilitated by the Foundation for the National Institutes of Health (www.fnih.org). The grantee organization is the Northern California Institute for Research and Education, and the study is coordinated by the Alzheimer's Therapeutic Research Institute at the University of Southern California. ADNI data are disseminated by the Laboratory for Neuro Imaging at the University of Southern California.

References

1. Siblini, W., Kuntz, P., Meyer, F.: A review on dimensionality reduction for multi-label classification. IEEE Trans. Knowl. Data Eng. **33**(3), 839–857 (2019)
2. Pappu, V., Pardalos, P.M.: High-dimensional data classification. In: Aleskerov, F., Goldengorin, B., Pardalos, P.M. (eds.) Clusters, Orders, and Trees: Methods and Applications. SOIA, vol. 92, pp. 119–150. Springer, New York (2014). https://doi.org/10.1007/978-1-4939-0742-7_8

3. Liu, H., Yu, L.: Toward integrating feature selection algorithms for classification and clustering. IEEE Trans. Knowl. Data Eng. **17**(4), 491–502 (2005)
4. Pan, M., Sun, Z., Wang, C., Cao, G.: A multi-label feature selection method based on an approximation of interaction information. Intell. Data Anal. **26**(4), 823–840 (2022)
5. Santos-Mayo, L., San-José-Revuelta, L.M., Arribas, J.I.: A computer-aided diagnosis system with EEG based on the P3b wave during an auditory odd-ball task in schizophrenia. IEEE. Trans. Biomed **64**(2), 395–407 (2016)
6. Liu, H., Setiono, R., et al.: A probabilistic approach to feature selection-a filter solution. ICML **96**, 319–327 (1996)
7. Sevilla-Salcedo, C., Imani, V., Olmos, P.M., Gómez-Verdejo, V., Tohka, J., Initiative, A.D.N., et al.: Multi-task longitudinal forecasting with missing values on Alzheimer's disease. Comput. Methods Programs Biomed. **226**, 107056 (2022)
8. Imani, V., Prakash, M., Zare, M., Tohka, J.: Comparison of single and multitask learning for predicting cognitive decline based on MRI data. IEEE Access **9**, 154275–154291 (2021)
9. Tuv, E., Borisov, A., Runger, G., Torkkola, K.: Feature selection with ensembles, artificial variables, and redundancy elimination. J. Mach. Learn. Res. **10**, 1341–1366 (2009)
10. Imani, V., Sevilla-Salcedo, C., Fortino, V., Tohka, J.: Multi-objective genetic algorithm for multi-view feature selection. arXiv preprint arXiv:2305.18352 (2023)
11. Mafarja, M.M., Mirjalili, S.: Hybrid whale optimization algorithm with simulated annealing for feature selection. Neurocomputing **260**, 302–312 (2017)
12. Zhu, X., Wu, X., Chen, Q.: Eliminating class noise in large datasets. In: Proceedings of the 20th International Conference on Machine Learning (ICML 2003), pp. 920–927 (2003)
13. Wang, Y., Ma, X., Chen, Z., Luo, Y., Yi, J., Bailey, J.: Symmetric cross entropy for robust learning with noisy labels. In: Proceedings of the IEEE/CVF International Conference on Computer Vision, pp. 322–330 (2019)
14. Zhou, X., Liu, X., Zhai, D., Jiang, J., Ji, X.: Asymmetric loss functions for noise-tolerant learning: theory and applications. In: IEEE Transactions on Pattern Analysis and Machine Intelligence (2023)
15. Gong, C., et al.: Class-wise denoising for robust learning under label noise. IEEE Trans. Pattern Anal. Mach. Intell. **45**(3), 2835–2848 (2022)
16. Natarajan, N., Dhillon, I.S., Ravikumar, P.K., Tewari, A.: Learning with noisy labels. In: Advances in Neural Information Processing Systems, vol. 26 (2013)
17. Deb, K., Pratap, A., Agarwal, S., Meyarivan, T.: A fast and elitist multiobjective genetic algorithm: NSGA-II. IEEE Trans. Evol. Comput. **6**(2), 182–197 (2002)
18. Shannon, C.E.: A mathematical theory of communication. Bell Syst. Tech. J. **27**(3), 379–423 (1948)
19. Ghosh, A., Kumar, H., Sastry, P.S.: Robust loss functions under label noise for deep neural networks. In: Proceedings of the AAAI Conference on AI, vol. 31 (2017)
20. Zhang, Z., Sabuncu, M.: Generalized cross entropy loss for training deep neural networks with noisy labels. In: Advances in Neural Information Processing Systems, vol. 31 (2018)
21. Tanaka, D., Ikami, D., Yamasaki, T., Aizawa, K.: Joint optimization framework for learning with noisy labels. In: Proceedings of the IEEE Conference on Computer Vision and Pattern Recognition, pp. 5552–5560 (2018)
22. Liu, Y., Guo, H.: Peer loss functions: learning from noisy labels without knowing noise rates. In: ICML, pp. 6226–6236. PMLR (2020)

23. Křížek, P., Kittler, J., Hlaváč, V.: Improving stability of feature selection methods. In: Kropatsch, W.G., Kampel, M., Hanbury, A. (eds.) CAIP 2007. LNCS, vol. 4673, pp. 929–936. Springer, Heidelberg (2007). https://doi.org/10.1007/978-3-540-74272-2_115
24. Mangasarian, O., Street N., William, W., Street, W.: Breast Cancer Wisconsin (Diagnostic). UCI Machine Learning Repository (1995)
25. Moradi, E., Pepe, A., Gaser, C., Huttunen, H., Tohka, J.: Machine learning framework for early MRI-based Alzheimer's conversion prediction in mci subjects. Neuroimage **104**, 398–412 (2015)
26. Gaser, C., Dahnke, R., Thompson, P.M., Kurth, F., Luders, E., Initiative, A.D.N.: CAT–A computational anatomy toolbox for the analysis of structural MRI data. bioRxiv, pp. 2022–06 (2022)
27. Marcus, D.S., Wang, T.H., Parker, J., Csernansky, J.G., Morris, J.C., Buckner, R.L.: Open access series of imaging studies (OASIS): cross-sectional MRI data in young, middle aged, nondemented, and demented older adults. J. Cogn. Neurosci. **19**(9), 1498–1507 (2007)

Improving Early Diagnosis: The Intersection of Lean Healthcare and Computer Vision in Cancer Detection

Mazdak Maghanaki, Mohammad Shahin, F. Frank Chen, and Ali Hosseinzadeh(✉)

The University of Texas at San Antonio, San Antonio, TX 78249, USA
{Mazdak.mohammadimaghanaki,Mohammad.Shahin,ff.chen,
ali.hosseinzadehghobadlou}@utsa.edu

Abstract. Cancer is a relentless adversary, and late detection only grants it more time to tighten its grip on lives and futures, underscoring the critical importance of early diagnosis. The integration of Lean Healthcare principles and Computer Vision technology is reshaping the landscape of cancer detection and diagnosis. This approach combines Lean's focus on efficiency and process optimization with Computer Vision's ability to analyze medical images, leading to more accurate, timely, and patient-centric cancer detection methods. This study embarks on a comprehensive investigation, utilizing the YOLO (You Only Look Once) v7 network for cancer detection and harnessing the PanNuke dataset—an extensive repository featuring 205,343 nuclei spanning 19 distinct tissue types. Concurrently, it delves into the discourse surrounding the integration of Lean Healthcare practices, illuminating a pathway to enhance the efficiency of cancer detection through the collaborative utilization of computer vision models and Lean Healthcare principles. By using the YOLO general-purpose object detection algorithm, potential cancer cases are identified successfully. The model achieves a high detection accuracy of 91.76%, Confirming that computer vision algorithms are a dependable tool for expediting cancer detection with high accuracy.

Keywords: Lean Healthcare · Computer Vision · Deep Learning · Cancer Detection · Healthcare 4.0

1 Introduction

Cancer is a leading global cause of death. Many diagnosed with cancer fear lengthy and toxic treatments, especially in later stages. Society seeks a proactive approach to detect cancer earlier, improving effectiveness and reducing side effects. Early cancer detection greatly improves patient prognosis, treatment success, and quality of life and Identifying cancer early boosts survival rates, reduces treatment intensity, and lowers costs [1]. Computer vision, a branch of AI, shows promise in early cancer detection by swiftly and accurately analyzing medical images like X-rays, MRIs, and CT scans. Its speed and precision reduce human error, enabling rapid diagnosis. Machine learning in computer vision can uncover subtle patterns and anomalies, aiding in early detection of cancers like breast, lung, and skin cancers [2].

K. Daimi and A. Al Sadoon (Eds.): ACR 2024, LNNS 956, pp. 404–413, 2024.
https://doi.org/10.1007/978-3-031-56950-0_34

The significant advancements in computer vision, empowered by AI techniques, have notably leveraged the capabilities of YOLO v7 network to achieve highly efficient and accurate object detection tasks in various applications, including medical imaging for cancer diagnosis [3]. YOLO v7 network has recently gained significant attention in the field of cancer detection, especially in the context of lung cancer [3]. Its remarkable ability to efficiently detect and localize objects, combined with its speed and accuracy, makes it a compelling choice for identifying and analyzing lung nodules within computed tomography images [4]. The implementation of YOLO v7 in the detection of cancers has provided a robust framework for assisting radiologists in the early diagnosis and tracking of lung cancer, thereby contributing to improved patient outcomes and survival rates [5]. This study utilizes the PanNuke dataset to detect and classify various cancer types. Divided into two sections, it focuses on the application of YOLO v7-driven object detection algorithms. Additionally, the integration of Lean Healthcare practices is emphasized, offering a pathway to improve cancer detection efficiency through the collaborative implementation of computer vision models and Lean Healthcare principles.

1.1 YOLO V7 and Healthcare 4.0

The utilization of YOLO v7 as a deep learning AI model in the context of Healthcare 4.0 highlights the synergy between advanced technological applications and the evolution of healthcare, facilitating precise diagnostics and personalized patient-centric solutions. Healthcare 4.0 is characterized by the seamless integration of digital technologies and data-driven insights into healthcare processes. This transformation empowers healthcare providers to offer more personalized, efficient, and effective care. Within the realm of Healthcare 4.0, two prominent subdivisions hold great potential for revolutionizing cancer detection: Lean Healthcare and Computer Vision [6]. Figure 1 illustrates the subdivisions within Healthcare 4.0.

1.2 Lean Healthcare and Computer Vision in Cancer Detection

Lean principles, often synonymous with manufacturing, offer valuable applications in healthcare settings, aiding in the elimination of waste [7]. Within the healthcare industry, Lean practices have the potential to drive efficiencies in various areas. These include optimizing billing procedures, minimizing medical errors, ensuring healthcare workers are equipped with the necessary tools to provide optimal care to patients and stakeholders, and, importantly, reducing wait times in emergency departments and medical offices [8].

The integration of Lean Healthcare principles with Computer Vision in the context of cancer detection is not only feasible but highly synergistic. By incorporating Lean methodologies into the development and deployment of Computer Vision algorithms, healthcare institutions can further improve the efficiency and accuracy of cancer diagnosis. Lean practices can enhance data annotation, model training, and the overall management of image data, resulting in more precise and timely detections [9]. Lean

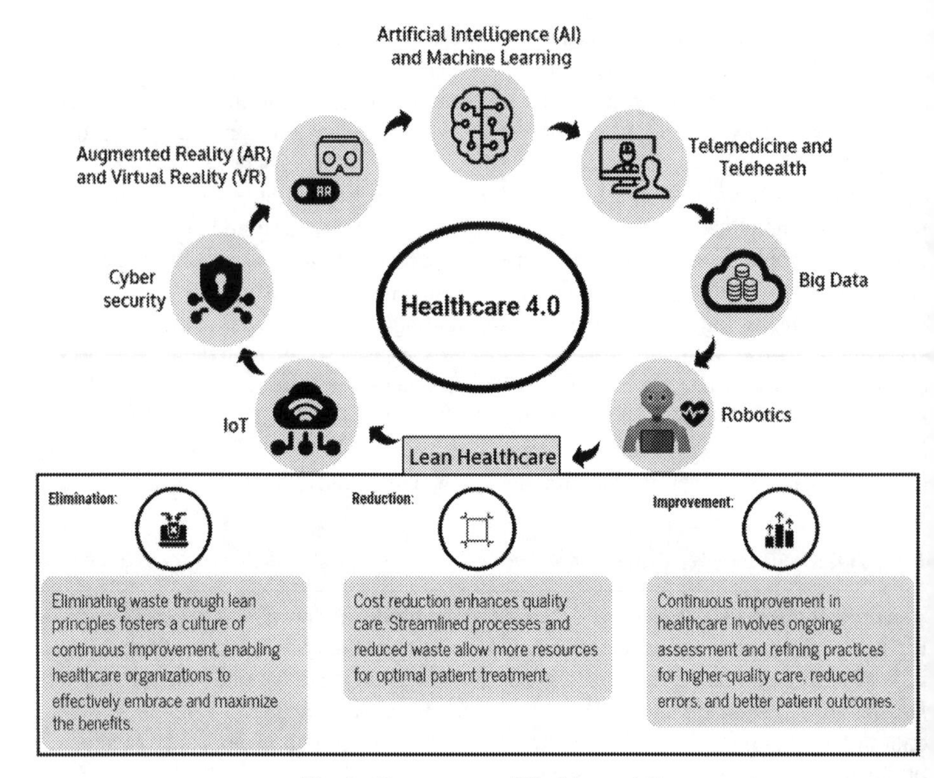

Fig. 1. Components of Healthcare 4.0

Healthcare can also play a pivotal role in addressing specific challenges in cancer detection via Computer Vision. For instance, it can optimize the workflow for radiologists and pathologists by prioritizing critical cases and minimizing unnecessary interventions [10]. Additionally, Lean methodologies can facilitate continuous improvement in algorithm performance, ensuring that Computer Vision systems remain up-to-date with the latest advancements in cancer diagnosis. Figure 2 illustrates the synergy between lean healthcare principles and computer vision technologies, emphasizing their role in improving cancer detection.

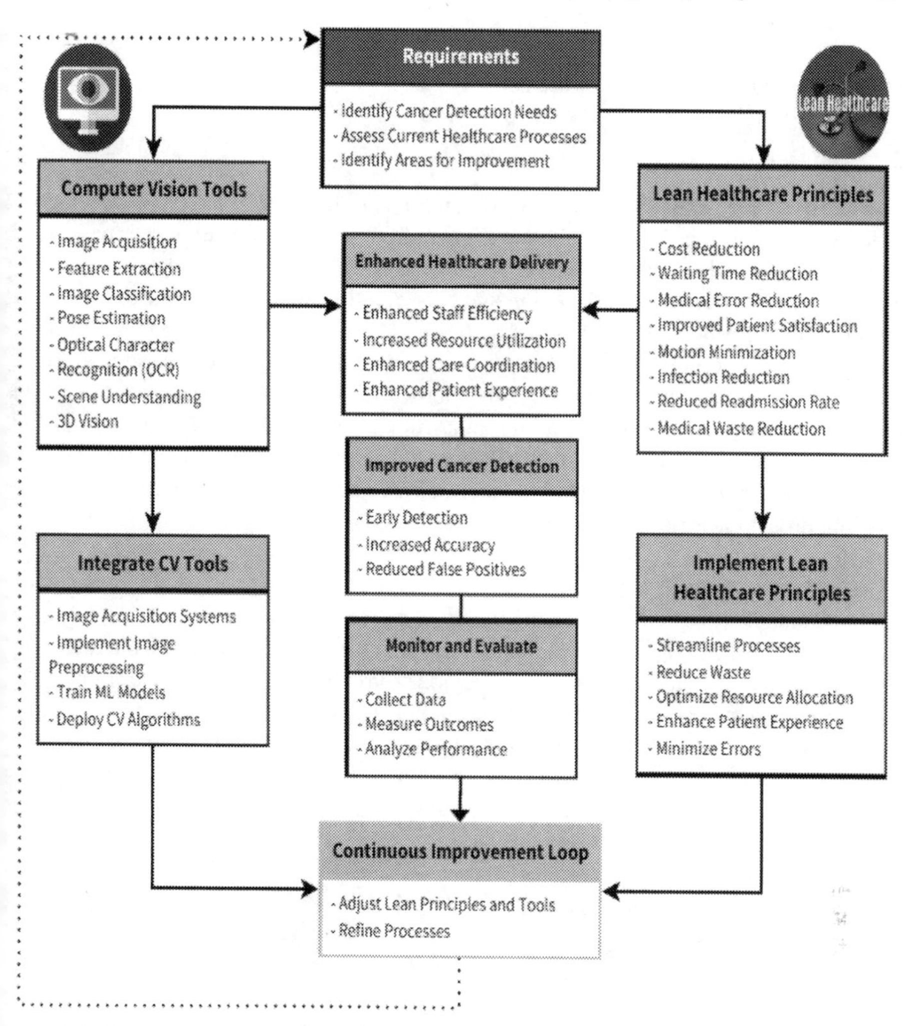

Fig. 2. Improving Cancer Detection Through Lean Principles and Computer Vision

2 Methodology

This study conducts a thorough investigation, making use of the YOLO (You Only Look Once) v7 network for cancer detection and tapping into the extensive PanNuke dataset [11], which encompasses 205,343 nuclei across 19 distinct tissue types. In parallel, it explores the discourse concerning the integration of Lean Healthcare practices, shedding light on a promising pathway to enhance the efficiency of cancer detection through the collaborative utilization of computer vision models and Lean Healthcare principles.

The selection of training epochs was informed by a comprehensive analysis of the model's convergence behavior. Balancing training time, computational resources, and the model's learning capacity, we determined the optimal number of epochs. This approach ensured the model achieved convergence without overfitting or underfitting, effectively learning the intricate features of the dataset.

2.1 Dataset

The PanNuke dataset [11], comprising 205,343 nuclei from 19 tissue types, is a meticulously crafted resource with instance segmentation and classification. Derived from 20,000+ whole slide images, it showcases diverse magnifications. This dataset serves as a benchmark for nucleus segmentation and classification in pathology images, promoting algorithm development. it focuses on multi-class nuclei classification and instance segmentation, offering comprehensive annotations and five distinct classes based on morphology and staining attributes. This dataset was curated by three board-certified pathologists using a custom annotation tool. They categorized nuclei into five classes: necrotic, connective (pertaining to soft tissues), neoplastic, inflammatory, and epithelial, with a fourth pathologist ensuring label validity and consistency. Figure 3 shows the labeling process across 19 tissue types. Figure 4 illustrates class distribution per tissue type.

The data underwent preprocessing to meet the YOLO model's requirements. This involved resizing images, normalizing pixel values, and augmenting the dataset. Image resizing standardized input dimensions, simplifying the training process while retaining crucial spatial information. Pixel value normalization enhanced the model's training convergence, preventing issues like vanishing gradients and facilitating faster convergence. Techniques such as random rotation, flipping, and brightness adjustments exposed the model to diverse variations in input data, enabling it to learn more robust and comprehensive features. The dataset was carefully split to ensure a balance between training

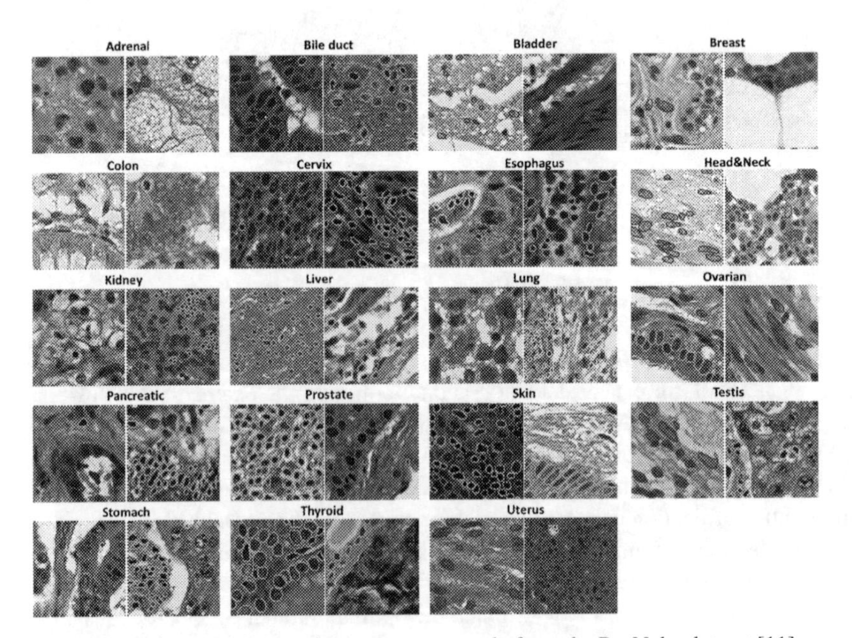

Fig. 3. Illustrating diverse tissue types, a sample from the PanNuke dataset [11]

and validation performance. 70% of the dataset was designated for training to enable the model to capture complex features and patterns effectively. A representative subset of 15% was reserved for validation purposes, allowing an assessment of the model's generalization ability and preventing overfitting. The remaining 15% of the dataset was used as the testing set, providing an unbiased evaluation of the model's performance on unseen data. After thorough analysis of the model's convergence, we settled on 27 training epochs, considering computational resources, training time, and the model's learning capability. This choice facilitated convergence without overfitting or underfitting, enabling effective learning of intricate dataset features.

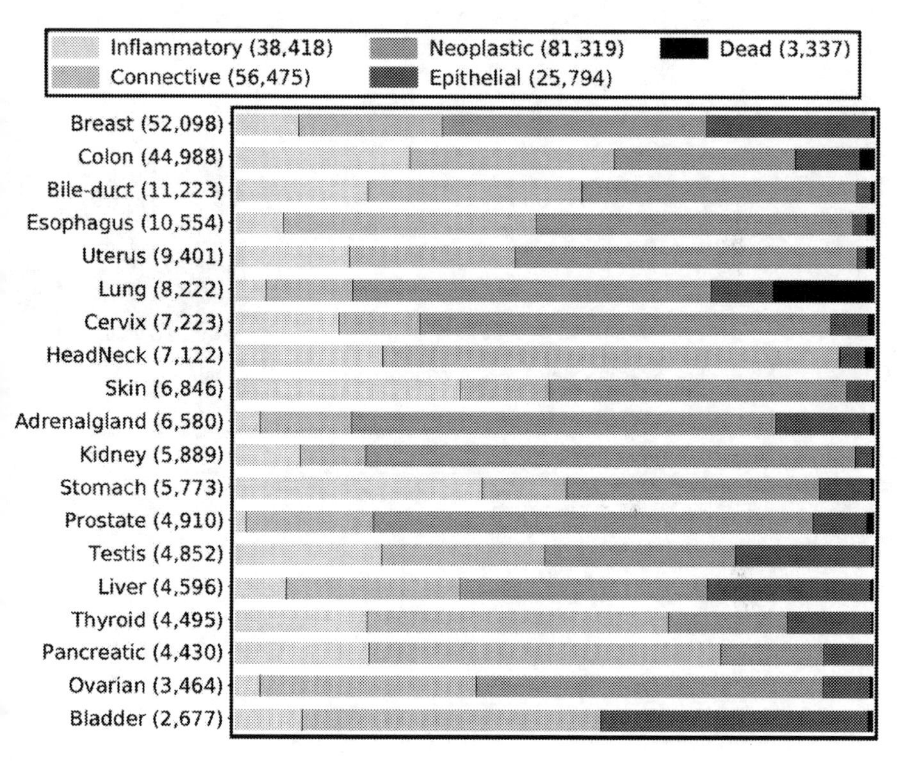

Fig. 4. Class statistics per tissue [11]

2.2 YOLO (You Only Look Once)

YOLO, a real-time object detection algorithm renowned for its remarkable speed and precision, distinguishes itself from other models like Mask R-CNN. YOLO's distinctive approach involves partitioning the input image into a grid of cells and subsequently predicting bounding boxes and class probabilities for each cell, all within the framework of a single Convolutional Neural Network (CNN) [12, 13]. YOLO v7 was selected for its strong history in object detection, showcasing a balance between precision and computational speed. Its architecture integrates anchor boxes and feature pyramid networks, enabling the model to effectively detect objects of varying sizes and proportions in intricate environments [14]. Figure 5 offers a visual depiction of YOLO v7's architecture, while Fig. 6 provides a graphical representation of its training loss across epochs.

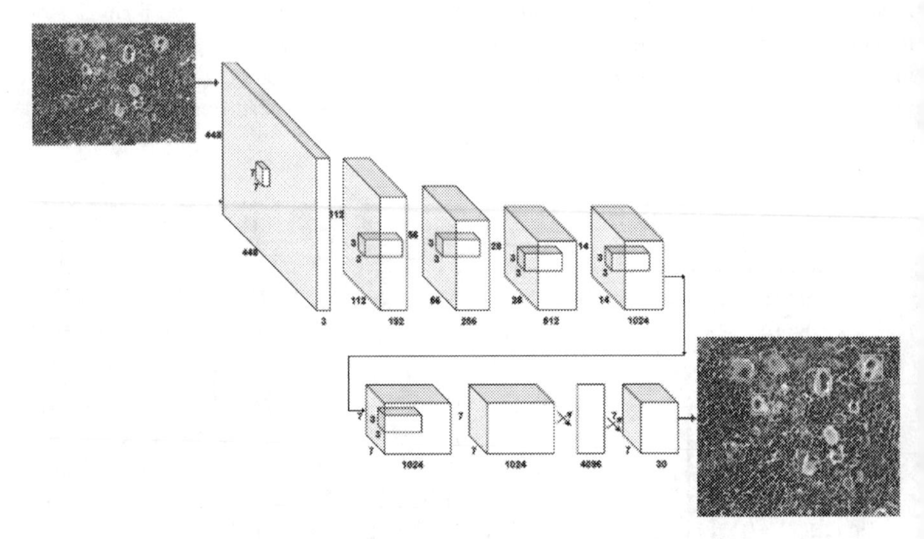

Fig. 5. The schematic architecture of YOLO v7 model

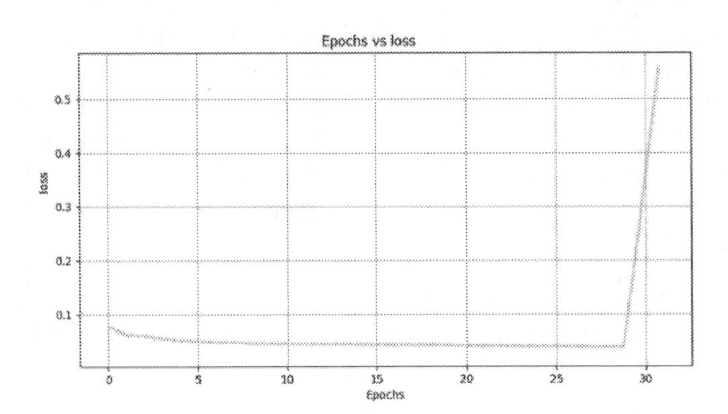

Fig. 6. The loss per epoch value for YOLO v7 model

3 Results and Discussion

The proposed method has been developed using the supervised learning algorithm Yolo (CNN architecture of deep learning). There were 22,733 tissue pattern images comprising 205,343 nuclei from 19 tissue types. 70% of the dataset was allocated for training, 15% for validation, and the remaining 15% for testing. A confusion matrix was used to evaluate the performance of our model. The performance of computer-based vision algorithms is determined based on the elements of their confusion matrix, which include True Positive (TP), False Positive (FP), False Negative (FN), and True Negative (TN). Additionally, several performance metrics for the classification model can be calculated from the confusion matrix, such as accuracy, precision, recall, and F1 score. These metrics can provide insights into the strengths and weaknesses of the model and/or the data used for training. Table 1 summarizes these values for YOLO v7 model, while Table 2 shows a summary of the average values of performance measurements. Figure 7 presents the performance measurement values for the model.

Table 1. TP, FP, TN, and FN results for YOLO v7

Custom Built Ml Model	Class Risk Level	TP	TN	FP	FN
YOLO v7	Neoplastic	20135	25148	3814	2354
	Inflammatory	6376	40040	2116	2919
	Connective	8171	37429	2256	3595
	Dead	433	49887	813	318
	Epithelial	5738	42702	1599	1412

Table 2. Average values of performance measurements

	Accuracy	Precision	Sensitivity	F1 score	Specificity	G-meanl
YOLO v7	91.76%	70.10%	73.10%	70.93%	94.18%	82.62%

Attaining a remarkable 91.76% detection accuracy, YOLO v7 underscores its pivotal role as a reliable instrument for expediting cancer detection. This achievement highlights how computer vision algorithms can significantly enhance the speed and cost-effectiveness of cancer detection processes.

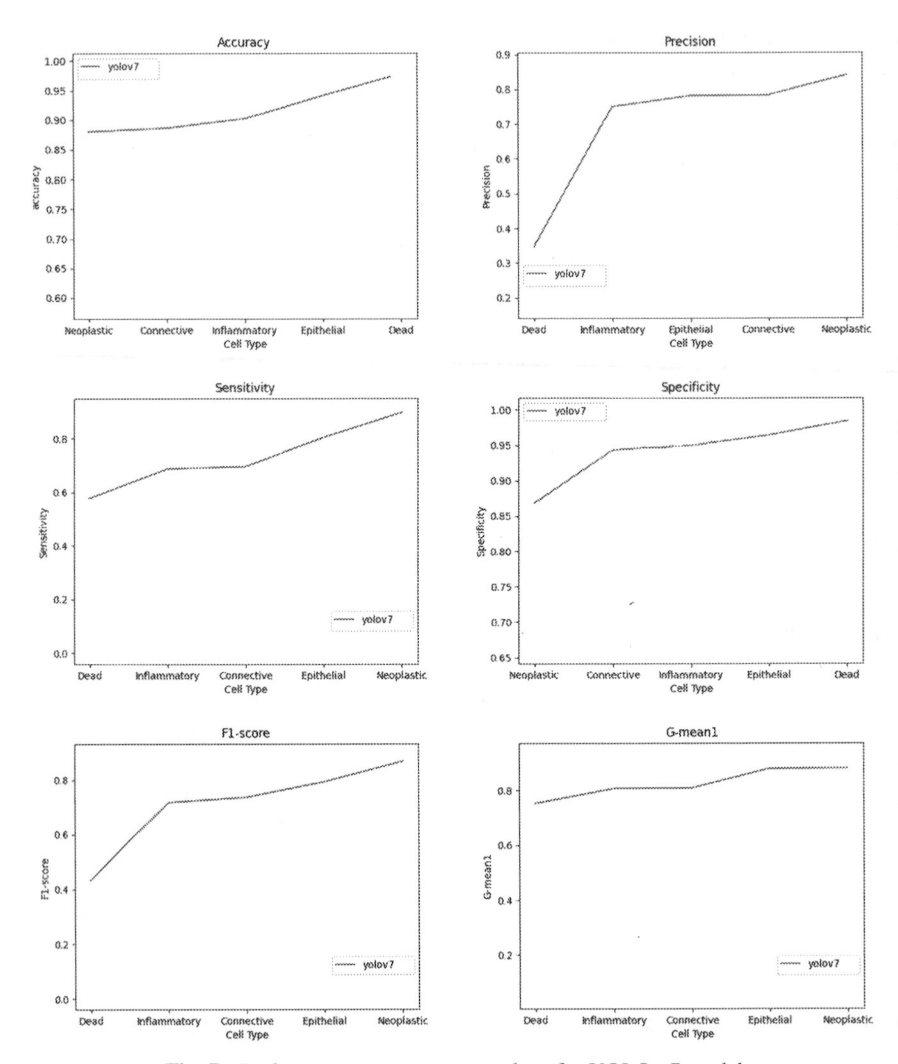

Fig. 7. Performance measurement values for YOLO v7 model

4 Conclusions

This study emphasizes the critical importance of early cancer diagnosis and presents a promising approach that combines Lean Healthcare principles with Computer Vision technology. By integrating Lean methodologies into the development and deployment of Computer Vision algorithms, healthcare institutions can significantly improve the efficiency and accuracy of cancer detection. The study utilized the YOLO v7 network and the extensive PanNuke dataset, achieving an impressive detection accuracy of 91.76%. These results affirm that computer vision algorithms are dependable tools for expediting cancer detection with high precision. This intersection of Lean Healthcare and Computer Vision holds great potential to enhance patient prognosis, treatment outcomes, and overall healthcare efficiency, offering a proactive solution in the fight against cancer.

Acknowledgments. The reported research work received partial financial support from Office of Naval Research MEEP Program (Award Number: N00014-19-1-2728), and Department of Energy/NNSA (Award Number: DE-NA0004003), as well as from the Lutcher Brown Distinguished Chair Professorship fund of the University of Texas at San Antonio.

References

1. Fitzgerald, R.C., Antoniou, A.C., Fruk, L., Rosenfeld, N.: The future of early cancer detection. Nat. Med. **28**(4), 666–677 (2022)
2. Tran, W.T., et al.: Personalized breast cancer treatments using artificial intelligence in radiomics and pathomics. J. Med. Imaging Radiat. Sci. **50**(4), S32–S41 (2019)
3. Mammeri, S., Amroune, M., Haouam, M. Y., Bendib, I., Corrêa Silva, A.: Early detection and diagnosis of lung cancer using YOLO v7, and transfer learning. Multimed. Tools Appl. (2023). https://doi.org/10.1007/s11042-023-16864-y
4. Ji, Z., et al.: ELCT-YOLO: an efficient one-stage model for automatic lung tumor detection based on CT images. Mathematics **11**(10), 2344 (2023). https://doi.org/10.3390/math11102344
5. Terven, J., Cordova-Esparza, D.: A Comprehensive Review of YOLO: From YOLOv1 and Beyond (2023). https://doi.org/10.48550/ARXIV.2304.00501
6. Li, J., Carayon, P.: Health care 4.0: a vision for smart and connected health care. IISE Trans. Healthc. Syst. Eng. **11**(3), 171–180 (2021)
7. Shahin, M., Chen, F.F., Bouzary, H., Krishnaiyer, K.: Integration of lean practices and industry 4.0 technologies: smart manufacturing for next-generation enterprises. Int. J. Adv. Manuf. Technol. **107**, 2927–2936 (2020)
8. Antony, J., Sunder M, V., Sreedharan, R., Chakraborty, A., Gunasekaran, A.: A systematic review of Lean in healthcare: a global prospective. Int. J. Qual. Reliab. Manag. **36**(8), 1370–1391 (2019)
9. Shahin, M., Chen, F.F., Hosseinzadeh, A., Koodiani, H.K., Shahin, A., Nafi, O.A.: A smartphone-based application for an early skin disease prognosis: Towards a lean healthcare system via computer-based vision. Adv. Eng. Inform. **57**, 102036 (2023). https://doi.org/10.1016/j.aei.2023.102036
10. Akmal, A., Greatbanks, R., Foote, J.: Lean thinking in healthcare–findings from a systematic literature network and bibliometric analysis. Health Policy **124**(6), 615–627 (2020)
11. Gamper, J., et al.: PanNuke Dataset Extension, Insights and Baselines, April 2020. https://doi.org/10.48550/arXiv.2003.10778
12. Jiang, P., Ergu, D., Liu, F., Cai, Y., Ma, B.: A review of YOLO algorithm developments. Procedia Comput. Sci. **199**, 1066–1073 (2022)
13. Shahin, M., Frank Chen, F., Bouzary, H., Hosseinzadeh, A.: Deploying convolutional neural network to reduce waste in production system. In: 51st SME North American Manufacturing Research Conference (NAMRC 51), vol. 35, pp. 1187–1195, August 2023. https://doi.org/10.1016/j.mfglet.2023.08.127
14. Shahin, M., Chen, F.F., Hosseinzadeh, A., Khodadadi Koodiani, H., Bouzary, H., Shahin, A.: Enhanced safety implementation in 5S+ 1 via object detection algorithms. Int. J. Adv. Manuf. Technol. 1–21 (2023)

Fast Artificial Intelligence Detecting Climate Change Effects in Imaging Data

Birgitta Dresp-Langley[1] (✉) and John M. Wandeto[2]

[1] CNRS UMR 7357 Strasbourg University, 67200 Strasbourg, France
birgitta.dresp@cnrs.fr

[2] Dedan Kimathi University of Technology, Nyeri, Kenya
john.wandeto@dkut.ac.ke

Abstract. Satellite images display visual data relating to natural or urban landscapes. In the course of time, they reveal structural alterations therein that may be a consequence of climate change. Capturing such visual data rapidly to make them available to citizens, professionals, and policymakers promotes awareness and assists decision making for action. We applied unsupervised Artificial Intelligence (AI) to the analysis of a time series of satellite images using Self-Organizing Maps (SOM). The Quantization Error (QE) in the map output is exploited as an indicator of change. Given the proven sensitivity of this neural network metric to intensity and polarity of image pixel contrast, and its proven selectivity to pixel colour, it is shown to capture critical changes in the water levels of Lake Mead across the years 1984–2008. The SOM-QE analysis is combined with statistical trend analysis to further highlight the magnitude and the direction of pixel contrast changes in specific regions of interest. We show that the structural change in the Lake Mead region is significantly correlated with demographic data for the same reference time period, translating the impact of human activities on the local environment. The results of this study show the usefulness of SOM-QE analysis as a parsimonious and reliable AI approach to the analysis of minimally pre-processed satellite images for rapid detection of environmental degradation as a consequence of human activities and climate change.

Keywords: Satellite Images · Climate Change · Landscapes · Structures · Water Levels · Change · Self Organizing Map (SOM) · Quantization Error · Public Data

1 Introduction

Identifying potentially relevant climate change or human activity-related phenomena by observing remotely sensed imaging data of earth states or landscapes at different moments in time [1] requires a reliable quantification of the critical changes. To show their evolution with time requires the ordering of discrete image data sets into meaningful time series [2]. This is facilitated in the case of time stamped images provided by satellites that observe Earth and other planetary bodies via remote sensors. These latter detect and record reflected or emitted energy, and provide not only a global perspective but also a wealth of data about Earth systems, enabling data-informed decision making based on

K. Daimi and A. Al Sadoon (Eds.): ACR 2024, LNNS 956, pp. 414–424, 2024.
https://doi.org/10.1007/978-3-031-56950-0_35

current and future states of the planet in image time series, generated through repetitive coverage at short temporal intervals. Also, as pointed out previously [3], a consistent quality of such imaging data can be ensured by minimal pre-processing. In this study here, extracts from a satellite image time series of a specific geographic Region Of Interest (ROI), Lake Mead Reservoir in the Nevada Desert of the United Stated of America, were analyzed. To quantify the effects of human activity and climate change on the water levels of the lake, we exploit a local change detection metric generated by the Self-Organizing Map (SOM), first introduced by Kohonen [4]. After pre-processing to guarantee consistency in scale and contrast intensity across images of the series, the resulting images were directly fed into the SOM without further annotation or additional, intermediate procedure of analysis. Our extensive and well-documented previous work [5–16] had permitted establishing that the Quantization Error (*QE*) in the SOM output, can be directly exploited as computational metric of critical local changes in images of one and the same location or object taken at different moments in time [6, 9], or temporal series of sensor data [7, 8, 10–16]. In this work here, we show simulations exploiting SOM-QE analysis [5] to demonstrate its statistically significant sensitivity to the spatial extent of local pixel contrast translating the effects of climate change and human activities on the water levels of Lake Mead Reservoir. NASA Landsat images of Lake Mead from the time period between 1984 and 2008 were chosen for this study. Lake Mead is a large reservoir on the main stem of the Colorado River, which flows through the Grand Canyon before reaching Lake Mead on the border between Arizona and Nevada. Lake Mead is surrounded by the Hoover Dam, which control floods, provides water irrigation, and produces hydroelectric power. Being one of the largest water reservoirs in the USA, the lake is a major source of supply for Nevada Arizona, and California. Over the last decades, climate change has led to hotter and drier conditions in Nevada that have accelerated the depletion of Lake Mead. Lake Mead's water source, the Colorado River, is supplied by snowmelt from the Colorado Rockies. Heat-trapping greenhouse gas emissions from the burning of fossil fuels and other human activities have warmed the planet, and the resulting temperature increase and changing precipitation patterns in the region have reduced snowpack and rain and dried out soils, contributing to lower water levels of Lake Mead, and other water sources, across the years. In the last year of the reference period of this study, nearly 20 million (now more) people in Las Vegas depended on the lake's supply. The reservoir also ensures water and energy supply for the many farms in the extensive land areas beyond Las Vegas, with a distance of 24 miles separating Lake Mead itself from the heart of Las Vegas and the Strip. The time period selected for this study is of particular interest insofar as it reveals the combined effects of climate change and a steep increase in human footprint on the water levels of the lake. In addition, major alterations of the surrounding natural landscape due to increasing global warming have been observed during that period. The results from the SOM-QE analysis exploited here are directly compared with the water level statistics from the Hoover Dam control room from the same years. The results and conclusions drawn from this study highlight SOM-QE analysis as an inexpensive, ready-to-use AI technology for visualizing potentially relevant temporal evolutions in pixel contents, relating to climate change effects and human impact on geographic ROI as illustrated here.

2 Materials and Methods

2.1 Image Input Processing

The 25 images of the geographic ROI, pre-processed and then submitted to SOM-QE analysis, were extracted from time-lapse animations of Lake Mead, Nevada, for a reference time period from 1984 to 2008, as captured by NASA Landsat sensors [17]. VLC, an open source media player, was used to generate static images from the time-lapse animations provided. The images are colour-coded, showing arid regions in brownish-green and healthy vegetation in red. Water is represented by black pixels. Sample copies of two of the 25 original satellite images are shown here below (Fig. 1).

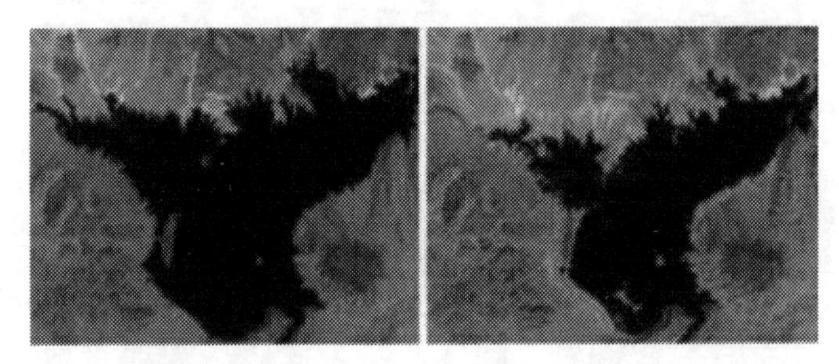

Fig. 1. Illustration of the first and the last two of the 25 images extracted from the NASA satellite time series, from the years 1984 (left) and 2008 (right) displaying the geographic ROI of this study.

Before running SOM-QE analysis on the image time series of this geographic ROI, all the images were pre-processed to ensure they are identically scaled and aligned. This was achieved by applying the method of co-registration using *StackReg* [18], which is a plug-in for *ImageJ*, an open source image processing program designed for scientific multidimensional image processing. The last image of the time series was used to anchor the registration. Control for variations in contrast intensity between images of the series was performed after registration. This was achieved by increasing the image contrast and by removing any local variations at different times of image acquisition [18–20]. For each extracted image, contrast normalization was ensured using

$$Ifinal = (I - Imin/Imax - Imin) \times 255 \tag{1}$$

The registered and normalized image taken in 2011 from each ROI was used to train a 4 by 4 SOM with a neighborhood distance of 1.2 and a learning rate of 0.2 for 10,000 iterations [5]. Since the original images used color to emphasize different areas on the maps, pixel-based RGB values are used as input features to the SOM. This ensures a pixel-by-pixel capture of detail and avoids errors due to inaccurate feature calculation which often occur with complex images [21].

2.2 SOM-QE Analysis

The Self-Organizing Map (a prototype is graphically represented in Fig. 2 for illustration) may be described formally as a nonlinear, ordered, smooth mapping of high-dimensional input data onto the elements of a regular, low-dimensional array [5–16].

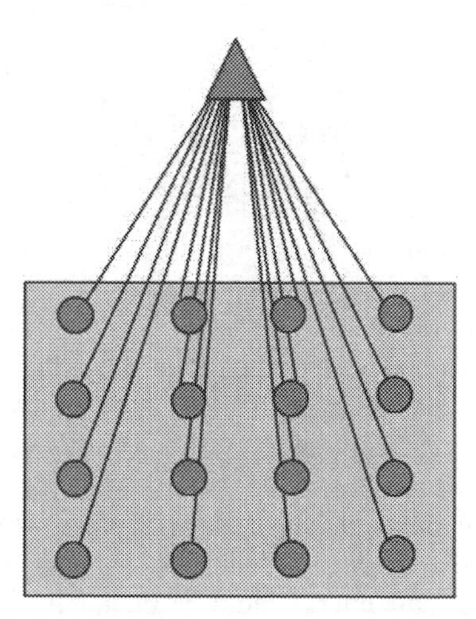

Fig. 2. Representation of the 4 × 4 SOM prototype with 16 models, indicated by the filled circles in the grey box. Each of these models is compared to the SOM input in an unsupervised winner-take-all learning process. The input vector corresponds to the RGB image pixel space.

It is assumed that the set of input variables can be defined as a real vector x, of n-dimensionality. A parametric real vector m_i of n-dimension is associated with each element in the SOM. Vector m_i is a model and the SOM is therefore an array of models. Assuming a general distance measure between x and m_i denoted by $d(x,m_i)$, the map of an input vector x on the SOM array is defined as the array element m_c that matches best (smallest $d(x,m_i)$) with x. During the learning process, the input vector x is compared with all the m_i in order to identify m_c. The Euclidean distances $\|x\text{-}m_i\|$ define m_c. Models topographically close in the map up to a certain geometric distance, indicated by h_{ci}, will activate each other to learn something from their common input x. This results in a local relaxation or smoothing effect on the models in this neigborhood, which in continuous learning leads to global ordering. SOM learning is represented by the equation

$$m(t+1) = m_i(t) + \alpha(t)h_{ci}(t)\lceil x(t) - m_i(t)\rceil \qquad (2)$$

where $t = 1, 2, 3\ldots$ is an integer, the discrete-time coordinate, $h_{ci}(t)$ is the neighborhood function, a smoothing kernel defined over the map points which converges towards zero with time, $\alpha(t)$ is the learning rate, which also converges towards zero with time and affects the amount of learning in each model. At the end of the *winner-take-all* learning process in the SOM, each image input vector x becomes associated to its best matching model on the map m_c. The difference between x and m_c, $\|x - m_c\|$, is a measure of how close the final SOM value is to the original input value and is reflected by the quantization error, QE. The average QE of all x (X) in an image is given by

$$QE = 1/N \sum_{i=1}^{N} \|X_i - m_{c_i}\| \tag{3}$$

where N is the number of input vectors x in the image. The final weights of the SOM are defined by a three dimensional output vector space representing each R, G, and B channel. The magnitude as well as the direction of change in any of these from one image to another is reliably reflected by changes in the QE. The SOM training process consisted of 1 000 iterations for a two-dimensional rectangular map of 4 by 4 nodes capable of creating 16 model observations from the data. The spatial locations, or coordinates, of each of the 16 models or domains, placed at different locations on the map, exhibit characteristics that make each one different from all the others. When a new input signal is presented to the map, the models compete and the winner will be the model the features of which most closely resemble those of the input signal. The input signal will thus be classified or grouped in one of models. Each model or domain acts like a separate decoder for the same input, i.e. independently interprets the information carried by a new input. The input is represented as a mathematical vector of the same format as that of the models in the map. Therefore, it is the presence or absence of an active response at a specific map location and not so much the exact input-output signal transformation or magnitude of the response that provides the interpretation of the input. To obtain the initial values for the map size, a trial-and-error process was implemented. Map sizes larger than 4 by 4 produced observations where some models ended up empty, which meant that these models did not attract any input by the end of the training. As a consequence, 16 models were sufficient to represent all the fine structures in the image data. Neighborhood distance and learning rate were constant at 1.2 and 0.2 respectively. These values were obtained through the trial-and-error method after testing the quality of the first guess, which is directly determined by the value of the resulting quantization error; the lower this value, the better the first guess. It is worthwhile pointing out that the models were initialized by randomly picking vectors from the training image. This allows the SOM to work on the original data without any prior assumptions about any level of organization within the data. This, however, requires starting with a wider neighborhood function and a higher learning-rate factor than in procedures where initial values for model vectors are pre-selected [17]. The approach is economical in terms of computation times, which constitutes one of its major advantages for rapid change *versus* no change detection on the basis of even larger sets of image data, prior to any further human intervention or decision making. The last image of the series from the time range here was used to train the SOM (4×4 neural network architecture with a 1.2 neighbourhood distance and a learning rate of 0.2 for 10,000 iterations). After training, SOM-QE analysis permits determining the QE in the map output for each of the 25 images of the series. The code used for implementing the SOM-QE is available [ref] in the "R-badged articles" series of the journal *Software Impacts*, a collection that presents software publications that have been verified for computational reproducibility by CodeOcean, a cloud-based computational reproducibility platform that helps the community by enabling sharing of code and data as a resource for non-commercial use. Certified papers have an attached Reproducibility Badge, a permanent Reproducible Capsule and are listed on the CodeOcean website.

3 Results

The QE data from the SOM analysis of the satellite images from the subsequent years of the study time period, with the water level statistics from these same years in feet above the sea level are summarized in Table 1 here below.

Table 1. SOM-QE data and water levels for the years of the study time period.

Year	SOM-QE	Water Level
1984	0,5534	1214,9100
1985	0,5544	1209,4600
1986	0,5478	1209,7400
1987	0,5459	1208,8400
1988	0,5407	1204,5600
1989	0,5356	1192,0000
1990	0,5352	1183,6900
1991	0,5208	1175,4300
1992	0,5204	1188,5900
1993	0,5238	1176,3900
1994	0,5211	1182,1800
1995	0,5276	1182,4000
1996	0,5280	1191,9800
1997	0,5383	1202,9300
1998	0,5448	1213,7100
1999	0,5442	1210,4100
2000	0,5338	1204,2200
2001	0,5077	1185,8000
2002	0,4900	1163,1700
2003	0,4953	1145,9300
2004	0,4603	1131,7600
2005	0,4657	1139,8700
2006	0,4607	1131,6600
2007	0,4725	1118,0000
2008	0,4588	1099,7200

When the QE is plotted as a function of the time of the image acquisition by Landsat (Fig. 3, left), we observe a decreasing QE for images of Lake Mead taken between the years 1984 and 1995, followed by an increase in the QE for images taken between the years 1995 and 2000, which is then followed by a sharp decrease for images taken between 2000 and 2008. The general trend is that of a decrease in QE as the years in which the images were taken progress. The Hoover Dam control room's water level statistics [22] given in yearly averages for the same time period are plotted for comparison (Fig. 3, right).

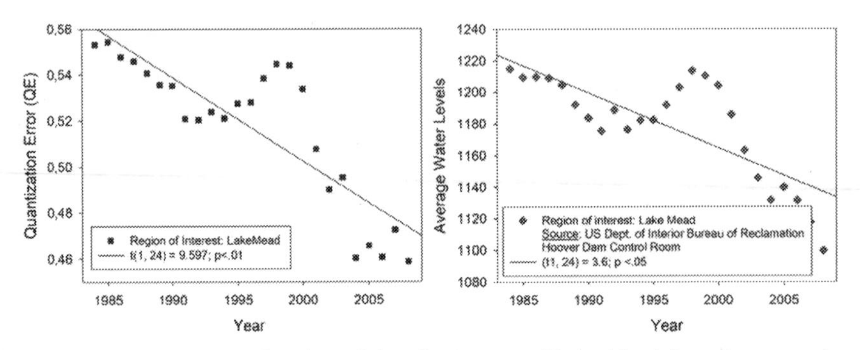

Fig. 3. The *QE* plotted as a function of time for images of Lake Mead from the years chosen (left), and the average water level estimates for these same years (right).

Linear regression analysis was then performed on these data. The correlation coefficient R^2 from this analysis gives an estimate of the part of variance in the data that is accounted for by a linear trend/fit. Statistical significance is determined by the probability that the linear adjustment sufficiently differs from zero on the basis of Student's distribution (t). The results from the comparison QE *versus* year of image acquisition reveal a statistically significant linear trend towards decrease in *QE* as a function of time. The linear regression coefficient ($R^2 = .75$) relating to this comparison, graphically shown in the fit on the left in Fig. 3, is statistically significant, with t (1, 24) = 9.59, $p < .01$. This significant downward trend in the *QE* from the SOM output directly translates, as shown previously in our work on cell imaging data [10], a highly meaningful decrease in the amount of black pixel contents, representing water in the study images here. The imaging differences captured by the neural network analysis thus directly translate different states of Lake Mead, as consistently reflected by data from public archives for these same years in terms of the Hoover Dam control room's water level statistics. For the comparison water level averages *versus* year of reference period, the linear trend analysis, graphically shown in the fit on the right of Fig. 3, also yields a statistically significant regression coefficient ($R^2 = .71$) with t (1, 24) = 3.60, $p < .05$. Table 2 gives a summary of these results for each comparison with the corresponding Degrees of Freedom (DF).

In the next analysis, the correlation between the *QE* distribution from the neural model (SOM-QE analysis) and the distribution reflecting the yearly water level averages was computed. Correlations are useful because they can indicate a predictive relationship between variables, which then can be further exploited in practice. To that effect we computed Pearson's correlation coefficient r, which mathematically determines statistical covariance. The probability p that the covariance of two observables is statistically significant is determined by the magnitude of the Pearson coefficient, which is directly

Table 2. Summary of the results from the linear trend analyses.

Comparison	DF	t	R^2	Probability (p)
QE *vs* Year	1, 24	9.59	.75	<.01
Water Level *vs* Year	1, 24	3.60	.71	<.05

linked to the strength of correlation, while its sign is directly linked to the direction of the covariance (positive or negative) of two variables.

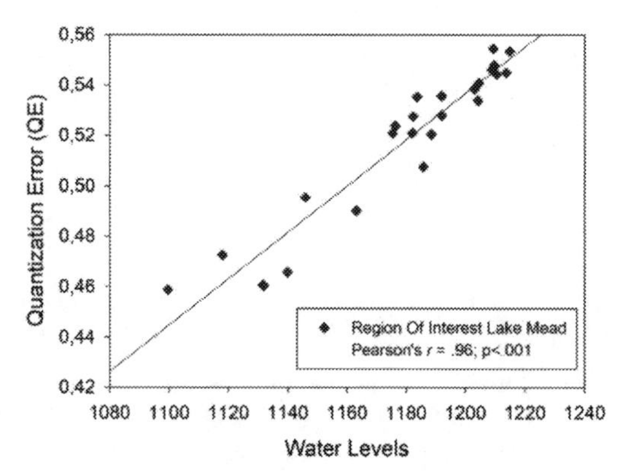

Fig. 4. Pearson correlation (r) between the QE data from the SOM satellite image analysis and Hoover Dam Control Room's yearly average water level estimates (in feet above sea level).

This analysis, performed on the paired distributions for QE and the average yearly water estimates, returned a statistically significant positive correlation ($r = .96$; $p < .001$) between the two variables. Outliers were not present in the data, which are represented graphically here above (Fig. 4). Further statistics from public archives [23] show a consistent increase in population estimates in thousands (Fig. 5, left), and in visitors in millions (Fig. 5, right) between the years 1984 and 1999 for Las Vegas and regions relying on the water and energy provided by Lake Mead. According to the Las Vegas population review website [24], the population estimates (Fig. 5, left) have remained relatively constant since 1999 while, according to the Las Vegas Convention and Visitors Authority [23], the visitor volume (Fig. 5, right) diminished considerably during the recent pandemic between 2019 and 2022. Recently, in March 2023, it once again reached the 40 million high from 2009 shown in the graph on the right here below.

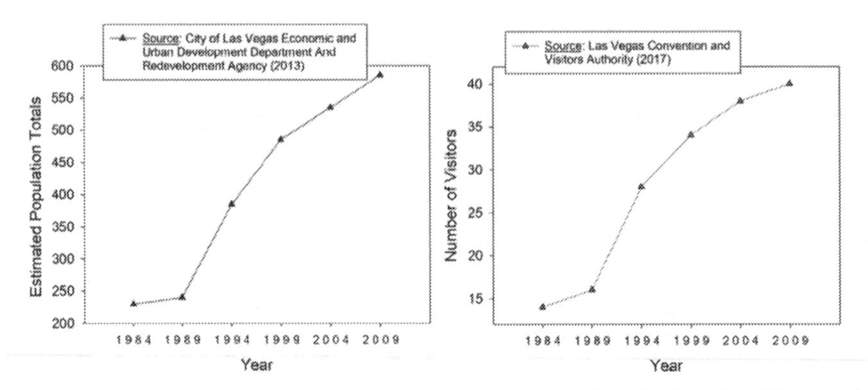

Fig. 5. Population estimates in thousands (left) and estimated number of visitors in millions (right) for the Las Vegas region consistent with a steeply increasing human impact on the water reservoir in the years given.

4 Conclusions

Using the example of satellite images of Lake Mead, USA, it is shown that the Quantization Error (*QE*) in the output of a SOM after unsupervised *winner-take-all* image pixel learning reliably signals changes in content relating to meaningful landscape changes as a consequence of human impact and climate change [1, 2]. The reference time period during which the satellite images for this study were taken was a time where both the human impact on Lake Mead and global warming were increasing steadily according to national statistics. The last image from the time series for this study was taken 15 years ago. In 2022, the water levels of Lake Mead reached drastically low levels in the summer, prompting fears that the much dreaded point where water levels are too low to flow downstream (*dead pool effect*) would occur much sooner than anticipated by experts. In the meantime, the lake's water levels have recovered a little in the summer in 2023 due to above-average precipitations and snowpack from the mountains melting. A meaningful interpretation of such and other environmental data in association with human impact measures, as shown here in this study example here, can be provided under the light of a consistent statistical co-variation with the *QE* from SOM-QE analysis of satellite imagery [5]. Other pixel colour-based approaches to the analysis of Earth images from satellites such as Landsat have been applied to study temporal changes relating to the effects of climate change like, for example, selective principal component analysis to study changes in blue ice extent in arctic regions [1]. SOM-QE analysis directly and automatically classifies such pixel color-coded image data, without any need of prior selection by a human. This highlights SOM-QE analysis as an inexpensive, ready-to-use AI technology making potentially relevant trends in climate change-related effects visible at a glance, without reference to prior knowledge or the need for image annotation by an expert.

References

1. Orheim, O., Lucchitta, B.: Investigating climate change by digital analysis of blue ice extent on satellite images of Antarctica. Ann. Glaciol. **14**, 211–215 (1990)
2. Furusawa, T., Koera, T., Siburian, R., et al.: Time-series analysis of satellite imagery for detecting vegetation cover changes in Indonesia. Sci. Rep. **13**, 8437 (2023)
3. Rosin, P.L., Ioannidis, E.: Evaluation of global image thresholding for change detection. Pattern Recognit. Lett. **24**, 2345–2356 (2003)
4. Kohonen, T.: MATLAB Implementation and Applications of the Self-Organizing Map. Unigrafia Oy Helsinki, Finland (2014)
5. Wandeto, J.M., Dresp-Langley, B.: SOM-QE ANALYSIS - a biologically inspired technique to detect and track meaningful changes within image regions. Softw. Impacts **17**, 100568 (2023)
6. Liu, R., Wandeto, J., Nageotte, F., Zanne, P., de Mathelin, M., Dresp-Langley, B.: Spatiotemporal modeling of grip forces captures proficiency in manual robot control. Bioengineering **10**, 59 (2023)
7. Dresp-Langley, B., Wandeto, J.M.: Unsupervised classification of cell-imaging data using the quantization error in a self-organizing map. In: Arabnia, H.R., Ferens, K., de la Fuente, D., Kozerenko, E.B., Olivas Varela, J.A., Tinetti, F.G. (eds.) Advances in Artificial Intelligence and Applied Cognitive Computing. Transactions on Computational Science and Computational Intelligence. LNCS, pp. 201–209. Springer, Cham (2021). https://doi.org/10.1007/978-3-030-70296-0_16
8. Dresp-Langley, B., Wandeto, J.M.: Human symmetry uncertainty detected by a self-organizing neural network map. Symmetry **13**, 299 (2021)
9. Dresp-Langley, B., Liu, R., Wandeto, J.M.: Surgical task expertise detected by a self-organizing neural network map (2021). https://doi.org/10.48550/arXiv.2106.08995
10. Dresp-Langley, B., Wandeto, J.M.: Pixel precise unsupervised detection of viral particle proliferation in cellular imaging data. Inform. Med. Unlocked **20**, 100433 (2020)
11. Wandeto, J.M., Dresp-Langley, B.: The quantization error in a self-organizing map as a contrast and colour specific indicator of single-pixel change in large random patterns. Neural Netw. **119**, 273–285 (2019)
12. Dresp, B., Nyongesa, H., Wandeto, J.M.: Vision-inspired automatic detection of water level changes in satellite images: the example of Lake Mead. Perception 48, ECVP Abstract Supplement (2019)
13. Wandeto, J.M., Dresp, B.: Ultrafast automatic classification of SEM image sets showing CD4 cells with varying extent of HIV virion infection. 7ièmes Journées de la Fédération de Médecine Translationnelle de Strasbourg, 25–26 May Strasbourg, France (2019)
14. Wandeto, J.M., Dresp-Langley, B.: The quantization error in a self-organizing map as a contrast and colour specific indicator of single-pixel change in large random patterns. Neural Networks 120, Special Issue in Honor of the 80th Birthday of Stephen Grossberg, pp. 116–128 (2019)
15. Wandeto, J.M., Nyongesa, H., Dresp-Langley, B.: Detection of smallest changes in complex images comparing self-organizing map to expert performance. Perception 46 ECVP Abstract Supplement (2017)
16. Wandeto, J.M., Nyongesa, H., Rémond, Y., Dresp-Langley, B.: Detection of small changes in medical and random-dot images comparing self-organizing map performance to human detection. Inform. Med. Unlocked **7**, 39–45 (2017)
17. NASA/Goddard Space Flight Center Landsat images from USGS Earth Explorer. ID: 10721, March 2012. http://svs.gsfc.nasa.gov/10721. Accessed 11 Aug 2023

18. The VLC media player source code. https://www.videolan.org/vlc/download-sources.html. Accessed 19 Aug 2023
19. Wieland, M., Pittore, M.: Performance evaluation of machine learning algorithms for urban pattern recognition from multi-spectral satellite images. Remote Sens. **6**, 2912–2939 (2014)
20. Schneider, C.A., Rasband, W.S., Eliceiri, K.W.: From NIH image to ImageJ: 25 years of image analysis. Nat. Methods **9**, 671 (2012)
21. Thévenaz, P., Ruttimann, U.E., Unser, M.A.: Pyramid approach to subpixel registration based on intensity. IEEE Trans. Image Process. **7**, 27–41 (1998)
22. US Department of Interior Bureau of Reclamation, Hoover Dam Control Room Statistics. https://www.usbr.gov/lc/region/g4000/hourly/mead-elv.html. Accessed 25 Oct 2023
23. Las Vegas Convention and Visitors Authority, Statistics. https://www.lvcva.com/. Accessed 20 Aug 2023
24. Las Vegas Population Review. https://worldpopulationreview.com/world-cities/las-vegas-population. Accessed 20 Aug 2023

A Web Application to Determine the Quality of Water Through the Identification of Macroinvertebrates

María-Isabel Cañar[1], Marcelo Flores[1,2(✉)], and Angélica Zea[1]

[1] Salesian Polytechnic University, Calle Vieja 12-30, Cuenca, Ecuador
mcanaru@est.ups.edu.ec, {mfloresv,azea}@ups.edu.ec
[2] Polytechnic University of Valencia, Camino de Vera s/n 46022, Valencia, Spain

Abstract. The quality of water present in rivers can be determined through the presence of certain types of aquatic macroinvertebrates.

This work shows the development of a mobile application that determines water quality through the identification of aquatic macroinvertebrates present in a river.

For the identification of macroinvertebrates, computer vision techniques were used, a convolutional neural network was trained using images of aquatic macroinvertebrates found in the Paute River basin (Cuenca - Ecuador) considering the analysis methods (ICA-NSF) and (BMWP/Col), to determine water quality.

The investigation further explores key performance metrics like precision, recall, F1-score, and support percentages.

The study extends its application to automated analysis of water quality indicators in organisms, utilizing computer vision techniques like OpenCV. This approach ensures instant, efficient information retrieval while maintaining ecological integrity. The integration of computer vision technologies opens ways to determine the quality of water in a river, in these places, without the need to transport samples to laboratories or know the types of macroinvertebrates that correspond to a certain level of water quality.

Keywords: computer vision · water quality · aquatic macroinvertebrates · mobile application · convolutional neural network

1 Theoretical Fundament

1.1 Bioindicators

Bioindicators are living organisms that are used to determine the current conditions of the water analyzed; they can be plants, animals, or microorganisms.

Each of them has specific characteristics that allow them to react to changes in the environment, such as pollution, soil alteration or climate change [1].

It can be deduced that bioindicators are living organisms or characteristics of an ecosystem that are used to measure environmental quality. Its presence or absence, as

K. Daimi and A. Al Sadoon (Eds.): ACR 2024, LNNS 956, pp. 425–435, 2024.
https://doi.org/10.1007/978-3-031-56950-0_36

well as its condition, are factors that indicate the state of an ecosystem and the influence of human actions on it. Bioindicators is a valuable tool for the evaluation and monitoring of environmental health either at a local or global level [2, 3].

In this study we focused on the use of bioindicators, with photographs of aquatic macroinvertebrates being the central component.

1.2 Aquatic Macroinvertebrates

They are considered aquatic organisms, clearly visible, they do not have a backbone, for example the larvae of insects, mollusks and crustaceans. Aquatic macroinvertebrates are sensitive to changes in the environment, such as pollution, temperature change or habitat alteration, and can be used as indicators of the current state of the aquatic ecosystem. They are excellent indicators of microbial activity and soil quality, which is important for agricultural production and land conservation. Furthermore, the presence of certain species of macroinvertebrates in the water may indicate the existence of contaminants from the air [4].

The study was carried out in the Sinincay River and eight essential points were considered to monitor the quality of the water, the first point analyzed is located in the sector called "Cochas".

Other points analyzed are: "El Chorro" sector, Parish Center, Daniel Durán, Chamana, Las Orquídeas, Camino a Patamarca, Industrial Park.

In the "Cochas" sector the water is considered slightly contaminated, this sector is located in the initial part of the river and there is little human intervention, the sectors of "El Chorro", "Daniel Duran", "Chamana", "Las Orquídeas", are places that are classified as having moderately contaminated water, while "Camino a Patamarca" and the "Industrial Park" present a highly contaminated water quality, an analysis that has its basis since these two final points analyzed receive water from At the other points, in these places there is the presence of human waste, the same that flows into the Sinincay River, added to this, the sand, the mud, increases the turbidity of the water.

The period in which the monitoring was carried out includes the months of June, July, and September of 2021, each month corresponding to the rainy, dry, and transition seasons [5].

In the analyzed locations it encounters various types of aquatic macroinvertebrates that adapt to the specific conditions present in the different river tracks.

1.3 Artificial Intelligence

Artificial Intelligence (AI) refers to the capability of a computer system to perform tasks that typically require human intelligence. This includes activities such as learning from experience (machine learning), understanding natural language, recognizing patterns, solving problems, and adapting to new situations. AI systems can be designed to perform specific tasks or exhibit general intelligence, simulating human cognitive functions like perception, reasoning, and decision-making. The goal of AI is to develop machines that can perform tasks intelligently, often surpassing human capabilities in certain domains.

1.4 Convolutional Neural Networks (CNN)

This type of network uses several convolutional layers, in addition, pooling layers and activation functions are used, all of this together to obtain relevant characteristics of the analyzed images. They are used for the detection of features in medical images and are also very useful in applications related to computer vision, such as image recognition and classification [7].

In a CNN, convolution is performed by sliding the filter over the input image and calculating the point-to-point product between the data obtained by the filter and the corresponding data from the region of the image covered by the filter, subsequently these products are added, and the result is placed in a new matrix known as a feature map.

In this study, we use convolutional neural networks, considered as the most common ideas to draw the analysis of images. These are some of the specialists who can recognize the complete patterns and specific characteristics of aquatic macroinvertebrates photographs. This application in this context allows a precise and efficient evaluation of the diversity and the state of the organisms present in the analyzed acoustic ecosystems.

1.5 Python

Python is a programming language that is widely used in industry, research, and education due to its ease of use, readability, and clear syntax. In Python, programs are written in plain text using a text editor and then executed using a Python interpreter.

Python excels in its ability to manage complex data structures and perform data analysis, machine learning, and image processing tasks. It is also required in creating web applications, **games,** and desktop applications. One of the most useful features of Python is its extensive library of predefined modules that provide additional functionality to programs [8].

In this investigation, we use Python libraries that provide a fundamental paper in the development of the code, facilitating the manipulation and analysis of acute macroinvertebrate images. The use of these libraries does not only optimize the programming process, but also allows an efficient implementation of algorithms related to the analysis of images, thus contributing to the robustness and precision of the project.

1.6 Flutter

Flutter is a framework created and powered by Google, used in the development of mobile applications that allows you to create high-quality cross-platform applications from a single code base. With its focus on widgets, native performance, hot reload, and an active community, Flutter is a great choice for developers looking to create fast, engaging, and highly customizable mobile apps [8].

2 Methodological Framework

2.1 Architecture Design

The completion of this project consists of several stages that will be detailed below:

Data acquisition: The images of aquatic macroinvertebrates, collected for analysis using a neural network, were taken in different sections of the Sinincay River, which belongs to the Paute River basin.

Back End: The collected images are used to train the CNN, once the network is trained using TensorFlow and Python, the results of both precision and loss are analyzed in the data sets corresponding to training and validation, if they are optimal they are exported the model in h5 format, then the h5 model is used together with "OpenCV" computer vision techniques to proceed with the analysis and classification of the images. Also, in the implementation of this process, the VS Code IDE is used.

Front End: The images corresponding to aquatic macroinvertebrates will be displayed in the web application with a brief description of their most representative characteristics. Through the mobile application you can also identify the species of aquatic macroinvertebrates to which the image captured by the camera belongs. Furthermore, using the inventor software, a prototype of a robot will be made where the CNN will be implemented in a small computer and, together with a camera, will have the ability to explore, capture, analyze and identify the macroinvertebrate. (see Fig. 1).

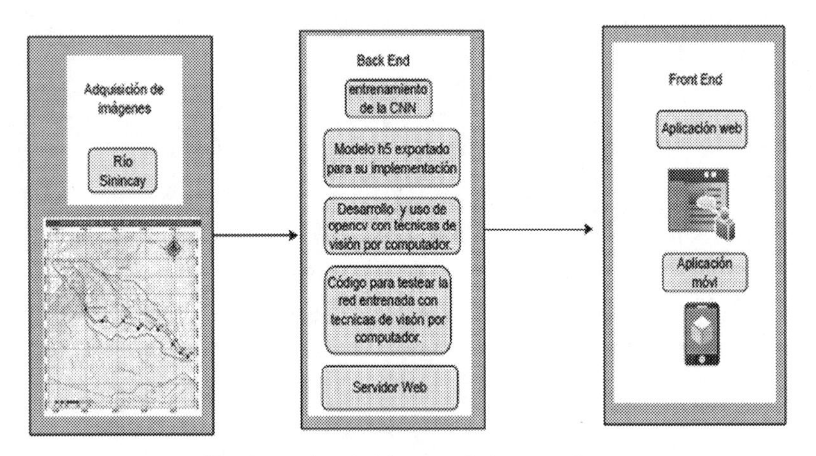

Fig. 1. Project architecture design. [Author]

2.2 Code Development for CNN Training

Import of libraries (matplotlib, NumPy, os, PIL, TensorFlow, pathlib, cv2), necessary in the implementation of the CNN.

Load the dataset, which is made up of 5002 images, sized at a height of 220 and a width of 220, the images are recognized in png format.

Select 80% of the dataset images for training, this corresponds to 4002 images.

Using the tf.keras.utils.image_dataset_from_directory function, a data set is created by including image files in a directory, segmenting the total data set into 7 image groups.

Select 20% of the dataset images for validation, this corresponds to 1000 images.

Using the tf.keras.utils.image_dataset_from_directory function, a data set is created by including image files in a directory, segmenting the total data set into 7 image groups, of which only 1000 images are used for validation.

Normalize and configure the data for training.

Develop the model, for the detection of macroinvertebrates a sequential model was used, made up of three Conv2D convolution blocks, in each of these blocks a maximum pooling layer called MaxPooling2D is integrated. After this, there is a fully connected layer known as Dense composed of 128 units and activated through the ReLu function.

Compile the model, using the Adam optimizer.

Train the model, adjusting the number of epochs.

Visualize the results of the network training, in the graph on the left you can see the resulting precision graphs, both from the training and validation data, while in the graph on the right you can see the loss graphs, both from the training and validation data.

The hyperparameters were selected considering the prevention of overtraining in the neural network.

2.3 Implementation of the Code for the Identification of Macroinvertebrates Using Computer Vision Techniques, Using OpenCV

Import of necessary libraries: The cv2 (OpenCV) libraries are imported for image processing, NumPy for matrix management, PIL for working with images, keras for loading and using a pre-trained model, os for operations related to the operating system and TensorFlow for calculation of predictions.

Model loading: A model previously trained using TensorFlow is loaded, which is located in the "./models" folder. The model is saved in variable models.

A video capture object is created using the device's default camera.

The main loop runs constantly, to end the 'q' key must be pressed.

The video frame is captured in the frame variable.

A copy of the original frame is made to draw contours.

Applying Gaussian blur to the frame, the frame is smoothed using a Gaussian blur filter with a kernel of size (7, 7) and a standard deviation of 1.

The smoothed frame is transformed to grayscale.

To obtain a binary image from the gray tone image, a thresholding process is carried out.

Using the Canny algorithm, the edges in the image are revealed in shades of gray.

Having the image in black and white, a dilation operation is executed using a kernel of size (5, 5).

3 Implementation and Analysis of Results

3.1 Display of the Online Platform Interface.

The Front-end comprises the web server interface, which can be viewed through the address (http:127.0.0.1:8000/index), locally. If it is run on a production server, the assigned public IP should be accessed from the browser.

To create the user interface of the web application, the Django framework was used, which is based on Python. Subsequently, to enter the interface in the command terminal, enter: "python manage.py.runserver".

When the server is deployed, the following interface is observed, where the image of the macroinvertebrate is chosen by clicking on the choose file box, loads the image, and performs an analysis indicating what kind of macroinvertebrate it belongs to, the level of water contamination, the sectors where they live, and some recommendations are also indicated that must be taken into account when consuming water (Fig. 2).

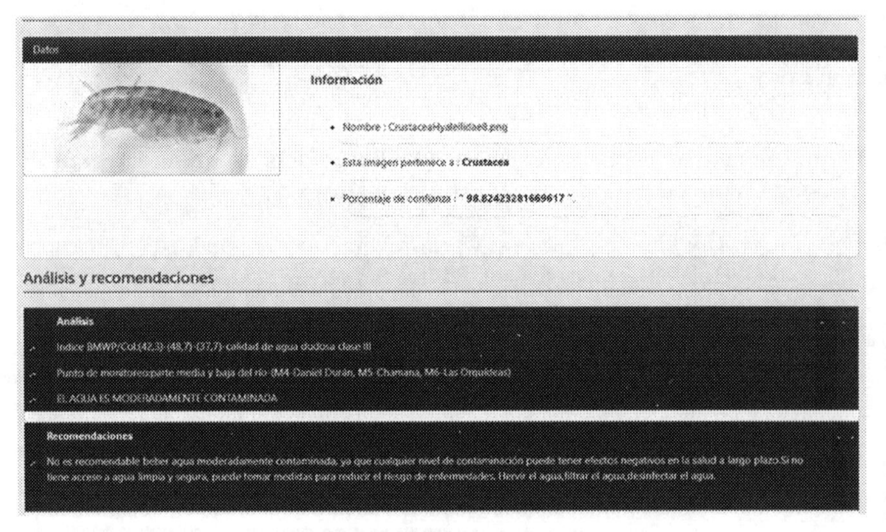

Fig. 2. Interface of the web application for the analysis of macroinvertebrates, with emphasis on those corresponding to the class Crustacea. [Author]

In the graphical interface, it is obvious that selecting the image shows a confidence level of 98%, indicating that the algorithm is incapable of handling excellent achievements with remarkable accuracy. This high level of precision, represented by the degree of confidence, suggests that the model is performing classifications with high precision, therefore reflecting the effectiveness and confidence of the implemented algorithm.

3.2 Analysis Carried Out on CNN

(See Tables 1, 2 and Fig. 3).

Table 1. Parameters entered for CNN analysis.

Parameters	Value
Batch_size	72
epochs	30

Table 2. Implementation of parameters in the sequential model for CNN analysis.

Symbol	Description	Settings
layers.Rescaling	Re-scaling of the input image	220x220
layers.Conv2D	2D Convolution	16,3, padding = 'same', activation = 'relu'
layers.MaxPooling2D	2D MaxPooling	
layers.Conv2D	2D Convolution	32,3, padding = 'same', activation = 'relu'
layers.MaxPooling2D	2D MaxPooling	
layers.Conv2D	2D Convolution	64,3, padding = 'same', activation = 'relu'
layers.MaxPooling2D	2D MaxPooling	
layers.Flatten	Flattening layer	
layers.Dense	Fully connected layer	128, activation = 'relu'
layers.Dense	Fully connected layer	num_classes

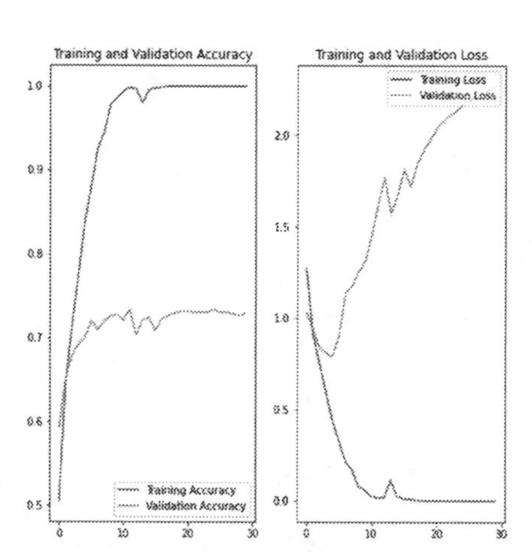

Fig. 3. Graph corresponding to the accuracy in training and validation (left). Graph corresponding to the loss in training and validation (right). [Author]

The graph corresponding to the precision in the training set and the validation indicate that there is overfitting or what is known as "overfitting" since they are deviated by wide margins, reaching approximately 74% precision in the data set belonging to the validation, while the accuracy of the training set increases proportionally with time. In the loss graph (right), corresponding to the training and validation data sets, there is a notable difference since in the validation loss data, as the epochs increase, there is greater loss of information.

Parameter configuration in the CNN using network improvement methods (data Augmentation and Dropout.) (Tables 3, 4 and 5, Fig. 4).

Table 3. Parameters entered for CNN analysis.

Parameters	Value
Batch_size	72
epochs	8

Table 4. Configuration-Data Augmentation

Parameters	Value
layers.RandomFlip	"horizontal_and_vertical"
layers.RandomRotation	0.1
Layers.RandomZoom	0.5

Improvement techniques were implemented in the network such as data augmentation and dropout. The improvement technique called data augmentation creates new data from existing data, this helps the model since it is exposed to more aspects and its learning capacity improves significantly. Another technique to reduce overfitting is the implementation of dropout, this consists of deactivating a layer, setting it to zero, several output units during the training stage. With these techniques implemented, it is observed that the graphs corresponding to the precision in training and validation indicates that there is 65% precision in the data belonging to the validation set, while the precision in the data belonging to the training set increases linearly with time. In the loss graph for both the training and validation data there is a notable improvement since the data loss decreases noticeably, reaching 0.72.

It is important to adjust and experiments to find a combination that balances the training time, the required memory, and the performance of the model in proven data.

If the number of times is excessively large, there is a risk of adjustment, where the model is adjusted too much to the training data and does not generalize well to the new data, Therefore, it is necessary to balance the parameters related to the times and the batch size.

Table 5. Implementation of parameters in the sequential model for CNN analysis.

Symbol	Description	Settings
layers.Rescaling	Re-scaling of the input image	220 × 220
layers.Conv2D	2D Convolution	16,3, padding = 'same', activation = 'relu'
layers.MaxPooling2D	2D MaxPooling	
layers.Conv2D	2D Convolution	32,3, padding = 'same', activation = 'relu'
layers.MaxPooling2D	2D MaxPooling	
layers.Conv2D	2D Convolution	64,3, padding = 'same', activation = 'relu'
layers.MaxPooling2D	2D MaxPooling	
Layers.Dropout	Drop Layer	0.2
layers.Flatten	Flattening layer	
layers.Dense	Fully connected layer	128, activation = 'relu'
layers.Dense	Fully connected layer	num_classes

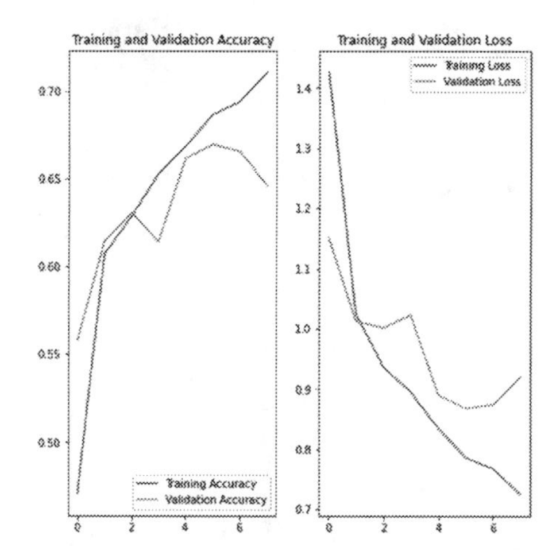

Fig. 4. Graph corresponding to the accuracy in training and validation (left). Graph corresponding to the loss in training and validation (right). Implementing network improvement techniques such as data augmentation and dropout. [Author]

3.3 Analysis of the CNN Confusion Matrix

In the confusion matrix of the data set corresponding to training, the main diagonal analysis was carried out, which represents the correct evaluations. In this context, the true positives were identified, which in this case are 1,348 images belonging to the class of insects that live in highly contaminated water. The true negatives, on the other hand, correspond to the other evaluations that do not belong to this class, but are in the diagonal matrix.

Additionally, false positives were identified in the vertical sense, which are images incorrectly classified as belonging to a specific class when they are not. False negatives were also identified in the horizontal sense, which are images incorrectly classified as if they did not belong to the class when they really do belong.

Also, the different percentages obtained in the analyzed parameters are observed, such as precision, recall, F1-score, and support. If you are looking for a classifier that minimizes false positives or keeps them at minimum levels, you should choose a classifier that offers greater accuracy. On the contrary, if a system is needed that reduces false negatives to a minimum, assigning most images to the corresponding species, a recall classifier would be chosen. Similarly, this graph shows the percentage of global precision obtained throughout the system (Figs. 5 and 6).

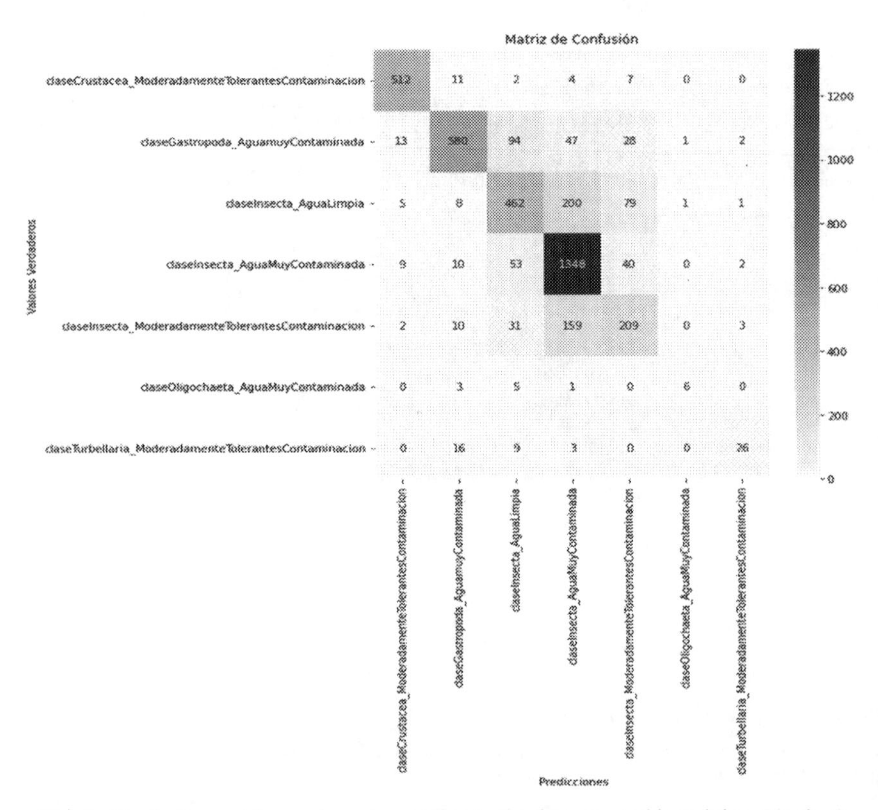

Fig. 5. Confusion matrix graph corresponding to the data set used in training. [Author]

In this work, computer vision techniques have been used in the implementation of a web application that allows determining the quality of water in a river through the identification of the macroinvertebrates present in the water. The application constitutes a tool that allows determining the water quality by personnel who do not know the types of macroinvertebrates that correspond to a certain level of water quality.

	precision	recall	f1-score	support
0	0.9464	0.9552	0.9508	536
1	0.9091	0.7582	0.8268	765
2	0.7043	0.6111	0.6544	756
3	0.7650	0.9220	0.8362	1462
4	0.5758	0.5048	0.5380	414
5	0.7500	0.4000	0.5217	15
6	0.7647	0.4815	0.5909	54
accuracy			0.7854	4002
macro avg	0.7736	0.6618	0.7027	4002
weighted avg	0.7857	0.7854	0.7801	4002

Fig. 6. Text summary including precision, recall, and F1 score for each macroinvertebrate class analyzed in the training data set [Author]

References

1. Fierro, P., Valdovinos, C., Vargas-Chacoff, L., Bertrán, C., Arismendi, I.: Ma-croinvertebrates and fishes as bioindicators of stream water pollution. Water Q. **2**, 23–38 (2017)
2. Hawksworth, D.L., Iturriaga, T., Crespo, A.: Líquenes como bioindicadores in-mediatos de contaminación y cambios medio-ambientales en los trópicos. Revista Iberoame-ricana de micología **22**(2), 71–82 (2005)
3. Alba-Tercedor, J.: Aquatic Macroinvertebrates. In: Ziglio, G., Flaim, G., Siligardi, M. (eds.) Biological Monitoring of Rivers, pp. 71–87. John Wiley, New York (2008)
4. Mora Campos, M.R., Tamay Heras, A.A.: Determinación del índice de calidad de agua mediante el monitoreo de macro invertebrados, parámetros fisicoquímicos y mi-crobiológicos en el río Sinincay, Cuenca-Ecuador (Bachelor's thesis) (2022)
5. Ponce Gallegos, J.C., et al.: Inteligencia artificial. Iniciativa Latinoame-ricana de Libros de Texto Abiertos (LATIn) (2014)
6. Chauhan, R., Ghanshala, K.K., Joshi, R.C.: Convolutional neural network (CNN) for image detection and recognition. In: 2018 First International Conference on Secure Cyber Computing and Communication (ICSCCC), pp. 278–282. IEEE, December 2018
7. Mirjalili, V., Raschka, S.: Python machine learning. Marcombo (2020)
8. Tashildar, A., Shah, N., Gala, R., Giri, T., Chavhan, P.: Application development using flutter. Int. Res. J. Mod. Eng. Technol. Sci. **2**(8), 1262–1266 (2020)

Analysis of Blood Smear Microscopic Images Using ML: DL

Hadia Mansouri[1] and Faouzi Benzarti[2(✉)]

[1] National School of Engineers of Tunis, SITI Laboratory, University of Tunis El Manar, University Campus Farhat Hached ElManar, Tunis, Tunisia
hadia.mansouri@enit.utm.tn

[2] High National School of Engineers of Tunis, SITI Laboratory, National School of Engineers of Tunis, University of Tunis, Tunis, Tunisia
faouzi.benzarti@enit.utm.tn

Abstract. Emerging AI technology intersects with several techniques simulating human cognitive processes that rely on creating algorithms that run in a dynamic computing environment. It is essential to put in place adequate tools of human intelligence. In this context, Machine Learning (ML) is becoming a real revolution that has greatly contributed to the generalization of AI. In principle, ML refers to a set of many methods aimed at automatically creating models from data. It allows computers to learn without being explicitly programmed to do so. Currently, ML occupies a growing interest in various field, such as: autonomous cars, smart cities, automatic checkouts, personal assistants, algorithmic finance, industrial robots, video games, medical diagnostics, scanners, etc. However, Our work focuses on the development of various machine learning techniques in application control especially medical process applications. The main objective is to implement a method for analyzing microscopic images of blood cells to fulfill tasks and facilitate human activity. More fundamentally, we developed a learning model to accelerate the process of diagnosing and detecting diseases with an accuracy rate that could exceed that of humans. Such analysis can be time-consuming and generate incorrect results for large-scale diagnostics. The process contains two essential phases: identification and classification of blood cells for the diagnosis and the prediction of certain abnormalities. First, we use convolution neural network CNN to extract blood image features and ML methods such as KNN, SVM, Bayes, for classification. Therefore, ML can help improve the performance, predictability, and accuracy of diagnostic systems for many diseases.

Keywords: AI · ML · blood cells · medical diagnostic process · ML techniques · blood disease detection

1 Introduction

Artificial intelligence (AI) has experienced a great development. It is considered to be a real innovation. By definition, AI is a set of concepts and technologies implemented to manufacture machines capable of simulating human intelligence. AI is the imitation

K. Daimi and A. Al Sadoon (Eds.): ACR 2024, LNNS 956, pp. 436–447, 2024.
https://doi.org/10.1007/978-3-031-56950-0_37

of human behavior using a machine that affects the creation or preservation of value. AI is real evolution. It includes various tools, of which machine learning (ML) is the best known (Fig. 1).

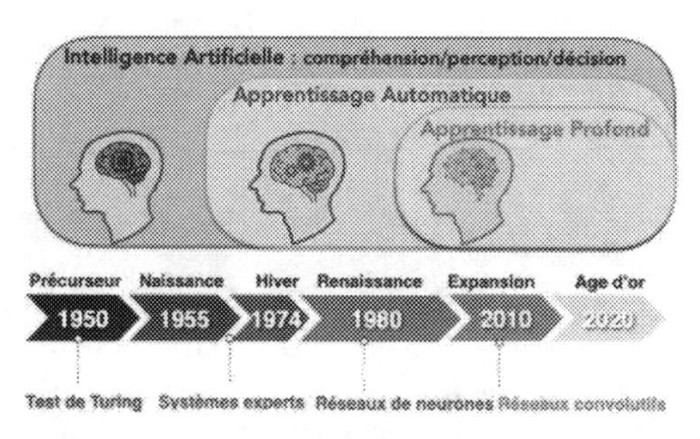

Fig. 1. Artificial Intelligence and its tools [1]

ML is a branch of AI in which machines are able to learn things automatically, predict outcomes more accurately without being programmed. It is implemented in the analysis, identification and decision-making without human intervention. ML is a term used daily everywhere: in the military, economic, financial, medical field, the last of which is the most studied [2].

ML is a subfield of AI combining many approaches to automatically create models from data [3–5] (Fig. 2).

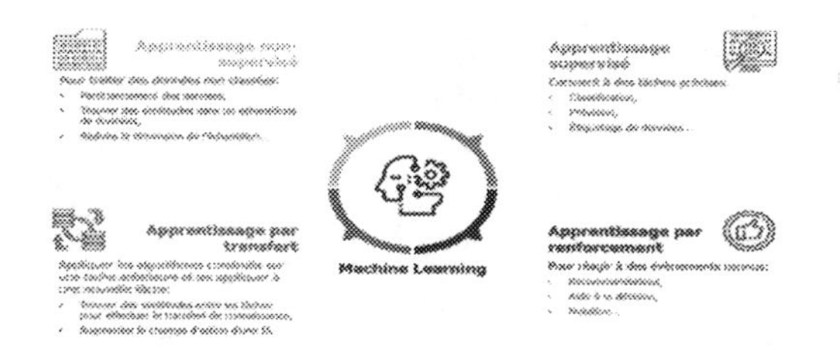

Fig. 2. Machine Learning approaches [6]

ML is a technology that always aims to make human life easier. It is present in various forms and in various applications: computer vision [7–9], audio recognition [10, 11], the development of AI [12], naturel language processing [13], robotics, facial recognition, image processing, medical learning. It is starting to be massively used in health.

It is in this perspective that this article falls. ML in application control; analysis of microscopic images of the blood smear using AI tools.

The blood smear is a test, a manual technique which makes it possible to spread blood on a glass slide stained with May Grunwald Giemsa (MGG), to give a qualitative estimate, to establish the leukocyte formula, to detect morphological anomalies of cells and determine other abnormalities of GR, GB, Plq (Fig. 3).

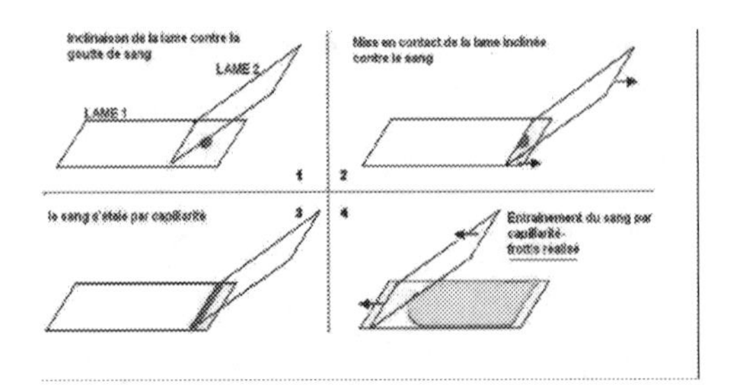

Fig. 3. The 4 steps for producing a blood smear [14]

Man has always been confronted with diseases. That it is about various categories according to the signs, the symptoms: respiratory, digestive, contagious, dangerous, light, curable, hematological diseases, from where the analysis of the images by the microscopists is a process of identification of some abnormalities but it can take time and generate incorrect results. In fact, the use of automated methods presents a need for a more precise and efficient diagnosis (an early diagnosis). Therefore, ML and its tools present a proposed solution to perform the learning process, save time, reduce workload and serve more patients.

2 Methodology

Early diagnosis of diseases increases the chances of treatment and survival of living beings. Some types of anomalies are difficult to identify at an early stage but with well-trained machine learning solutions they can be accurately detected.

In this work, we develop a solution based on a rigorous method of systematic analysis of blood smear microscopic images from a well-defined process.

According to the ISO9001:2000 standard, the process is a set of interrelated or interactive activities that transform inputs into outputs. These elements can be material objects or information. Like many image analysis tools, we focus on deep learning (a type of AI derived from ML where the machine is able to learn itself, relies on an artificial neural network s inspired by the human brain), especially CNN (it has the ability to automatically extract features from images [15]. The main advantage of CNN is automatic feature detection without any human supervision), involving the two most known: GoogleNet (one of the first CNN architectures which is based on several very small convolutions in order to drastically reduce the number of parameters [16, 17]), AlexNet (the first application of convolutional networks in computer vision [18, 19]). More convolution, more depth, therefore obtaining a better result. The proposed process has three phases: pre-processing, learning and classification.

The first phase presents the database, it is the acquisition, is used to prepare the set of images to be processed. The second phase is learning; and as its name suggests is a set of tools to acquire knowledge, knowledge. It is a process used to establish a diagnosis which is able to associate a class with a list of symptoms, observations. It consists of four steps: "Teaching" = providing information; "Learn" = perceive information; "Knowing" = evoking information, constructing meaning; "Return" = apply knowledge.

During this step, we specify the image, identify its characteristics from where we use transfer learning (it is one of the research fields of machine learning which is used to transfer knowledge from a one or more source tasks to one or more target tasks. It aims to reuse a pre-trained deep learning model and adopt it to a specific problem with a smaller number of images.

For the last step, we classify the image in order to make a decision, then, we compare these two models: GoogleNet, AlexNet with those of automatic learning such as: SVM, KNN, Tree in order to evaluate the classification performance for each of them for a set of data in this step, we have included supervised and unsupervised learning algorithms.

3 Results

The implementation of a model based on CNN particularly on transfer learning is presented in the following figure:

We start with the database presentation. It was a set of microscopic images of blood cells, contains a total of 410 images which will be expanded into 9957 images. The size of the images is 320 * 240 pixels which has been modified according to the architecture used (for GoogleNet: 224 * 224; AlexNet: 227 * 227).

For the implementation of the model, transfer learning was used. More specifically, two architectures were chosen: GoogleNet and AlexNet. Starting with the first architecture, we first loaded the microscopic images to the network (Fig. 4):

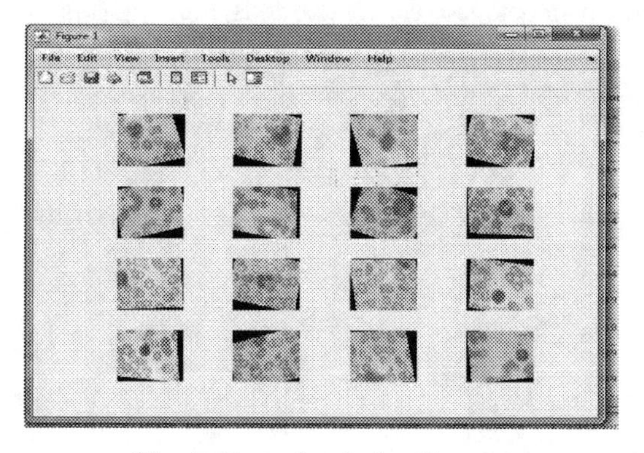

Fig. 4. Example of mixed images

Then, the data was split into 70% images for processing and 30% for validation. Then, the network architecture and its detailed information were presented (Fig. 5).

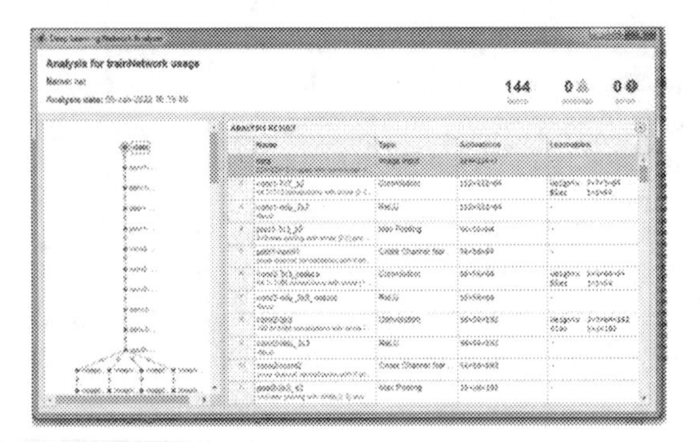

Fig. 5. Visualization of GoogleNet architecture

Afterwards, we resized the data to (224 * 224 * 3). The convolutional layers of the network aim to extract image features. So we replaced these two existing layers in the proposed algorithm:: "loss3-classifier" and "output" which include information on the extraction features of a 25 min recycle a pre-trained network to classify new images. Thus, the last layer (CFC) was replaced by a new one with a number of outputs equal to the number of database classes. The network was ready to be trained on the new database. After the visualization of the architecture, we specified the training options during the training phase. To speed up the learning in the new layers, we based on the learning speed parameters. We launched training, carried out the training and then we assessed the training parameters: precision, periods, duration (Fig. 6).

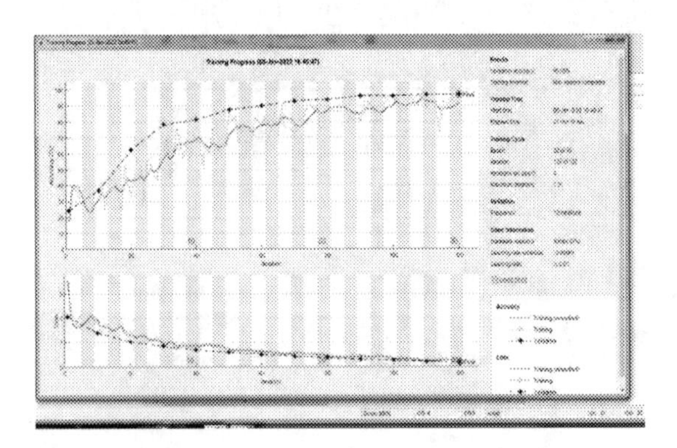

Fig. 6. GoogleNet Formation Progression

During the progression, the accuracy was 96.88% at the 30 epochs of the validation. The training lasted 41 min 17 s for 30 epochs. After training, the images were identified by cell types. Subsequently, the images were classified into images of a healthy or diseased individual (Figs. 7 and 8).

For the second architecture, we do the same as the GoogleNet method. First, image loading and data splitting were performed (Fig. 9).

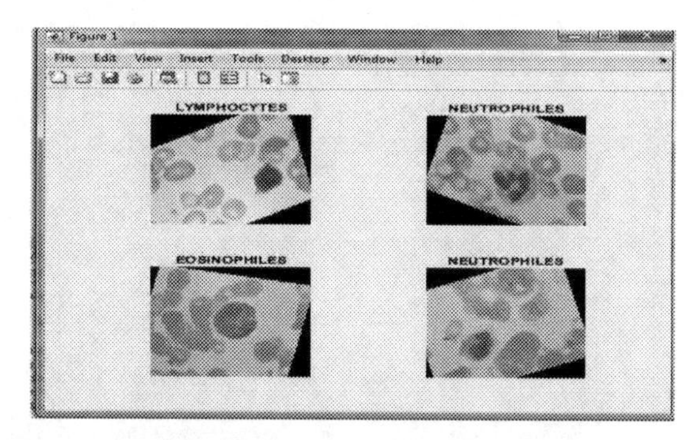

Fig. 7. Results obtained by GoogleNet network (identification)

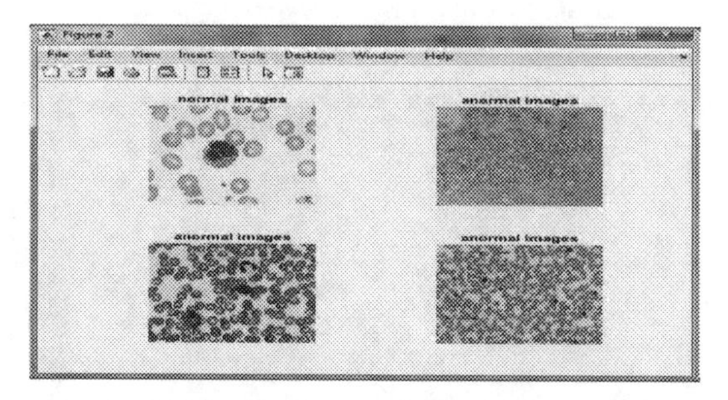

Fig. 8. Results obtained by GoogleNet network (classification)

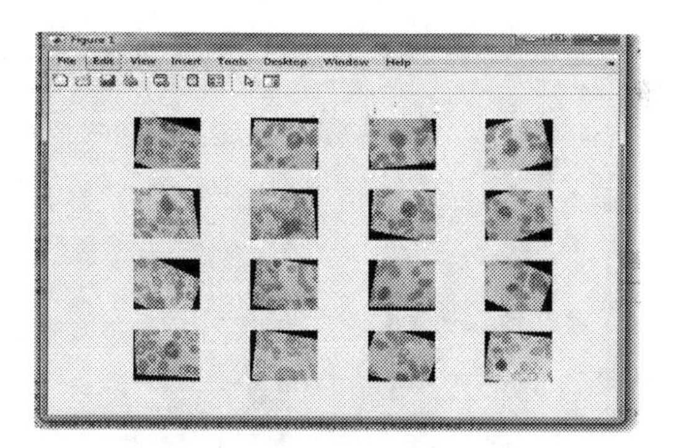

Fig. 9. Loading Microscopic Images

Then, the presentation of the architecture and the resizing of the inputs (227 * 227 * 3), also followed by each convolutional layer by a linear rectified unit (Fig. 10).

Then the launch of the training and obtaining the evaluation parameters. After the progression of the training, the accuracy was 64.84% at the 6 epochs of the validation with training duration of 25 min 50 s (Fig. 11).

After reviewing the data, the images were identified and categorized (Figs. 12 and 13).

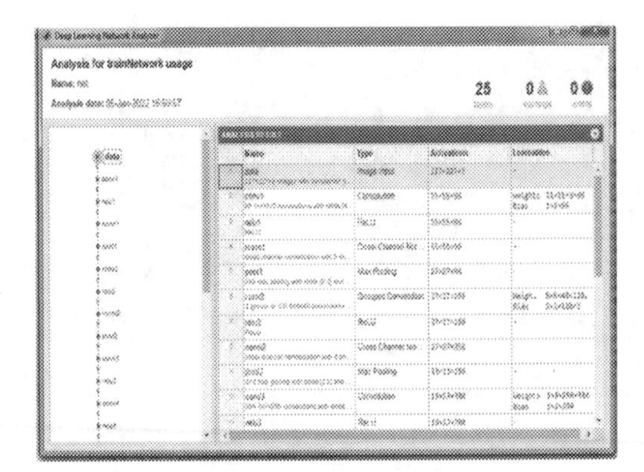

Fig. 10. Visualization of AlexNet architecture

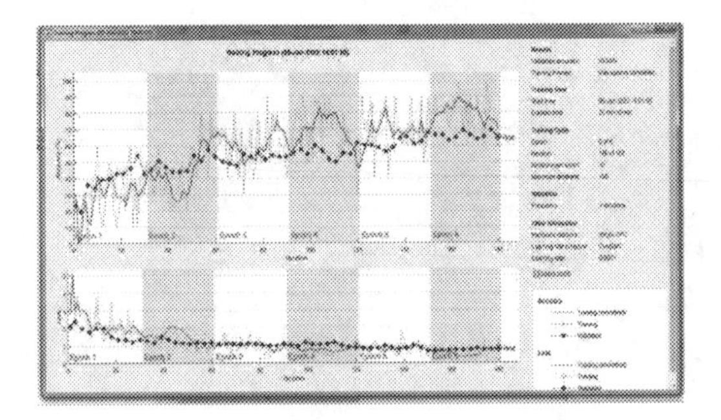

Fig. 11. AlexNet Pre-Trained Accuracy

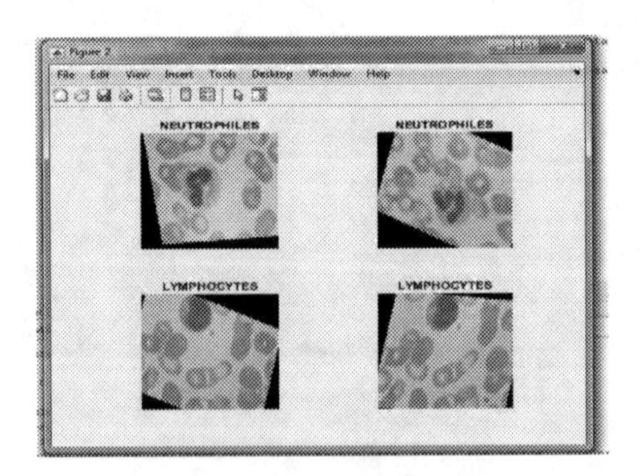

Fig. 12. Results obtained by AlexNet network (identification)

As well as the use of TL architectures, datamining software tools were used to analyze and classify the data (Fig. 14).

Orange Datamining software is used to analyze the data and compare them with those obtained by the two transfer learning architectures. (Figs. 15, 16, 17 and 18).

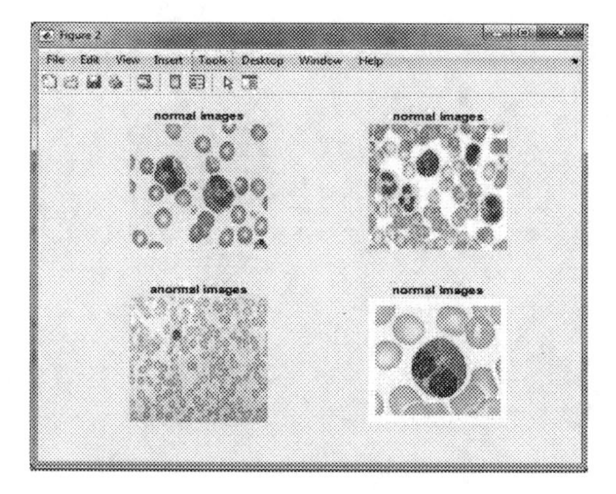

Fig. 13. Results obtained by AlexNet network (classification)

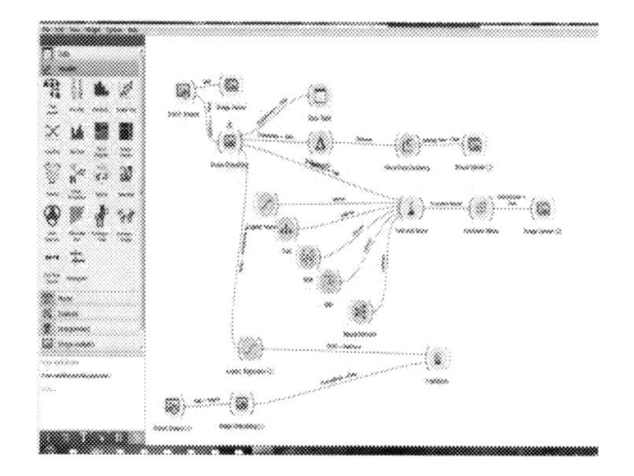

Fig. 14. Image analysis model by orange datamining

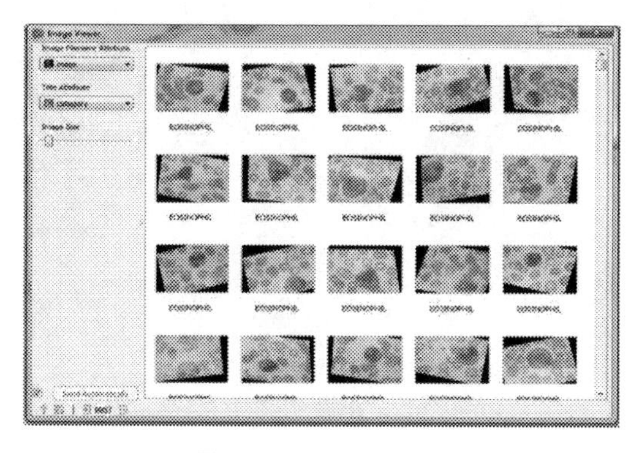

Fig. 15. Image display

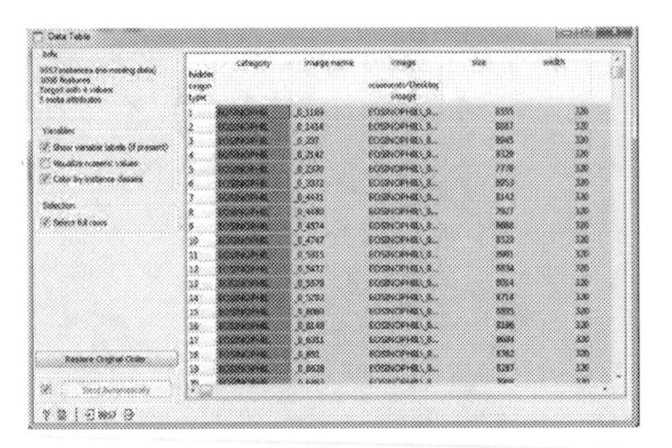

Fig. 16. Data visualization

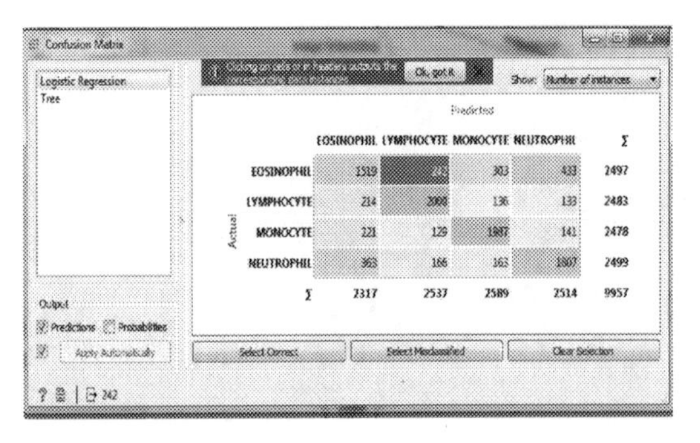

Fig. 17. Evaluation of results

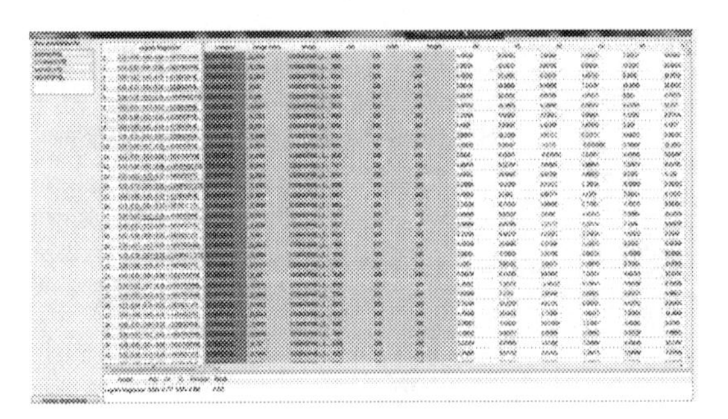

Fig. 18. Data prediction

4 Discussion

To validate the results obtained and determine the parameters, we compared the two pre-trained models with other classification tools such as Tree and SVM.

Tree's accuracy that we could achieve was 77.3%. The accuracy obtained from SVM is 58.8% (Table 1).

Table 1. Comparison of the accuracy of different classification techniques

Technical	Precision (%)
GoogleNet	96,88
AlexNet	64,84
Tree	59,1
SVM	58,8

From the previous table, it can be seen that the CNN model based on GoogleNet has established the highest accuracy rate compared to other models such as AlexNet, Tree, SVM. This implies that convolutional neural networks are able to learn characteristics suitable for a specific problem from the given information (Fig. 19).

Evaluation Results

Model	AUC	CA	F1	Precision	Recall
kNN	0.976	0.900	0.898	0.902	0.900
Tree	0.689	0.542	0.542	0.542	0.542
SVM	0.910	0.679	0.689	0.714	0.679
Neural Network	0.995	0.947	0.947	0.947	0.947
Logistic Regression	0.919	0.734	0.733	0.732	0.734

Fig. 19. Results obtained by orange datamining

According to the previous figure, we notice that the neural network model is the most efficient compared to the other models.

Therefore, the use of pre-trained model for classification can accelerate training and improve learning performance. First, the images were transformed into grayscale as shown in the appendix. Next, the data was normalized to fit the sizes of the GoogleNet and AlexNet entries. Then, we divided the data into 70% for training and 30% for testing. After standardization, fully connected layers were adapted to existing classes. Finally, we compared the results obtained with other techniques in order to test the performance of each classifier.

5 Conclusions

Disease detection is not a new subject, but the new idea is that the application of machine learning in medical diagnosis is becoming an autonomous discipline with its own measurement tools and its own control procedures.

In this article, a model based on deep learning has been proposed to classify blood cells: GR, GB, Plq… from a set of microscopic images. In addition, some machine learning technologies including SVM, Tree, KNN technique were used to compare their performance.

The usefulness of ML in medical applications reflects that ML can be integrated into every step of the analysis process, from preprocessing to decision making.

A deep learning model based on convolutional neural network (CNN) was applied as a diagnostic tool to classify blood cells from the microscopic images, adapting as a model used, the pre-trained model.

Thus, in this work, we presented a methodological framework to better understand the different AI tools in a systematic and coherent way in order to analyze the microscopic images of the blood smear that can affirm the presence of disease and classify the different types.

Therefore, the proposed methodology will help microscopists to diagnose phenomena more quickly and efficiently. In the future, a new architecture will be developed to increase detection performance.

References

1. https://www.google.com/url?sa=i&url=https%3A%2F%2Fwww.sciencedirect.com%2Fscience%2Farticle%2Fpii%2FS1957255720300407&psig=AOvVaw0vCUTs4LUgAQqlKr6SPz2e&ust=1672652683985000&source=images&cd=vfe&ved=0CBAQjRxqGAoTCKjakKq0ivwCFQAAAAAdAAAAABDoAw
2. Math Works. Pourquoi le Deep Learning EST important (2017). https://fr.mathworks.com/discovery/deep-learning.html
3. McCulloch, W.S., Pitts, W.: A logical calculus of the ideas immanent in nervous activity. Bull. Math. Biophys. **5**(4), 115–133 (1943)
4. Hinton, G., et al.: Deep neural networks for acoustic modeling in speech recognition. IEEE Signal Process. Mag. **29** (2012)
5. Goldberger, J., Roweis, S., Hinton, G., Salakhutdinov, R.: Neighbourhood components analysis. Adv. Neural. Inf. Process. Syst. **17**, 513–520 (2005)
6. https://www.google.com/url?sa=i&url=https%3A%2F%2Fwww.digitalcorner-wavestone.com%2F2018%2F08%2Fintelligence-artificielle-decryptage-dune-singularite-technologique-preoccupante%2F&psig=AOvVaw0vCUTs4LUgAQqlKr6SPz2e&ust=1672652683985000&source=images&cd=vfe&ved=0CRxqGAoTCKjakKq0ivwCFQAAAAAdAAAAABDYAw
7. Parkhi, O.M., Vedaldi, A., Zisserman, A.: Deep face recognition. In: Proceedings of the British Machine Vision (2015)
8. He, K., et al.: Deep residual learning for image recognition. arXiv e-prints, arXiv:1512.03385 (2015)
9. Szegedy, C., et al.: Going deeper with convolutions. In: The IEEE Conference on Computer Vision and Pattern Recognition (CVPR) (2015)
10. Waibel, A., et al.: Phoneme recognition using time-delay neural networks. IEEE Trans. Acoust. Speech Signal Process. **37**(3), 328–339 (1989). https://doi.org/10.1109/29.21701. ISSN0096-3518
11. Amodei, D., et al.: Deep speech 2: end-to-end speech recognition in English and mandarin. In: Proceedings of The 33rd International Conference on Machine Learning, sous la dir. de Maria Florina BALCAN et Kilian Q. WEINBERGER, t. 48. Proceedings of Machine Learning Research, New York, NY, USA, pp. 173–182. PMLR (2016). http://proceedings.mlr.press/v48/amodei16.html
12. Silver, D., et al.: Mastering the game of Go without human knowledge. Nature **550**(7676), 354 (2017)

13. https://www.google.com/url?sa=i&url=https%3A%2F%2Fsvt.ac-versailles.fr%2FIMG%2Farchives%2Fbosvt%2Ffrottis.html&psig=AOvVaw0RSiAxtes6CdQQ8P3nHVZX&ust=1672652516580000&source=images&cd=vfe&ved=0CBAQjRxqFwoTCOj3947BivwCFQAAAAAdAAAAABAE
14. L'italien, R., Lord Dubé, H.: Hématologie, deuxième édition, Sainte-Foy (Québec), Le Griffon d'argile, p. 434 (1998). https://www.biron.com/fr/glossaire/frottis-sanguin/
15. Lecun, Y., Bengio, Y.: Convolutional networks for images, speech, and time-series. Handb. Brain. Theor. Neural Network. **3361**(10), 255–258 (1995)
16. Szegedy, C., et al.: Going deeper with convolutions. In: Proceedings of the IEEE Conference on Computer Vision and Pattern Recognition, pp. 1–9 (2015)
17. Srivastava, N., Hinton, G., Krizhevsky, A., Sutskever, I., Salakhutdinov, R.: Dropout a simple way to prevent neural networks from overfitting. J. Mach. Learn. Res. **15**, 1929–1958 (2014)
18. He, K., Zhang, X., Ren, S., Sun, J.: Deep residual learning for image recognition. In: Proceedings of CVPR (2016)
19. Krizhevsky, A., Sutskever, I., Hinton, G.E.: ImageNet classification with deep convolutional neural networks. Adv. Neural. Inf. Process. Syst. **25**, 1097–1105 (2012)

Networking and Communication

Study of Sober and Efficient LoRaWAN Networks

Lemia Louail(✉) and Jean-Philippe Georges

Université de Lorraine, CNRS, CRAN, 54000 Nancy, France
{lemia.louail,jean-philippe.georges}@univ-lorraine.fr

Abstract. The Internet of Things (IoT) is a rapidly evolving and expanding field, with more and more devices being connected. The proliferation of these devices, coupled with the widespread deployment of networks, has ushered in an era of unprecedented connectivity and data-driven applications.

While these advancements promise revolutionary benefits for society and industry, their environmental implications have become a subject of growing concern.

This paper presents a study that highlights the different metrics that need to be prioritized to obtain a sober and efficient LoRaWAN network. These metrics, such as the distance, the transmission power, and the spreading factor, will be examined through extensive simulations that recover data for analysis and evaluation of the network's environmental impact and quality of service. The work focuses on the deployment of gateways in a LoRaWAN network and the configuration of gateways to limit environmental impact while guaranteeing a sufficient level of QoS.

Keywords: Green Networking · IoT architecture · LoRaWAN · QoS · Energy Efficiency · CO_2 emissions

1 Introduction

Future networks, including IoT (Internet of Things), IIoT (Industrial Internet of Things), and 5/6G networks, will be the backbone of digital ubiquity. To support new control strategies or enable specific applications, these networks must be able to automatically reconfigure. In this type of network, the dynamics of traffic, mobility, QoS (Quality of Service) requirements, and the environment are all highly dynamic [1].

One of the most used protocols in these future networks is LoRaWAN (Long Range Wide Area Network). It is a wireless communication protocol for low-power, long-range communication between IoT devices. It operates on the sub-gigahertz frequency bands, typically using an unlicensed spectrum, allowing efficient and long-range communication with low power consumption. LoRaWAN is particularly well-suited for applications where devices need to send small amounts of data periodically, such as sensor data from environmental monitoring or asset tracking devices [2,3].

K. Daimi and A. Al Sadoon (Eds.): ACR 2024, LNNS 956, pp. 451–464, 2024.
https://doi.org/10.1007/978-3-031-56950-0_38

With more and more devices being connected to such networks, the environmental and social footprint of communication networks has emerged as a major issue in the deployment of communication infrastructures. This aspect must not be limited to only minimizing energy consumption; it should also take into account the infrastructure as a whole and other metrics, including energy efficiency, the various sources of pollution such as the mode of production of energy, radio-frequency pollution, and/or the carbon footprint [4].

We note that, in this context, energy consumption and energy efficiency are related concepts, but they refer to different aspects of energy use. Energy consumption refers to the total amount of energy used by a specific device or system over a given period. It measures the actual quantity of energy consumed to operate a particular application, process, or system. On the other hand, energy efficiency refers to how effectively a device or a system converts the input energy into useful output. It quantifies how well energy is utilized to perform a specific task or provide a certain level of service. High energy efficiency means that a system or device can achieve the desired output with minimal energy input, resulting in less waste and lower energy costs.

In this paper, we focus on the deployment of gateways in a LoRaWAN network and the configuration of gateways to limit environmental impact while guaranteeing a sufficient level of QoS. This deployment may depend on certain metrics such as distance, Transmission Power (TP), and Spreading Factor (SF).

The remainder of this paper is organized as follows. Section 2 presents the related works. Section 3 details the study in which we highlight the different metrics that need to be prioritized to obtain a sober and efficient LoRaWAN network with the different simulations. Section 4 summarizes the obtained results. Finally, Sect. 5 concludes the work.

2 Related Works

LPWAN (Low Power Wide Area Network) is a wireless communication network designed to provide long-range and low-power connectivity for IoT devices and other applications. LPWAN technology is well-suited for scenarios where devices need to transmit small amounts of data over long distances while conserving battery life [5,6].

LoRaWAN is one of the most popular LPWAN technologies. A LoRaWAN network usually works as follows. The IoT devices (end devices) with built-in sensors/actuators collect data and/or perform tasks. They periodically send small data packets to the LoRaWAN network. The Gateways serve as a bridge between the end devices and the central network server. They receive data from nearby end devices and forward it to the server. The LoRaWAN Network Server controls the communication between end devices and applications. It receives data from gateways, performs security checks, and forwards the information to the appropriate application server. Moreover, it is capable of returning configuration updates or commands to the end devices. The Application Server is responsible for processing and interpreting the data received from the network server. A star-of-stars topology is used for communication between end devices and gateways, with each end device connecting to one or more gateways. Multiple data rates are supported by the LoRaWAN protocol, enabling devices to modify their communication speed in response to various conditions including available power or distance from the gateway [2,3].

LoRaWAN can be used to influence metrics such as Spreading Factor (SF) or Transmission Power (TP) to reduce environmental impact, as shown by [3,7–9], and [10].

[11] presented NB-IoT, an Energy Efficient Narrowband Internet of Things protocol. NBIoT achieves energy efficiency by employing low-power modes, low data rates, and efficient signaling techniques in its architecture. It is particularly well-suited for IoT applications that require long-lasting, low-power connectivity over extended ranges. The paper discussed various practical applications, including smart agriculture, smart cities, and healthcare, which benefit from NBIoT's energy-saving capabilities. The authors of [5] presented a comparative study of the two technologies, LoRaWAN and NB-IoT.

[9,12] presented a study showing that saving energy does not necessarily lead to a lower cost or environmental footprint of the network. They demonstrated that energy consumption and ecological footprint can conflict with each other as constrained optimization objectives. The authors in [9] employed an Integer Linear Programming (ILP) to understand network behavior with varying objective functions that can rely on several metrics to improve the network's financial cost, time-on-air, connection quality, and battery lifespan. Another solution to reduce carbon emissions is to put certain devices on standby by increasing certain parameters, such as SF and TP. [12] highlighted the significant reduction in carbon emissions if some nodes were put on standby, forcing other nodes to transmit over greater distances and therefore use more energy. [12] also demonstrated that to have a more sustainable network, we need to take into account the location of the gateway to minimize carbon emissions.

[7,13], and [14] presented different studies concerning the use of energy recovery devices to reduce carbon emissions. The energy efficiency of some networks, such as a 5G Green network, was analyzed through various energy-efficient technologies like energy harvesting, resource allocation, massive MIMO, device-to-device network, spectrum sharing, and ultra-dense networks for 5G green. [7] proposed an algorithm to estimate the system power consumption. The energy demand must also power another data transmission technology since the Gateway must forward the packets received by the End Nodes to the LoRaWAN Network Server. On the other hand, [14] focused on the fact that the cost should not increase as compared with the data rate provided since 5G networks use massive MIMO technology that deals with the introduction of a large number of antennas and enormous base stations.

One of the main missions of QoS is to allocate network resources fairly To achieve this, [15] proposed using game theory to enable a better quality of experience (QoE) when allocating network resources. The implementation of certain methods, such as Massive MIMO and Device to Device (D2D) communications, presented by [5,15,16], would also reduce latency and interferences while saving equipment battery life.

[17] surveyed the new architectural changes related to green 6G networks which additionally provides a brief overview of many possible technologies including THz communication, edge intelligence, ubiquitous 3D coverage, and Blockchain.

Defining and deploying network architecture also helps to improve network energy efficiency. [5] detailed LPWAN architecture to enable long-range communications. This study discussed different topologies and their advantages, such as the most widespread star topology, tree topology for a longer range but more nodes, and mesh topology with minimal delay but more energy consumption.

[18] mapped different metrics such as functional stability, performance, compatibility/interoperability, usability, reliability, security, maintainability/modularity/scalability, and portability and identified reliability, performance, functional stability, security, compatibility/Interoperability and maintainability/scalability as QoS metrics in IoT architectures.

According to [19], there could be differences in the QoS settings between the core network and the access network. Moreover, end devices typically have to notify network devices of their QoS requirements. For this, the authors developed a QoS-aware selection scheme for multi-radio access technologies (M-RAT). The IoT nodes with M-RAT can connect to one or more access points simultaneously and the optimization problem is executed independently at each node to determine the best access device.

The aim of [20] was to reduce the environmental footprint of IoT systems by examining how the layers of the Internet of Things architecture are arranged into perception, transport, processing, network, and application layers. They identified the power-hungry components as sensing, communicating, processing, and communicating across layers. The authors recalled different techniques to optimize energy consumption (such as multi-hop) in transmission over long paths. The sensors' operation can be geared toward scheduling, which turns them off when not in use, or toward data centers, which use dedicated algorithms to balance the load.

[21] analyzed the problem of green networking from the sustainability point of view. Besides energy-aware routing, authors propose pollution-aware routing with new metrics like the percentage of non-renewable energy usage and CO_2 emission factor. The proposed algorithm provides optimal control and data planes for these metric types and enables different routers' scheduling and link bandwidth adaptations while ensuring scheduling and adoption priority according to traffic demand requirements. The impact of the proposed algorithm enabling green routing was assessed for three different metrics.

The authors in [21] proposed a pollution-aware routing alongside an energy-aware routing. The main idea was to route data through different paths based on environmental factors such as carbon emissions and the non-renewable energy usage percentage of a node. The proposed approach tried to reduce CO_2 emissions or the usage percentage of non-renewable energy in the total network. This routing can be applicable only for geographically diverse, distributed network architectures where every node has different means of energy production. The results showed that the proposed pollution-aware routing approach reduced CO_2 emissions by 20% compared with energy-based routing and by 36% compared with shortest-path routing.

All these studies serve to highlight the lack of research on potential network architecture enhancements that could reduce their negative impact on the environment and guarantee acceptable QoS. Table 1 summarizes the notions addressed in each related work to show that there are few works dealing with the environment, QoS, and architecture at the same time. Articles dealing with all three notions often skim over one of them.

Table 1. Summary of related works

Metrics	Related works															
	[5]	[7]	[8]	[9]	[10]	[11]	[12]	[13]	[14]	[15]	[16]	[17]	[18]	[19]	[20]	[21]
Environment		X		X	X	X	X	X	X						X	X
QoS	X		X			X		X	X	X	X		X	X		
Network Architecture			X				X		X	X		X		X		

In this paper, we focus on the deployment of gateways in a LoRaWAN network and the configuration of gateways to limit environmental impact while guaranteeing a sufficient level of QoS.

3 Sober and Efficient LoRaWAN Network Simulation and Evaluation

In this work, we simulate a LoRaWAN network to determine a sober and efficient network architecture. The idea is to optimize a shared budget for the network, including QoS-related metrics and pollution-related metrics. We use LoRaWAN gateways since they are widely used in both literature and simulation software such as NS3. We use the GW SX1272 gateway model, following [24], in order to have sufficient data to carry out the various measurements during calculations and simulation.

To assess QoS and environmental impact, we need to define analysis metrics for each category. For QoS, we focus on Energy Efficiency (EE) of the network. For the environmental impact, we consider carbon emissions. These metrics will be evaluated for different SF (Spreading Factor) values and different TP (Transmission Power) values. These measurements aim to enable analyzing and evaluating the most optimal SF and TP for configuring LoRaWAN gateways, and thus determine the soberest and most efficient network configuration. Carbon emissions will be computed based on the results of the simulation, taking into account the energy consumption of a gateway and the CO_2 emissions per kWh of electricity produced in France.

[3] presented various simulation tools for a LoRaWAN network. In our study, we will use the NS-3 Network Simulator software [25]. It is a discrete-event network simulator for Internet systems, intended mainly for research and teaching purposes. It is also free open-source software, which allows getting feedback from other users. As shown in Fig. 1, we placed 10 Gateways (GW), and 10 end devices (ED). The GWs are full black circles. The EDs are the empty circles placed randomly within a perimeter between 5 and 10 km. The duration of the simulation is 6 h, and the EDs send messages every second to the nearest gateway.

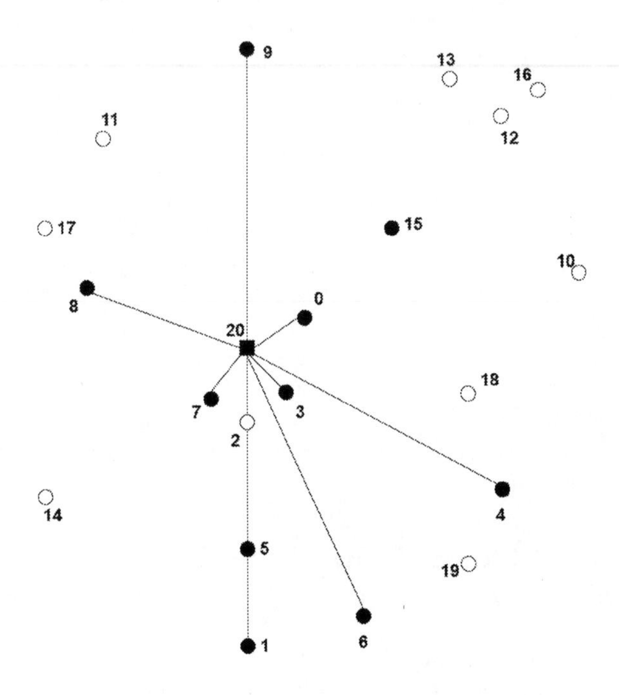

Fig. 1. Positioning Gateways and End Devices in the network

First, we evaluate the percentage of packets received for SF $\in [7, 12]$, using different distances between 5 and 10 km.

By computing the number of messages received out of the number sent, we obtain the probability of success for different SF values, as shown in Tables 2 and 3.

Table 2. QoS for different SF in a range of 5 km

Side Length 5 km			
SF	Packets sent	Packets received	%
7	21606	19352	89.6%
8	21098	21087	99.9%
9	11773	11689	99.2%
10	6620	6604	99.7%
11	2949	2879	97.6%
12	1660	1489	89.7%
auto	21555	21462	99.5%

Table 3. QoS for different SF in a range of 10 km

Side Length 10 km			
SF	Packets sent	Packets received	%
7	21606	4102	18.9%
8	21098	8560	40.6%
9	11773	4950	42.0%
10	6620	4154	62.7%
11	2949	1842	62.5%
12	1660	1201	72.3%
auto	21555	8280	91.7%

The number of messages sent drops when the FS is increased because the latter implies a longer message transmission time. For a range of distance of 5 km, the percentage of messages received remains relatively homogeneous. There is no significant difference between the different SFs in terms of QoS. We can, therefore, use a fixed SF on the gateways for shorter distances. However, it is preferable to adjust the SF to the distance between the ED and the GW over longer distances. This difference in the percentage of success can be explained by the maximum transmit/receive distance for each FS according to NS3. By placing a gateway at a fixed location and increasing the distance for one ED, we can find the maximum transmit/receive distance for each FS. The maximum distance is shown in Table 4.

Table 4. Maximum transmit/receive distance for each SF

SF	7	8	9	10	11	12
Distance (meters)	4216	4914	5727	6675	7779	9066

To compute the energy consumption, we use the formula proposed by [22] as follows.

$$E = V \times I \times ToA \quad (1)$$

Where:
E is the consumed energy in Joules. V is the Supply Voltage in Volt. I represents the Current Voltage in mA. ToA is the Time on Air.

[23] gives the ToA for each SF (see Table 5), as well as the current consumption I in transmission and standby (see Table 6), and the supply voltage which is $V = 3.3$ V.

Table 5. Time on Air (ToA) corresponding to each SF [23]

SF	7	8	9	10	11	12
Sensitivity (dBm)	−123.0	−126.0	−132.0	−134.5	−137.0	
Time on Air (ms)	61.7	113.2	205.8	370.7	659.5	1318.9

Table 6. Current consumption of SX1272 for packet transmission and sleep mode for transmit power 10 dBm [23]

State	Packet Transmission	Sleep Mode
Current consumption	31 mA	100 nA

The measurements are performed on a Gateway SX1272, which is the same model as the one we are using in the NS3 simulator.

After performing the calculations, we obtain the energy consumption for each SF as shown in Table 7.

Table 7. Energy consumption for each SF

SF	7	8	9	10	11	12
Energy consumption (Joule)	0.0063119	0.0115804	0.0210533	0.0379226	0.0674669	0.1349235

To estimate the power consumption for each SF, we run a simulation to measure the remaining battery. An end device will send a packet of size 23 bytes every 10 s, during 3600 s (1 H), to a gateway located 300 m away. The SF is set for each simulation, and the energy expenditure per transmission is adapted to each SF. Standby and Sleep modes remain the same, Standby consumes 0,0014 J and Sleep mode consumes 3.2999999999999996e−07 J The battery capacity is 10000 J.

Table 8. Battery left after the simulation for each SF

SF	7	8	9	10	11	12
Battery left	9999.16	9998.16	9997.19	9995.25	9991.82	9983.49

Table 8 shows a clear reduction in remaining battery life as soon as the SF is increased.

Modifying the TP has little effect on battery levels.

As shown in Table 9, [24] gives the actual power consumption of each TP, enabling the computation of the power consumption of each SF-TP combination using the calculation presented in [22].

Once this consumption is obtained, it is possible to modify the simulation parameters to obtain the battery level remaining after each simulation. The

Table 9. Energy consumption for each TP

TP (dBm)	2	3	4	5	6	7	8	9	10	11	12	13	14
I_{tx} (mA)	24	24	24	25	25	25	25	26	31	32	34	35	44

Table 10. Energy consumed and battery left after the simulation for each SF-TP combination

SF	TP	E(J)	Battery left (J)	SF	TP	E(J)	Battery left (J)
7	2	0.00488664	9999.25	10	2	0.0293594399	9996.28
	4	0.00488664	9999.25		4	0.0293594399	9996.28
	6	0.00509025	9999.24		6	0.030582750	9996.13
	8	0.00509025	9999.24		8	0.030582750	9996.13
	10	0.00631191	9999.16		10	0.037922609	9995.25
	12	0.006922740	9999.12		12	0.04159254	9994.80
	14	0.008958840	9999.00		14	0.05382564	9993.33
8	2	0.00896544	9998.47	11	2	0.0522324	9993.52
	4	0.00896544	9998.47		4	0.0522324	9993.52
	6	0.009339	9998.43		6	0.054408750	9993.25
	8	0.009339	9998.43		8	0.054408750	9993.25
	10	0.01158036	9998.16		10	0.06746685	9991.65
	12	0.01270104	9998.02		12	0.0739959	9990.85
	14	0.016436640	9997.58		14	0.0957594	9988.19
9	2	0.01629936	9997.76	12	2	0.10445688	9987.20
	4	0.01629936	9997.76		4	0.10445688	9987.20
	6	0.0169785	9997.68		6	0.108809250	9986.67
	8	0.0169785	9997.68		8	0.108809250	9986.67
	10	0.02105334	9997.19		10	0.13492347	9983.49
	12	0.023090760	9996.95		12	0.147980580	9981.89
	14	0.029882160	9996.13		14	0.19150428	9976.59

simulation duration is set to 1 h. The other parameters remain unchanged. After simulation, we obtain the results shown in Table 10.

We note that the difference is insignificant for TP $\in [2, 8]$ regarding energy consumption. However, higher consumption is observed for TP $\in [10, 14]$.

After this data collection, we compute the energy efficiency of the network. [22] provides a formula for calculating energy efficiency as a function of packet size, probability of success, bandwidth, and energy required.

$$EE = \frac{Payload\ in\ bits \times p_s}{BW \times E_i} \tag{2}$$

Where EE is the Energy Efficiency; p_s is the Probability of success; BW is the Bandwidth; and Ei is the Energy expended.

We note that, in this study, the bandwidth used is 125 kHz, and the packet size is 23 bytes.

Calculations are made for each SF-TP combination. The obtained results for the 5 km range are shown in Table 11. The results for the 10 km range are presented in Table 12.

Table 11. Energy Efficiency for 5 km range for each SF-TP combination

SF	TP	EE_i (bits/Hz/J)	SF	TP	EE_i (bits/Hz/J)	SF	TP	EE (bits/Hz/J)
7	2	0.2699	9	2	0.0896	11	2	0.0275
	4	0.2699		4	0.0896		4	0.0275
	6	0.2591		6	0.0860		6	0.0264
	8	0.2591		8	0.0860		8	0.0264
	10	0.2089		10	0.0694		10	0.0213
	12	0.1905		12	0.0632		12	0.0194
	14	0.1477		14	0.0488		14	0.0150
8	2	0.1640	10	2	0.0499	12	2	0.0126
	4	0.1640		4	0.0499		4	0.0126
	6	0.1574		6	0.0479		6	0.0121
	8	0.1574		8	0.0479		8	0.0121
	10	0.1269		10	0.0387		10	0.0098
	12	0.1157		12	0.0353		12	0.0089
	14	0.0894		14	0.0273		14	0.0069

These results show that energy efficiency depends more on energy emission than it depends on distance and QoS. There is little change between SF12–TP14 at 5 km and SF12–TP14 at 10 km: 0.0069 and 0.0056. And much more difference between SF7–TP14 and SF12–TP14 at 5 km: 0.1477 and 0.0069.

It is, therefore, preferable to have a low SF-TP before trying to influence the distance between the gateways.

Now that we have the various elements for measuring energy consumption, we can evaluate the different combinations of SF-TP and distance in terms of environmental impact.

To evaluate the environmental effect of the different combinations of parameters, we compute the Carbon emissions. We use the Eco2mix website [26], which allows the retrieving of a CSV file listing the CO_2/kWh rate over an hour. The battery level (in Joules) is retrieved every second and divided by 3,600,000 to obtain the value in kWh. Once this conversion is done, we simply multiply the obtained values to obtain the carbon emission of each combination. The obtained results (see Table 13) show that the Carbon emissions increase significantly when increasing the SF and the TP.

Table 12. Energy Efficiency for 10 km range for each SF-TP combination

SF	TP	EE (bits/Hz/J)
7	2	0.0569
	4	0.0569
	6	0.0546
	8	0.0546
	10	0.0440
	12	0.0401
	14	0.0310
8	2	0.0666
	4	0.0666
	6	0.0640
	8	0.0640
	10	0.0516
	12	0.0470
	14	0.0363
9	2	0.0379
	4	0.0379
	6	0.0364
	8	0.0364
	10	0.0293
	12	0.0267
	14	0.0207
10	2	0.0314
	4	0.0314
	6	0.0301
	8	0.0301
	10	0.0243
	12	0.0222
	14	0.0171
11	2	0.0176
	4	0.0176
	6	0.0169
	8	0.0169
	10	0.0136
	12	0.0124
	14	0.0096
12	2	0.0101
	4	0.0101
	6	0.0098
	8	0.0098
	10	0.0079
	12	0.0072
	14	0.0056

Table 13. CO_2 emissions for each SF-TP combination

SF	TP	CO_2 emissions (g CO_2 eq)
7	2	6.2500957854305l9e−06
	4	6.250095785430519e−06
	6	6.250287356338799e−06
	8	6.250287356338799e−06
	10	7.208141762450261e−06
	12	7.122222222192908e−06
	14	0.000520833333334929
8	2	1.2666954022967112e−05
	4	1.2666954022967112e−05
	6	1.3277681992339594e−05
	8	1.3277681992339594e−05
	10	1.5882088122605805e−05
	12	1.684013409959827e−05
	14	0.0012759611111109724
9	2	1.8919731800748735e−05
	4	1.8919731800748735e−05
	6	1.9875766283514806e−05
	8	1.9875766283514806e−05
	10	2.404070881226659e−05
	12	2.6123659003839038e−05
	14	0.002038361111110578
10	2	3.133668582374516e−05
	4	3.133668582374516e−05
	6	3.272452107279256e−05
	8	3.272452107279256e−05
	10	4.0104693486596233e−05
	12	4.384032567050866e−05
	14	0.0034996277777784857
11	2	5.5211973180087945e−05
	4	5.5211973180087945e−05
	6	5.772729885055737e−05
	8	5.772729885055737e−05
	10	7.12702107279665e−05
	12	7.80411877394475e−05
	14	0.006178616666667169
12	2	0.00010917356321836579
	4	0.00010917356321836579
	6	0.00011377452107281265
	8	0.00011377452107281265
	10	0.00014076427203064184
	12	0.00015447624521073186
	14	0.01224604999999188

4 Results Summary

Figure 2 summarizes the study of this work by showing the effect of the Spreading Factor (SF) and the Transmission Power (TP) on both the Energy Efficiency (EE) and the CO_2 emissions of the LoRaWAN network. The orange circles represent the EE and the blue circles the CO_2 emissions. The size of each circle reflects the value of its metric.

It is important to remember that the goal is to have high Energy Efficiency but low CO_2 emissions which implies that we are looking for SF and TP values that give the biggest orange circle and the smallest blue circle.

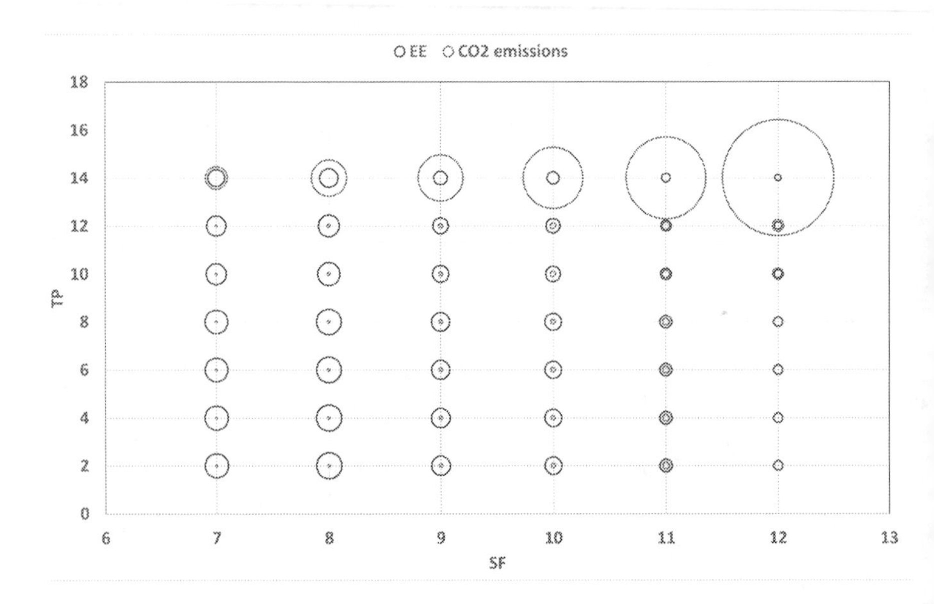

Fig. 2. EE and CO_2 emissions corresponding to each SF and TP combination

The combination of an SF $\in$ [7,8] with a TP $\in$ [2,8] generates the highest Energy Efficiency and the lowest CO_2 emissions for our LoRaWAN network.

5 Conclusion

The Internet of Things (IoT) is a rapidly evolving and expanding field, with more and more devices being connected. However, there is a valid concern about how this expansion may affect the environment. For this reason, this paper highlights the lack of research on potential network architecture enhancements that could reduce their negative impact on the environment and guarantee acceptable quality of service.

We present a series of simulations that illustrate the various metrics to focus on in order to achieve sober and efficient LoRaWAN networks. These different metrics, such as distance, transmission power (TP), and spreading factor (SF), are studied through extensive simulations that recover data for analysis and evaluation of the network's environmental impact and quality of service. This goal was achieved by combining an SF $\in$ [7,8] and a TP $\in$ [2,8] according to the obtained results.

References

1. Meira, J., et al.: Industrial internet of things over 5G: a practical implementation. Sensors **23**(11), 5199 (2023)
2. Jouhari, M., Saeed, N., Alouini, M.S., Amhoud, E.M.: A survey on scalable LoRaWAN for massive IoT: recent advances, potentials, and challenges. IEEE Commun. Surv. Tut. **25**(3), 1841–1876 (2023)
3. Almuhaya, M.A., Jabbar, W.A., Sulaiman, N., Abdulmalek, S.: A survey on LoRaWAN technology: recent trends, opportunities, simulation tools and future directions. Electronics **11**(1), 164 (2022)
4. Alsharif, M.H., Jahid, A., Kelechi, A.H., Kannadasan, R.: Green IoT: a review and future research directions. Symmetry **15**(3), 757 (2023)
5. Ogbodo, E.U., Abu-Mahfouz, A.M., Kurien, A.M.: A survey on 5G and LPWAN-IoT for improved smart cities and remote area applications: from the aspect of architecture and security. Sensors **22**(16), 6313 (2022)
6. Mekki, K., Bajic, E., Chaxel, F., Meyer, F.: A comparative study of LPWAN technologies for large-scale IoT deployment. ICT Exp. **5**(1), 1–7 (2019)
7. Sherazi, H.H.R., Piro, G., Grieco, L.A., Boggia, G.: When renewable energy meets LoRa: a feasibility analysis on cable-less deployments. IEEE Internet Things J. **5**(6), 5097–5108 (2018)
8. Dawaliby, S., Bradai, A., Pousset, Y.: Distributed network slicing in large scale IoT based on coalitional multi-game theory. IEEE Trans. Netw. Serv. Manage. **16**(4), 1567–1580 (2019)
9. Rady, M., Georges, J.P., Lepage, F.: Can energy optimization lead to economic and environmental waste in LPWAN architectures? ETRI J. **43**(2), 173–183 (2021)
10. Clemm, A., Westphal, C.: Challenges and opportunities in green networking. In: 2022 IEEE 8th International Conference on Network Softwarization (NetSoft), June 2022, pp. 43–48. IEEE (2022)
11. Popli, S., Jha, R.K., Jain, S.: A survey on energy efficient narrowband internet of things (NBIoT): architecture, application and challenges. IEEE Access **7**, 16739–16776 (2018)
12. Alvarado-Alcon, F.J., Asorey-Cacheda, R., Garcia-Sanchez, A.J., Garcia-Haro, J.: Carbon footprint vs energy optimization in IoT network deployments. IEEE Access **10**, 111297–111309 (2022)
13. Al-Nedawe, B.M., Alhumaima, R.S., Ali, W.H.: On the quality of service of next generation green networks. IET Netw. **11**(1), 1–12 (2022)
14. Sofi, I.B., Gupta, A.: A survey on energy efficient 5G green network with a planned multi-tier architecture. J. Netw. Comput. Appl. **118**, 1–28 (2018)
15. Gandotra, P., Jha, R.K.: A survey on green communication and security challenges in 5G wireless communication networks. J. Netw. Comput. Appl. **96**, 39–61 (2017)
16. Huang, J., Xing, C.C., Shin, S.Y., Hou, F., Hsu, C.H.: Optimizing M2M communications and quality of services in the IoT for sustainable smart cities. IEEE Trans. Sustain. Comput. **3**(1), 4–15 (2017)

17. Huang, T., Yang, W., Wu, J., Ma, J., Zhang, X., Zhang, D.: A survey on green 6G network: architecture and technologies. IEEE Access **7**, 175758–175768 (2019)
18. White, G., Nallur, V., Clarke, S.: Quality of service approaches in IoT: a systematic mapping. J. Syst. Softw. **132**, 186–203 (2017)
19. Asad, M., Basit, A., Qaisar, S., Ali, M.: Beyond 5G: hybrid end-to-end quality of service provisioning in heterogeneous IoT networks. IEEE Access **8**, 192320–192338 (2020)
20. Tahiliani, V., Dizalwar, M.: Green IoT systems: an energy efficient perspective. In: 2018 Eleventh International Conference on Contemporary Computing (IC3), August 2018, pp. 1–6. IEEE (2018)
21. Hossain, Md.M., et al.: Energy, carbon and renewable energy: candidate metrics for green-aware routing? Sensors **19**(13), 2901 (2019)
22. Gupta, G., Van Zyl, R.: Energy harvested end nodes and performance improvement of LoRa networks. Int. J. Smart Sens. Intell. Syst. **14**(1), 1–15 (2021)
23. Narieda, S., Fujii, T., Umebayashi, K.: Energy constrained optimization for spreading factor allocation in LoRaWAN. Sensors **20**(16), 4417 (2020)
24. Loubany, A., Lahoud, S., Samhat, A.E., El Helou, M.: Improving energy efficiency in LoRaWAN networks with multiple gateways. Sensors **23**(11), 5315 (2023)
25. Henderson, T.R., Lacage, M., Riley, G.F., Dowell, C., Kopena, J.: Network simulations with the ns-3 simulator. In: SIGCOMM Demonstration, vol. 14, no. 14, p. 527 (2008)
26. Eco2Mix. https://www.rte-france.com/eco2mix. Accessed Nov 2023

User Controlled Routing Exploiting PCEPS and Inter-domain Label Switched Paths

Leonardo Boldrini[1(✉)], Matteo Bachiddu[2], Ralph Koning[3], and Paola Grosso[1]

[1] MNS Group, University of Amsterdam, Amsterdam, The Netherlands
{l.boldrini,p.grosso}@uva.nl
[2] NETGroup, Politecnico di Torino, Turin, Italy
[3] SIDN Labs, Arnhem, The Netherlands
ralph.koning@sidn.nl

Abstract. The UPIN project tackles the security issue of the Internet at its root, by providing more transparency and control over the network to the end user. Traffic Engineering is required to create paths across multiple domains following constraints set by the user. We present here the feasibility of using the Path Computation Element Communication Protocol Secure (PCEPS) to accomplish the goal of traffic steering - hence control - across multiple domains. Specifically, we leverage on IPv4 Segment Routing (SR) and a modified version of the Netphony Path Computation Element (PCE) to build a multi domain Label Switched Path (LSP) according to a user's request. We present a proof of concept where we verify the correctness of the operation of the modified PCE code.

Keywords: PCEPS · PCEP · UPIN · Segment Routing · Path Control

1 Introduction

The Internet is today a global infrastructure that supports a wide range of services and products on which all companies and governments depend on [1]. This dependence is often based on systems produced and managed by entities in other countries, which generates in several circumstances political and economical concerns. As a result, we are observing the emergence of more concerns regarding digital autonomy and greater attention over control of data. The Responsible Internet was proposed to address these problems and provide a higher degree of trust and sovereignty for users of the Internet [2]. Ideally users should understand what the network is capable of, what problems may arise with their data in transit, and ultimately, make responsible decisions on how should the network deal with their data.

The User-driven Path verification and control in Inter-domain Networks (UPIN) project [3] addresses these needs. Its main goal is to provide more transparency and control over the network to end users.

K. Daimi and A. Al Sadoon (Eds.): ACR 2024, LNNS 956, pp. 465–478, 2024.
https://doi.org/10.1007/978-3-031-56950-0_39

The research we present here focuses on the control aspects of the communication, and in particular, on the problem of inter-domain control. In a multi domain setup, different operators are in charge of setting up different portions of a path. If the user requires from the network specific services, all network operators need to decide together how to steer traffic in order to satisfy this request.

To accomplish its goal the UPIN framework that we present here adopts and integrates three technologies that have seen significant attention in the networking research community, as attested by the numerous publication on this topic: Segment Routing (SR), Path Computation Elements (PCEs) and the associated Path Computation Element Communication Protocol Secure (PCEPS) [4], that exploits Transport Layer Security (TLS) across domains. We will describe these in more detail in Sect. 2.

With this work we intend to answer the following questions: "Can we accomplish SR-MPLS path computation across multiple domains using Path Computation Elements (PCEs)?", and more specifically: "Can PCEPS be used for this purpose?".

Our contributions are as follows:

- we evaluated a number of PCEs implementation to identify the best suited; we concluded that Netphony is the implementation to adopt;
- we modified the communication between PCEs to support the creation of paths across domains by defining and exchanging a set of global labels in a secure fashion by means of PCEPS;
- we evaluated our changes in a prototype testbed by creating SR paths across two domains.

Our implementation and subsequent experiment prove that it is possible to adopt SR-MPLS and PCEPS to enable user control over network services.

2 Background

In order to understand our work, we need to briefly introduce the technologies we rely on, namely Segment Routing, Path Computation Elements and PCEPS.

2.1 Segment Routing

In the current Internet architecture, every router makes forwarding decisions based on each packet's destination. In contrasts source routing is a paradigm where "... the source of internet packets specifies the complete internet route." [5].

The source routing concept has been implemented in the Segment Routing paradigm [6]. The actual path to be taken is specified as a list of segments, via segment identifiers (SIDs). Segments can be of four types: node, adjacency, prefix and anycast. A node segment represents a specific network node and the adjacency segment represents the link between two nodes; the prefix segment represents an IP prefix, anycast segments are used for anycast traffic. In this paper we use node segments that represent routers. Segment Routing helps network operators with distributing the traffic more efficiently and makes rerouting possible in case of failures. We rely on SR to provide users with a mechanism to identify services running on certain network nodes that they want and steer traffic through them, e.g. users can specify that their traffic needs to be evaluated by a firewall or an intrusion detection system.

Segment Routing can be implemented as an extension of MPLS in SR-MPLS [7,8]. In SR-MPLS, the segments are specified by the MPLS labels. An MPLS label is 20-bit long and it can represent any of the SID types. When an MPLS label represents a specific SID, this information can be distributed within a domain by an Interior Gateway Protocol (IGP). A Segment Routed Label Switched Path (SR-LSP) is a path through an SR-MPLS network. This path is unidirectional. We had presented a single domain implementation of SR-MPLS to steer traffic according to specific constraints in [9].

Because we use an IGP to distribute SID information within a domain, none of this information is available for other domains, hence it is not possible to create a multi domain SR-LSP following this method. Furthermore, the pool of MPLS labels available within a domain can be the same for each domain, so the simple solution of distribution of SIDs across domains is not feasible. This is also a security feature for network operators, as they don't want to expose to other domains their SIDs and what they use them for. For all of these reasons, we set out to identify ways to construct a multi domain SR-LSP by signaling between Path Computation Elements that belong to different network domains.

2.2 Path Computation Elements

A Path Computation Element (PCE) is a network element that is capable of computing a network path or route based on a network graph, and of applying computational constraints during the computation [10]. This follows the paradigm of Constraint-based Shortest Path First (CSPF). The information based on which a PCE computes a path is stored in the Traffic Engineering Database (TED), which contains the topology and resource information of the domain. The TED may be fed by Interior Gateway Protocol (IGP) extensions or potentially by other means.

A PCE can be either stateful or stateless; in a stateful setup, the PCE keeps memory not only of topology and resource information contained in the TED, but also of all the paths it has already computed, and will remove this information if the path is no longer needed or available. The drawback of this approach is that all information available to the PCE needs to be up to date, resulting in heavy control plane overhead. On the other hand, a stateless PCE does not keep state of the paths it has already computed, it instead uses the information available in the TED to compute a new path. Every new path is then processed independently of the others. We use stateful PCEs because we need to keep track of already computed local paths in order to signal to other domains which portion of a multi domain path to use. PCEs traditionally communicate between each other using Path Computation Element Communication Protocol (PCEP). More recently, PCEPS has been introduced as a more secure version of PCEP [4].

2.3 PCEP and PCEPS

The Path Computation Element Communication Protocol (PCEP) allows to communicate network paths [11] among PCEs. It was originally designed for MPLS and Generalized Multi-Protocol Label Switching (GMPLS) networks to facilitate communications between PCEs. It identifies the operation between a PCE and a client, called Path Computation Client (PCC). PCEP defines a specific set of requests. Each session consists of a Transmission Control Protocol (TCP) connection that can be secured via SSL or TCP-MD5. Table 1 summarizes the types of PCEP messages available and that we use in our Proof of Concept.

Table 1. Message types available in PCEP.

Message type	Description
PCReq	The PCC requests a path to the PCE
PCRep	The PCE responds to the PCC with a path
PCUpd	The PCE updates a path on the PCC
PCNtf	The PCE sends a notification to the PCC
PCErr	The PCE or the PCC sends an error

In PCEP, a Label Switched Path (LSP) is set up by a PCC sending a path computation request. The PCE response message contains the path or an error message, in case no path was found. The PCE can send an update message containing a new label stack for an LSP in case it needs to update the corresponding path. If the connection between the PCE and the PCC is lost, the PCC will minimize traffic disruptions. If it can no longer reach the PCE, it will remove the installed paths.

Our goal is to push SR-LSPs to the routers in the network. The path is pushed out by the PCE to the PCC as an Explicit Route Object (ERO). In PCEP, support for segment routing was added as per RFC 8664 as segment routing EROs (SR-EROs) [12]. Previous work [13,14] have demonstrated the viability of using PCEP and BGP-LS in the MPLS data plane to construct paths, making them a good starting point for our implementation.

The Path Computation Element Communication Protocol Secure (PCEPS) was presented in RFC 8253 as an addition of Transport Layer Security (TLS) to provide a secure transport for PCEP [4]. TLS provides a secure transport channel above layer 4 bringing many security features: peer authentication, message confidentiality, message authentication and integrity, protection against replay and filtering attacks [15]. Only one new message type, other than the ones presented in Table 1, needs to be added in order to implement PCEPS, which is the StartTLS message. The other regular PCEP messages are sent over the new established TLS channel. New errors are encapsulated inside the PCErr message in order to signal problems occuring in the TLS connection.

The initiation of a PCEPS session between a PCE and PCC happens in 4 phases:

- initialization and establishment of a TCP connection; this phase is no different from what happens in regular PCEP;
- both peers (PCE/PCC) send a StartTLS message to initiate TLS;
- negotiation of TLS parameters and establishment according to the TLS procedure;
- PCEP messages can now be sent in a secure fashion over TLS, starting with PCEP Open messages.

By modifying all the PCEs in our implementation to run PCEPS, we ensure that every message that is exchanged across different network domains benefits from the security features that come with TLS. This way, we can provide a secure transmission of the SR-EROs that cross inter-domain links and carry information about what path their data will go through.

Although PCEPS was introduced in RFC 8253 as a more secure version of PCEP, it has not been standardized neither widely used as PCEP is not usually deployed across different domains. However, our implementation requires all the security improvements that PCEPS brings in order to send sensitive information for users across domains.

3 The UPIN Framework

The technologies we described briefly in the previous section support the creation of the UPIN [3] framework.

The UPIN project provides the concrete implementation for the Responsible Internet, namely transparency, controllability and accountability for the users of the network infrastructure [1,3,16].

The UPIN framework consists of the folloing components: a Domain Explorer, Path Controller, Path Tracer, Path Verifier, and Frontend [3,16]. Every component plays a specific role in managing a domain. The Domain Explorer obtains metadata about properties of the network, such as security and environmental details. It stores information on the nodes in the network. The Path Controller sets forwarding rules based on what the user has asked. The Path Tracer gathers measurements on the traffic in the UPIN domain. Its goal is to store important details for the possible verification. The Path Verifier analyzes measurements from the Path Tracer to verify whether the desires of the user are satisfied. If the path traverses a non-UPIN enabled domain, there is no way for the Path Verifier to be certain whether the intent is satisfied over the full path. The Frontend allows for the communication between the user and the domain. A useful implementation of the Frontend within the scope of UPIN can be found in [2]. Through the Frontend, a user can see what services or Virtual Network Functions (VNFs) are available in the network, and which paths can be taken to reach the desired destination. A user can then request a specific path to be taken, following a set of constraints that can include for example which VNFs to traverse (e.g. a firewall), or which jurisdictions the whole path can traverse.

In this paper we use PCEs to perform the functions of the Path Controller of the UPIN framework.

We leverage on SR and PCEs so that we can steer traffic of every user through different paths, following their requests. We focus on the path creation, including the intermediate elements to be traversed, therefore addressing the real goals of a Responsible Internet.

4 PCE Evaluation

There are many PCE implementations available and we wanted to evaluate the one most suitable for adoption in UPIN. We considered the following:

- *OpenDaylight(ODL).* The PCE developed in this automation platform supports Segment Routing, stateful paths, binding labels, objective functions and include route objects;
- *NorthStar.* The SDN controller developed by Juniper Networks contains a PCE that supports stateful paths, binding labels and segment routing extensions;
- *Netphony-PCE.* The PCE developed by Telefonica supports segment routing extensions, stateful paths and is open source.
- *ONOS.* This is an open-source network operating system that can provide the control plane in an SDN. It supports the PCEP southbound interface to communicate to network devices.
- *IOS XR.* In this network operating system developed by Cisco there is support for version 2 of PCEP and the relevant SR extensions.

We evaluated all of the above with respect to a number of essential features for inclusion in UPIN.

- **Open source**: we want access to the code for extension possibilities. The main extension we want to implement is the use of PCEPS for path creation across domains, as well as the security that comes with TLS. Open source is the ideal option but we evaluated also easily obtainable closed source PCEs;
- **Hierarchical-PCE (H-PCE)**: for inter-domain path creation we want to avoid to have a central PCE that controls all domains. H-PCEs introduce a child-PCE and a parent-PCE, where the child-PCE is responsible for intra-domain control, while the parent-PCE takes care of inter-domain PCE communication;
- **Stateful**: a stateful PCE will maintain knowledge of the paths that were computed in the past; this allows us to propagate back path requests across the domain to create the full path;
- **SR support**: our implementation of UPIN relies at the moment on VNFs that are reachable by their label number; hence we need support for SR to build a SR-MPLS multi domain path;

- **Protocol support**: we want the PCE to support traffic engineering protocols such as OSPF-TE or ISIS-TE, as well as BGP-LS. This is needed to communicate information and instructions to the routers.

Table 2 shows the features supported by the PCE implementations we considered. Based on this evaluation, we decided to use Netphony as base PCE implementation. Netphony has most features we need and, being open source, it allows us to implement the RFCs and extensions that we require, namely the implementation of PCEPS. OpenDaylight and ONOS could also be an option; they both miss support for H-PCE but this could be potentially implemented; however the code base for both is larger than Netphony-PCE and more complex to manage.

Table 2. PCE evaluation based on the required features.

	ODL	Northstar	Netphony	ONOS	IOS XR
Open source	Yes	No	Yes	Yes	No
H-PCE	No	No	Yes	No	No
SR support	Yes	Yes	Yes	Yes	Yes
Stateful	Yes	Yes	Yes	Yes	Yes
OSPF-TE	No	Yes	Yes	Yes	Yes
BGP-LS	Yes	Yes	Yes	Yes	Yes
ISIS-TE	No	Yes	No	Yes	Yes

Initially, Netphony implemented older drafts of the multiple RFCs about PCEs. However, the backend library that this PCE uses for implementing various protocols, called netphony-network-protocols, has a more recent development version. We implemented the non-draft RFCs that we needed to be able to communicate with FRR, as that is the software of our routers. This process led us to change certain objects that were either moved or renamed from drafts to RFCs. As an example, the Type Length Value (TLV) encoding of sub-objects in the PCEP messages got overhauled in the standardized RFCs [11,17].

5 Inter-domain Paths with Global Labels

SR-MPLS requires the definition of a block range for the SID selection within a single domain. To set up a multi domain path, we need also to define a range of global labels which will be exchanged only across the inter-domain links. This range needs to be disjoint of the single domain range, to ensure no ambiguity in path selection.

Global labels sent across domains carry information on paths used by users and this might have privacy implications. Therefore, securing the exchange of these labels was a primary requirement of our setup. This is the main reason that led us to implement PCEPS for inter-domain communication.

Each domain configures a static export for the whole global range towards the other domain. A PCE can then build a path using one of these global labels. The global labels will be replaced by the locally significant labels once the packets reach the next domain.

We implement an SR-MPLS algorithm in Netphony based on RFC5441 [18] and an Internet-draft on PCEP extensions for stateful Inter-Domain tunnels [19]. RFC5441 discusses how to perform the Backwards Recursive Path Computation (BRPC) procedure. It discusses how paths are computed through multiple domains, as well as the relevant extensions needed to the PCEP. [19] extends stateful paths to inter-domain deployments. In all these scenarios, the domain discovery and resolving is left to the implementation. This led us to delve into related works and propose our idea.

RFC8685 [20] proposes that PCEs communicate via a Hierarchical Path Computation Element (H-PCE). They propose the use of one central parent PCE that connects to each child PCE. This method creates a single point of failure and assumes one entity in control of the whole network. We propose instead to use a distributed setup, where each PCE only has to maintain a connection to the PCEs of the neighbouring domains.

Segment Routing Traffic Engineering (SR-TE) policies are stateful. This means that we need to keep a list of policies that are active. With our approach, all this needs to be done in the PCE.

In our implementation, when a PCE receives a computation request from a PCC, the PCE resolves the source and the destination. If one of them is not present in the TED, a *no path possible* error is sent back to the PCC. If both endpoints are present in its domain, the PCE computes the local path.

If the destination is not in the local domain but exists in the TED, and the TED has an entry to reach the PCE of the corresponding domain, a request will be forwarded to the external PCE via PCEPS. When a domain forwards a request, it waits for a response. If it gets a *no path possible* response, this is sent back to the requestor. If it receives a partial path, it computes a path from the start to the router that borders the other domain and appends this to the received path. This total path gets sent back to the requestor. This happens in compliance with the Backwards Recursive Path Computation as described in [18].

If the PCE has no stored information on either the source nor the destination, but both are present in the reachability manager, the PCE forwards the request to the PCE that contains the destination node, and then sends back the partial path to the requestor.

Our algorithm takes the shortest route possible between two nodes. It performs the shortest path algorithm on the graph to get a node list. For each node in this node list, we perform a lookup in the TED to find the corresponding SID.

6 Proof of Concept

We built a proof of concept to verify that our implementation worked correctly and was able to build multi-domain paths while exchanging only secure PCEPS messages across domains.

Our setup topology is shown in Fig. 1. This includes two domains, controlled by one PCE each. A domain is composed of four SR capable routers, a client that acts as a host to generate and receive traffic, and the modified Netphony PCE. We use the latest version of Netphony PCE: 1.3.3. For the routers, we use Free Range Routing version 8.3.1, which at the time of testing was the latest available. Because we haven't modified FRR, routers in our setup use regular PCEP and not PCEPS. The clients are hosted on Ubuntu 22.04 based machines.

We focused our work on the SR-MPLS data plane, the implementation of Segment Routing in IPv4. Therefore, in our setup, MPLS labels will correspond to SIDs and a path will consist of a set of these labels [9]. In [9] we also investigated how we can map these SIDs to VNFs present in one domain, loaded in specific hosts. This allowed us to compute a path where traffic was going through VNFs present in one domain. The setup that we present now is compatible with this feature, but for the sake of this multi-domain proof of concept, we haven't loaded any VNF in our system. SR can be used with IPv6 as well and that remains for now a future direction of research.

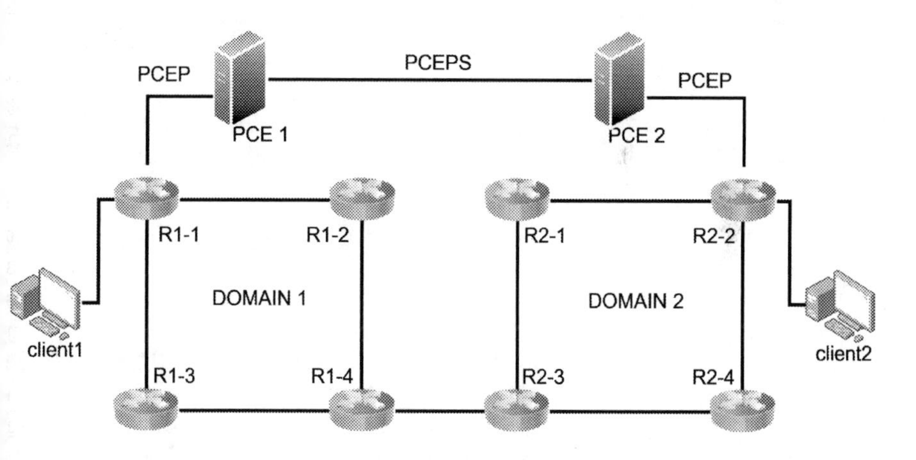

Fig. 1. Setup topology with two domains, each containing four routers and its own PCE. The two PCEs connect direclty and exchange PCEPS messages on this link.

In our proof of concept, once the TLS communication has been established, all PCEs need to support two types of requests:

- local destination requests, i.e. the PCE receives a path request for an endpoint that is located in its domain;
- remote destination requests, i.e. the request received by the PCE is for a destination in a different domain.

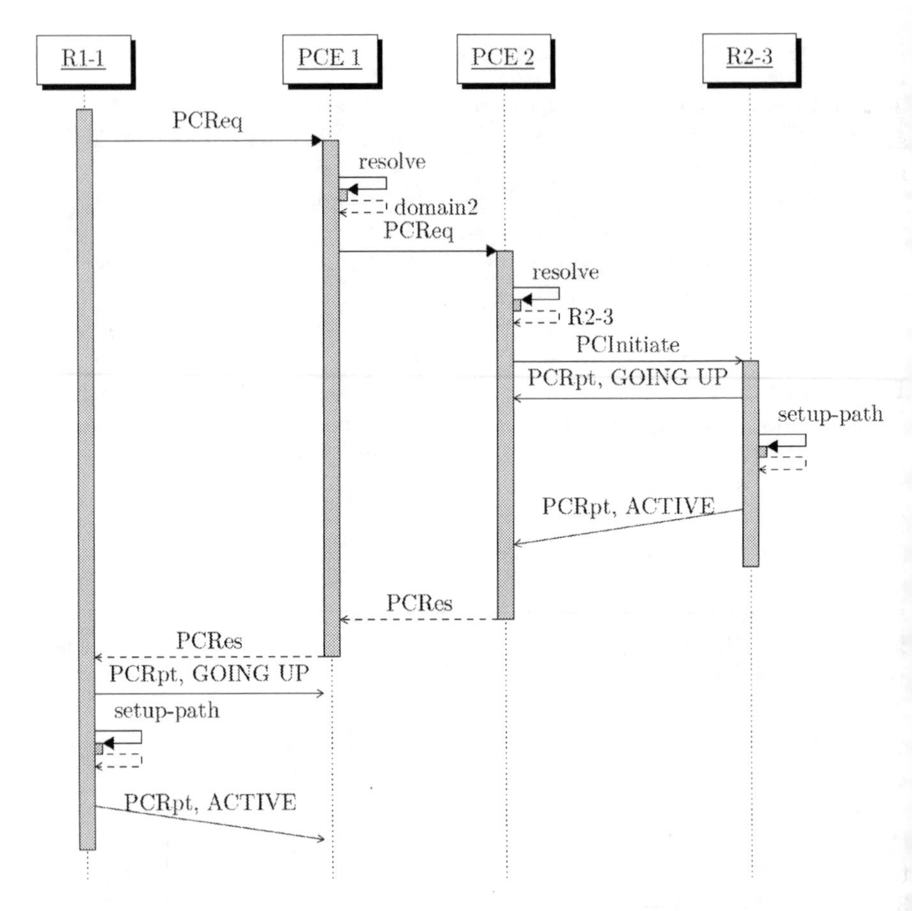

Fig. 2. PCEP and PCEPS messages exchange for multi domain path provisioning. Routers only support PCEP, while PCEs support both and use PCEPS between each other.

All our software, configuration of routers and the code of the PCEs is available and can be found in the following repository [21].

The first exchange of messages across domains happens between the PCEs, as described in 2.3. Once the TLS establishment between the PCEs is completed, PCEPS messages can be exchanged. Because FRR does not support PCEPS, we implemented in our modified Netphony PCE an option for allowing the use of regular PCEP with legacy devices that require it. Our PCEs then establish a TLS channel between them and use regular PCEP with routers in their own domains. We analyze now the PCEP and PCEPS messages that are exchanged to create the multi domain path.

When a router needs to reach a destination in a remote domain, it sends a *remote destination request* to its own PCE and this one forwards the request to the corresponding remote PCE on top of the TLS communication. The remote

PCE receives it as a *local destination request* as this destination is present in its own domain. The receiving PCE then provisions a global label at its border router and sends this back to the requesting domain. The global label acts as a stitching label: it is appended at the egress router of the first domain and removed and modified at the ingress router of the following domain.

Our goal is to steer traffic from client1 in Domain 1 to client2 in Domain 2 through inter-domain SR-LSPs that are created by the exchanging secure PCEPS messages between the PCEs and regular PCEP between a PCE and its routers. Within a domain, we need to use an IGP which enables passing the segment routing information between local network elements. The two clients are not in the same domain, so when client1 sends the first packet to R1-1, the only router it is directly connected to, R1-1 has no information on how to reach client2. In order to set up this path, there needs to be communication between R1-1 and PCE 1, between R2-3 and PCE 2, as well as between the two PCEs. This is shown in Fig. 2 where we illustrate the whole chain of messages needed to set up such a path across domains. The chain of messages is illustrative also for other cases where source and destination clients attach to different routers than the ones in our test setup.

The first PCEP message (*PCReq)* is sent from R1-1 to the PCE of its domain, PCE 1. Note that here R1-1 acts as a PCC. PCE 1 resolves the endpoint location and determines that the endpoint is in Domain 2. This corresponds to the *remote destination request.* In this case PCE 1 initiates a PCEPS PCReq to the PCE of the destination domain, PCE 2, over a TLS channel. This will be a *local destination request* from the perspective of PCE 2.

PCE 2 resolves the endpoint location, it computes the path that goes from the Area Border Router (ABR) R2-3 to R2-2, where the prefix that corresponds to client2 is injected into the routing domain. PCE 2 then sends a *PCInitate* R2-3. R2-3 informs PCE 2 on the state of the path with a PCRpt message, and once R2-3 has calculated the path to client2, it informs PCE 2 with another *PCRpt.* PCE 2 can now respond to PCE 1 over the TLS channel with the global label sent to the ABR. PCE 1 computes the path towards the ABR that got assigned this global label and sends this as a *PCRes* back to R1-1. R1-1 computes the path to R2-3 through R1-4 and informs PCE 1 with a *PCRpt.*

We verified the correct operations of this path setup across domains by looking at the Label Information Base (LIB) in all relevant routers: R1-1, R1-4, R2-3 and R2-2. All the correct SIDs are added to incoming packets. The path between R1-1 and R1-4 is chosen by the IGP, either through R1-2 or R1-3, and a similar situation happens in Domain 2. We could confirm that the correct forwarding entries were installed in all routers, hence that our software implementation supports creation across domains, while using only PCEPS across domains, the ultimate goal of this work.

7 Discussion

We encoutered a few limitations in our implementation that need to be addressed in future work.

At the time of writing there are no devices that officially support PCEPS, hence we started our work with determining which PCE software was extendable to implement this protocol. However, also FRR doesn't support PCEPS. Therefore we had to implement our modified Netphony PCE to be able to set up a PCEPS session with other PCEs as well as regular PCEP with routers.

Furthermore, we only used a pool of 10 global labels per direction, and only between two domains. This poses challenges in the amount of requests from users that can be served within an ISP with this setup and how many domains we can connect to each other. In all these cases, we need to use one unique label to avoid collisions. The scalability remains a challenge due to the limited number of 20-bit MPLS labels available. Ideally, we would like to have the possibility for two PCEs to negotiate a union of free labels and use them on the inter-domain link in an on-demand fashion. The limited amount of labels may be overcome by using SRv6 instead of SR-MPLS; this should be further investigated.

The PCEP protocol still leaves many details about inter-PCE communication open, especially with regard to the PCUpdate and PCReport messages. This means that signaling that one path needs to be deployed is possible, but informing the other party that the path is no longer needed requires more coordination.

The use of stateful PCEs increases the overall control plane overhead, so it is necessary to investigate how the performance of our implementation scales in more complex networks.

The PCE requires reachability information. Ideally, the PCE receives a full Border Gateway Protocol (BGP) feed of each border, but each locally configured route-policy also needs to be replicated towards the PCE to aid the route selection. RFC8821 [22] discusses possible extensions to the PCEP protocol for this. One option proposed is transmitting the next-hop information within the PCEP response.

Furthermore, we chose Free Range Routing (FRR) as the router stack on top of Linux. Yet this has had some limitations: the PCEP implementation of FRR is still experimental and not completely upstreamed at time of testing.

Finally, at the time of writing, a new draft adds support to deploy bidirectional paths. To prevent asymmetric routing it would be beneficial if the return traffic uses the same path. The implementation and design of this are out of scope for this paper.

8 Conclusion

The aim of this research was to investigate possibilities and limitations of PCEPS to set up a multi-domain path to allow for user-driven path control. We explored several aspects of this protocol, specifically focusing on what devices support it, how we can implement it in devices that don't support in natively, and finally analyzing its feasibility in a virtualized multi-domain environment. Our software consists of a modified version of the Netphony PCE that allows for the instantiation of PCEPS sessions, that we use to maintain safe the data about what multi-domain path is requested by a user. This is an important milestone in our investigation on the consequences that shifting control from operators to end users of a network has on its security.

Acknowledgment. This research received funding from the Dutch Research Council (NWO) under the project UPIN.

References

1. Hesselman, C., et al.: A responsible internet to increase trust in the digital world. J. Netw. Syst. Manage. **28**(4), 882–922 (2020)
2. Meijer, A.R., Boldrini, L., Koning, R., Grosso, P.: In: 2022 IEEE/ACM International Workshop on Innovating the Network for Data-Intensive Science (INDIS). IEEE (2022)
3. Bazo, R., Boldrini, L., Hesselman, C., Grosso, P.: In: Proceedings of the ACM SIGCOMM 2021 Workshop on Technologies, Applications, and Uses of a Responsible Internet, pp. 8–13 (2021)
4. Lopez, D., de Dios, O.G., Wu, Q., Dhody, D.: PCEPS: Usage of TLS to Provide a Secure Transport for the Path Computation Element Communication Protocol (PCEP). RFC 8253 (2017). https://doi.org/10.17487/RFC8253
5. Sunshine, C.A.: Source routing in computer networks. ACM SIGCOMM Comput. Commun. Rev. **7**(1), 29–33 (1977)
6. Filsfils, C., Previdi, S., Ginsberg, L., Decraene, B., Litkowski, S., Shakir, R.: Segment Routing Architecture. RFC 8402 (2018). https://doi.org/10.17487/RFC8402
7. Bashandy, A., Filsfils, C., Previdi, S., Decraene, B., Litkowski, S., Shakir, R.: Segment Routing with the MPLS Data Plane. RFC 8660 (2019). https://doi.org/10.17487/RFC8660
8. Xu, X., Bryant, S., Farrel, A., Hassan, S., Henderickx, W., Li, Z.: MPLS Segment Routing over IP. RFC 8663 (2019). https://doi.org/10.17487/RFC8663
9. Portegies, C., Kaat, M., Grosso, P.: In: 2021 24th Conference on Innovation in Clouds, Internet and Networks and Workshops (ICIN), pp. 1–5 IEEE (2021)
10. Farrel, A., Vasseur, J.P., Ash, J.: A path computation element (PCE)-based architecture. Tech. rep. (2006)
11. Vasseur, J., Roux, J.L.L.: Path Computation Element (PCE) Communication Protocol (PCEP). RFC 5440 (2009). https://doi.org/10.17487/RFC5440
12. Sivabalan, S., Filsfils, C., Tantsura, J., Henderickx, W., Hardwick, J.: Path Computation Element Communication Protocol (PCEP) Extensions for Segment Routing. RFC 8664 (2019). https://doi.org/10.17487/RFC8664
13. Rzym, G., Wajda, K., Chołda, P.: SDN-based WAN optimization: PCE implementation in multi-domain MPLS networks supported by BGP-LS. Image Process. Commun. **22**(1), 35–48 (2017)
14. Dugeon, O., Guedrez, R., Lahoud, S., Texier, G.: In: 2017 20th Conference on Innovations in Clouds, Internet and Networks (ICIN), pp. 143–145. IEEE (2017),
15. Dowling, B., Fischlin, M., Günther, F., Stebila, D.: A cryptographic analysis of the TLS 1.3 handshake protocol. J. Cryptol. **34**(4), 37 (2021)
16. Boldrini, L., Bazo, R., Hesselman, C., Grosso, P.: In: ICT Open 2021 (2021)
17. Minei, I., Crabbe, E., Sivabalan, S., Ananthakrishnan, H., Dhody, D., Tanaka, Y.: RFC 8697 Path Computation Element Communication Protocol (PCEP) Extensions for Establishing Relationships between Sets of Label Switched Paths (LSPs) (2020)

18. Vasseur, J., Zhang, R., Bitar, N., Le Roux, J.: A backward-recursive PCE-based computation (BRPC) procedure to compute shortest constrained inter-domain traffic engineering label switched paths. Tech. rep. (2009)
19. Dugeon, O., Meuric, J., Lee, Y., Ceccarelli, D.: PCEP Extension for Stateful Inter-Domain Tunnels. Internet-Draft draft-ietf-pce-stateful-interdomain-03, Internet Engineering Task Force (2022).https://datatracker.ietf.org/doc/draft-ietf-pce-stateful-interdomain/03/. Work in Progress
20. Zhang, F., Zhao, Q., de Dios, O.G., Casellas, R., King, D.:Path Computation Element Communication Protocol (PCEP) Extensions for the Hierarchical Path Computation Element (H-PCE) Architecture (2019)
21. Boldrini, L.: PCEPS Proof of concept (2023). https://bitbucket.org/leoboldrini/workspace/projects/PCEPS
22. Wang, A., Khasanov, B., Zhao, Q., Chen, H.: PCE-Based Traffic Engineering (TE) in Native IP Networks. RFC 8821 (2021). https://doi.org/10.17487/RFC8821

Performance Evaluation of Multi-hop Multi-branch AF Relaying Cooperative Diversity Network

Arwa Sh. Aqel and Mamoun F. Al-Mistarihi(✉)

Jordan University of Science and Technology, Irbid, Jordan
mistarihi@just.edu.jo

Abstract. The amplify-and-forward relaying method is used in the proposed work to examine the cooperative diversity system's multi-hop multi-branch relaying performance. This paper proposes a best-path selection combining reception technique that enables the destination to choose the best route based on bit error rate (BER), outage probability (OP) or signal-to-noise ratio (SNR) at the receiving antenna's output. Furthermore, closed-form formulas for the system's BER and OP are presented taking into account Nakagami-m fading channels and additive white Gaussian noise, assuming independent non-identical slow flat fading channels. Plotting the simulation results was done using various fading parameters.

Keywords: Cooperative diversity · multi-hop · multi-branch · amplify-and-forward relaying · Nakagami-m fading channel · best-path selection combining · Signal to Noise Ratio · bit error rate · outage probability

1 Introduction

In conventional wireless communications, a single antenna is used at the source, and another single antenna is used at the destination. But in some cases, this signal is scattered many paths to reach the destination due to obstructions such as hills, canyons and buildings. This causes problems such as fading, cut-out, and intermittent reception. And then, a reduction in data speed and an increase in the probability of errors. The use of multiple antennas at the transmitter and the receiver to transmit a signal, eliminates the problems caused by multipath effects.

With the growing demand for high data rates, enhancing transmission capacity and energy efficiency in wire-less communication, novel approaches and methods are required [1, 2]. Multipath, fading, and distortion are only a few of the difficulties that wireless communication must overcome using various ways to diversity techniques. A cooperative relaying system is an excellent technique for dealing with multipath fading in a wireless channel [3, 4].

Cooperative diversity is a strategy that uses cooperative multiple antennas in wireless multi-hop networks to increase total network channel capacity for any given set of bandwidths by decoding the combined signal of the relayed signal and the direct

K. Daimi and A. Al Sadoon (Eds.): ACR 2024, LNNS 956, pp. 479–493, 2024.
https://doi.org/10.1007/978-3-031-56950-0_40

signal. Whereas a traditional single hop system employs direct transmission, in which a receiver decodes information completely based on the direct signal and considers the relayed signal to be interference, but cooperative diversity considers the other signal to be contribution.

In other words, cooperative diversity decodes information from the combined signal of the direct signal and the relayed signal. As a result, cooperative diversity is an antenna diversity that employs distributed antennas on each node in a wireless network. Another definition of cooperative diversity is user cooperation that takes into account the reality that each user relays the signal of the other user, whereas cooperative diversity is also achievable by multi-hop relay networks.

The simplest and most basic cooperative relaying scheme consists of three nodes, which are source, relay, and destination, where each relay forwards a replica of its received signal to the next hop. Therefore, several works proposed different approaches and techniques to utilize the unlicensed spectrum for mobile communication [5–8].

In an effort to minimize the effects of fading, cooperative diversity is applied by transmitting independent copies of the signal. Selection Combining (SC) [9], Equal Gain Combining (EGC) [10], and Maximum Ratio Combining (MRC) [11] are the three most frequently used combining diversity approaches SC is the simplest technique due to its low cost and complexity.

The process of selecting one or more relays is one of the most important elements to include in a cooperative relaying system. Since relaying demands more receiving actions than direct source to destination transmission, relay selection must be efficient [12–14]. Relay schemes are classified into three categories:

1. Amplify-and-Forward (AF), in which the relay amplifies and sends the received signal from the source to the destination [15].
2. Decode-and-Forward (DF), in which the relay decodes and re-encodes the received signal from the source before forwarding it to the destination [15, 16].
3. Compress-and-Forward (CF), in which the relay compresses the received signal from the source and transfers it to the destination without decoding [17].

2 Related Works

Several works studied the cooperative relaying networks to analyze its performance based on the type of the relay and the combining diversity approaches are introduced. The authors in [18–20] studied the ABER of multi hops AF relay-based systems via Nakagami-m fading channels in channel connections. Also, the ABER with mixed DF and AF relays with BPSK and QPSK modulation techniques over Rayleigh fading channels using best path selection is calculated in [21].

In [22], for a Dual-hop DF Incremental Relaying system via Nakagami-m fading channels with the existence of multiple L distinguishable interferers positioned close to the destination, the system's BER improves as the Nakagami order grows and there are fewer interferers. In addition, the BER of the system is analyzed in [23] using Rayleigh fading channels with a range of adjacent L non-indistinguishable interferers. On a cooperative communication system, hybrid relay selection selects the relay used between AF and DF relays. It depends upon the highest SNR value achieved when switching between AF and DF choices [24].

A cooperative relay network, on the other hand, is a promising technology for enhancing outage performance in wireless communications [25]. Dual Hop Differential Amplify-and-Forward relaying system is derived as OP performance using Post-Detection Selection combining reception technique in [26] where the receiver uses the previous received sample in each branch as the estimate of the current fading gain in that branch. A homogeneous Poisson point approach is used to explain the random distribution of femtocell base stations and macrocell users in a 5G heterogeneous network in order to satisfy the extremely high data rate requirements of forthcoming 5G communications. As part of the performance study, the energy effectiveness, network throughput, and OP are all analyzed in [27].

The studies of [28–31] evaluated the performance of dual-hop and multi-hop multi-branch cognitive relay systems of OP via independent and non-identical Rayleigh, Nakagami-m and Rician fading channels, both with and without selection diversity and direct path broadcasting to the destination.

[32] demonstrated that the system with multiple relays outperforms the system in a single relay with regard to both symbol error probability and OP on Rayleigh fading channels. The efficiency of a dual-hop differential AF relay network was examined in [33, 34] as BER and OP performance through Nakagami-m fading channels with a post-detection SC approach. Furthermore, the performance of this system is investigated in [35] under the assumption of an M-ary phase-shift keying modulation.

[36] presented a DF-IR system, and it has been recognized that as the Nakagami order decreases and co-channel interference increases, the system's OP becomes substantially impeded. Furthermore, in [37], using a similar system design on Rayleigh fading channels, increasing co-channel interferences will increase the BER and OP, reducing overall system efficiency.

In this study, we present a cooperative multi-hop multi-branch relaying network. We assume that each link follows the AF relaying protocol. The protocol employs $N_i - 1$ (out of $(N_i - 1)$) of the relays and one of the branches at a time. The switching of the M branches is caused by the destination having one feedback toggling bit (such as, for a toggle state bit $= 1$ and for a hold state bit $= 0$) to keep one of the branches active and the others put on hold until a request from the destination is received. The criterion on the receiver for sending the feedback bit is a type of measurement of the SNR at the receiving antenna output, the BER, or the OP where the receiver has a single antenna. Then, the best multi-hop path can be selected at the destination side. Consequently, the proposed system investigates both the exact ABER and the OP performance.

The remainder of this article is organized as follows. Section 3 presents our proposed system model. In Sect. 4, the system BER and outage performance expressions are derived as exact formulas. Plotted simulation results and discussion are presented in Sect. 5. A summary of this paper's conclusion is provided in Sect. 6.

3 System Model

Figure 1 depicts the system model of a relaying cooperative with multi-hop multi-branch. It consists of a total of M branches, each of them consists of N_i hops between the source node (S) and the destination node (D). $L = \sum_{i=1}^{M}(N_i - 1)$ is the total number of relays in the network as a result. Over a slow flat Nakagami-m fading channel, all nodes transmit data. The channel coefficient between each two of nodes is given by h_{ij}, where $i = 1, 2, \ldots, M$ and $j = 1, 2, \ldots, N_i$. Additionally, it is assumed that each link is mutually independent and uncorrelated. They have an additive white Gaussian noise (AWGN) terms with a zero mean and equal variance N_o. Also, there is no line of sight between nodes S and D.

At the receiver, the best route to the destination is chosen by a selection combining technique.

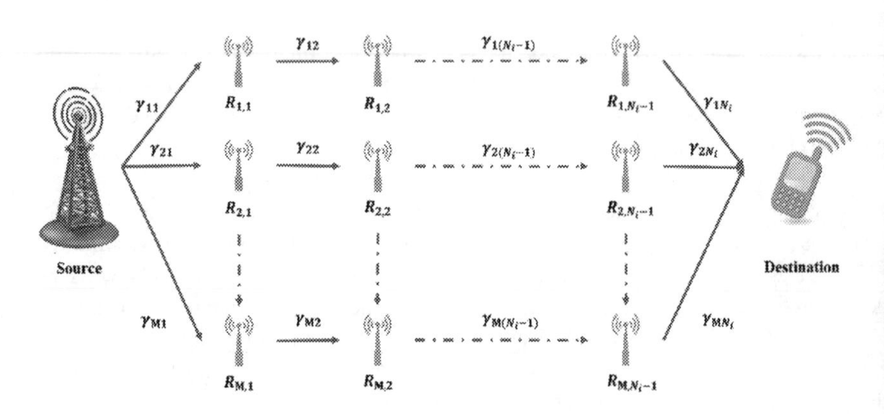

Fig. 1. System model.

4 Performance Analysis

In this section, we calculate the ABER and OP of the proposed model.

4.1 Bit Error Rate

Based to the suggested system model, the total of all error sources caused by the use of all branches defines the ABER $P_b(\gamma_b)$ of a multi-hop multi-branch network.

$$P_b(\gamma_b) = \sum_{i=1}^{M} P_r(\gamma_{RDi} > \gamma_{RD\forall\ell})P_{ri}(e), \quad \ell = 1, 2, \ldots, M, \quad \ell \neq i \tag{1}$$

where,

$$P_r(\gamma_{RDi} > \gamma_{RD\forall\ell}) = \prod_{\substack{\ell = 1 \\ \ell \neq i}}^{M} P_r(\gamma_{RDi} > \gamma_{RD\ell}) \tag{2}$$

$$P_{ri}(e) = P_{rSR_{i1}R_{iN_i-1}}(e)P_{xi}(e) + \left(1 - P_{rSR_{i1}R_{iN_i-1}}(e)\right)P_{rRDi}(e) \tag{3}$$

Here, $P_r(\gamma_{RDi} > \gamma_{RD\ell})$ is the probability that the SNR γ_{RDi} is greater than $\gamma_{RD\ell}$ which means selecting the ith branch for transmission, $P_{rSR_{i1}R_{iN_i-1}}(e)$ is the bit error probability at the $(N_i - 1)$ relay for the ith branch, $P_{rRDi}(e)$ is the bit error probability at the destination correctly for the ith branch and $P_{xi}(e)$ is the error propagation probability with the worst-case value, $P_{xi}(e) < 0.5$, for the ith branch [18].

The selection of multi branches for transmission is determined by the SNR measurements at the output of the receiving antenna to make the branch with the highest SNR stay in the working state and the other branches stay hold off until a request from the destination is turned on. The average SNR γ_{ij} at the input of the jth hop in the ith branch with taking into account the effect of the path loss [38] is defined as:

$$\overline{\gamma}_{ij} = \frac{E_s}{N_0}\left[\frac{d_{SD}}{d_{ij}}\right]^{\alpha} \tag{4}$$

In which, E_s is the energy of transmitted signal, h_{ij} is the channel fading coefficient of the jth hop in the ith branch, d_{SD} is the distance between the source and the destination, d_{ij} is the distance from $(j - 1)^{th}$ hop to j^{th} hop in the ith branch and α is the path loss exponent.

To get the BER $P_{rSR_{i1}R_{iN_i-1}}(e)$ at the $(N_i - 1)$ relay for the ith branch, the probability density function (PDF) of the equivalent received SNR at the input of the $(N_i - 1)$ relay for the selected branch have to be determined. The equivalent received SNR γ_{eq,N_i-1} of the $(N_i - 1)$ relay is expressed as:

$$\gamma_{eq,N_i-1} = \left[\prod_{j=1}^{N_i-1}\left(1+\frac{1}{\gamma_{ij}}\right) - 1\right]^{-1} \tag{5}$$

Instead of using the exact value of γ_{eq,N_i-1}, , a tight upper bound is employed to describe the PDF of (5) in a more mathematically tractable manner.

$$\gamma_{eq,N_i-1} \le \gamma_i = \min\left(\gamma_{i1}, \gamma_{i2}, \ldots, \gamma_{i(N_i-1)}\right) \tag{6}$$

where, $\min(x, y)$ indicates the smallest value of x and y.

The PDF of a continuous random variable γ_i can be expressed as the derivative of its cumulative distribution function (CDF) $F_{\gamma_i}(\gamma)$. Since, the received SNR at the input of each relay is independent random variable for all M branches. Then,

$$F_{\gamma_i}(\gamma) = 1 - \prod_{k=1}^{N_i-1}\left[1 - F_{\gamma_{ik}}(\gamma)\right] \tag{7}$$

And,

$$f_{\gamma_i}(\gamma) = \sum_{j=1}^{N_i-1}\left(\prod_{\substack{k=1 \\ k \neq j}}^{N_i-1}\left[1 - F_{\gamma_{ik}}(\gamma)\right] f_{\gamma_{ij}}(\gamma)\right) \tag{8}$$

For every path, the fading channel coefficient is represented by a Nakagami-m random variable. As a result, the SNR γ_{ij} has a gamma distribution [39, 40] with a PDF and CDF, respectively, are given by:

$$f_{\gamma_{ij}}(\gamma) = \frac{1}{\Gamma(m_{ij})}\left(\frac{m_{ij}}{\overline{\gamma}_{ij}}\right)^{m_{ij}} \gamma^{m_{ij}-1} e^{-\frac{m_{ij}}{\overline{\gamma}_{ij}}\gamma} \tag{9}$$

$$F_{\gamma_{ij}}(\gamma) = \frac{\gamma\left(m_{ij}, \frac{m_{ij}}{\overline{\gamma}_{ij}}\gamma\right)}{\Gamma(m_{ij})} \tag{10}$$

where, m_{ij} is the Nakagami-m fading parameter related to the jth hop of the ith branch and $\gamma(\alpha, x)$ is the lower incomplete gamma function.

Now, the average bit error probability at the $(N_i - 1)$ relay for the ith branch $P_{rSR_{i1}R_{iN_i-1}}(e)$ is expressed by averaging the conditional bit error probability $P(\rceil/\gamma)$ over the PDF of γ_i.

$$P_{rSR_{i1}R_{iN_i-1}}(e) = \int_0^{\infty} P(\rceil/\gamma) f_{\gamma_i}(\gamma) d\gamma \tag{11}$$

where,

$$P(\rceil/\gamma) = a\,\mathrm{erfc}\left(\sqrt{b\gamma}\right) \tag{12}$$

where, a and b are the coefficients that determine the modulation scheme that is used. For BPSK $\left(a = \frac{1}{2}, b = 1\right)$ and for QPSK $\left(a = \frac{1}{2}, b = \frac{1}{2}\right)$.

Therefore,

$$P_{rSR_{i1}R_{iN_i-1}}(e) = \frac{2a}{\pi}\sum_{j=1}^{N_i-1} \frac{1}{\Gamma(m_{ij})}\left(\frac{m_{ij}}{\overline{\gamma}_{ij}}\right)^{m_{ij}} \int_0^{\frac{\pi}{2}}\int_0^{\infty} \gamma^{m_{ij}-1} e^{-\left(\frac{b}{\sin^2\theta}+\frac{m_{ij}}{\overline{\gamma}_{ij}}\right)\gamma} \prod_{\substack{k=1 \\ k\neq j}}^{N_i-1}\left[\frac{\Gamma\left(m_{ik}, \frac{m_{ik}}{\overline{\gamma}_{ik}}\gamma\right)}{\Gamma(m_{ik})}\right] d\gamma\, d\theta \tag{13}$$

$P_{rSR_{i1}R_{iN_i-1}}(e)$ can be determined as follows:

$$P_{rSR_{i1}R_{iN_i-1}}(e) = \frac{2a}{\pi}\sum_{j=1}^{N_i-1}\left(\frac{1}{\Gamma(m_{ij})}\left(\frac{m_{ij}}{\overline{\gamma}_{ij}}\right)^{m_{ij}}\left[\sum_{t=0}^{\sum_{\substack{k=1\\k\neq j}}^{N_i-1}(m_{ik}-1)} \sum_{\sum_{\substack{k=1\\k\neq j}}^{N_i-1} n_k = t}\left(\prod_{\substack{k=1\\k\neq j}}^{N_i-1}\frac{(m_{ik}-1)!\left(\frac{m_{ik}}{\overline{\gamma}_{ik}}\right)^{n_k}}{n_k!\,\Gamma(m_{ik})}\frac{\Gamma(m_{ij}+t)}{\left(\sum_{k=1}^{N_i-1}\frac{m_{ik}}{\overline{\gamma}_{ik}}\right)^{m_{ij}+t}}\right)\right.\right.$$

$$\times\left[\frac{\pi}{2}\left(1-\sqrt{\frac{\left(\prod_{k=1}^{N_i-1}\overline{\gamma}_{ik}\right)b}{\left(\sum_{k=1}^{N_i-1}\left(m_{ik}\prod_{\substack{l=1\\ l\neq k}}^{N_i-1}\overline{\gamma}_{i\ell}\right)\right)+\left(\prod_{k=1}^{N_i-1}\overline{\gamma}_{ik}\right)b}}\right)\right]^{m_{ij}+t} \quad (14)$$

where, $n_k = 0, 1, \ldots, (m_{ik} - 1)$.

The average bit error probability at the destination for the ith branch $P_{rRDi}(e)$ can be determined as in [41], then,

$$P_{rRDi}(e) = \frac{2a}{\pi}\left[\frac{\pi}{2}\left(1-\sqrt{\frac{\overline{\gamma}_{RDi}b}{m_{RDi}+\overline{\gamma}_{RDi}b}}\right)\right]^{m_{RDi}} \quad (15)$$

Because the path with the highest SNR at the destination is used to determine which is the best way. It is assumed that the random variable Y is:

$$Y = \gamma_{RDi} - \gamma_{RD\ell}, \quad i, \ell = 1, 2, \ldots, M, \quad i < \ell \quad (16)$$

Accordingly, this indicates that when $\gamma_{RDi} > \gamma_{RD\ell}$, the signal is transmitted by the ith branch, and when $\gamma_{RD\ell} > \gamma_{RDi}$, the ℓth branch is chosen.

In order to calculate the probability of selecting the best branch for transmission for the two cases $\gamma_{RDi} > \gamma_{RD\ell}$ and $\gamma_{RD\ell} > \gamma_{RDi}$, the PDF of (16) $f_Y(\gamma)$ have to be determined. It can be computed as in the manner shown in [41]. Then,

$$f_Y(\gamma) = \frac{1}{\Gamma(m_{RDi})\Gamma(m_{RD\ell})}\left(\frac{m_{RDi}}{\overline{\gamma}_{RDi}}\right)^{m_{RDi}}\left(\frac{m_{RD\ell}}{\overline{\gamma}_{RD\ell}}\right)^{m_{RD\ell}} \times \begin{cases} e^{\frac{m_{RD\ell}}{\overline{\gamma}_{RD\ell}}\gamma}\sum_{k=0}^{m_{RD\ell}-1}\binom{m_{RD\ell}-1}{k}\frac{\Gamma(m_{RDi}+k)(-\gamma)^{m_{RD\ell}-k-1}}{\left(\frac{m_{RDi}}{\overline{\gamma}_{RDi}}+\frac{m_{RD\ell}}{\overline{\gamma}_{RD\ell}}\right)^{m_{RDi}+k}}, & y \leq 0 \\ e^{-\frac{m_{RDi}}{\overline{\gamma}_{RDi}}\gamma}\sum_{k=0}^{m_{RDi}-1}\binom{m_{RDi}-1}{k}\frac{\Gamma(m_{RD\ell}+k)\gamma^{m_{RDi}-k-1}}{\left(\frac{m_{RDi}}{\overline{\gamma}_{RDi}}+\frac{m_{RD\ell}}{\overline{\gamma}_{RD\ell}}\right)^{m_{RD\ell}+k}}, & y > 0 \end{cases} \quad (17)$$

Assume $\overline{\gamma}_{RDi} = \overline{\gamma}_{RDl} = \overline{\gamma}_{RD}$. Then, one can obtain a general expression of the probability of selecting the ith branch for transmission as in [41]. As a result, $P_r(\gamma_{RDi} > \gamma_{RD\ell})$ is given by:

$$P_r(\gamma_{RDi} > \gamma_{RD\ell}) = \frac{2am_{RD\ell}{}^{m_{RD\ell}}}{\pi\Gamma(m_{RDi})\Gamma(m_{RD\ell})}\sum_{k=0}^{m_{RDi}-1}\binom{m_{RDi}-1}{k}\frac{m_{RDi}{}^{k}}{(m_{RDi}+m_{RD\ell})^{m_{RD\ell}+k}}\Gamma(m_{RDi}-k)\,\Gamma(m_{RD\ell}+k)\times\left[\frac{\pi}{2}\left(1-\sqrt{\frac{\overline{\gamma}_{RD}b}{m_{RDi}+\overline{\gamma}_{RD}b}}\right)\right]^{m_{RDi}-k}, \quad i, \ell = 1, 2, \ldots, M, \ell \neq i \quad (18)$$

The closed-form formulation of BER in multi-hop multi-branch AF relaying system $P_b(\gamma_b)$ can now be obtained as in (19) by replacing (2), (3), (14), (15) and (18) into (1).

$$
\begin{aligned}
P_b(\gamma_b) &= \sum_{i=1}^{M}\Bigg[\prod_{\substack{\ell=1\\ \ell\neq i}}^{M}\Bigg[\frac{2\,a\,m_{RD\ell}{}^{m_{RD\ell}}}{\pi\Gamma(m_{RDi})\,\Gamma(m_{RD\ell})}\sum_{k=0}^{m_{RDi}-1}\binom{m_{RDi}-1}{k}\frac{m_{RDi}{}^{k}\,\Gamma(m_{RDi}-k)\,\Gamma(m_{RD\ell}+k)}{(m_{RDi}+m_{RD\ell})^{m_{RD\ell}+k}}\Bigg[\frac{\pi}{2}\Bigg(1-\sqrt{\frac{\bar{\gamma}_{RD}\,b}{m_{RDi}+\bar{\gamma}_{RD}\,b}}\Bigg)\Bigg]^{m_{RDi}-k}\Bigg] \\
&\times\Bigg[\frac{2a}{\pi}\sum_{j=1}^{N_i-1}\Bigg(\frac{1}{\Gamma(m_{ij})}\bigg(\frac{m_{ij}}{\bar{\gamma}_{ij}}\bigg)^{m_{ij}}\Bigg[\sum_{t=0}^{\sum_{k=1,k\neq j}^{N_i-1}(m_{ik}-1)}\ \sum_{\sum_{k=1,k\neq j}^{N_i-1}n_k=t}\Bigg(\prod_{\substack{k=1\\ k\neq j}}^{N_i-1}\frac{(m_{ik}-1)!\left(\frac{m_{ik}}{\bar{\gamma}_{ik}}\right)^{n_k}\Gamma(m_{ij}+t)}{n_k!\,\Gamma(m_{ik})\left(\sum_{k=1}^{N_i-1}\frac{m_{ik}}{\bar{\gamma}_{ik}}\right)^{m_{ij}+t}}\Bigg)\Bigg[\frac{\pi}{2}\Bigg(1 \\
&-\sqrt{\frac{\left(\prod_{k=1}^{N_i-1}\bar{\gamma}_{ik}\right)b}{\left(\sum_{k=1}^{N_i-1}\left(m_{ik}\prod_{\substack{\ell=1\\ \ell\neq k}}^{N_i-1}\bar{\gamma}_{i\ell}\right)\right)+\left(\prod_{k=1}^{N_i-1}\bar{\gamma}_{ik}\right)b}}\Bigg)\Bigg]^{m_{ij}+t}\Bigg]\Bigg)P_{xi}(e) \\
&+\Bigg(1 \\
&-\frac{2a}{\pi}\sum_{j=1}^{N_i-1}\Bigg(\frac{1}{\Gamma(m_{ij})}\bigg(\frac{m_{ij}}{\bar{\gamma}_{ij}}\bigg)^{m_{ij}}\Bigg[\sum_{t=0}^{\sum_{k=1,k\neq j}^{N_i-1}(m_{ik}-1)}\ \sum_{\sum_{k=1,k\neq j}^{N_i-1}n_k=t}\Bigg(\prod_{\substack{k=1\\ k\neq j}}^{N_i-1}\frac{(m_{ik}-1)!\left(\frac{m_{ik}}{\bar{\gamma}_{ik}}\right)^{n_k}\Gamma(m_{ij}+t)}{n_k!\,\Gamma(m_{ik})\left(\sum_{k=1}^{N_i-1}\frac{m_{ik}}{\bar{\gamma}_{ik}}\right)^{m_{ij}+t}}\Bigg)\Bigg[\frac{\pi}{2}\Bigg(1 \\
&-\sqrt{\frac{\left(\prod_{k=1}^{N_i-1}\bar{\gamma}_{ik}\right)b}{\left(\sum_{k=1}^{N_i-1}\left(m_{ik}\prod_{\substack{\ell=1\\ \ell\neq k}}^{N_i-1}\bar{\gamma}_{i\ell}\right)\right)+\left(\prod_{k=1}^{N_i-1}\bar{\gamma}_{ik}\right)b}}\Bigg)\Bigg]^{m_{ij}+t}\Bigg]\Bigg)\Bigg)\frac{2a}{\pi}\Bigg[\frac{\pi}{2}\Bigg(1 \\
&-\sqrt{\frac{\bar{\gamma}_{RD1}\,b}{m_{RDi}+\bar{\gamma}_{RDi}\,b}}\Bigg)\Bigg]^{m_{RDi}}\Bigg]\Bigg]
\end{aligned}
\tag{19}
$$

For BPSK $\left(a=\frac{1}{2}, b=1\right)$ and for QPSK $\left(a=\frac{1}{2}, b=\frac{1}{2}\right)$.

4.2 Outage Probability

Information theory employs the Shannon–Hartley theorem to determine the maximum bit/sec channel capacity C that may be used to transmit data via a communication channel with a given bandwidth of B Hz while noise is there. This formula is $C=\mu B\log_2(1+\gamma)$. Here, the pre-log factor $\mu=\frac{1}{2}$ is due to the relay working under half-duplex mode, which requires two time slots to transfer data from the source to the destination. Additionally, a normalized bandwidth B of 1 Hz is specified for the system.

Therefore, the mutual information I of the proposed system model where the best-path selection is employed, can be expressed as follows:

$$I = \frac{1}{2}\log_2(1 + \gamma_{max}) \tag{20}$$

where, γ_{max} is the maximum of all M branches' total end-to-end SNR.

The opportunity that the mutual information of channel I goes under the necessary threshold spectral efficiency R (bps/Hz) is defined as the OP of the system P_{out}. So, the data rate must be lower than the channel information rate in order to guarantee dependable connections.

Therefore,

$$P_{out}(x) = P_r(I \leq R) \tag{21}$$

Then (21) can be expressed as:

$$P_{out}(x) = P_r(\gamma_{max} \leq x) = F_{\gamma_{max}}(x) \tag{22}$$

where,

$$\gamma_{max} = \max(\gamma_1, \gamma_2, \ldots, \gamma_M) \tag{23}$$

Since, γ_i for all M branches are mutually independent random variables. Then

$$F_{\gamma_{max}}(x) = \prod_{i=1}^{M} F_{\gamma_i}(x) = P_{out}(x) \tag{24}$$

The total end-to-end SNR of the ith branch γ_i can be approximated as:

$$\gamma_i = \min\left(\gamma_{i1}, \gamma_{i2}, \ldots, \gamma_{iN_i}\right) \tag{25}$$

Therefore, the CDF of (25) can be expressed as:

$$F_{\gamma_i}(x) = 1 - \prod_{j=1}^{N_i}\left[1 - F_{\gamma_{ij}}(\gamma)\right] \tag{26}$$

$P_{out}(x)$ can then be rewritten as follows:

$$P_{out}(x) = F_{\gamma_{max}}(x) = \prod_{i=1}^{M}\left[1 - \prod_{j=1}^{N_i} \frac{\Gamma\left(m_{ij}, \frac{m_{ij}}{\overline{\gamma}_{ij}}x\right)}{\Gamma\left(m_{ij}\right)}\right] \tag{27}$$

where, $x = 2^{2R} - 1$.

5 Numerical Results

To illustrate the efficiency of the proposed model, the obtained expressions of BER and OP are shown in this part analytically under BPSK and QPSK modulation schemes. The Monte Carlo simulation results are confirmed with the analytical ones.

In Fig. 2, the performance of BER versus SNR is shown with various modulation schemes; BPSK and QPSK. Here, the network consists four branches with four hops for each branch. The Nakagami-m parameters for all channels are assumed to be $m = 2$. Comparison of the BER curves shows that BPSK has the better performance of the proposed system than the other. For example, at $P_e = 10^{-10}$, the performance with BPSK offers a SNR of about 7 dB over QPSK. Additionally, by increasing the SNR for the same modulation scheme, the performance will be improved.

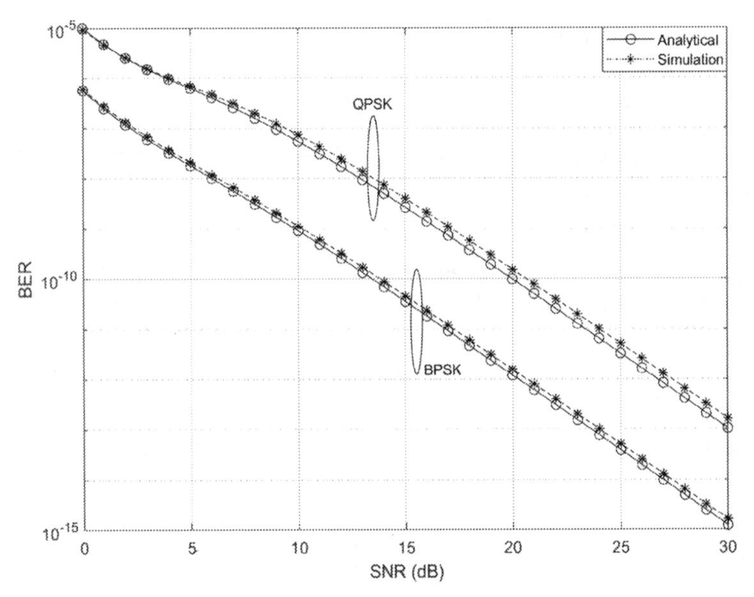

Fig. 2. The BER of the system using $M = 4, N = 4, m = 2$ for BPSK and QPSK.

On other hand, with using $N = 3, m = 2$ and QPSK modulation scheme, one observes in Fig. 3 that when the number of branches M is increased, the system performance will be better. Increasing the number of branches means increasing the transmitted signal copies that will arrive on different branches to the destination to select the best one. Since, the different branches undergo independent fading, then if one branch undergoes a deep fade, another branch may have strong signal. Therefore, $M = 6$ has the best performance. When $M = 2$, the performance is confirmed with [41] in terms of OP.

In Fig. 4, the performance of outage probability versus SNR is shown with various spectral efficiency $R = 3, 4, 5$ bps/Hz. Here, the network consists four branches with four hops for each branch. The Nakagami-m parameters for all channels are assumed to be $m = 2$. Comparison of the outage probability curves shows that $R = 3$ bps/Hz has the

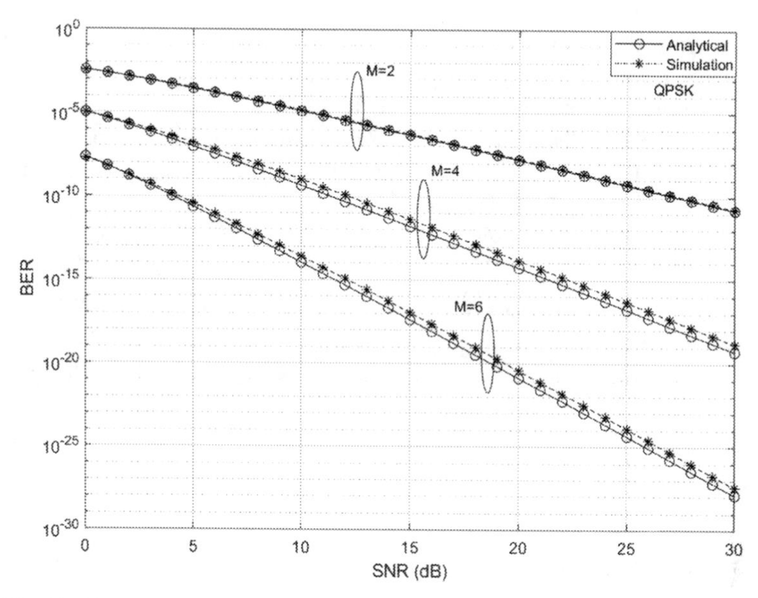

Fig. 3. The BER of the system using $N = 3, m = 2$ for QPSK with $M = 2, 4, 6$.

better performance of the proposed system than the others. Additionally, by increasing the SNR for the same spectral efficiency, the performance will be improved.

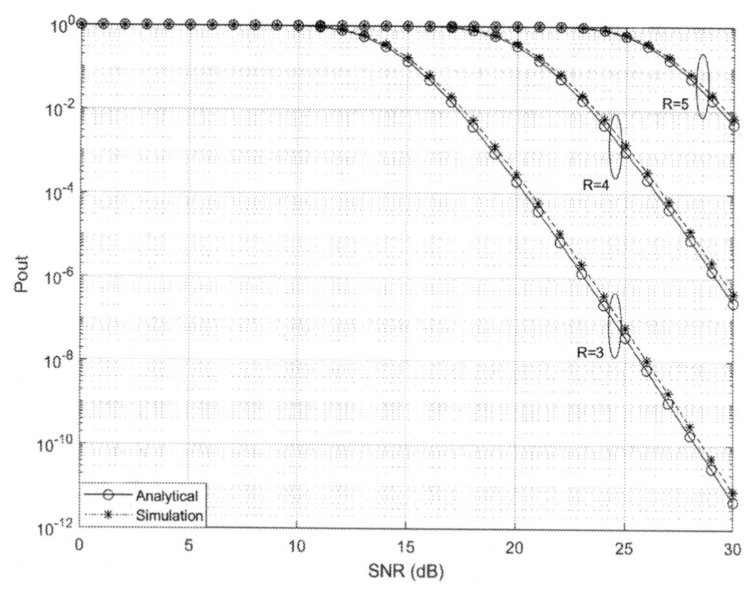

Fig. 4. The outage probability of the system using $M = 4, N = 4, m = 2$ for $R = 3, 4, 5$ bps/Hz.

With increasing the number of hops in each branch and the other variables remain constant, the outage probability will be decrease. This is because the relays will be continuously amplifying its received signal and forward it to another node in the network to arrive the destination. That means the presence of more relays or hops will decrease the probability of the system to be in out of service. This is presented in Fig. 5 with $M = 2$, $m = 2$ and spectral efficiency $R = 5$ bps/Hz. When $N = 3$, the performance is confirmed with [41] in terms of OP.

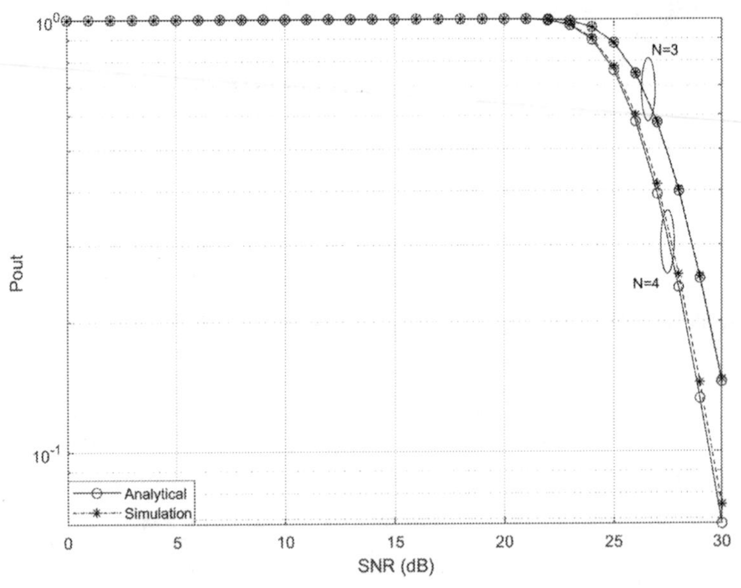

Fig. 5. The outage probability of the system using $M = 2, m = 2, R = 5$ bps/Hz with $N = 3, 4$.

6 Conclusion

This research evaluates the BER and OP performance analysis of cooperative networks using a diversity technique over independent non-identical Nakagami-m slow flat fading channels. The system model is evaluated using the best-path selection combining technique with a multi-hop multi-branch AF relaying protocol that enables the destination to choose the best route based on bit error rate, outage probability or signal-to-noise ratio at the receiving antenna's output. The efficiency of the proposed model is demonstrated by Monte Carlo simulation results, which are verified by the analytical ones under BPSK and QPSK modulation schemes. The presence of more branches and more relays or hops will decrease the probability of the system to be in out of service and therefore will enhance the performance of the system. Since, different branches undergo independent fading, then if one branch undergoes a deep fade, another branch may have strong signal.

References

1. Agiwal, M., Roy, A., Saxena, N.: Next generation 5G wireless networks: a comprehensive survey. IEEE Commun. Surv. Tutor. **18**(3), 1617–1655 (2016)
2. Asshad, M., Khan, S.A., Kavak, A., Küçük, K., Msongaleli, D.L.: Cooperative communications using relay nodes for next-generation wireless networks with optimal selection techniques: a review. IEEJ Trans. Electr. Electron. Eng. **14**, 658–669 (2019)
3. Ju, J., Duan, W., Sun, Q., Gao, S., Zhang, G.: Performance analysis for cooperative NOMA with opportunistic relay selection. IEEE Access **7**, 131488–131500 (2019)
4. Huang, R., et al.: Performance analysis of NOMA-based cooperative networks with relay selection. China Commun. **17**(11), 111–119 (2020)
5. Alhulayil, M., López-Benítez, M.: Methods for the allocation of almost blank subframes with fixed duty cycle for improved LTE-U/Wi-Fi coexistence. In: 2019 IEEE International Conference on Wireless Networks and Mobile Communications (WINCOM), pp. 1–6. IEEE, Fez (2019)
6. Alhulayil, M., López-Benítez, M.: Static contention window method for improved LTE-LAA/Wi-Fi coexistence in unlicensed bands. In: 2019 IEEE International Conference on Wireless Networks and Mobile Communications (WINCOM), pp. 1–6. IEEE, Fez (2019)
7. Alhulayil, M., López-Benítez, M.: Dynamic contention window methods for improved coexistence between LTE and Wi-Fi in unlicensed bands. In: 2019 IEEE Wireless Communications and Networking Conference Workshop (WCNCW), pp. 1–6. IEEE, Marrakech (2019)
8. Alhulayil, M., Lopez-Benitez, M.: LTE/Wi-Fi coexistence in unlicensed bands based on dynamic transmission opportunity. In: 2020 IEEE Wireless Communications and Networking Conference Workshops (WCNCW), pp. 1–6. IEEE, Virtual Conference (2020)
9. Sahu, H.K., Sahu, P.R., Mishra, J.: ABEP of SSK with SWIPT at relay and generalised selection combining at the destination over rayleigh fading. In: 2020 National Conference on Communications (NCC), pp. 1–6. IEEE, Kharagpur (2020)
10. Hashemi, H., Haghighat, J., Eslami, M., Hamouda, W.A.: Analysis of equal gain combining over fluctuating two-ray channels with applications to millimeter-wave communications. IEEE Trans. Veh. Technol. **69**(2), 1751–1765 (2020)
11. Olyaee, M., Eslami, M., Haghighat, J.: Performance of maximum ratio combining of fluctuating two-ray (FTR) mmWave channels for 5G and beyond communications. Trans. Emerg. Tel Tech. **30** (2019)
12. Asam, M., Zeeshan, H., Tauseef, J., Kashif, G., Aleena, A.: Novel relay selection protocol for cooperative networks. arXiv preprint (2019)
13. Onalan, A.G., Salik, E.D., Coleri, S.: Relay selection, scheduling, and power control in wireless-powered cooperative communication networks. IEEE Trans. Wirel. Commun. **19**(11), 7181–7195 (2020)
14. Guo, K., et al.: Performance analysis of hybrid satellite-terrestrial cooperative networks with relay selection. IEEE Trans. Veh. Technol. **69**(8), 9053–9067 (2020)
15. Saniar, M.N., Anggraini, N.P., Arifin, Moegiharto, Y.: Evaluation of the PTS PAPR reduction technique with the Hammerstein-wiener predistortion model in amplify-and-forward (AF), decode-and-forward (DF) relaying systems over asymmetric channels. In: 2021 International Electronics Symposium (IES), pp. 87–91. IEEE, Surabaya (2021)
16. Li, B., Yang, J., Yang, H., et al.: Decode-and-forward cooperative transmission in wireless sensor networks based on physical-layer network coding. Wirel. Netw. (2019)
17. Huang, C., Chen, G., Gong, Y., Wen, M., Chambers, J.A.: Deep reinforcement learning-based relay selection in intelligent reflecting surface assisted cooperative networks. IEEE Wirel. Commun. Lett. **10**(5), 1036–1040 (2021)

18. Magableh, A.M., Jafreh, N.: Exact expressions for the bit error rate and channel capacity of a dual-hop cooperative communication systems over Nakagami-m fading channels. J. Franklin Inst. **355**(1), 565–573 (2018)
19. Asshad, M., Khan, S.A., Kavak, A., Küçük, K.: Performance Analysis of multi-node cooperative network with amplify and forward relay protocol. In: 1st International Informatics and Software Engineering Conference (UBMYK), pp. 1–4. IEEE, Ankara (2019)
20. Bouteggui, M., Merazka, F.: Performance analysis of sub-optimal transmit and receive antenna selection amplify and forward cooperative communication. IET Commun. **13**(20), 3537–3546 (2019)
21. Al-Zoubi, S., Mohaisen, R., Al-Mistarihi, M.F., Khatalin, S.M., Khodeir, M.A.: On the outage probability of DF relay selection cooperative wireless networks over Nakagami-m fading channels. In: IEEE 7th International Conference on Information and Communication Systems (ICICS). IEEE, Irbid (2016)
22. Al-Mistarihi, M.F., Mohaisen, R., Darabkh, K.A.: Closed-form expression for BER in relay-based DF cooperative diversity systems over Nakagami-m fading channels with non-identical interferers. In: Galinina, O., Andreev, S., Balandin, S., Koucheryavy, Y. (eds.) NEW2AN ruSMART 2019 2019. LNCS, vol. 11660, pp. 700–709. Springer, Cham (2019). https://doi.org/10.1007/978-3-030-30859-9_61
23. Al-Mistarihi, M.F., Mohaisen, R., Darabkh, K.A.: BER analysis in relay-based DF cooperative diversity systems over rayleigh fading channels with non-identical interferers near the destination. In: International Conference on Advanced Communication Technologies and Networking (CommNet). IEEE, Rabat (2019)
24. Agaiby, R.: Performance evaluation of multi–hop multi–branch hybrid AF/DF relaying networks (2020)
25. Wan, H., Høst-Madsen, A., Nosratinia, A.: Compress-and-forward via multilevel coding. In: IEEE International Symposium on Information Theory (ISIT), pp. 2024–2028. IEEE, Paris (2019)
26. Magableh, A., Al-Mistarihi, M.F., Mohaisen, R.: Closed-form expression for bit error rate in relay-based cooperative diversity systems over multipath fading channels with interference. In: 9th International Wireless Communications and Mobile Computing (IWCMC). IEEE, Sardinia (2013)
27. Abidrabbu, A.M., Al-Mistarihi, M.F.: Performance analysis of 5G heterogeneous networks under the impact of aggregate interference over Nakagami-m fading channels. Trans. Emerg. Telecommun. Technol. (ETT) (2022)
28. Khodeir, M.A., Al-Mistarihi, M.F., Ibrahem, L.N.: Performance evaluation of cognitive relay networks for end user mobile over mixed realistic channels. IET Commun. **17**, 228–245 (2022)
29. Shurman, M.M., Al-Mistarihi, M.F., Alhulayil, M.: Performance analysis of amplify-and-forward cognitive relay networks with interference power constraints over Nakagami-m fading channels. IET Commun. **10**(5), 594–605 (2016)
30. Bastami, A.H., Kazemi, P.: Cognitive multi-hop multi-branch relaying: spectrum leasing and optimal power allocation. IEEE Trans. Wireless Commun. **18**(8), 4075–4088 (2019)
31. Fathollahi, H., Madani, M.H.: Performance analysis of multi-hop multi-branch amplify-and-forward cooperative communication over Rician fading channels. J. Circ. Syst. Comput. **29**(09), 2050148 (2020)
32. Al-Mistarihi, M.F., Sharaqa, A., Mohaisen, R., Abu-Alnadi, O., Abu-Seba, H.: Performance analysis of multiuser diversity in multiuser two-hop amplify and forward cooperative multi-relay wireless networks. In: 35th Jubilee International Convention on Information and Communication Technology, Electronics and Microelectronics (MIPRO), pp. 647–651. IEEE, Opatija (2012)

33. Al-Mistarihi, M.F., Harb, M.M., Darabkh, K.A., Aqel, A.Sh.: On the performance analysis of dual hop relaying systems using differential amplify-and-forward along with post-detection selection combining techniques over nakagami-m fading channels. Trans. Emerg. Telecommun. Technol. (ETT) (2020)
34. Harb, M.M., Al-Mistarihi, M.F.: Dual hop differential amplify-and-forward relaying with selection combining cooperative diversity over Nakagami-m fading channels. In: IEEE 8th International Conference on Communication Software and Networks (ICCSN), pp. 225–228. IEEE, Beijing (2016)
35. Al-Mistarihi, M.F., Aqel, A.S., Darabkh, K.A.: BER analysis in dual hop differential amplify-and-forward relaying systems with selection combining using M-ary phase-shift keying over Nakagami-m fading channels. In: Galinina, O., Andreev, S., Balandin, S., Koucheryavy, Y. (eds.) NEW2AN ruSMART 2019 2019. LNCS, vol. 11660, pp. 688–699. Springer, Heidelberg (2019). https://doi.org/10.1007/978-3-030-30859-9_60
36. Al-Mistarihi, M.F., Mohaisen, R., Darabkh, K.A.: Performance evaluation of decode and forward cooperative diversity systems over Nakagami-m fading channels with non-identical interferers. Int. J. Electr. Comput. Eng. (IJECE) **10**(5), 5316–5328 (2020)
37. Al-Mistarihi, M.F., Mohaisen, R., Darabkh, K.A.: On the performance of relay-based decode and forward cooperative diversity systems over rayleigh fading channels with non-identical interferers. IET Commun. **13**(19), 3135–3144 (2019)
38. Hayajneh, A.M., Khodeir, M.A., Al-Mistarihi, M.F.: Incremental-relaying cooperative-networks using dual transmit diversity and decode and forward relaying scheme with best relay selection. In: 37th Jubilee International Convention on Information and Communication Technology, Electronics and Microelectronics (MIPRO). IEEE, Opatija (2014)
39. Alhulayil, M., Al-Mistarihi, M.F., Shurman, M.M.: Performance analysis of dual-hop AF cognitive relay networks with best selection and interference constraints. Electronics **12**(1), 124 (2022)
40. Ibrahem, L.N., Al-Mistarihi, M.F., Khodeir, M.A., Alhulayil, M., Darabkh, K.A.: Best relay selection strategy in cooperative spectrum sharing framework with mobile-based end user. Appl. Sci. **13**(14), 8127 (2023)
41. Aqel, A.Sh., Al-Mistarihi, M.F.: Performance analysis of dual-hop dual-branch amplify-and- forward relaying cooperative diversity system using best-path selection technique over Nakagami-m fading channels. Trans. Emerg. Telecommun. Technol. (ETT) (2023)

Cloud and Mobile Computing

An Overview of Infrastructure as Code (IaC) with Performance and Availability Assessment on Google Cloud Platform

Hongyu Wang, Brian Kishiyama, David Lopez, and Jeong Yang(✉)

Department of Computational, Engineering, and Mathematical Sciences, Texas A&M University-San Antonio, San Antonio, TX, USA
{hwang04,bkish01,david.lopez}@jaguar.tamu.edu,
jeong.yang@tamusa.edu

Abstract. This paper presents the results of an exploratory study on the performance and availability of two prominent Infrastructure as Code (IaC) tools - Google Cloud Deployment Manager and Terraform. The Deployment Manager is native to Google Cloud Services while Terraform is not. The study assesses the deployment and management of cloud resources by using these tools, and examines their integration benefits, flexibility, and multi-cloud capabilities. It highlights Terraform's consistently faster resource destruction times compared to Google Cloud Deployment Manager, as evidenced by tests using the Linux 'time' command, providing insights into their operational efficiency and adaptability in cloud environments. Our findings indicate that the native Google Cloud Deployment Manager better integrates with its resources. In contrast, Terraform is versatile, provides better flexibility and deploys faster. Its independence is more useful in working with various cloud environments – and is not limited to GCP. Additionally, to gain insight, this study discusses the benefits and inherent challenges associated with IaC. This paper underlines the significance of technical expertise in effectively leveraging these tools for cloud infrastructure management.

Keywords: Cloud Infrastructure as Code · IaC · Google Cloud Deployment Manager · Terraform · Cloud Computing · Performance Analysis · Availability Assessment · Cloud Resource Management · Multi-Cloud Strategy · Google Cloud Platform · GCP

1 Introduction

Organizations deal with large volumes of data relying on computing resources. Cloud Computing is growing and expanding with businesses. Businesses rely on Cloud Computing resources to become more efficient and profitable in a competitive market. With large enterprises, many cloud resources are needed. They need to be coordinated and deployed quickly and efficiently. Infrastructure as Code (IaC) is a tool to address this. IaC is a modern approach to handling computing infrastructure by automating tasks and treating infrastructure configurations as code. It is a valuable tool for improving scalability, reducing manual work, ensuring consistency, and enhancing infrastructure management in cloud environments.

K. Daimi and A. Al Sadoon (Eds.): ACR 2024, LNNS 956, pp. 497–514, 2024.
https://doi.org/10.1007/978-3-031-56950-0_41

This paper explores advantages of IaC, as discussed from various sources, that shed light on the numerous benefits to organizations. Its approach involves managing and provisioning computing infrastructure through machine-readable script files, deviating from traditional methods dependent on physical hardware configuration or interactive tools. The concept of IaC emerged as a solution to challenges in manual infrastructure management, addressing issues like inconsistencies, configuration drift, and scalability difficulties. It emphasizes the need for a standardized and automated approach to configuration management, aligning with the principles of DevOps practices that encourage collaboration and efficiency. Early IaC tools like Puppet and Chef, and later tools like Ansible and SaltStack, played significant roles in establishing IaC as a preferred methodology. The rapid growth of cloud computing and the start of platforms like Terraform further drove the adoption of IaC, making it a standard practice for organizations seeking streamlined and consistent infrastructure deployment and management [4].

Although IaC is a useful tool, there are many challenges in its implementation. IaC tools are complex and should be understood to implement them effectively. Some developers are unable to harness the full potential of IaC due to its complexity [41]. In addition to possessing knowledge of IaC, an understanding of Cloud Computing Platforms and its resources is required. There seems to be a steep learning curve in the implementation of IaC.

Mostly, when it comes to challenges, IT staff need extensive knowledge and training. If qualified staff are non-existent, experts need to be consulted. The required experts need to be versed in Cloud platforms, IaC tools, multiple programming languages, and data security. Overall, cloud services along with IaC tools allow business operations to grow.

The rest of the paper is organized as follows: Section 2 Related Work summarizes some of the recent works in terms of the benefits and challenges of using IaC and suggested solutions to the challenges. This includes the aspects of security related concerns. Section 3 talks about IaC tools that are available in cloud, focusing on two IaC tools, Google's Cloud Deployment Manager and Terraform. Section 4 shares the experimental results on Terraform as an IaC tool on GCP. Section 5 provides the analysis of the performance and availability of the two IaC Tools, and Sect. 6 concludes the paper.

2 Related Work

Table 1 outlines an overview of the main benefits and associated challenges, including security concerns, related to utilizing the Infrastructure as Code (IaC). Each of these is discussed with detailed descriptions for better understanding.

2.1 Benefits of Using IaC

Automatic Scaling and Reduced Manual Effort: IaC empowers organizations to leverage automatic scaling, an asset for managing fluctuating traffic patterns. It allows for the automated provisioning and configuration of servers, facilitating quick and cost-effective scaling to handle varying workloads. Furthermore, IaC decreases the need for manual tasks, streamlining processes and enhancing efficiency. This automation minimizes repetitive manual work, leading to better resource management and reduced operational costs.

Table 1. Benefits, challenges, and security concerns of utilizing IaC.

Benefits	• Automatic Scaling and Reduced Manual Effort • Monitoring, Troubleshooting, and Disaster Recovery • Automation and Rapid Provisioning • Consistency and Reliability • Flexibility, Reduced Costs, and Enhanced Collaboration • Vendor Neutrality and Performance Assurance • Support for Continuous Integration and Continuous Deployment (CI/CD), Innovation, and Quality Assurance
Challenges	• Difficulty of testing the code • Readability and Polyglot • Difficulty of learning IaC • Inability to find staff • Large and complex infrastructure • Lack of Synchronization or Inconsistency • Requires time and coordination of resources • Runtime automation expected • Validation and verification
Security	• Improper configuration • Shared Security Model chart • Developers need access to privileged systems • Not understanding policies, guidelines, or best practices

Monitoring, Troubleshooting, and Disaster Recovery: IaC enhances monitoring and troubleshooting in cloud-automated infrastructure. Automated tools simplify the identification and resolution of server issues, resulting in improved performance and higher availability. Additionally, IaC simplifies disaster recovery by automating infrastructure provisioning and configuration. Streamline recovery efforts in case of disasters or outages, reducing downtime and associated costs.

Version Control, Auditing, and Compliance: IaC provides organizations with valuable version control and auditing capabilities, enabling them to track changes to their infrastructure over time. This feature is particularly important for compliance and security, as it ensures transparency and accountability in infrastructure management. By embedding best practices and security policies into infrastructure code, IaC contributes to compliance and mitigates security risks, reducing potential threats.

Automation and Rapid Provisioning: IaC supplies organizations with automation and rapid provisioning capabilities for IT infrastructure. This translates to faster, more efficient, and cost-effective deployment of cloud applications. It simplifies the setup, configuration, and management of infrastructure resources, leading to quicker development, testing, and production deployments. This speed and efficiency are crucial for organizations striving to stay competitive in dynamic markets [4].

Consistency and Reliability: IaC ensures consistency and reliability in infrastructure environments over time. Treating infrastructure as code gets rid of configuration drift, reducing the risk of inconsistencies that can lead to security vulnerabilities and operational errors. This consistency enhances infrastructure security and streamlines troubleshooting, fostering operational excellence.

Flexibility, Reduced Costs, and Enhanced Collaboration: IaC's flexibility allows organizations to scale infrastructure resources according to their needs. This agility is valuable for businesses in fast-paced environments or with fluctuating workloads. Moreover, IaC can lead to cost savings by optimizing resource utilization, reducing manual labor, and preventing over-provisioning. Additionally, IaC encourages collaboration among different teams, fostering a DevOps culture and enhancing cooperation between development, operations, and quality assurance teams.

Vendor Neutrality and Performance Assurance: IaC practices and tools are cloud-agnostic, allowing organizations to use them with various cloud service providers. This flexibility prevents vendor lock-in and enables organizations to choose the best cloud resources for their specific requirements. IaC can also ensure performance guarantees for cloud-deployed applications, particularly crucial for applications with changing workload needs. It provides the ability to adjust infrastructure resources on-demand, optimizing performance and cost-effectiveness.

Support for Continuous Integration and Continuous Deployment (CI/CD), Innovation, and Quality Assurance: IaC seamlessly integrates with CI/CD pipelines, enabling automated testing, deployment, and monitoring of applications. This contributes to faster and more reliable software delivery, allowing organizations to respond promptly to market demands. IaC also supports innovation by simplifying and expediting the deployment of new technologies, including emerging trends like Internet of Things (IoT), machine learning, and edge computing. Furthermore, IaC encourages quality assurance practices such as static analysis and testing for infrastructure code, enhancing infrastructure reliability and stability [41].

2.2 Challenges of Using IaC

While IaC offers many benefits for businesses, there are many challenges when implementing in a cloud environment. Some of the challenges are detailed below for a compressive understanding.

Testing the code is one of the main problems [15]. For developers, testing the code is difficult because there is no platform to test it. There is not an integrated development environment (IDE) specific to IaC.

Readability and Polyglot is another problem when implementing IaC [15]. Polyglot is programming by using different coding languages to increase functionality and efficiency [24]. For example, Java, JavaScript, and HTML can be mixed to create an application. Regarding cloud infrastructures, resources that are utilized are not required to conform to a specific programming language. Due to different languages, a specialist with extensive knowledge is often needed [15].

Learning IaC is a challenge as it is complex and not simple to learn and implement. Using IaC tools such as Terraform requires learning a new language. There is a steep learning curve, especially when learning IaC for the first time. Users will also need to know how resources integrate into the infrastructure, how to use them appropriately, and how to program resources into an IaC model [27].

The inability to find staff with technical expertise is another challenge related to IaC. Technical knowledge is needed to write and maintain the code for the many resources in the infrastructure [17]. Some organizations prefer their own in-house staff for their networks. But they may not find capable staff and will need to find and pay consultants [7].

Challenges increase if managers expect their IT staff to implement IaC and are not aware that technical expertise is needed for its implementation. IaC is a powerful and useful tool and cannot be put into practice with minimal resources [39]. When organizations rely on in-house staff and do not hire consultants, all features of IaC are not fully implemented [17]. Some parts of IaC are too complex for developers to enact. Staff may try to learn about the tools and associated APIs by reading the documentation. However, the documentation is not always up to date, or it is incomplete. So, developers will need to search for answers elsewhere [29]. Stack Overflow, Terraform community, and other blogs are alternatives to documentation.

Developers should also study and know about the array of IaC tools, such as Terraform, Ansible, Chef, CloudFormation, etc. There are differences among the tools. Some are more advanced and complex but work better in certain situations. Similarly, developers will need to be aware that different APIs may exist on one platform but not on another.

Large and complex infrastructures create issues or challenges. More resources mean more potential problems. As infrastructures grow, the complexity of IaC programs also increases. Collaboration, versioning, testing, security, integration, and automation are needed. Improper implementation means that the infrastructure does not deploy, or it deploys with security vulnerabilities [31].

Merging an existing framework with new technology is another challenge. "Adoption discrepancies" arise [41]. Transformations and the task of interrelating objects and dependencies in IaC code need to be written. This takes time, preparation, and coordination of involved teams. This issue is not only for organizations who are implementing newer technology, but for organizations that merge with other organizations.

Lack of Synchronization or Inconsistency is another challenge with IaC. This occurs when different versions of tools are developed and implemented. A new tool may not be compatible with other tools or components in the system [15]. Inconsistency may also arise when resources are updated [29]. In large systems, more resources translate into more updates in the system. When updates cause inconsistencies in the system, the system will not function properly or not function at all. If the system cannot operate, the updates are then reversed. The resources do not get updates. So, the system does not operate at peak efficiency, or a vulnerability is not patched [29]. The lack of synchronization occurs because some resources are dependent on the behavior of other resources [8, 27].

For large infrastructures, with many resources, it is difficult for one person to track all resources. However, IaC provides tagging such that resources could relate to a specific group. It is essential to track resources and should be required; otherwise, vulnerabilities could result. Some resources, however, are missed, not tagged at all, or improperly tagged. Untagged resources end up as "ghost" resources [21] which become challenges because they are hard to detect and hard to provide a visualization of what is happening in the cloud.

Verification and Validation is also a challenge. Verification and Validation is a process that ensures the infrastructure optimally meets its defined goals without errors. Verifying changes is not available in modern IaC programs [32]. Before IaC, users relied on feedback to validate the changes in the infrastructure. Most IaC tools do not provide a visualization feature, so it is difficult to see the effects of changes. The lack of visibility can also lead to deployment errors [30].

2.3 Security as a Challenge

Staff may create security vulnerabilities; IaC is safer since it uses less human interaction. Also, the infrastructure uses the Internet and outside attackers exist. Meaning, security is needed when IaC is adopted. Communication, proper use of security assessment tools, and auditing needs to be employed [40]. The principle of least privilege should be enforced, and Identity Access Management (IAM) should be used to enforce access [21]. Security tools are important to maintain but affect the system's operation. Security is affected by several factors.

Improper configuration is a security challenge. Bad Configurations are caused by human input errors, not properly configuring the resources and infrastructure, making changes to applications with unintended behavior, and manually editing resources at a cloud terminal [21, 27]. According to Google Cloud Platform, most cloud security breaches are the result of misconfigurations. This is expected to increase [13]. In another study, by a private company, Ponemon reports that the top threat to sensitive data is caused by employee mistakes. The second biggest threat is system failure, while the third biggest threat is hackers. Normally, the IaC process is automated, and configuration is not an issue. However, some steps need to be executed manually because not all actions are fully automated and for some reason cannot be automated [29]. For example, generation of the parent code is a manual task. Whenever humans are involved, the parent code needs to be checked for technical errors; otherwise, there could be errors [27].

Shared Security Model chart is important to know who is responsible for what, or what is being protected in speaking of responsibilities of the cloud provider and of the cloud user. Cloud users need to know their responsibilities and that the cloud provider's responsibilities of securing an infrastructure do not include everything [7].

Developers need access to privileged systems; although, this creates risk to mission critical systems. Some developers use scripts to execute the infrastructure instead of working in the physical system's configuration. These configurations should not be written into IaC; it is not recommended [27]. In addition, developers need to be aware that deployment application configuration settings can overwrite infrastructure configurations when deployed - this can cause issues [29].

Not understanding policies, guidelines, or best practices leads to lack of security. Developers who do not understand policies, guidelines or best practices will either not implement them or improperly implement them. This leads to vulnerabilities. In one study, Verdet et al. checked to see if best practices related to security policies of Infrastructure as Code were implemented. They looked at Terraform and checked GitHub repositories in their research. They found several areas that were insufficient such the lack of encryption, lack of logging and monitoring, using outdated features, and lack of security access policy configuration [38]. Lack of encryption ensures confidentiality such that data cannot be read. Logging and monitoring shows patterns of network activity and can identify areas that are possibly compromised. Using outdated features could mean that a system has not received the latest security updates or patches. Updating is often disabled since it may cause incompatibility among resources. Finally, if security access is not properly configured, unauthorized users can access internet resources. For example, when setting up secure shell (ssh) protocol, the default IP address (0.0.0.0/0) is set to allow access to any user. IP addresses should be configured to allow only IT staff into its resources. Overall, developers need to know how to appropriately set up their infrastructure for services rendered and ensure that it is secure.

2.4 Suggested Solutions to Challenges

IaC is complex, and expertise is needed for its utilization. We address solutions to the challenges other than previously stated. To address the challenges of IaC, developers need to research the type of tools that are offered by each platform and how to effectively implement them. It is recommended for users who are using Cloud platforms along with the various tools to understand the various platforms and the specific tools that are offered. To deal with the lack of IaC understanding, online training classes are offered. Udemy offers Infrastructure as Code courses that include Terraform, Azure, and AWS [37].

KodeKloud, launched in 2019, also offers IaC training. Learning IaC involves Linux, Shell Scripts, Dockers, Terraform, Ansible, etc. [19]. Another class is offered by Koenig. They are tailored towards Azure IaC certification which is a "professional qualification that validates an individual's capability to manage cloud and on-premises infrastructure through code" [20]. This course is designed for individuals who possess an understanding of networking, cloud infrastructures, Azure services, software development, programming, code deployment, version control, and DevOps.

Terraform offers many tutorials and its own certification [35]. The tutorials include subjects regarding AWS, Azure, Docker, GCP, Oracle Cloud Infrastructure, Terraform Cloud, CLI, Configuration Language, Modules, Provision, State, HashiCorp Products, SaaS Providers, Kubernetes, Machine Images, Networking, Policy, Security, CDK, etc.

Textbooks are also available to help understand IaC and can be found at bookstores. To combat outdated information in documentation, developers should know that there are other places to obtain current information. This includes Stack Overflow, Terraform community, and other blogs for solutions.

Developers should also know how to protect data while in the cloud. GCP, as an example, allows client-side encryption. Current encryption schemes could be implemented to provide security.

Client-side encryption should not be overlooked as it can protect data in cloud servers. The cloud is susceptible to attacks, and researchers advise that data should be encrypted before it is uploaded to an outsourced server [6, 22, 25, 38]. An independent research company, Ponemon Institute, reports that 38% of respondents report encrypting data before sending it to the cloud - in 2021. Furthermore, 60% send sensitive data to the cloud whether encrypted or not - an indication that the benefits of the cloud outweigh the risks of data breaches [12]. There are current encryptions schemes to always protect data, i.e. in transit, at rest, and in use. Searchable encryption and Confidential Computing protect data while in use.

Searchable Encryption (SE) came about in 2000 when Song et al. stated that data should not be decrypted in untrusted servers [33]. They proposed a search scheme to search encrypted data in use. Since then, many searchable schemes have developed, such as homomorphic encryption. Homomorphic Encryption (HE) is also an encryption scheme but not native to GCP. HE allows addition and multiplication on encrypted data. With some HE schemes, i.e., Fully Homomorphic Encryption schemes, we can now perform unlimited addition and multiplication operations on encrypted data. This is the latest of the encryptions schemes that was developed by Dr. Craig Gentry in his PhD dissertation in 2009 [36]. SE schemes provide protection of data such that plaintext is never exposed, even for operations such as searching, updating, deleting, creating, adding, multiplication, etc.

Confidential Computing (CC) is implemented via GCP and appears effective; Google is part of the Confidential Computing Consortium under the Linux Foundation. The Confidential Computing Consortium is a combination of "hardware vendors, cloud providers, and software developers to accelerate the adoption of Trusted Execution Environment technologies and standards" [10].

By default, GCP encrypts data when at rest and in transit. It offers encryption for data in use via CC [14]; however, this is not a default feature. If implemented, CC allows data to be always protected. Both SE and CC use software to implement encryption. Unlike SE, CC requires specialized hardware. Both provide confidentiality, but CC also provides integrity. Finally, SE data is always encrypted, but CC decrypts data while in the CPU to perform its operations. With CC, however, only the authorized application can access the CPU. If an attack is detected, the operations cease.

Overall, there are many security challenges to address. Best practices could be used as a comprehensive guide to set up the IaC and ensure all security concerns are addressed. These guidelines help organizations persevere, and can be found at various websites, such as GitGuardian [23], GCP, and Terraform.

3 IaC Tools on Cloud

In the rapidly evolving field of cloud computing, Infrastructure as Code (IaC) stands as a pivotal development, introducing tools that automate and streamline the management of cloud-based infrastructure. These tools are diverse, each tailored to specific requirements of cloud service deployment and management. Before focusing on the specific IaC tools that are the subject of this study, some other tools are examined here.

Ansible by Red Hat is an influential open-source automation tool, known for its simplicity and agentless architecture. It effectively automates cloud provisioning, application deployment, and intra-service orchestration [1]. Chef emerges as a powerful automation platform, adept at transforming infrastructure into code, particularly suited for large-scale environments [2]. Puppet is renowned for its declarative approach to infrastructure definition, widely utilized for configuration management and automating the provisioning of infrastructure [3]. Additionally, AWS CloudFormation and Azure

Resource Manager (ARM) offer specialized IaC solutions for their respective platforms. CloudFormation provides a unified language to model and provision resources in Amazon Web Services [5], while ARM is key to Microsoft Azure, facilitating the definition and deployment of infrastructure via a JSON template [26].

Code (IaC) tools have significantly revolutionized the way which manage and provision cloud resources. While there is a variety of IaC tools available, each offering unique features and functionalities tailored to specific cloud environments and user requirements. Selecting an appropriate IaC tool is often dictated by factors such as the specific cloud platform, the complexity of the infrastructure, scalability requirements, and the organization's comfort with the tool's language and architecture. Two tools have gained substantial attention for their robust capabilities in managing cloud resources: Google Cloud Deployment Manager and Terraform.

Google Cloud Deployment Manager [9] is a native management service specifically designed for Google Cloud Platform (GCP). It provides an efficient way to deploy, manage, and maintain GCP resources using declarative templates. The key advantage of using Google Cloud Deployment Manager lies in its tight integration with GCP services, allowing for seamless and optimized management of GCP resources. It enables users to define all the resources needed for their application in a declarative format using YAML, Python, or Jinja2. This integration ensures that users can leverage the latest GCP features and services, making it an ideal choice for projects heavily reliant on GCP.

Terraform, developed by HashiCorp, stands out for its ability to manage multi-cloud and hybrid-cloud environments. Unlike Google Cloud Deployment Manager, Terraform is not tied to a single cloud provider. Instead, it offers extensive support for several providers including Google Cloud, AWS, Microsoft Azure, and many others. This multi-provider support makes Terraform an exceptionally versatile tool, allowing users to manage a diverse range of resources across different environments using a single configuration language [18]. Terraform's approach to infrastructure management is declarative, enabling users to specify what the desired state of their infrastructure should be, and the tool then works to achieve that state. This ability to handle complex, distributed environments efficiently makes Terraform a preferred choice for organizations seeking flexibility and scalability across various cloud platforms.

This study focused on Google Cloud Deployment Manager and Terraform due to their distinct yet complementary capabilities. Google Cloud Deployment Manager offers specialized, in-depth management of GCP's resources, making it an excellent case study for GCP-centric deployments. Terraform, on the other hand, provides a broader perspective with its capacity to handle multiple cloud providers, presenting a more holistic view of IaC's potential in diverse cloud environments. Together, they represent a comprehensive spectrum of IaC's applicability in cloud resource management – from single-cloud to multi-cloud scenarios. This paper aims to explore the details of the tools, offering insights into their operational mechanisms, performance, and suitability for different cloud infrastructure management needs.

3.1 Google Cloud Deployment Manager

Google Cloud Deployment Manager stands as a dynamic service engineered to streamline and automate the provisioning and orchestration of Google Cloud resources. Users can craft templates and configurations, which the Deployment Manager utilizes to instantiate a variety of resources, including virtual machine instances and cloud storage buckets, thereby easing the developer's workload [34].

Introduced in 2013 as an integral part of the Google Cloud Platform (GCP), Deployment Manager marked Google's strategic initiative toward providing users with a robust and extensible framework to effectively govern cloud infrastructure. Since its inception, Deployment Manager has evolved, receiving regular enhancements to embrace a broader range of GCP services and resource types. Key developments include the implementation of cross-project deployments, enabling the unified management of resources across the expanse of GCP projects. Further refinement of the tool's configuration and templating syntax has empowered users to create more intricate, modular, and sustainable deployment architectures [9].

Interoperability with other core Google Cloud offerings, such as Cloud Monitoring and Cloud Logging, has been achieved, ensuring a cohesive and integrated user experience. The advent of type providers has been a significant milestone, broadening Deployment Manager's reach to encompass custom resource types and to extend its governance to include third-party and select Google Cloud services outside its native purview. Deployment Manager has emerged as a pivotal instrument within the Google Cloud arsenal, encouraging users to incorporate IaC principles into their workflows. Enhanced versioning of templates and configurations now underpins change management, bolstering the maintenance of sophisticated deployments.

Google's commitment to community engagement has spurred the growth of an open-source ecosystem around Deployment Manager, incentivizing template sharing and collaborative development. The platform's integration with GitHub simplifies the template import process, further nurturing a culture of collective innovation. As of April 2023, Deployment Manager continues to play a vital role in Google Cloud's infrastructure management suite. Nonetheless, the cloud landscape is characterized by its perpetual progression, with new tools and functionalities regularly surfacing. Among these, HashiCorp's Terraform has gained traction as a preferred IaC tool within the GCP community, distinguished for its versatility across multiple cloud environments.

3.2 Terraform

Terraform, the brainchild of HashiCorp, is an acclaimed open-source tool that embodies the principles of infrastructure as code (IaC), enabling users to construct and manage data center infrastructure with ease using its native HashiCorp Configuration Language (HCL), or optionally JSON for those who prefer it [18]. Unveiled to the public in July 2014, Terraform was envisioned as a breakthrough tool that could guarantee the safe, predictable, and incremental evolution of infrastructure. By utilizing HCL, it facilitated the expression of infrastructure designs with a clarity that resonated well within the IT community.

Its ascent in popularity was catalyzed by the burgeoning IaC movement, which Terraform rode to prominence. Its key selling point was its agnostic approach to infrastructure provisioning, offering support for a vast array of cloud providers and thereby promoting a multi-cloud strategy. This versatility made it an attractive choice for organizations keen on avoiding vendor lock-in and those wishing to orchestrate a diverse range of resources across various platforms. The fostering of a vibrant community has been central to Terraform's growth. HashiCorp has actively encouraged open contributions and the exchange of modules. To this end, the Terraform Registry was established, serving as a nexus for the community to publish and disseminate modules widely.

With the release of Terraform 0.10 in August 2017, a new era of modularity commenced as it introduced the decoupling of providers from Terraform's core binary. This enabled providers to evolve independently, facilitating a more dynamic and responsive development ecosystem. The launch of Terraform 0.12 in May 2019 introduced pivotal language enhancements, enriching the tool with more expressive capabilities and a more sophisticated type of system. The debut of Terraform 1.0 in June 2021 was a watershed moment, symbolizing its maturation into a stable and comprehensive tool. The 1.x series promises enduring compatibility and stability, reinforcing its reliability for users. Continual enhancements mark Terraform's evolutionary journey, with HashiCorp routinely augmenting its capabilities. Terraform Cloud and Terraform Enterprise offer specialized solutions tailored for team collaboration and governance, expanding Terraform's utility in enterprise settings.

Terraform's stature in the DevOps domain is underpinned by its simplicity, extensive provider support, and its adeptness at managing an array of resources spanning IaaS, PaaS, and SaaS services. As it streamlines infrastructure deployment across varied environments, Terraform's role in automating modern data centers is likely to remain indispensable.

4 Evaluation of Challenges on GCP

Since we had access to Google Cloud Platform (GCP), we evaluated Terraform as an IaC tool. Terraform is not native to GCP and we look at its integration. Specifically, we used GCP labs to assist in Terraform implementation. In this evaluation, we set up a small infrastructure to test the IaC code and learn about Terraform. Because of its complex structure, time and effort is required as we observed some of the challenges that developers may face.

We started with the study of GCP's IaC code related to Terraform. We executed and tested it, but errors arose. Troubleshooting took time as errors needed to be pinpointed to the correct section of the code and fixed. Mostly, altering and testing small parts of the code, or commands, section by section is an option that we utilized. We eventually found resolutions and could see how these problems would amplify with larger projects.

Difficulties of learning and using different programming languages existed. When trying to fix errors in the labs, knowledge of HashiCorp Configuration Language (HCL) is needed. Since we did not have access to an expert, we studied HCL. This included research into different versions of the code. Terraform allows users to specify the version of code, which allowed us to change and test versions to eliminate errors.

In addition to code and version research, our troubleshooting included seeking resources such as comments from other lab users and using the Command Line Interface help command. Obtaining knowledge of the file system also proved helpful. As errors arise, troubleshooting included the reviewing of programming files such as the main.tf (terraform) file and associated files, such as the variable.tf file.

Part of our troubleshooting included the Terraform registry. This registry exists to help develop an infrastructure when provisioning resources. So, developers should use codes that have already been tested and used – rather than writing their own. For our existing infrastructures, we made comparisons between GCP's lab code and Terraform's registry code found at [35]. The comparison provided insight into how the code should be written and where to place it in a specific file. We concluded our experiment by successfully running Terraform inside of GCP.

5 Performance Analysis

This section presents the results of the comparative analysis of two IaC tools, Google Cloud Deployment Manager and Terraform, in terms of performance and availability of their service. When analyzing their performance and availability, it's important to check their individual design principles and operational strengths. Through the analysis, we intend to examine their capabilities through the execution of sample code, thereby providing a practical basis for comparison.

The selection of Google Cloud Platform (GCP) and its Deployment Manager, along with Terraform for this study, is influenced by GCP's notable high computing capabilities and its robust network infrastructure, which benefits Google's global network [28]. GCP is particularly favored for its developer-centric approach, offering deep integration with open-source technologies and harnessing Google's innovative tech expertise. This makes GCP, coupled with its native Deployment Manager and the versatile Terraform, a compelling choice for the study's focus on cloud computing tools.

Google Cloud Deployment Manager is inherently optimized for managing Google Cloud Platform (GCP) resources, leveraging direct access to GCP's APIs for potentially swifter deployment cycles within the GCP ecosystem. Its integration into Google Cloud's framework may offer reduced operational latency due to the absence of intermediary processes. On the other hand, Terraform's architecture is built for versatility, enabling it to interface with a myriad of providers such as GCP, AWS, and Azure.

5.1 Performance Analysis on Creating and Destroying a Virtual Machine

Virtual Machines (VMs) are software based and act like physical computers that execute programs and perform other computing operations. The starting steps for using Google Cloud Deployment Manager and Terraform involve setting up the necessary configurations to create and destroy VMs. This includes defining the VM specifications, such as the machine type, zone, and image to be used, in configuration files. For Deployment Manager, this is done using YAML templates, while Terraform uses HCL (HashiCorp Configuration Language). Both tools require authentication and appropriate permissions set within Google Cloud, ensuring seamless interaction with GCP's APIs for resource management. These preliminary steps are crucial for the effective execution of subsequent commands to deploy and remove VMs.

The comparison of Google Cloud Deployment Manager and Terraform was conducted in the us-central-1 zone, chosen for its low latency relative to the experiment's location. Executions were carried out via Google Cloud Shell, with the Linux 'time' command measuring the deployment and destruction durations of resources. Each tool underwent five consistent test runs. The study utilized Google Cloud SDK 453.0.0 and Terraform v1.6.3. For simplicity and validity, VMs were uniformly set to "g1-small" with a "debian-11" image, and default network settings. The creation and destruction scripts are available at this GitHub repository: https://github.com/walkon1007/IaC_sample.git.

Terraform had much faster deployment times, as shown in Fig. 1. In every run, Terraform completed the creation process significantly faster than Google Deployment Manager. The creation times for Terraform are consistently around the 13-s, while Google Deployment Manager's times are roughly double or more, ranging from approximately 27 to over 49 s.

Figure 2 presents the time comparison on destroying a virtual machine on those two tools. Again, the data presented here leads to the conclusion that resource destruction on Google Cloud using Terraform is consistently faster compared to the use of Google Cloud Deployment Manager. For each run count, the time taken in seconds for Terraform is less than that for Google Cloud Deployment Manager. The difference in time ranges from a few seconds to over 10 s in some instances.

Therefore, for tasks focused on resource destruction speed on Google Cloud, Terraform appears to be the more efficient tool. The conclusion here is that Terraform not only performs more efficiently in terms of creation of resources but also in the destruction of resources on Google Cloud, showing a consistency over Google Deployment Manager in terms of speed.

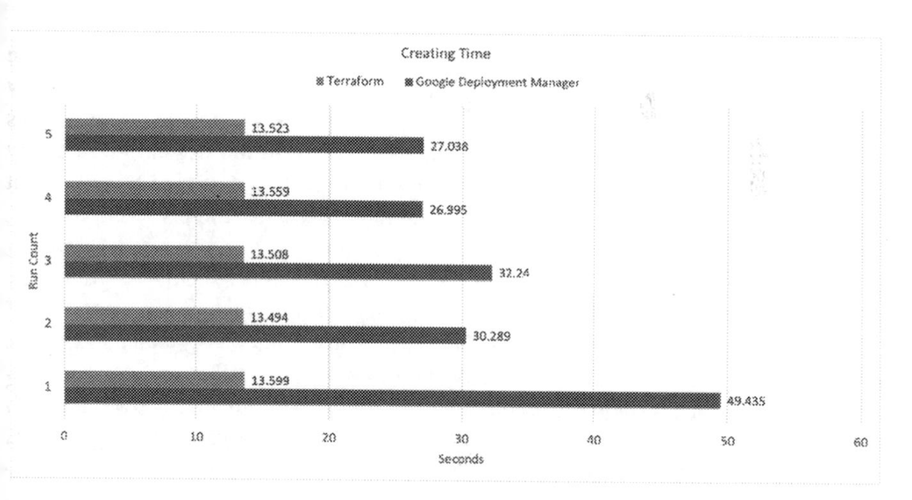

Fig. 1. Time Comparison Creating a Virtual Machine.

5.2 Analysis of Results

The superior performance of Terraform in resource creation and destruction times, as demonstrated in the study, provides valuable insights for best practices in Infrastructure

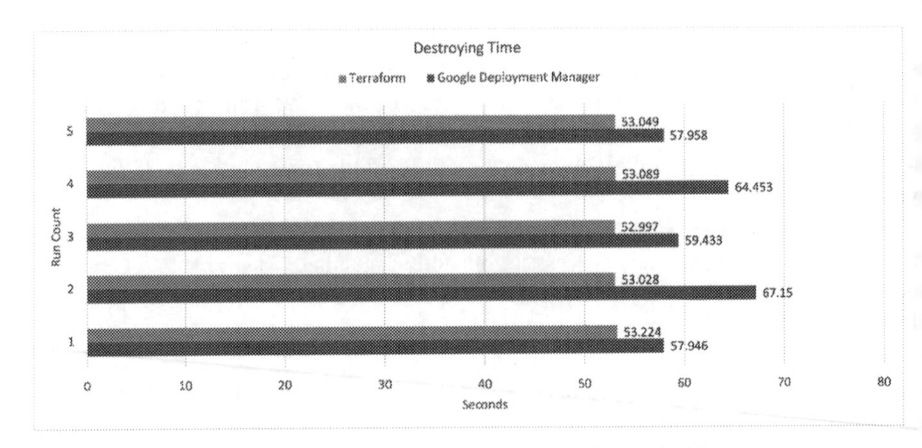

Fig. 2. Time Comparison Destroying a Virtual Machine.

as Code (IaC). This efficiency is attributed to Terraform's design, which optimizes the management of state changes and resource dependencies [26]. The study's results suggest that for tasks requiring frequent and rapid changes to cloud resources, Terraform could be more effective. Such findings can guide organizations in choosing IaC tools that align with their operational needs, particularly in dynamic cloud environments where quick resource turnaround is essential.

Overall, Google Cloud Deployment Manager exhibits superior performance for GCP-specific deployments due to its native integration, whereas Terraform's strength lies in its ability to manage complex, heterogeneous environments. This gives us insights on the cost of increased execution times during the planning and application phases. Regarding availability, the Deployment Manager's reliance on GCP's infrastructure means its uptime is as robust as the cloud services it orchestrates. Terraform's decentralized nature and community-driven development model offer a different kind of resilience; it is not confined by the operational status of any cloud service [11] and can pivot to managing resources across different clouds during an outage [16].

The decision between Deployment Manager and Terraform should be guided by the specific requirements of the cloud environment in question, the importance of multi-cloud strategy, and the preferred balance between community-driven and vendor-supported tooling. The insights presented here are derived from the execution of standardized sample code, which is essential for an empirical assessment. Such an approach not only yields quantitative data on performance metrics but also qualitatively informs the reliability and robustness of each tool in dynamic cloud environments.

5.3 Limitation

The availability of Google Cloud Deployment Manager is linked to the operational status of GCP services. Consequently, any disruptions within GCP could directly affect the tool's functionality. Nevertheless, being a native service, it provides immediate updates corresponding to the latest GCP offerings, ensuring alignment with new features and services as they emerge.

On the other hand, Terraform operates independently of any single cloud provider's infrastructure. It does rely on a robust community and HashiCorp's stewardship for updates and maintenance. However, the open-source version lacks an official cloud SLA (Service-Level Agreement). Organizations requiring guaranteed uptime can turn to HashiCorp's managed services, Terraform Cloud and Terraform Enterprise, both of which do offer SLAs.

The comparative analysis limits only two IaC tools, thus further analysis with other tools can be done. The performance analysis mainly involved the time comparisons on creating and destroying a virtual machine in each of the two IaC tools, Google Cloud Deployment Manager and Terraform. It may not necessarily reflect the performance of executing other resources, questioning further consideration for additional experiments needed.

6 Conclusion

IaC is a cloud environment tool that offers many benefits to businesses. Benefits include automation, consistency, cost savings, and agility. IaC improves efficiency and expedites the deployment of software applications and services. Several IaC tools exist in the marketplace. Google provides Deployment Manager as its version which works well in a Google Cloud Environment. There are third party IaC tools that work in Cloud Environments such as Terraform. It works well in single cloud environments, such as in Google Cloud, or in versatile or multi-cloud environments. It is not uncommon to see multiple resources from multiple cloud vendors used in an organization's cloud infrastructure. For instance, cloud resources can be combined and coordinated from Google Cloud, AWS, and Azure.

Although IaC has many advantages and is used in cloud infrastructures, they grow towards complexity. This complexity leads to challenges in the utilization of IaC. Challenge exists such as in testing the code, learning IaC and multiple programming languages, the inability to find qualified staff to implement IaC, merging platforms into an IaC platform, synchronization of resources used in the infrastructure, and automating all tasks. Security is also a challenge in IaC infrastructures. If not properly configured, vulnerabilities arise. To combat the challenges, learning about IaC in the Cloud environments is essential. There are online training modules to assist in learning IaC as well as research journals and books. In addition, Cloud platforms, such as GCP, and IaC tools, such as Terraform offer training. Organization's need to acknowledge that the implementation of IaC requires technical expertise and is complex.

We leveraged Google Cloud Manager and Terraform, two IaC tools. We focused on their performance and availability within the context of Google Cloud Platform (GCP). For the performance, we deployed a standardized compute instance on GCP using both tools. We measured deployment and destroyed times. Our findings indicate that Google Cloud Deployment Manager exhibits native integration benefits. But Terraform performs faster deployment capabilities. In comparison, Terraform's versatile multi-cloud capabilities offer broader flexibility and independence from single-vendor cloud service fluctuations. We are not immune to the steep learning curve of all involved technologies. Further research is needed with other Cloud platforms such as AWS and

Azure. Additionally, further research could include other IaC tools, such as Ansible, Chef, Puppet, Crossplane, Vagrant, Saltstack, Pulumini, etc. We limited our research to Terraform and Google Cloud Deployment Manager due to the requirement of extensive knowledge.

References

1. Ansible Documentation (2023). https://docs.ansible.com/ansible/latest/index.html. Accessed 3 Dec 2023
2. Chef Infra Documentation (2023). https://docs.chef.io/. Accessed 3 Dec 2023
3. Puppet Documentation (2023). https://puppet.com/docs/puppet/latest/. Accessed 3 Dec 2023
4. Alonso, J., Piliszek, R., Cankar, M.: Embracing IaC through the DevSecOps philosophy: concepts, challenges, and a reference framework. IEEE Softw. **40**(1), 56–62 (2023). https://doi.org/10.1109/MS.2022.3212194
5. Amazon Web Services. AWS CloudFormation User Guide. Amazon Web Services (2021). https://docs.aws.amazon.com/AWSCloudFormation/latest/UserGuide/Welcome.html
6. Amorim, I., Costa, I.: Leveraging searchable encryption through homomorphic encryption: a comprehensive analysis. Mathematics **11**(13), 2948 (2023). https://doi.org/10.3390/math11132948
7. Aviv, I., Gafni, R., Sherman, S., Bertha, A., Sterkin, A., Bega, E.: Cloud infrastructure from python code-breaking the barriers of cloud deployment (2023)
8. Basher, M.: DevOps: an explorative case study on the challenges and opportunities in implementing Infrastructure as code (2019). https://urn.kb.se/resolve?urn=urn:nbn:se:umu:diva-161048
9. Google Cloud. Google Cloud Deployment Manager documentation (2023). https://cloud.google.com/deployment-manager/docs. Accessed 6 Nov 2023
10. ConfCompCons. About – Confidential Computing Consortium (2023). https://confidentialcomputing.io/about/
11. de Carvalho, L.R., de Araujo, A.P.F.: Performance comparison of terraform and cloudify as multicloud orchestrators (2020). https://doi.org/10.1109/CCGrid49817.2020.00-55
12. Entrust. 2021 Global Encryption Trends Study (2021). https://www.entrust.com/lp/en/global-encryption-trends-study
13. GCP. Shared responsibilities and shared fate on Google Cloud | Architecture Framework (2023). https://cloud.google.com/architecture/framework/security/shared-responsibility-shared-fate
14. GCP_CC. Encryption for Cloud Security (2023). https://cloud.google.com/security/encryption
15. Guerriero, M., Garriga, M., Tamburri, D.A., Palomba, F.: Adoption, support, and challenges of infrastructure-as-code: insights from industry (2019). https://doi.org/10.1109/ICSME.2019.00092. ISSN: 2576-3148
16. Gupta, M., Chowdary, M.N., Bussa, S., Chowdary, C.K.: Deploying hadoop architecture using ansible and terraform (2021). https://doi.org/10.1109/ISCON52037.2021.9702299
17. Hasan, M.R., Ansary, M.S.: Cloud infrastructure automation through IaC (infrastructure as code). Int. J. Comput. (IJC) **46**(1), 34–40 (2023)
18. HashiCorp. Automate Infrastructure on Any Cloud. https://developer.hashicorp.com/terraform. Accessed 23 Feb 2023
19. KodeKloud. Infrastructure as Code (IaC) Training Roadmap | Kodekloud (2023). https://kodekloud.com/learning-path/iac

20. Koenig. Master Azure Infrastructure as Code (IaC) - Comprehensive Online Course (2023). https://www.koenig-solutions.com/azure-infrastructure-as-code-training
21. Langford, M.: Top 5 infrastructure as code (IaC) security challenges (2023). https://www.trendmicro.com/en_sg/devops/22/g/infrastructure-as-code-iac-security.html. Section: best practices
22. Lin, J.-K., Lin, W.-T., Wu, J.-L.: Flexible and efficient multi-keyword ranked searchable attribute-based encryption schemes (2023). https://doi.org/10.3390/cryptography7020028
23. May, C.J.: Best Practices for Scanning and Securing Infrastructure as Code (IaC) [cheat sheet included] (2023). https://blog.gitguardian.com/infrastructure-as-code-security-best-practices-cheat-sheet-inclu
24. McKenzie, C.: What is polyglot programming? | Definition from TechTarget (2015). https://www.techtarget.com/searchsoftwarequality/definition/polyglot-programming
25. Song, F., Qin, Z., Xue, L., Zhang, J., Lin, X., Shen, X.: Privacy-preserving keyword similarity search over encrypted spatial data in cloud computing. IEEE Internet Things J. **9**(8), 6184–6198 (2022). https://doi.org/10.1109/JIOT.2021.3110300
26. Levan, M.: Compare Google cloud deployment manager vs. terraform on GCP (2020). https://www.techtarget.com/searchcloudcomputing/tip/Compare-Google-Cloud-Deployment-Manager-vs-Terraform-on-GCP. Accessed 01 Nov 2024
27. Nedeltcheva, G.N., Xiang, B., Niculut, L., Benedetto, D.: Challenges towards modeling and generating infrastructure-as-code. In: Companion of the 2023 ACM/SPEC International Conference on Performance Engineering (ICPE 2023 Companion), pp. 189–193. Association for Computing Machinery, New York (2023). DOI:https://doi.org/10.1145/3578245.3584937
28. Google Cloud. Google Cloud Global Locations (2023). https://cloud.google.com/about/locations
29. Pingen, I.R.: A reflection on the perceived benefits of infrastructure as code (2021)
30. Qiu, Y., et al.: Simplifying cloud management with cloudless computing. Resource **7**, 8 (2023)
31. Qwiklabs. Google Cloud Skills Boost (2023). https://www.cloudskillsboost.google
32. Sokolowski, D., Salvaneschi, G.: Towards reliable infrastructure as code (2023). https://doi.org/10.1109/ICSA-C57050.2023.00072
33. Song, D.X., Wagner, D., Perrig, A.: Practical techniques for searches on encrypted data. In: Proceeding 2000 IEEE Symposium on Security and Privacy, S&P 2000, Berkeley, CA, USA, pp. 44–55. IEEE Computer Society (2000). https://doi.org/10.1109/SECPRI.2000.848445, http://ieeexplore.ieee.org/document/848445/. ISBN 978-0-7695-0665-4
34. Sullivan, D.: Deploying applications with cloud launcher and deployment manager (2019). https://doi.org/10.1002/9781119564409.ch16
35. Registry Terraform. Terraform-google-modules/network/google | firewall-rules Submodule | Terraform Registry (2023). https://registry.terraform.io/modules/terraform-google-modules/network/google/6.0.0/submodules/firewall-rules
36. Gentry, C.: Fully homomorphic encryption using ideal lattices. In: Proceedings of the Forty-First Annual ACM Symposium on Theory of Computing (STOC 2009), Bethesda, MD, USA, pp. 169–178. Association for Computing Machinery, New York (2009). https://doi.org/10.1145/1536414.1536440
37. Udemy. Top Infrastructure as Code Courses Online – Updated (2023). https://www.udemy.com/topic/infrastructure-as-code/
38. Verdet, A., Hamdaqa, M., Da Silva, L., Khomh, F.: Exploring security practices in infrastructure as code: an empirical study (2023)
39. Wang, Z., et al.: Efficient location-based skyline queries with secure r-tree over encrypted data. IEEE Trans. Knowl. Data Eng. **35**(10), 10436–10450 (2023). https://doi.org/10.1109/TKDE.2023.3253883

40. Guest Writer. Infrastructure as Code: Challenges and How to Deal With Them (2022). https://www.iotforall.com/infrastructure-as-code-challenges
41. Zhang, Y., Rahman, M., Wu, F., Rahman, A.: Quality assurance for infrastructure orchestrators: emerging results from ansible (2023). https://doi.org/10.1109/ICSA-C57050.2023.00073

Determination of Pareto-Optimal Solutions to the Problem of Multicriteria Selection

Sergiy Shevchenko(✉)

National Technical University, Kharkiv Polytechnic Institute, Kharkiv, Ukraine
serhii.shevchenko@khpi.edu.ua

Abstract. The problem of multi-criteria selection with the construction of a Pareto-optimal subset of solutions is considered. The presence of a set of criteria requires the construction of procedures that ensure the determination of adequate evaluations of alternative solutions. Well-known approaches to justifying solutions to selection problems suggest using a comparison of selection options based on selected criteria and the criteria themselves. Most of these approaches are on the use of expert assessments to determine the merits of individual options based, but their application can be appropriate only in the absence of reliable data on the actual characteristics of the alternatives considered. These approaches often rely on assumptions that may not hold. This is the possibility of comparisons, the use of fixed scales to determine the level of preferences, assumptions about the linear dependence of evaluations according to criteria in different ranges of values, the use of unreliable samples, etc. The article proposes an approach to the formation of solutions to the choice problem based on the construction of a criterion that determines the assessment of the approximation of solution candidates to the virtual example. Mathematical models were of the dependence of evaluations by criteria on the characteristics of the objects of comparison built. The results of determining the architecture of the virtual data processing system from cloud providers from the positions of a number of criteria are given. The results obtained indicate the feasibility of applying the proposed approach to solve a wide range of selection problems.

Keywords: Selection Problems · Multi-criteria Optimization · Decision-maker Virtual Data Processing System · Cloud Computing

1 Introduction

Decision-making procedures are on solving selection problems based, which involve obtaining and analyzing generalized assessments of the decisions made, based on a set of selected criteria. Establishing the greatest correspondence of the selection option to the selected criteria among the applicants corresponds to the content of the selection tasks. The urgency of the need to reliably solve these issues for a wide range of practical applications requires the development of appropriate theoretical foundations and information technologies as part of decision support subsystems.

K. Daimi and A. Al Sadoon (Eds.): ACR 2024, LNNS 956, pp. 515–526, 2024.
https://doi.org/10.1007/978-3-031-56950-0_42

The criteria chosen to justify decisions determine the preferences of the decision-maker (DM), and in general should characterize the quality and effectiveness of decision options, taking into account the influence of external factors that are of significant importance for decision-making. In addition, the requirements for the level of technical and economic indicators of applicants and the conditions of their use should be defined in the criteria.

Traditionally, in order to determine the best alternatives in a number of developments, it is proposed to apply a series of comparisons with the formation of appropriate evaluations of choice alternatives according to selected criteria and levels of importance of the relevant criteria. Among these approaches, the method of analyzing hierarchies [1] is well-known. Based on the specified comparisons, the final result of the evaluation of alternative solutions is formed. Such approaches to the formation of solutions to similar problems are, as a rule, based on the use of expert assessments, the use of which can increase the uncertainty of decisions and which are expedient to use in the absence of objective data on the characteristics and feasibility of choosing certain options for solutions, in the presence of uncertainty about the preferences of the DM in relation to acceptable characteristics applicants and selected criteria. There are also well-known approaches to the formation of solutions to choice problems, built using fuzzy logic, which in turn should also use either expert evaluations or some a priori information about choice options. Therefore, it can be noted that these approaches to obtaining reasonable results for solving the choice problem are based on a number of assumptions that may not be fulfilled, which their authors mostly do not report, or the possibilities and areas of their adequate application are quite limited.

2 Literature Review

Currently, the number of publications devoted to the design processes of complex systems and technologies, which use procedures for multi-criteria evaluation of decisions made, is growing rapidly.

The most well-known approach to multi-criteria evaluation of decisions is considered to be the "Analityc hierarchy process" (AHP) [1–3]. The method allows you to determine the priorities of individual alternative solutions under consideration, based on the received expert evaluations on the set of selected performance criteria. For comparisons, a linguistic scale is used, which corresponds to fixed weighting factors. The method has many assumptions and therefore can be effectively used in limited settings. Not ensuring full consideration of all circumstances and peculiarities of decision-making conditions [4]. But the simplicity of its application has led to quite wide implementation [5, 6]. There are many approaches to improving the AHP, which should eliminate some of its shortcomings and take into account the conditions of application [7]. There are approaches built on using the advantages of solving a problem with one criterion. For this, the form of presentation of the original problem is replaced by combining all criteria into one common one. Another option is to define the main criterion with the transfer of all others to the composition of restrictions [8–10]. These approaches are appropriate, as a rule, for certain classes of practical problems with compatible criteria. The presence of conflicting criteria requires the formation of mechanisms for finding compromise solutions based on the adoption of some agreement on the ratio of evaluations of criteria values. Such tasks are practically the most common. Developments involving additional research into decision-making conditions with the construction of a Pareto-optimal subset are devoted to their solution. But at the same time, the determination of an acceptable decision option relies exclusively on the DM [9].

The association of the authors of similar developments led to the creation of the International Society on Multiple Criteria Decision Making (MCDM) [10].

3 Methodology

3.1 A Statement of the Task

Formation of the Pareto-optimal subset of solutions is mostly proposed to be performed based on the use of the concession method. The essence of the method is to find a compromise solution by making some concessions based on the values of individual criteria and determining the appropriate sequence of a subsets of Pareto-optimal solutions.

This work is devoted to the formation of an approach for optimizing the solution of the problem of multi-criteria selection in the considered range of issues. It is necessary to find a better option for solving the problem of choosing among possible alternative solutions based on the values of estimations the selected criteria.

When determining the level of advantages of individual applicants according to some criteria over others, it is necessary to formalize the process of comparisons according to individual criteria and ensure the formation of indisputable final evaluations of the effectiveness of applicants.

3.2 B Construction of Pareto-Optimal Subset

An approach to the construction of a Pareto-optimal subset of solutions to the multi-criteria selection problem is presented as a result of constructing a sequence of decision options with the best agreed ratios of the values of the current selected criteria and taking into account the limitations of available resources. This approach makes it possible to form a decision as a composition, which is built on the basis of comparisons of the characteristics of the applicants according to the evaluations of the values of the selected criteria, taking into account their importance and the amount of resources needed to achieve a certain level of evaluations.

We will assume that the choice variants are represented by a set of (allowable solutions) **P**, the elements $X \in \mathbf{P} = \{X_1, X_2, \ldots, X_m\}$ of which determine possible applicants. A set of characteristics and parameters is known for each variant $X = \{x_j\}$, $j \in \boldsymbol{J} = \{1, 2, \ldots, n\}$, the values of which make it possible to assess its attractiveness from the standpoint of the selected criteria.

To compare the applicants, we will use the evaluations of the values of the selected criteria $f_k(X, Y)$, which will be considered local criteria and which together form a vector

$$F(X, Y) = \{f_k(X, Y)\}, X \in \mathbf{P}, Y \in \mathbf{D}_k, k \in \mathbf{K}. \tag{1}$$

The use of choice variants is determined by vectors $Y \in \mathbf{D} = \bigcup_k \mathbf{D}_k$, the set of which reflects acceptable characteristics of applicants in the form of a set of conditions and limitations.

The sequence of the specified local criteria will be divided into two subsets $\mathbf{K} = \mathbf{K}_1 \cup \mathbf{K}_2$. A subset $\mathbf{K}_1$ is formed by the criteria, on the basis of which it is possible to assess the level of the main construction concepts and the architecture of the candidates for selection using promising technologies that create conditions for supporting economically feasible demand, and allow to determine the level of the basic characteristics of the applicants. The subset $\mathbf{K}_2$ includes the criteria by which it is possible to obtain evaluations of the results of the preliminary selection of applicants according to the criteria $\mathbf{K}_1$ in the form of their preferences in a certain direction according to the criteria of this subset, which are determined by the architecture and concept of their construction. We will assume that the sequences of subsets $\mathbf{K}_1$ and $\mathbf{K}_2$ can be ordered according to the level of their importance for the decision-maker.

Determination of estimations values of criteria's for variants of comparison on the given local criteria can be carried out on the basis of construction and use of mathematical models, which with an acceptable level of adequacy reproduce dependences of estimations on characteristics of candidates at selection and take into account conditions of use. According to the assumptions made, the criteria of the first group can be those that determine either the cost indicators of the applicants depending on the conceptual and architectural features of their construction and conditions of use, or criteria that allow assessing the overall level of technological advantages of the applicants depending on their cost characteristics and application features.

Then we will assume that the following mathematical models can be built, which allow to find

$$\left(X_k^*, Y_k^*\right) = Arg \max_{X \in \mathbf{P}, Y \in \mathbf{D}_k}[\min]\{f_k(X, Y)\},\ k \in \boldsymbol{K}. \tag{2}$$

The use of mathematical models (1) allows obtaining a subset of Pareto-optimal solutions $\mathbf{P}^* \subseteq \mathbf{P}$ as a result of the following sequence of calculations:

1. Let $\alpha = 1$, $\mathbf{P}^* = \varnothing$.
2. Let's denote $\tilde{\mathbf{P}} = \mathbf{P}$, $\beta = 1$.
3. Let's define $\left(X_{\alpha\beta}^*, Y_{\alpha\beta}^*\right) = Arg \max\limits_{X \in \tilde{\mathbf{P}}, Y \in \mathbf{D}_k}[\min] f_\beta(X, Y)$, $\mathbf{K}_1 = \mathbf{K}_1 \backslash \beta$.
4. Let's define $\forall k \in \mathbf{K}_2 : f_{\alpha\beta k} = f_k\left(X_{\alpha\beta}^*, Y_{\alpha\beta}^*\right)$, $\mathbf{P}^* = \mathbf{P}^* + X_{\alpha\beta}^*$.
5. Let's redefine $\tilde{\mathbf{P}} = \tilde{\mathbf{P}} \backslash \left\{X_{\alpha 1}^*, X_{\alpha 2}^*, \ldots, X_{\alpha i}^*\right\}$, $i \in \overline{1, \beta}$.
6. If $\mathbf{K}_1 \neq \varnothing$ then $\beta = \beta + 1$, go to point 3.
7. If $\tilde{\mathbf{P}} \neq \varnothing$ then $\alpha = \alpha + 1$, go to point 2.
8. $\mathbf{P}^*$ – subset of Pareto-optimal solutions, $\mathbf{P}^* \subseteq \mathbf{P}$.

The redefinition of the set can be realized by introducing additional constraints in the area of definition of the corresponding criterion, leading to the exclusion of the previous solution from the given sequence of calculations, and obtaining concessions on the criterion based on the introduction of restrictions on the number of resources determining the value of the criterion.

The given calculation process can be graphically represented as a decomposition of a multi-criteria selection problem based on a set of local criteria with successive concessions when constructing a subset of Pareto-optimal solutions $\forall X \in \mathbf{P}$ (see Fig. 1).

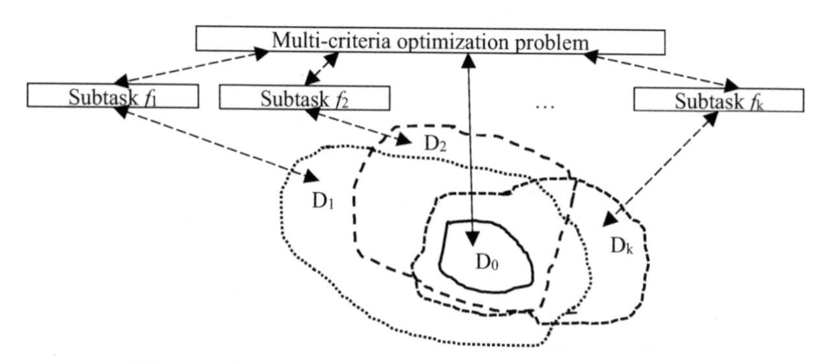

Fig. 1. Decomposition of a multi-criteria selection problem.

It should be noted that the comparison of evaluations of criteria values, which have different physical content and orientation, could not be implemented without the introduction of new measurement scales, the shortcomings of which were noted above. Analysis and clarification of the possibilities of using such scales with objective justifications requires conducting research and forming evaluation mechanisms, which, as a result of the application of additional transformations, contribute to increasing the level of uncertainty of the obtained results and reducing their reliability.

An approach that is free from the mentioned shortcomings should be considered the application of normalization of the relative values of the criteria by bringing them to some common range, for example (0, 1), and carrying out an adequate transformation by using common direction of optimization. Without loss of generality, the search for maximum values can be chosen as such a direction.

For comparisons of applicants, we will build a virtual sample, which corresponds to the best values of local criteria among the choice variants, and estimates of their values together create a vector F_0. Then, the comparison of the applicants with the virtual sample corresponding to F_0, should identify the applicant with advantages having the best values of the characteristics among the choice variants.

After carrying out transformations and normalization of the vector F_0 according to the above provisions, we will get a vector of the following form

$$F_0^* = \{1, 1, \ldots, 1\}. \quad (3)$$

If we consider the space formed by local criteria $\{f_1, f_2, \ldots, f_d\}$, then the feasibility of choosing an applicant $X \in \mathbf{P}$ can be determined by the degree of approximation of the normalized vector of values estimates according to the selected criteria $F(X, Y)$ and the vector of estimates of the virtual sample F_0^* based on the calculation of the scalar product of these vectors.

Considering the values of the components of the vector F_0^*, the evaluation of approximation of the candidate's of choice $X \in \mathbf{P}$ to the virtual specimen will have the following form

$$\left(F(X, Y), F_0^*\right) = \sum_{k \in \mathbf{K}} f_k(X, Y). \tag{4}$$

Thus, the selection of the applicant that best meets all the selected criteria can be performed based on the results of solving the following problem

$$X^* = Arg \max_{X \in \mathbf{P}, Y \in \mathbf{D}} \left(F(X, Y)_0, F_0^*\right) = Arg \max_{X \in \mathbf{P}^*, Y \in \mathbf{D}_k} \sum_{k \in \mathbf{K}} f_k(X, Y). \tag{5}$$

The proposed procedure is finite due to the finiteness of the sets $\mathbf{D}_k$ and $\mathbf{P}$, the elements of which are compared according to the values of the defined global criterion (2). Applicants that best meet all of the selected criteria can be found by the procedure in step (3) in the above calculation sequence.

If there is data on the importance (significance) of local criteria obtained, for example, on the basis of expert evaluations with subsequent normalization, their level can be taken into account when normalizing the evaluation values of the criteria themselves. At the same time, the content of the calculations does not change.

As an example of the application of the proposed approach, consider the process of multi-criteria selection of a variant of the architecture of a virtual data processing system from a cloud computing provider.

Virtual data processing tools from cloud computing providers are offered in a fairly wide range of types of information services and technologies and occupy a constantly growing part of the information processing market. The constant attention of users to productivity, quality, technical and economic characteristics and the list of cloud data processing services requires the formation of reasonable approaches to the objective assessment of the benefits and risks of using these technologies.

The formation of a subset of effective solutions to the selection problem involves the selection of appropriate criteria for evaluating the effectiveness of the processes of using virtual resources based on the given processing tasks and their characteristics, as well as taking into account the influence of the main factors that change the level of evaluations of applicants according to local criteria. These factors, first of all, should include the shares of the volumes of common resources, their distribution and redistribution, which create the possibility of forming a subset of effective solutions.

We will consider performing calculations when determining solutions to multi-criteria selection problems using the example of forming the architecture of a virtual data processing system in a cloud computing environment.

The effectiveness of such solutions is due to the determination of the cost of information services, technologies and the amount of resources of modern high-performance computer systems with the necessary software for data processing only for the immediate time of calculations or use.

Based on the customer's need for data processing procedures, it is possible to choose the virtual system architecture that best meets the processing requirements and selected criteria.

The task of choosing a cloud computing provider for the performance of specified volumes of data processing work can be represented by a mathematical model of task discrete programming with a vector criterion in the following formulation.

We will assume that the volumes of computing work $\Omega_t = \{\omega_{rt}\}$ that require the use of computing resources $r \in \mathbf{R}$ are known at the time $t \in T$. The data from the cloud service provider contain multiple architecture options for building a virtual data processing system $\mathbf{P}$, resource characteristics of virtual machines, their cost, and current status $W_t \in \mathbf{W}$. It is necessary to choose the best version of the architecture $X_t \in \mathbf{P}$, to find the components of the control vector $Y_t \in \mathbf{D}_R$, which, as part of a set of admissible solutions, determine the initialization of components of computing resources, the distribution of data processing volumes, ensure the change of virtual system states and the execution of data processing.

The evaluation of the effectiveness of the options for building a virtual data processing system is determined according to the selected local efficiency criteria in the composition of the vector by the following mathematical models

$$f_k(X_t, Y_t, \Omega_t, W_t) \to \max[\min], \tag{6}$$

$$X_t \in \mathbf{P}, Y_t \in \mathbf{D}_R, W_t \in \mathbf{W}. \tag{7}$$

Building a system with the best ratios of the values of the vector efficiency criterion F from the standpoint of the Pareto-optimality principle corresponds to the search for the best choices.

Considering the importance of individual criteria makes it possible to search for solutions to the problem with the formation of a sequence of applicants according to the proposed approach and to obtain evaluations for the next variant of the architecture according to the current criterion, reducing the number of alternatives for the analysis. Such a process of calculations takes the form of constructing solutions in accordance with the selected criteria.

The formalization of relations (6)–(7) for the task of choosing the architecture of a virtual data processing system in a cloud environment involves the construction of mathematical models, on the basis of which solutions can be determined that meet the set goals and allow obtaining evaluations according to the selected criteria.

We will consider virtual systems of the following type (see Fig. 2).

It can be noted that the data input/output and storage subsystems are determined mainly by parameters that are not essential when choosing the architecture of a virtual data processing system, as they are determined mainly by compliance with the characteristics of processing tasks with the required throughput and cost of use. The processing subsystem has the greatest impact on the performance and efficiency of the system, and its performance requirements must be met by the characteristics of all other subsystems.

To demonstrate the content of the approach to building multi-criteria solutions, we consider the problem of determining the composition and characteristics of a set of virtual machines based on the calculation of estimates of the selected criteria of data processing processes. As a basic mechanism for determining the criteria scores, a mathematical model of an optimization problem of type (6)–(7) with Boolean variables is chosen to form dependencies between the amount of task data processing and the characteristics of

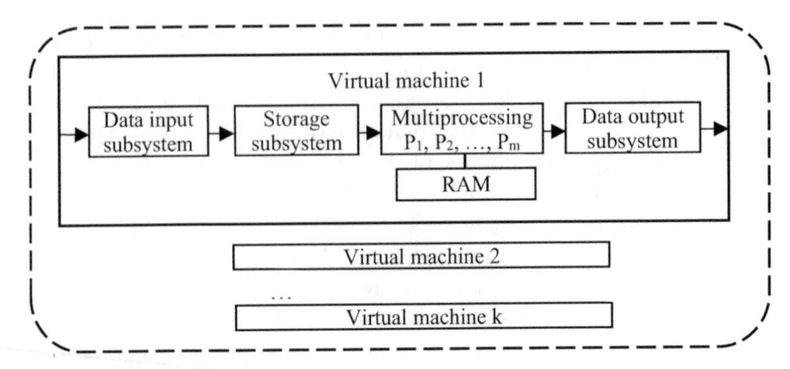

Fig. 2. Virtual data processing system.

virtual machines. To determine solutions to optimization problems with the distribution of tasks and resources, the What'sBest package was used [11].

The solution to the problem determines the distribution of processing tasks between virtual machines, taking into account the parameters of processing processes, the amount of computing resources, and the following criteria

$f_1(X, Y) \rightarrow \min$ – Cost of computing;
$f_2(X, Y) \rightarrow \min$ – Processing time;
$f_3(X, Y) \rightarrow \min$ – Waiting time;
$f_4(X, Y) \rightarrow \min$ – Reliability of calculations;
$f_5(X, Y) \rightarrow \min$ – Utilization of resources;
$f_6(X, Y) \rightarrow \min$ – Losses from waiting;
$f_7(X, Y) \rightarrow \min$ – Number of virtual machines.

We will use the following data to determine the value estimates according to the above criteria according to the concepts of providing services from cloud providers:

$C_i^{(r)}$ – specific cost of using computing resources of the r-th type of the i-th provider, $r \in \mathbf{R}_i$, $i \in \mathbf{I}$; $\theta_i^{(r)}$ – the average execution time of the r-th type of operation by the resources of the i-th provider, $r \in \mathbf{R}_i$, $i \in \mathbf{I}$; $p_j^{(r)}$ – the average number of operations of the r-th type for the j-th software module, $j \in \mathbf{J}$.

Then for $t \in T$

$$f_1(X_t, Y_t) = \sum_{i \in I} \left(\sum_{j \in J} \sum_{r \in R} C_i^{(r)} \theta_i^{(r)} p_j^{(r)} x_{ij}^{(r)} + \sum_{r \in R} A_r y_{ir}^{(in)} \right) \rightarrow \min \tag{8}$$

$$f_2(X_t, Y_t) = \sum_{i \in I} \left(\sum_{j \in J} \sum_{r \in R} \theta_i^{(r)} p_j^{(r)} x_{ij}^{(r)} + \sum_{r \in R} \tau_r y_{ir}^{(in)} \right) \rightarrow \min \tag{9}$$

where $X_t = \left\{ x_{ir}^{(r)} \right\}$, $Y_t = \left\{ y_{ir}^{(in)} \right\}$ are vectors with logical variables that determine the allocation and initialization of processing operations; A_r – initialization cost of the r-th resource; τ_r – initialization time of the r-th resource.

Architecture options are represented by types of virtual machines with corresponding characteristics.

The estimation of the waiting time $f_3(X, Y)$, taking into account the information about the presence of a normal or arbitrary law of the distribution of processing execution time, can be obtained by modeling the random processes of receipt of tasks and their processing.

An assessment of the reliability of the system architecture $f_4(X, Y)$ can be obtained based on the analysis and consideration of the structure of the processing system, its subsystems that have serial-parallel connections according to the main stages of data processing, the type of components and their reliability, Fig. 3. The data input subsystem, data storage subsystem, RAM subsystem, processor processing subsystem, and information output subsystem are considered. It is believed that the processing subsystem is multiprocessor and, together with the OS, provides parallel processing, which increases performance and reliability. Then an estimate of the reliability of the system can be obtained in the form of the probability of failure of the serial-parallel stages of processing by the corresponding subsystems with known estimates of the probability of failure of the components guaranteed by the manufacturers.

The assessment of the level of utilization of computing resources $f_5(X, Y)$ is performed according to the determination of their balances after optimization according to the criteria $f_1(X, Y)$, $f_2(X, Y)$, $f_4(X, Y)$ and concessions according to the determined shares of the levels of use of available resources.

The estimate of losses from waiting time $f_6(X, Y)$ is determined by the waiting time and the value of the lost profit that will be lost as a result of waiting.

The estimation of the number of virtual machines $f_7(X, Y)$ is determined when forming decisions according to the criteria $f_1(X, Y)$, $f_2(X, Y)$, $f_4(X, Y)$ as a necessary value to ensure the existence of solutions to the corresponding problems.

3.3 C Results and Discussion

To demonstrate the performance of such calculations without advertising of famous brands, conditional data were selected that reflect the existing relationships of objects and their characteristics, the real values of which can be found on the websites of cloud service providers.

Data about processing tasks to be executed are characterized by information about the execution conditions, contain general characteristics of program modules and volumes of data used in solving problems with the stages of data entry, processing and output of results. For example calculations, the number of operations in tasks was determined depending on the size of program modules, the expected composition of elementary operations of various types, the volume of data to be processed, and taking into account the dependencies of the structure of processing processes.

Taking into account the accepted approaches of providers to determine the cost of providing computing services and resources, data on the cost of using the time of processors, RAM devices, input-output subsystems (IOS), initializing and performing calculations is used. The data on the technical characteristics of virtual machines includes information about the types and number of processors, their performance, RAM amounts, types, number and throughput of input/output devices, machine state (working, not working), initialization time.

Table 1 presents normalized evaluations of criteria for options for constructing a virtual system when using “Processing cost” -> min as the first significant criterion and choosing the optimization direction according to the criterion “Number of VMs” -> min. In accordance with the data in Table 1 the best option that meets all the criteria is option V03.

Figure 3 shows graphical dependences of criteria evaluations on the variants of virtual system construction when using “Processing Time” -> min as the first significant criterion and choosing the optimization direction by the criterion “Number of VMs” -> max, taking into account other criteria significance levels.

The results obtained also make it possible to establish the distance between the choice options, which creates conditions for a more detailed analysis of their characteristics.

Table 1. Normalized estimates of options for building a virtual system by criteria.

Variants	f_1	f_2	f_3	f_4	f_5	f_6	f_7	Normalized scalar product
V01	1,0000	1,0000	0,0000	0,0000	1,0000	0,0000	1,0000	0,80782
V02	0,9965	0,9965	0,4865	0,0000	0,5652	0,6186	1,0000	0,77457
V03	0,7680	0,7680	0,6492	0,8461	0,5652	0,6874	0,5000	1,00000
V04	0,4378	0,4378	0,9025	1,0000	0,5652	0,9244	0,0000	0,87651
V05	0,7645	0,7645	0,7691	0,8461	0,3913	0,8856	0,5000	0,86048
V06	0,6242	0,6242	0,8593	0,8461	0,3043	0,9599	0,5000	0,82678
V07	0,4734	0,4734	0,9797	0,8461	0,2174	0,9857	0,5000	0,95559
V08	0,2106	0,2106	0,9966	0,8461	0,1304	0,9977	0,5000	0,85213
V09	0,0662	0,0662	0,9996	1,0000	0,0435	0,9998	0,0000	0,67889
V10	0,0000	0,0000	1,0000	1,0000	0,0000	1,0000	0,0000	0,64802

Based on the values of the generalized criterion, it can be argued that in these conditions the optimal option, providing the best combination of assessment values for the selected criteria, taking into account their significance levels, is option V07.

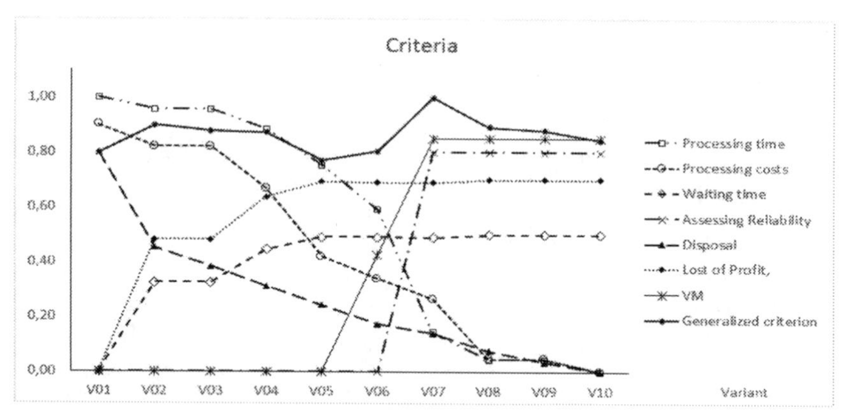

Fig. 3. Estimates of selection variants with the first criterion of "Processing time" -> min. Changing the direction of the criterion "Number of VM" -> max.

4 Conclusions

Multi-criteria choice problems are a common class of problems in many practical situations. Numerous developments are dedicated to their solution, which should be implemented in automated decision support systems. Existing approaches to the solution of such problems do not always allow determining reasonable and transparent solutions with adequate consideration of conditions in various spheres of activity, quality criteria of solutions and their evaluation procedures. The adequacy of comparisons of options by criteria is lost when using subjective approaches and violating a number of assumptions that were the basis of the justifications for the relevant multi-criteria evaluation procedures. (1) The paper proposes an approach that allows for the formation of Pareto-optimal subsets of solutions to multi-criteria selection problems with the ordering of applicants by iterative concessions according to the selected criteria. The determination of the best applicants from this set is based on the calculation of the values of the proposed criterion, which allows you to choose the best option that most closely matches the selected criteria and conditions of its use.

The given example of a multi-criteria evaluation of options for building a virtual data processing system allows us to draw conclusions about the possibility of applying this approach to solving a wide range of problems of justifying the choice as part of operational management systems for dynamic productions and service processes.

References

1. Saaty, T.: A scaling method for priorities in hierarchical structures. J. Math. Psychol. **15**(3), 234–281 (1977)
2. Saaty, T.: Decision making with the analytic hierarchy process. Int. J. Serv. Sci. **1**(1), 83–98 (2008)
3. Saaty, T., Shang, J.: An innovative orders of-magnitude approach to AHP-based mutli-criteria decision making: prioritizing divergent intangible humane acts. Eur. J. Oper. Res. **214**(3), 703–715 (2011)

4. Podinovski, V., Podinovskaya, O.: An approach of the criteria importance theory to decision making problems with hierarchical criterial structures. Autom. Doc. Math. Linguist. **48**(1), 1–5 (2014)
5. Solangi, Y.: Assessing and overcoming the renewable energy barriers for sustainable development in Pakistan: an integrated AHP and fuzzy TOPSIS approach. Renew. Energy **173**, 209–222 (2021)
6. Zhang, H.: The analysis of the reasonable structure of water conservancy investment of capital construction in China by AHP method. Water Resour. Manage **23**, 1–18 (2009)
7. Ayhana, M.: Fuzzy AHP approach for supplier selection problem: a case study in a gearmotor company. Int. J. Manag. Value Supply Chains (IJMVSC) **4**(3), 11–23 (2013)
8. Podinovski, V.: Potential optimality in multicriterial optimization. Comput. Math. Math. Phys. **54**, 429–438 (2014)
9. Odu, G., Charles-Owaba, O.: Review of multi–criteria optimization methods – theory and applications. OSR J. Eng. (IOSRJEN) **3**(10), 1–14 (2013)
10. International Society on MCDM (Multiple Criteria Decision Making). http://www.mcdmsociety.org. Accessed 21 June 2023
11. LINDO® Software for Integer Programming, Linear Programming, Nonlinear Programming, Stochastic Programming, Global Optimization. https://www.lindo.com/. Accessed 15 May 2023

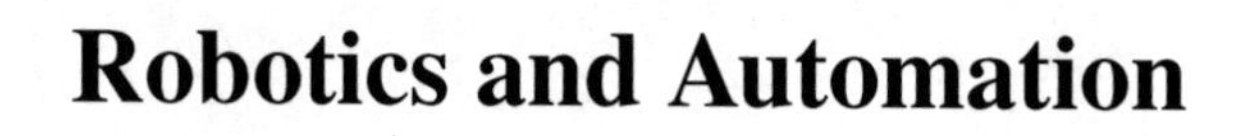

Robotics and Automation

A Quadcopter Development for Security Purposes

Yusra Obeidat(✉) and Rana Daoud

Electronics Engineering Department, Yarmouk University, Irbid, Jordan
yusra.obeidat@yu.edu.jo

Abstract. The use of technology has increased in the recent years especially during the spread of Covid-19 disease all around the world. There was a great need of developing a new system to ensure that people follow the public safety rules to prevent the spread of the disease. The main goal of this work is to create a quadcopter (commonly referred to as a drone) intended for outdoor security applications. The drone includes an implementation of the mask detection that can detect if people wear masks during disease spread. The drone is controlled using Xbox controller, and an Arduino Duo is used as a main Microcontroller for the drone. Raspberry pi is used at the image processing side to recognize people and detect whether they wear masks or not. The required components and how to select them are discussed in details in this work. The drone can be manually operated via the LORA network. Additionally, a Raspberry Pi functions as a server for streaming data and video to a monitoring station's website. This allows for real-time monitoring and alerts in the event of individuals not wearing face masks or the detection of a person of interest within the designated search area. Notably, the drone developed in this project has demonstrated the capability to achieve vertical flight up to 20 m and cover horizontal distances ranging from 60 to 70 m.

Keywords: Drone · Quadcopter · Image processing · Mask detection · Security · Covid-19

1 Introduction

UAV (Unmanned Aerial Vehicle) is a type of aircraft that can fly without any human pilot, crew, or passengers on board [1–3]. UAV is commonly known as a drone, it can be self or wirelessly controlled without any human intervention. It can be used for security, military, monitoring, civil, mapping, hobbies or even rescue purposes [1–8]. There are two main types of drones that are widely used, the first type is drone with fixed wings and the other type is drone with rotary wings. The fixed wings drone is used widely in military and aerial mapping applications because of its high flight speed, and it can fly at high altitude [9]. On the other hand, the rotary wing drones can fly near the earth and can be used for maneuvering in confined spaces [10]. A Rotary wing drone could be a single rotor which is called helicopter or multirotor which is named by the number of motors it contains. If the drone contains four motors then it is called quadcopter, if it has six motors

K. Daimi and A. Al Sadoon (Eds.): ACR 2024, LNNS 956, pp. 529–542, 2024.
https://doi.org/10.1007/978-3-031-56950-0_43

it is called hexacopter, and so on [11]. The drone can be used for security purposes where sensors and camera can be connected to the drone to discover unusual circumstances or conditions in the flying area [12]. It can be used to monitor people such as checking if they wear masks to prevent the spread of diseases such as Covid-19, it can also be used to search for wanted or lost persons [13]. The drone can reconnaissance tour, take pictures, and process them, identify the violators, and report that to the command center. Another possible use for the drone is to predict weather conditions and various natural changes [14]. A group of students at RCC INSTITUTE OF INFORMATION TECHNOLOGY designed a drone based on Arduino microcontroller for search & rescue operations as well as for remote package delivering operations [15]. They used ESP32 to control the drone over the internet, the pressure, temperature and humidity sensors values in their system were streamed and displayed through WIFI. Another group of students from the Department of Electronics & Communication from L.D. College of Engineering have built a drone for general purposes. They have used Proportional-Integral-Derivative (PID) controller for the stabilization, and a ZigBee module was used to send information from the sensors. This paper presents the design and implementation of a quadcopter that can be used to detect wearing masks during the spread of a disease, as well as for face recognition to find wanted or lost people. This drone was designed to be controlled for flying properly, and it is now under development to make it fully automated and self-flying within a specific area and will be able to detect and avoid obstacles. Deep learning algorithms such as single shot multi-box detector (SSD) is used to detect faces and decide whether people wear masks or not [16]. The drone we designed in this work was able to fly a vertical distance of up to 20 m and a horizontal distance of about 60–70 m.

2 Design and Methods

In this work, we have designed a drone operated through an Xbox controller, with Arduino serving as the primary drone controller. Raspberry Pi is utilized for image processing, specifically for recognizing individuals and determining if they are wearing masks. This section will cover the designs and operations of the main parts of the autopilot system including the quadcopter, the PID controller, the Inertial Measurement Unit (IMU), and LORA module.

2.1 Quadcopter Design

The Quadcopter designed in this work contains four rotors and a control system that is used for guiding and controlling the overall flight, this system is called the Autopilot system. There are several commercial and open-source systems that could be used such as Pixhawk and Navio2 [17–20]. These two systems are cheap and easy to use to control several types of drones. The user can set a mission to the autopilot that contains several locations to flight in between them, it can take-off and land to a specific location with all the control options being controlled from the cockpit by the user. In this work. We have used Navio2 because its Hardware Attached on Top (HAT) of raspberry pi that can be reached through the internet. We have also used an Arduino due microcontroller to control the drone manually. An x-shape quadcopter is implemented in this work, two of the motors must be rotated in clockwise direction while the other two must be rotated in the opposite direction, and the speed of each motor must be controlled to ensure a zero total sideways momentum at the drone.

A suitable propeller is selected for motors where propeller dimensions are measured in inches and written as "9545", this means that the propeller is 9.5 inch in length and 4.5 inch in width. An outrunner brushless DC motors are used because of many advantages such as very good speed-torque characteristic, higher efficiency, low noise, great dynamic response, and high speed. The speed and direction of each brushless DC motor are controlled by an electronic speed controller (ESC). A Li-po battery is used to drive the motors because it has a very high capacity and can provide a high current for a long time and ensure long flight time.

Ecalc.ch website was used to calculate and estimate the efficiency and flight time of the drone. Considering all of the components types and variables, we put them into the website as shown in Fig. 1 and we achieved the results of the estimated characteristics for the drone as shown in Fig. 2.

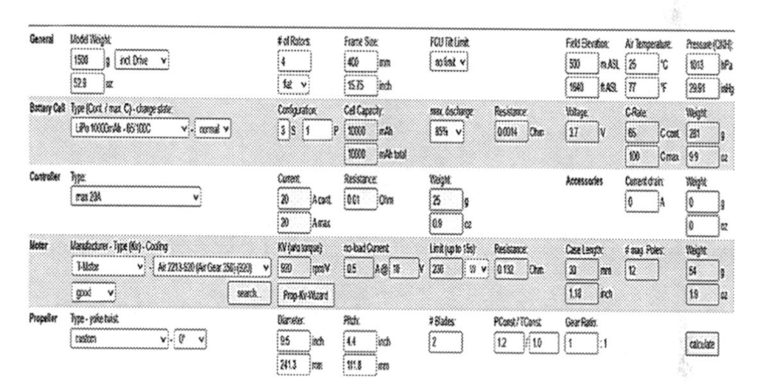

Fig. 1. Ecalc setup of the expected components

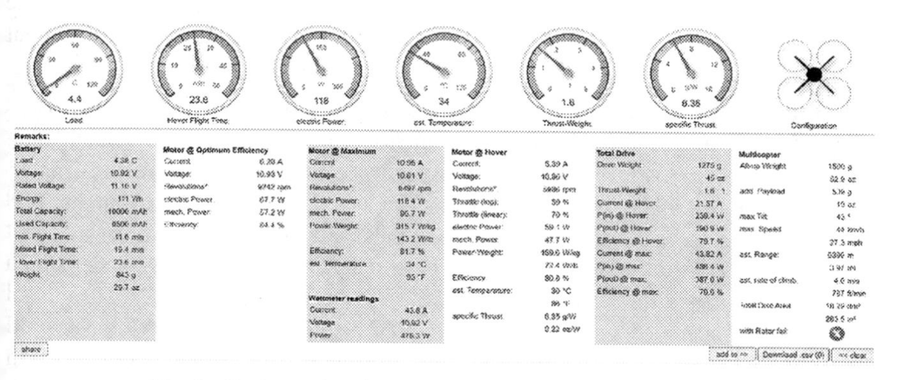

Fig. 2. Ecalc results with estimated flight time, thrust and more

The estimation time of the components we chose for our drone is 23.6 min which is very good compared to the commercial quadcopters, and the estimated weight of the drone is 1500 g. Figure 3 shows the range estimator for our drone, where the green area is the best range, and it shows that the flight time is 20 min at an air speed of 25 km/h for about 8500 m of range.

2.2 PID Controller

In this work we have used a proportional–integral–derivative controller (PID controller) as a control loop feedback mechanism. PID algorithm consists of three basic coefficients: proportional, integral, and derivative which are changed to get optimal response. The entire idea of this algorithm revolves around manipulating the error. PID controller calculates an error value as the difference between a measured process variable and a desired setpoint. It can be understood as a controller that takes the present, the past, and the future of the error into consideration [23].

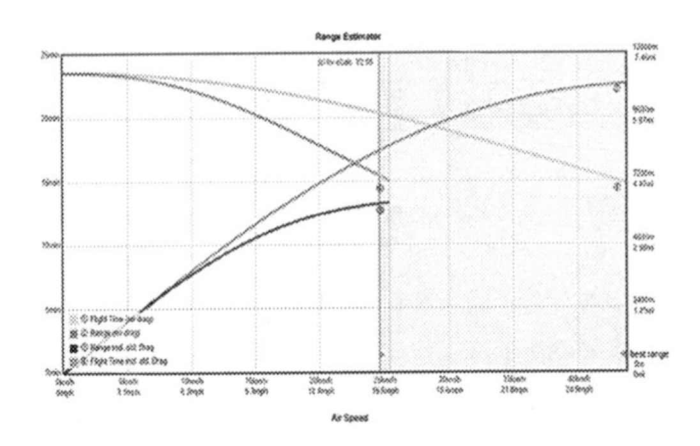

Fig. 3. The range estimator of the drone

The block diagram illustrated in Fig. 4 outlines the functioning of the PID controller. In this diagram, the variable 'e' symbolizes the tracking error, which represents the disparity between the input and the actual output – in our case, this pertains to roll, pitch, and yaw. This error signal 'e' is directed to the PID controller, which computes both the derivative and the integral of this error signal.

The signal 'u' is subsequently determined as the sum of the proportional gain (Kp) multiplied by the magnitude of the error, the integral gain (Ki) multiplied by the integral of the error, and the derivative gain (Kd) multiplied by the derivative of the error. This 'u' signal is then transmitted to the device, leading to the generation of a new output. This fresh output is fed back to the sensor, initiating the calculation of a new error signal 'e' once more. The controller takes this updated error signal and reevaluates its derivative and integral, perpetuating this iterative process.

A proportional controller (Kp) has the effect of reducing the rise time but not completely eliminating the steady-state error. An integral control (Ki) serves to eradicate the steady-state error, although it may potentially worsen the transient response. A derivative control (Kd) bolsters system stability, reduces overshoot, and enhances transient response.

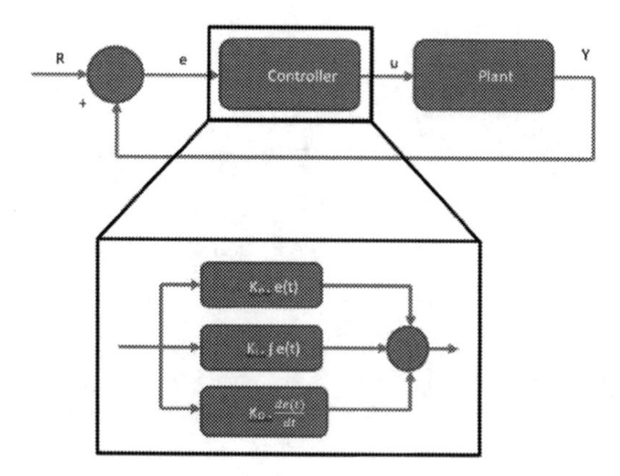

Fig. 4. The block diagram of PID controller [23].

2.3 Inertial Measurement Unit (IMU)

The Inertial Measurement Unit (IMU) that is used in this project is GY-951 which contains a microcontroller that reads the data from three sensors (Magnetometer, Gyroscope, and accelerometer) and make a fusion between them to give (Roll, Pitch, Yaw).

2.4 Lora (E220-900t22d)

The drone designed in this work is controlled over internet using LORA because it can send data for long rang. LoRaWAN gateways can transmit and receive signals over a distance of over 10 km in rural areas and up to 3 km in dense urban areas. LoRa E220-900T22D module used in this project can send and receive data through UART TTL.

Before the use of the module, both of the transmitter and receiver were reconfigured to make them sending and receiving at the same channel and the same baud rate. The configuration of LORA module is shown in Fig. 5.

3 Implementation

The technical details of the drone implementation are included in the following sections.

3.1 Control System

The drone designed in this work is controlled with a camera to monitor a specific area and the project will be developed to make it autonomous system without any human intervention.

Xbox controller was connected to the computer by USB to control the drone. We have used python as a processing language to read the data from the controller through USB where each of the buttons need to be named as shown in Fig. 6.

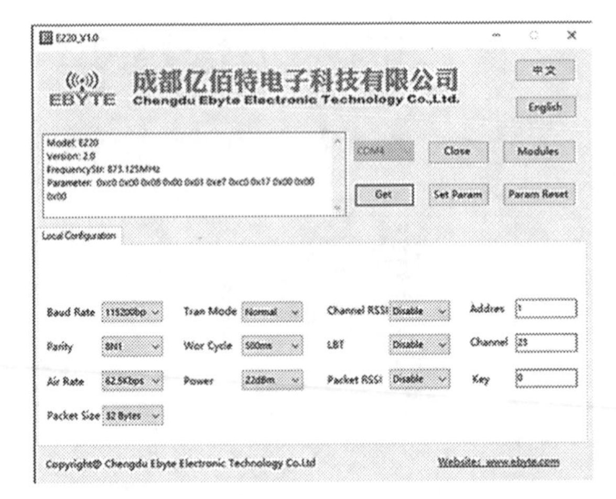

Fig. 5. LORA configuration for the drone Implementation

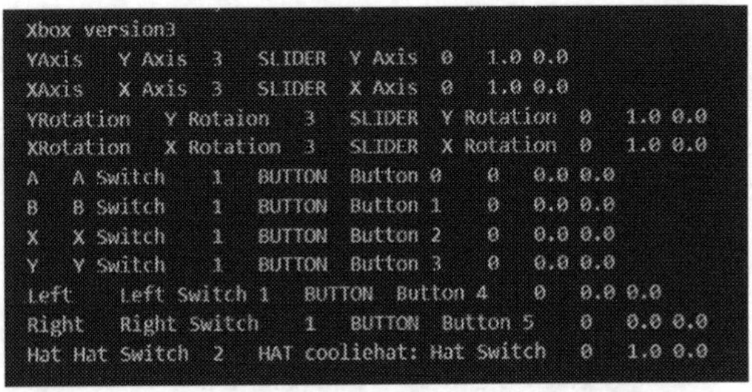

```
Xbox version3
YAxis    Y Axis   3   SLIDER  Y Axis  0   1.0 0.0
XAxis    X Axis   3   SLIDER  X Axis  0   1.0 0.0
YRotation   Y Rotaion   3   SLIDER  Y Rotation  0   1.0 0.0
XRotation   X Rotation  3   SLIDER  X Rotation  0   1.0 0.0
A   A Switch    1   BUTTON  Button 0    0   0.0 0.0
B   B Switch    1   BUTTON  Button 1    0   0.0 0.0
X   X Switch    1   BUTTON  Button 2    0   0.0 0.0
Y   Y Switch    1   BUTTON  Button 3    0   0.0 0.0
Left    Left Switch 1   BUTTON  Button 4    0   0.0 0.0
Right   Right Switch    1   BUTTON  Button 5    0   0.0 0.0
Hat Hat Switch  2   HAT cooliehat: Hat Switch   0   1.0 0.0
```

Fig. 6. Controllers Buttons names and description file

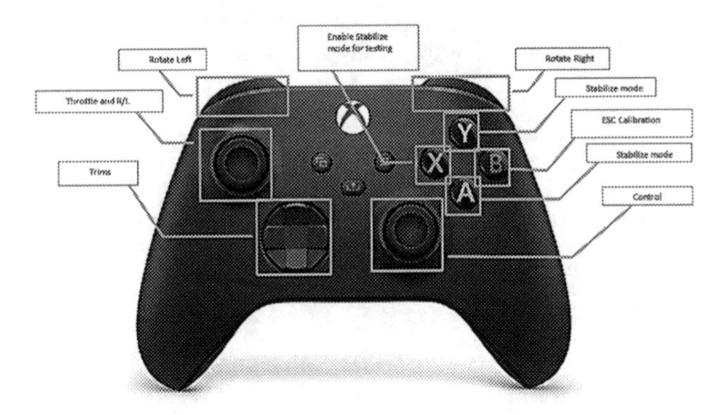

Fig. 7. Xbox Controller buttons functions.

After that a library called GCP (Game Control Plus) is used to read each value; for example, Y Axis value if from −1 to 1, and it is converted from 0 to 100 before sending. The controller switches function used are shown in Fig. 7.

After acquiring the switch values, these values need to be transmitted as a message to the drone. To achieve this, a comprehensive message encompassing all the switch values is constructed. This message incorporates a distinct header, facilitating the recipient's ability to identify the initiation of the message and extract the values of each button. The header that indicates the message's commencement has the following format: '81 A1 xx xx xx xx xx xx xx xx xx xx xx xx xx xx', where '81 A1' serves as the message header, and 'xx' represents the individual switch values.

These values are then conveyed via the LORA network, using a UART TTL module for data transmission. This setup obviates the need for a dedicated microcontroller to handle data transmission. Alternatively, a USB/TTL converter can be utilized, establishing a direct connection between the computer and the module to transmit data. The system's control architecture is depicted in Fig. 8.

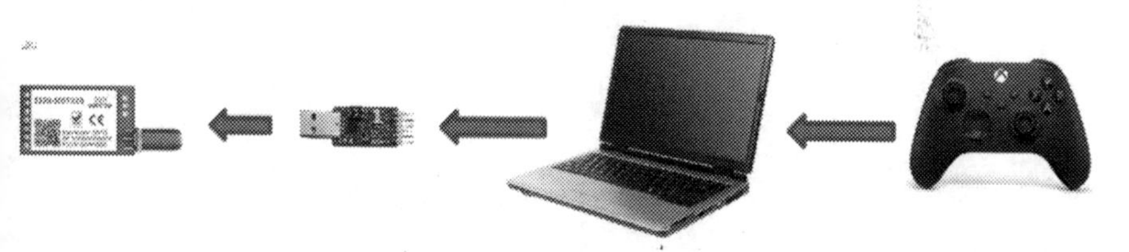

Fig. 8. Xbox controller side

Figure 9 shows the block diagram for the main code that we used to control the drone, some other components will be added such as laser and barometer to measure the altitude of the drone.

The Inertial Measurement Unit (IMU) serves as a feedback system for the PID Controller. It transmits data in the form of messages, and it's crucial that this data is transmitted rapidly without any delays. To ensure this swift data transfer, it's not advisable to utilize a library. Instead, the data needs to be read and parsed in a manner similar to Xbox controller data. Therefore, IMU data is sent in the following format: '#YPR = xx.xx,xx.xx,xx.xx', where '#YPR' serves as the header, and 'xx.xx' represents the values of Roll, Pitch, and Yaw.

This process is somewhat different because the data length can vary, and its length is unknown. The code begins by searching for the main header. Once found, it searches for the commas within the message. The Roll value appears after the header and before the first comma, Pitch is located between the first and second comma, and Yaw is after the second comma.

The reference values for Roll and Pitch are both set to zero. The range for Roll and Pitch values is between –180 and 180. When the drone's stabilization mode is activated, it initiates the stabilization process after take-off.

Additionally, an Ultrasonic sensor is employed to detect and avoid obstacles. The time difference between sending and receiving ultrasonic waves must be factored into the control system. To address this, a timer is used to begin counting when the trigger is applied, ensuring it doesn't interrupt the main code.

Furthermore, Electronic Speed Controllers (ESCs) utilize PWM (pulse width modulation) for control. Initially, the ESCs require calibration. Calibration, in this context, involves determining the maximum and minimum values of PWM signals that govern the motors. Each ESC needs calibration each time it is powered on, and the process involves:

1. Sending the maximum PWM value that the controller can provide.
2. Powering up the ESCs.
3. Sending the minimum PWM value that the controller can provide.

The motors will emit a beep sound, indicating their current ESC mode. The motors used are Air920, which have a 920 kV rating. As previously mentioned, two of the motors rotate clockwise, while the other two rotate counter-clockwise.

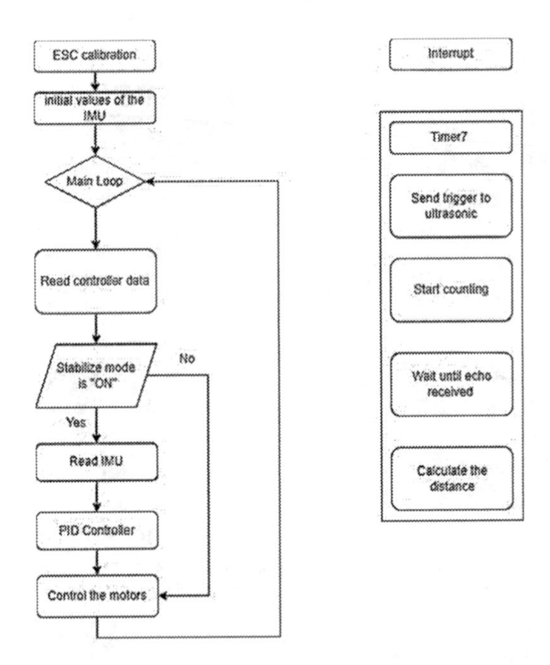

Fig. 9. The block diagram for the code function

3.2 Calibration and Tuning

It is practically unattainable to create a drone that achieves perfect balance, meaning that all components are positioned in a way that centers the mass at the drone's geometric center. Additionally, achieving a 100% alignment between the IMU and the drone is also an impractical goal. Therefore, PID tuning becomes a necessary step to determine the most suitable gain values for ensuring the drone's stability, even when subjected to factors like added weight or changing weather conditions.

Furthermore, two distinct calibration processes are essential. The first type is referred to as 'Trims calibration,' and its purpose is to ensure that the drone takes off vertically. This calibration is a manual process, allowing for adjustments during flight as needed. Trims calibration can be performed using the controller's trim buttons. The second type of calibration is used to rectify any misalignment between the IMU and the drone. It addresses the issue of potential misalignment between the IMU's orientation and that of the drone itself.

The tuning of the PID controller's gains, specifically Kp, Ki, and Kd, is carried out to regulate the drone's response. A calibration and testing platform is employed for this purpose. The drone is affixed to this platform, allowing it to move freely to assess its responses. Accordingly, the gains are adjusted, either increased or decreased, based on the observed responses. The complete block diagram for the drone developed in this project is shown in Fig. 10.

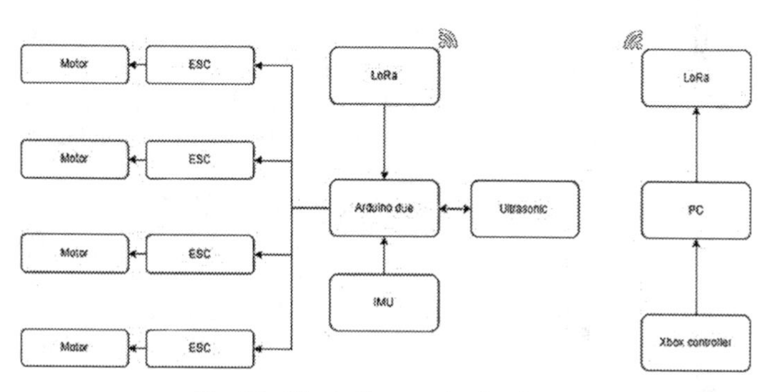

Fig. 10. Block diagram for the drone.

3.3 Mask Detection

An image processing technique was utilized to determine whether individuals were wearing masks, and it would issue a notification if they were not. The primary tools employed in this algorithm are TensorFlow and OpenCV, both of which are well-established libraries in the Python programming ecosystem.

The mask detection process in this project makes use of a Convolutional Neural Network (CNN) and involves three key image processing steps: convolution, pooling, and flattening.

When computers interpret images, they perceive them as arrays of numbers. In grayscale images, each number falls within the range of 0 to 255, while colored images are represented as 3D tensors with three channels (Red, Green, and Blue), with each channel's numbers also ranging from 0 to 255.

In any machine learning (ML) algorithm, the model must undergo training using a dataset before it can begin making predictions with new data. For this purpose, we downloaded our dataset from Kaggle, which includes numerous images of people both wearing and not wearing masks.

During the convolution step, each feature generates a feature map, and this feature map is systematically moved across the entire image to assess its similarity to the image's features. All feature maps traverse the image, ultimately classifying the features within smaller, overlapping sections of the image.

In the pooling step, certain pixels are replaced by their maximum, minimum, or average values. This pooling process helps reduce the image's dimensions while retaining its most significant features, allowing the computer to recognize the image more effectively.

The flattening step occurs after the image is resized to a manageable size with its essential features, eliminating noise and unwanted details. Pixels are restructured to make them compatible with input to the neural network, which is then trained as previously mentioned.

3.4 Raspberry Pi

The Raspberry Pi operates on its own operating system, allowing it to function in a specialized environment without requiring connection to an external computer for programming. It can be self-programmed using the Python language. In this project, Raspberry Pi is employed for the image processing applied for mask detection, and data streaming to the ground station.

Raspberry Pi is utilized to stream data to the ground station, enabling the real-time monitoring of the drone's location and the camera feed used for face mask detection. It serves as a server where a simple website is created to display the drone's current location and the camera's output. To determine the drone's location, a GPS module is employed. This module is connected via UART and retrieves the location data, including latitude and longitude, which is then stored in a text file. A JavaScript code reads the file's content and displays the data on a map.

It's worth noting that enabling UART is a crucial step to allow data reception from the GPS module, and this can be achieved by editing the config.txt file and adding specific values as follows:

dtparam = spi = on.
dtoverlay = pi3-disable-bt.
core_freq = 250.
enable_uart = 1.
force_turbo = 1.

GPS messages are rich in information pertaining to satellites, their statuses, speeds, and more. However, for our purposes, we only require the latitude and longitude values. These values can be extracted either manually or by utilizing specialized libraries designed to handle GPS messages, such as pynmea2, which we will employ in this context.

To install pynmea2, at the terminal type:
sudo pip install pynmea2.

4 Results and Discussion

An example of results of Image processing that is implemented on raspberry pi is shown in Fig. 11. If the detected person doesn't wear mask or if he wears mask but it does not cover his nose this will be detected as "No mask detected", but if he wears a mask that covers his nose and mouth this will be detected as "Mask detected".

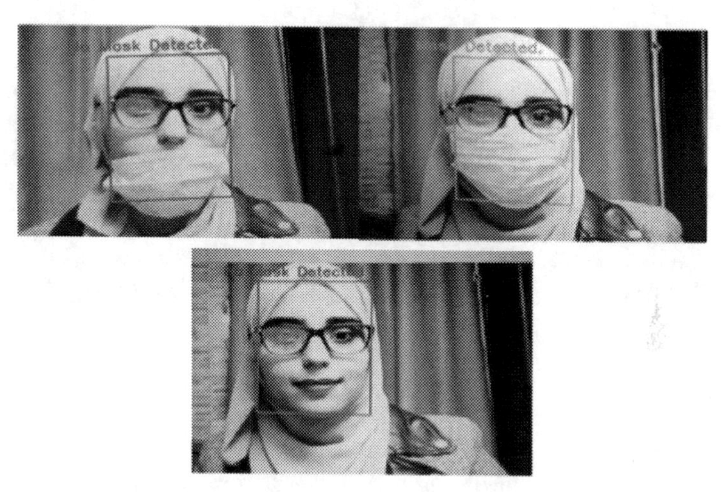

Fig. 11. Example of the results of the mask detection

The web site created for this work contains three main pages, the first one is the private login page as no one can login to the website except the main user. After logged in, the main page welcoming page will open it and does not contain any control or viewing options. There are 4 tabs in the main page: The first one is "statue" which contains the map to show the location of the drone in real time. The second tab is "control" tab that contains the reading of sensors from the drone and some other options for the pilot to use for extra control. The other two taps are not important, one of them contains the admin contact information, the second one is a logout tab to logout from the website.

Figure 12a shows the final designed drone. After several crashes and failures attempt, we lost several propellers and several landing gears, and we spent long time to do tuning and calibration. At the end the drone becomes stable and was able to flight successfully without any issues. Three testing and tuning stages were done, the first one was on the testing platform to check the overall functionality and the initial or suggested gains. The second one uses a rope to tie the drone to do tuning and make adjustment to the required gains to ensure that the drone will not be crashed. The last one was on controlling the real flight without using the rope to make sure that the drone is stable and can fly without any problem. Figure 12b shows the drone in the flying field of MARS ROBOTICS, Irbid, Jordan. Figure 12c shows that our drone is flying in the air were it was able to fly a vertical distance of up to 20 m and a horizontal distance of about 60–70 m.

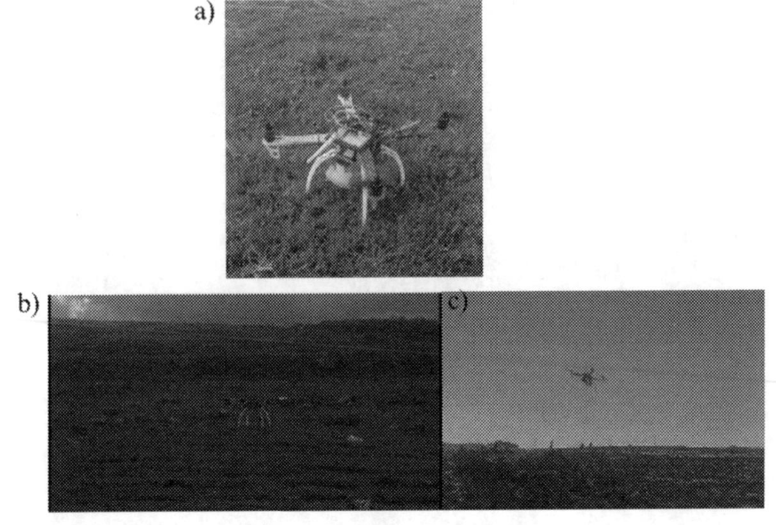

Fig. 12. a) The final designed drone. b) The drone in the flying field. c) the drone flying in the air

5 Conclusion

In this work, we have designed a drone that can be used as an outdoor system for security purposes. The drone was able to fly a vertical distance of up to 20 m and a horizontal distance of about 60–70 m.The image processing that is used for mask detection works successfully but its not efficient to use raspberry pi because it needs high processing power to make a real time image processing. There is other alternatives such as "jetson nano" which is a mini-computer like raspberry pi and its special for ML and DL applications. In future, we will use NVIDIA® Jetson Nano™ minicomputer because it is small and powerful for running multiple neural networks in parallel for applications like image classification, object detection, segmentation, and speech processing. Moreover, using the drone in public area is not that easy in Jordan because it needs security approval, we will apply to get the approval from the Jordanian military intelligence to use our drone in public areas to find missing people or to check if people wear masks or not.

References

1. Dietrich, B., Iff, S., Profelt, J., et al.: Development of a Local air surveillance system for security purposes: design and core characteristics. Eur. J. Secur. Res. **2**, 71–81 (2017). https://doi.org/10.1007/s41125-017-0015-7
2. Yao, H., Qin, R., Chen, X.: Unmanned aerial vehicle for remote sensing applications—a review. Remote Sensing **11**(12), 1443 (2019). https://doi.org/10.3390/rs11121443
3. Kim, J., Kim, S., Ju, C., Son, H.I.: Unmanned aerial vehicles in agriculture: a review of perspective of platform, control, and applications. IEEE Access **7**, 105100–105115 (2019). https://doi.org/10.1109/ACCESS.2019.2932119
4. Liu, Y., Dai, H.-N., Wang, Q., Shukla, M.K., Imran, M.: Unmanned aerial vehicle for internet of everything: opportunities and challenges, Comput. Commun. (2020)

5. Rahman, M.F.F., Fan, S., Zhang, Y., Chen, L.: A comparative study on application of unmanned aerial vehicle systems in agriculture. Agriculture **11**(1), 22 (2021).https://doi.org/10.3390/agriculture11010022
6. Zuo, Z., Liu, C., Han, Q.-L., Song, J.: Unmanned aerial vehicles: control methods and future challenges. IEEE/CAA J. Automatica Sinica **9**(4), 601–614 (2022). https://doi.org/10.1109/JAS.2022.105410
7. Mohsan, S.A.H., Khan, M.A., Noor, F., Ullah, I., Alsharif, M.H.: Towards the unmanned aerial vehicles (UAVs): a comprehensive review. Drones. **6**(6), 147 (2022). https://doi.org/10.3390/drones6060147
8. Reddy Maddikunta, P.K,. et al.: Unmanned aerial vehicles in smart agriculture: applications, requirements, and challenges. IEEE Sensors J. **21**(16),17608–17619 (2021). https://doi.org/10.1109/JSEN.2021.3049471
9. Mulero-Pázmány, M., et al.: Development of a fixed-wing drone system for aerial insect sampling. Drones. **6**(8), 189 (2022). https://doi.org/10.3390/drones6080189
10. Nurrohaman, M.F., Titalim, B.A., Utama, T.H., Adiprawita, W.: Design and Implementation of on-board hybrid generator for rotary wing drone. I/n: 2019 International Conference on Electrical Engineering and Informatics (ICEEI), Bandung, Indonesia, pp. 310–314 (2019). https://doi.org/10.1109/ICEEI47359.2019.8988811
11. Ucgun, H., Yuzgec, U., Bayilmis, C.L A review on applications of rotary-wing unmanned aerial vehicle charging stations. Inter. J. Adv. Rob. Syst. **18**(3) (2021). doi:https://doi.org/10.1177/17298814211015863
12. Svanström, F., Alonso-Fernandez, F., Englund, C.: Drone Detection and tracking in real-time by fusion of different sensing modalities. Drones. **6**(11), 317 (2022). https://doi.org/10.3390/drones6110317
13. Kumar, A., Sharma, K., Singh, H., Naugriya, S.G., Gill, S.S., Buyya, R.: A drone-based networked system and methods for combating coronavirus disease (COVID-19) pandemic. Future Gener Comput Syst. **115**, 1–19 (2021). https://doi.org/10.1016/j.future.2020.08.046. Epub 2020 Sep 3. PMID: 32895585; PMCID: PMC7467876
14. Gao, M., Hugenholtz, C.H., Fox, T.A., et al.: Weather constraints on global drone flyability. Sci. Rep. **11**, 12092 (2021). https://doi.org/10.1038/s41598-021-91325-w
15. Bhattacharjee, A., Hazra, A., Sar, S.K.: Under the Supervision of ARIJIT GHOSH. Quadcopter Control Using Arduino Microcontroller, RCC Institute of Information Technology, Kolkata (2018)
16. Kumar, A., Zhang, Z.J., Lyu, H.: Object detection in real time based on improved single shot multi-box detector algorithm. J Wireless Com. Netw. **2020**, 204 (2020). https://doi.org/10.1186/s13638-020-01826-x
17. Solidakis, G.N. ,et al.: An Arduino-based subsystem for controlling UAVs through GSM. In: 2017 6th International Conference on Modern Circuits and Systems Technologies (MOCAST), Thessaloniki, Greece, pp. 1–4 (2017). https://doi.org/10.1109/MOCAST.2017.7937656
18. Rajpoot, A.S., Gadani, N., Kalathia, S.: Development of Arduino Based Quadcopter. Inter. Adv. Res. J. Sci. Eng. Technol. **3**(6) (2016)
19. Sandhu, P.S.: Development of ISR for quadcopter. Inter. J. Res. Eng. Technol. (IJRET) **03**(04), 185–186 (2014)
20. Quadcopter Dynamics, Simulation, and Control (26 January 2010)
21. Khajure, S., Surwade, V., Badak, V.: Quadcopter design and fabrication. Inter. Adv. Res. J. Sci. Eng. Technol. (IARJSET) 3(20) February 2016

22. Mengistie, T.T., Kumar, D., Covid-19 face mask detection using convolutional neural network and image processing. In: 2nd International Conference for Emerging Technology (INCET). Belagavi, India 2021, pp. 1–7 (2021). https://doi.org/10.1109/INCET51464.2021.9456288
23. Knospe, C.: PID control. IEEE Control. Syst. Mag. **26**(1), 30–31 (2006). https://doi.org/10.1109/MCS.2006.1580151

Posters

Towards a Scalable Spiking Neural Network

Rasha Karakchi(✉) and Jacob Frierson

University of South Carolina, Columbia, SC 29208, USA
karakchi@cec.sc.edu, jacobtf@email.sc.edu

Abstract. Spiking Neural Network (SNN) is the biological-brain model that has the capability of solving complex problems related to pattern recognition and character classification. Each neuron fires an output based on the discrete spikes that are collected from its predecessors which results in changing the ionic level or the membrane potential in the neuron. Once the level reaches a threshold, the neuron transmits signal to its successors. Transmitting data among neurons is a data-dependency problem because each neuron depends on receiving signals from its surrounding neurons at the current time and transmitting it into next neurons. Due to this high level of dependency, scaling up spiking neural network (represented by increasing number of neurons and hidden layers) is a real challenge. In hardware, the number of neurons is limited by the hardware (device) capacity and the number of internal wires available to connect between neurons. In this paper, we examine the main factors that significantly impact the scalability of spiking neural networks in hardware through implementing a spiking neural network model using the hardware description language SystemVerilog. Through evaluating the design on Alveo U55 high performance compute FPGA card, we found that the highest number of neurons that we can map on the hardware is 128 neurons per hidden layer and the higher number of synapses is 384,000 per hidden layer.

Keywords: Spiking Neural Network · Leaky Integrate-and-Fire · Scalability · FPGA · Accelerators

1 Introduction

Spiking Neural Network (SNN) is the third generation of timing-based Artificial Neural Networks (ANNs) [1] where information is stored in the timing of spikes and its behavior is similar to the biological neurons in human brain. Like Convolutional Neural Networks (CNNs), spiking neural network consists of a set of neurons that run in parallel. Each network consists of an input layer, hidden layers, and an output layer where each layer includes a set of neurons. More neurons in the network demands a higher level of parallelism and more power consumed [2], therefore, traditional computers represented by Von-Neumann architectures such as CPUs and GPUs struggle to execute such applications efficiently for large datasets. For this reason, recent research has shifted towards domain-specific architectures or accelerators that can be designed specifically for special purposes [2]. FPGAs are two-dimensional arrays which consist of a massive number of

K. Daimi and A. Al Sadoon (Eds.): ACR 2024, LNNS 956, pp. 545–547, 2024.
https://doi.org/10.1007/978-3-031-56950-0_44

processor elements (processors) where all can run in parallel and can be customized to perform different functions [3]. This allowed FPGAs to be well-suited for neural network applications where each processor element can be programmed as a neuron. Achieving higher accuracy in neural networks is related to the number of neurons and the hidden layers the network consists of. The more neurons are utilized for training, the higher accuracy is achieved, therefore, scaling up the network is crucial to achieve better performance. However, there is a real challenge for neural network scalability in the hardware. One of the major factors which significantly impacts scaling up spiking neural network in FPGAs is the wire limitation, which is neglected in most of prior work [4]. As shown in Fig. 1a, neurons are connected to their surroundings through wires which makes it limited by the internal connections and hardware resources. In this paper, we measure the limitation in number of wires (or synapses) represented by registers and number of processor elements (or neurons) represented by the configuration blocks through implementing a fully connected spiking neural network and evaluated it on Alveo U55 high performance compute FPGA card. We study the trade-off between the number of neurons in each hidden layer and the number of hidden layers which, in turn, affects the number of synapses in the network.

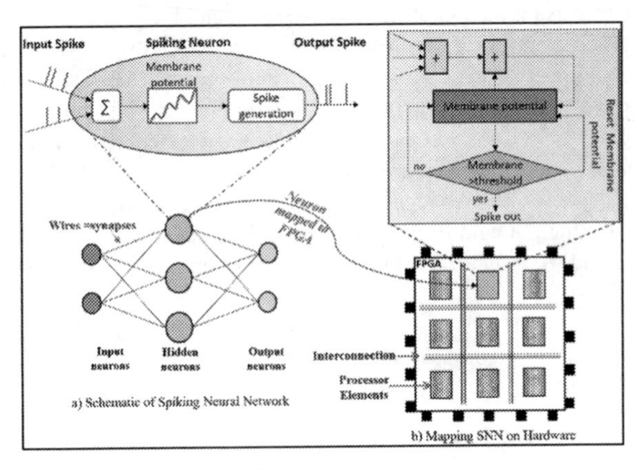

Fig. 1. Proposed SNN model and its Implementation

2 Proposed Design and Implementation

2.1 Proposed Spiking Neural Network (SNN) Model

We designed our SNN model based on Leaky Integrate-and-Fire (LIF) approach where neurons transmit information only when a membrane potential reaches the threshold as shown in Fig. 1a. When the membrane potential reaches the threshold, a neuron generates and fires a signal into its successors, which in turn affects their potential based on this received signal. To model the membrane potential of biological neurons, each neuron in a SNN maintains and updates internal state with a neuron update function. The function combines the weighted pulses arriving on the synapses with the current state and produces a series of spikes to send downstream.

2.2 Implementation of SNN Model on FPGA

FPGA is a two-dimensional array of logical elements called configurable logic blocks (CLBs) which communicate with each other through internal interconnections as shown in Fig. 1b. We programmed the FPGA to serve as a spiking neural network model by mapping every neuron to a set of CLBs that represent a processor element using the hardware description language SystemVerilog.

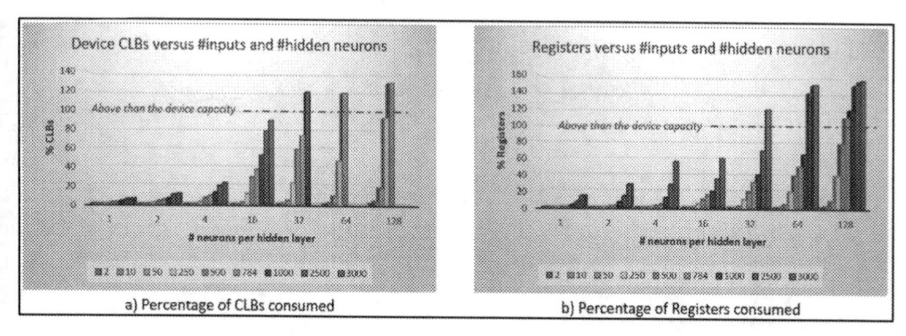

Fig. 2. Percentage of CLBs and registers consumed.

3 Evaluation and Conclusion

We designed our model as a parameterized model where we can vary the number of neurons and hidden layers. We set the weight width to 32-bit and membrane potential width to 48-bit. We set the number of output neurons to 10 while we set the inputs and the neurons in the hidden layer as parameters. Figure 2 shows the hardware resources consumed to implement 9 different models based on the 9 input values starting from the trivial 2 inputs up to 3000 inputs. As shown in Fig. 2 a and b, if we increase the number of hidden neurons to 500 inputs for 128-input model (last blue bar), the design will not fit on the device because it consumes more than 100% of the device capacity (same for the registers in Fig. 2b).

References

1. Gupta, A., Lyle, L.N.: Hebbian learning with winner take all for spiking neural networks. In Proceedings of the International Joint Conference on Neural Networks, Atlanta, GE, USA, pp. 1054–1060 (2009)
2. Bouvier, M., et al.: Spiking neural networks hardware implementations and challenges: a survey. ACM J. Emerging Technol. Comput. Syst. (JETC) **15**(2), 1–35 (2019)
3. Hu, Y., Liu, Y., Liu, Z.: A survey on convolutional neural network accelerators: GPU, FPGA and ASIC. In: Proceedings of the 14th International Conference on Computer Research and Development (ICCRD), Shenzhen, China, pp.100–107 (2022)
4. Li, J., et al.: FireFly: A High-Throughput and Reconfigurable Hardware Accelerator for Spiking Neural Networks, arXiv preprint arXiv:2301.01905, (2023)

Driving Through Crisis: A Comparative Analysis of Road Accidents Before, During, and After the Pandemic

Balakiran Neelam, Chandra Ponnathota, Manikanta Tumu, and Samah Senbel(✉)

Sacred Heart University, Fairfield, CT, USA
{neelamb,ponnathotac,tumum2}@mail.sacredheart.edu,
senbels@sacredheart.edu

Abstract. The COVID-19 pandemic has triggered unprecedented changes worldwide, influencing various facets of daily life. This study focuses on the state of Connecticut, conducting a meticulous analysis of road accidents to discern patterns and trends before, during, and after the pandemic. Leveraging comprehensive datasets from the Connecticut Department of Transportation, we employ statistical methodologies to unveil the dynamics shaping road safety in the face of the crisis. Our study was done using the R programming language and it identifies intriguing shifts in accident rates over the studied periods. Contrary to conventional expectations of decreased traffic leading to safer roads during lockdowns, our findings indicate a nuanced relationship. We explore three factors: frequency of accidents, spatial distribution of accidents in the different towns and the severity of the accidents. By incorporating real-world facts and figures, this study provides a granular understanding of how the pandemic has influenced road safety in the state.

Keywords: COVID-19 · Road Accidents · Data Analytics · Traffic patterns · Road safety

1 Introduction and Related Work

The COVID-19 pandemic, an unparalleled global crisis, ushered in transformative changes across all facets of society, from public health to daily routines. The aim of this research is to conduct a comprehensive comparative examination of road accidents in the state of Connecticut before, during, and after the pandemic. By scrutinizing extensive datasets obtained from the Connecticut Department of Transportation, we seek to identify patterns and contributing factors that have shaped the landscape of road safety during this critical period.

The impact of the COVID-19 pandemic on road safety has been the subject of increasing research interest. Several studies have documented a decrease in road accidents during the early stages of the pandemic, when lockdowns and travel restrictions were in place. For example, a study by Zhang et al. [4] found that road accidents in China decreased by 50% in the first two months of the pandemic. Similarly, a study by

K. Daimi and A. Al Sadoon (Eds.): ACR 2024, LNNS 956, pp. 548–551, 2024.
https://doi.org/10.1007/978-3-031-56950-0_45

Faggian et al. [1] found that road accidents in Italy decreased by 35% in the first month of the pandemic.

However, other studies have found that the impact of the pandemic on road safety is more complex. For example, a study by Lacey et al. [2] found that the number of major injury crashes in Alabama increased during the pandemic, even though the total number of miles driven decreased. The study attributed this increase to speeding, DUI, and weekend driving. Similarly, a study by Schulz et al. [3] found that the number of single-vehicle crashes in Germany increased during the pandemic.

2 Background

Our dataset provides a comprehensive exploration of traffic accidents in the state of Connecticut from 2017 to 2023. The dataset's main components include a unique crash identifier and a binary distinction for fatal cases, shedding light on the severity spectrum. Geospatial context is added through 'Latitude' and 'Longitude" coordinates, offering a visual representation of incident distribution across Connecticut. Temporal analysis is guided by the 'Date' and 'Time' attributes, revealing notable dates with the highest and lowest crash frequencies. The year-wise breakdown unveils that 2019 witnessed the highest number of accidents, totaling 8462 accidents, while 2020, heavily influenced by the pandemic, recorded 3582 incidents, the lowest in our dataset.

In summary, this dataset is a valuable resource for understanding and mitigating the impact of traffic accidents, especially in the context of the COVID-19 pandemic. Its multifaceted attributes, coupled with the temporal and contextual dimensions, provide a nuanced foundation for predictive modelling and evidence-based decision-making in the realm of road safety. We used the R programming language to analyze this rich dataset, and our findings are presented in the next section.

3 Method

We start with a simple analysis of the number of crashes in Connecticut before, during, and after the pandemic. Figure 1 shows the number of crashes in each year in our dataset, note that the data for 2023 is for only 5 months (January-May). We observe that the annual number of crashes per year was just above 8000 per year approximately. The number dropped sharply to 3582 crashes in 2020 during the pandemic, and then slowly rose to pre-pandemic levels over the next two years. This is clearly due to fewer cars on the road in 2020 and 2021 due to online work and education.

Next, we analyzed the location of those accidents in the pandemic year compared to the other years in the dataset (2017 to June 2023). Table 1 shows the top 10 towns in both groups, and the percentage drop of accidents in 2020. The table matches the size of the towns in Connecticut, with bigger towns having more traffic and therefore more accidents. However, the pandemic year showed a different pattern. In general accident numbers dropped and the 2020 accidents report about 60% of accidents in all six years. The town of Waterbury, an industry hub in the centre of CT, had the least drop in accidents during the pandemic with 267 accidents, 77% of an average year. On the other hand, the town of Norwalk had the largest drop in traffic and accidents a 43% drop in accidents.

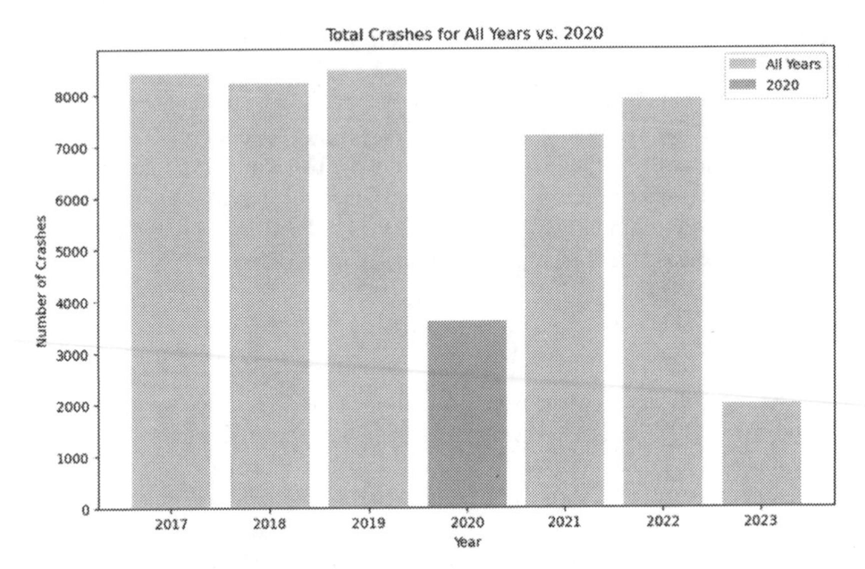

Fig. 1. Number of crashes per year

Table 1. Top10 car crash towns

Top 10 towns with the most crashes		Top 10 towns with the most crashes in 2020		Percent
Town	Annual # of Crashes	Town	Annual # of Crashes	
New Haven	462	New Haven	285	61.68%
Bridgeport	396	Waterbury	267	**77.61%**
Hartford	395	Bridgeport	262	66.16%
Waterbury	344	Hartford	242	61.26%
Stamford	259	Stamford	132	50.96%
Norwalk	213	Danbury	103	52.28%
Danbury	197	Norwalk	92	**43.19%**
Fairfield	124	West Haven	83	62.85%
Hamden	120	Meriden	81	68.07%
Meriden	119	New Britain	75	63.53%

Table 2 shows the severity of those car crashes for all years in our dataset as well as that of 2020 alone. There are three levels of severity recorded: Property damage only, injury of any type, and fatal. From the table, we observe that accidents in 2020 were less severe with a larger percent being "property damage only", 73.5% compared to 71.5% for all years, and a lower percentage for accidents with injury of any type, 25.9% compared to 28.5% in all years. Fatal accidents remain rare in all years.

Table 2. Crash severity in 2020

Crash Severity	All years	2020
Property Damage Only	71.1%	73.5%
Injury of any type (Serious, minor, possible)	28.5%	25.9%
Fatal (kill)	0.4%	0.6%

4 Conclusion

We compared accident data in 2020 with accident data in the period immediately before the pandemic (2017–2019) and after the pandemic (2021–2023) to study the effect if the pandemic on three issues: frequency of car crashes, severity of car crashes, and location of car crashes. The frequency of car crashes was around 8000+ accidents annual before the pandemic, and it dropped to less than half in the pandemic year, and was slow to rebound post-pandemic, reflecting the slow 2-year recovery from the pandemic. Looking into the major towns data for the state, we notice another interesting observation: the town of Waterbury was unique in the fact that it had the lowest drop in accident rate over the pandemic, and on the other hand, the waterside town of Norwalk had the biggest drop in accident rate. The severity of the crashes was also affected by the pandemic with a bigger percentage of accidents being a property damage only rather than an injury. In conclusion, our study shows that the effect of the pandemic was not only in a decrease in the number of car crashes, but also a decrease in the severity of those accidents and a different spatial accident distribution compared to previous years.

References

1. Faggian, M., Read, R.: COVID-19 pandemic and reduced road accidents: a natural experiment on traffic safety. Nat. Commun. **11**(1), 1–5 (2020)
2. Lacey, J.A., Bissell, C., Jones, M.R.: How did the COVID-19 pandemic affect road crashes and crash outcomes in Alabama? J. Trans. Safety Health **16**(3), 245–255 (2022)
3. Schulz, S., Koch, M., Senser, F.: Impact of the first COVID lockdown on accident- and injury-related pediatric intensive care admissions in Germany—a multicenter study. Children **9**(12), 1958 (2022)

An Approach to Mitigate CNN Complexity on Domain-Specific Architectures

Rasha Karakchi(✉) and Noah Robertson

University of South Carolina, Columbia, SC 29208, USA
karakchi@cec.sc.edu, noahhr@email.sc.edu

Abstract. Deep learning Convolutional Neural Network (CNN) is a powerful tool for feature extraction, edge detection and image classification. However, the training system of the networks has become increasingly complex due to the continuous growth in dataset which significantly impacts the computational time and energy consumption. In domain-specific platforms, this system is bounded by another level of limitation which is the hardware resources and the I/O resources. Using Gabor filter as a preprocessing layer can eliminate the redundant features and unnecessary information which results in much fewer memory used and less computation involved. In this paper, we propose a preprocessing layer which consists of Gabor kernel that serves as a weight kernel for CNNs and convolutional kernel that produces the features. We implemented the two kernels using the hardware description language Verilog that targets Xilinx FPGA devices. We designed a novel Gabor kernel based on the reconfigurability of FPGA by utilizing the BlockRAM (BRAMs) to store Gabor parameters, SRAM-based memory to store the input image and Digital Signal Processing (DSPs) for convolutional computation. We evaluated the design on Virtex 5 FPGA device using a 64×64 image, and we measured the performance of the Gabor kernel and convolutional kernel individually and found that Gabor kernel spend ~0.1 μs to produce the weight kernel and convolutional unit spends ~0.8 μs to find features.

Keywords: Convolutional Neural Network · Reconfigurability · Gabor Filter · FPGA · Accelerators

1 Introduction

Deep learning Convolutional Neural Networks (CNNs) have widely been used to solve problems related to machine learning and computer vision [1]. However, the large-scale structure and the associated training complexity present CNNs as one of the most compute-intensive workloads across all modern computing platforms [2]. This results in slowing down the computation process and lowering the overall performance. Domain-specific platforms such as Field-Programmable Gate Arrays (FPGAs) are well-known for their suitability to execute CNNs efficiently because of their high level of parallelism and the large number of Digital Signal Processing (DSPs) available on the chip [3]. However, the exponential growth in data size has made many of the existing designs

K. Daimi and A. Al Sadoon (Eds.): ACR 2024, LNNS 956, pp. 552–555, 2024.
https://doi.org/10.1007/978-3-031-56950-0_46

and methodologies ineffective and hardware resources not enough for CNN's operation. Therefore, reconfigurable computing technology has leveraged to utilize all types of memory built-in on such devices and exploit the capability of reconfigurability (reuse components) [4]. Gabor filter is a linear filter which executes two exponential functions as illustrated in Eq. 1. In this paper, our goal is to mitigate CNN complexity through designing a preprocessing layer representing a parameterizable partially reconfigurable Gabor kernel.

$$g(x, y, \lambda, \theta, \psi, \sigma, \gamma) = exp(-\frac{x'^2 + \gamma^2 y'^2}{2\sigma^2})exp(i(2\pi\frac{x'}{\lambda} + \psi)) \quad (1)$$

2 Proposed Approach

Our research contribution involves a novel design for Gabor kernel and the convolutional kernel using Verilog language which target Virtex 5 FPGA device. We designed Gabor kernel as a parameterizable accelerator that represents the weight kernel (window) which will be created based the given parameters. As shown in Fig. 1, the accelerator itself consists of three main units that run consecutively: *pi_sinx_siny* (orange), *Gaussian* (light blue) and *sinusoidal* units (green). The Gaussian function is represented by the real part $x' = x\cos\theta + y\sin\theta$ and the imaginary part $y' = -xsin\theta + ycos\theta$. Each unit executes a part of Gabor kernel function (Eq. 1) and implemented using DSP components on FPGA. We used Taylor series to execute Cosine, Sine, Exp functions. *ParRAM* component (dark blue) is Block RAM that is used to store the parameters' values where each parameter is located in a specific address of the memory as shown in Table 1. The input buses to *ParRAM* represents the addresses (add) of each parameter in the BRAM. Our convolutional unit performs the 2D convolution operation [11] based on Eq. 2. As shown in Fig. 2, the unit reads the small matrix of weight generated by the Gabor-Kernel unit. The kernel slides over the 2D input image matrix performing an elementwise multiplication with the part of input it is currently on, then summing up the results into a single output pixel as shown in Fig. 2a. The kernel repeats this process for every location it slides over, converting a 2D matrix of features into yet another 2D matrix of features (shown in Fig. 2c).

3 Evaluation and Conclusion

We tested our design on 64×64 image and set up Gabor parameters as shown in Table 1. Gabor kernel design spent about 100 ns to generate the weight kernels and about 800 ns for the convolutional kernel to generate the features. This is a preliminary work that targets CNN complexity growth in respect to data growth. The results we obtained are promising, therefore for future work we plan to explore the following. We plan to test the design on actual benchmarks and compare it with state-of-the-art methods. We also plan to expand the design to support multi-scale and multi-directional Gabor filters.

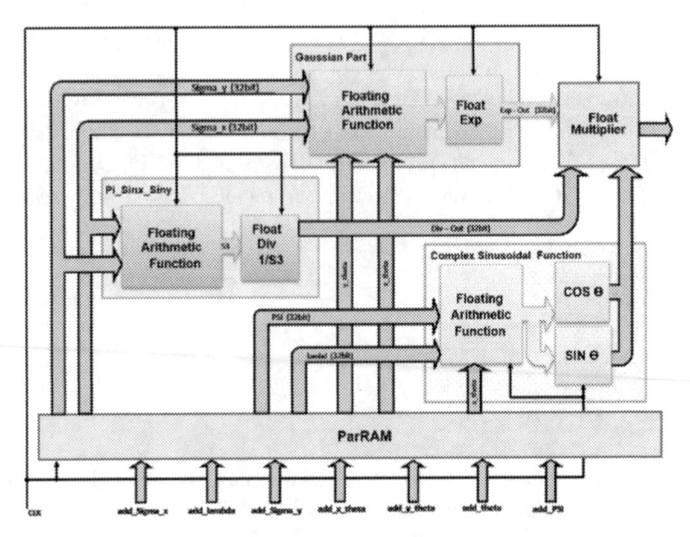

Fig. 1. Implementation of Gabor-Kernel Architecture

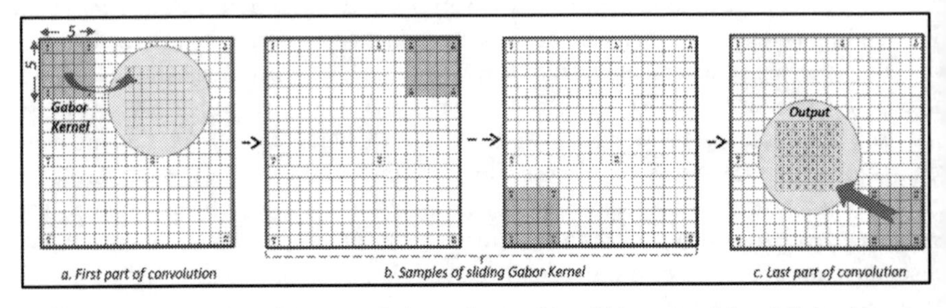

Fig. 2. The operation of 2D convolution unit on a 64 × 64 image and 5 × 5 Gabor kernel

Table 1. ParRAM addresses and values.

Assigned parameters	Assigned addresses	Values used for testing
$\propto\_x$	0	0.1
$\propto\_y$	1	1
θ,	2	0,45
λ	3	5,7
φ	4	0
γ	5	0.5
x_theta	6–30	(−2.7) – (2.7)
y_theta	31–55	(−0.6512) – 0.6512

References

1. Chai, J., Zeng, H., Li, A., Ngain, E.W.: Deep learning in computer vision: a critical review of emerging techniques and application scenarios. Mach. Learn. Appl. **6**, 100134 (2021)
2. Glorot, X., Bengio, Y.: Understanding the difficulty of training deep feedforward neural networks. In: Proceedings of the International Conference on Artificial Intelligence and Statistics. JMLR Workshop and Conference Proceedings (2010)
3. Basalama, S., Sohrabizadeh, A., Wang, J., Guo, L., Cong, J.: FlexCNN: an end-to-end framework for composing CNN accelerators on FPGA. ACM Trans. Reconfigurable Technol. Syst. **16**(2), 1–32 (2023)
4. Kim, H., Choi, K.K.: A reconfigurable CNN-based accelerator design for fast and energy-efficient object detection system on mobile FPGA. IEEE Access **11**, 59438–59445 (2023)

Posters Abstracts

Exploration of TPUs for AI Applications

Diego Sanmartín Carrión(✉), Vera Prohaska, and Oscar Diez

IE University, 28029 Madrid, Spain
{dsanmartin.ieu2020,vprohaska.ieu2020}@student.ie.edu,
odiezg@faculty.ie.edu

Abstract. Tensor Processing Units (TPUs) are specialized hardware accelerators for deep learning developed by Google. This poster aims to explore TPUs in cloud and edge computing focusing on its applications in AI. An in-depth overview of TPUs is presented, highlighting their unique architectural design tailored to neural network computations. The architecture is dissected to reveal how it differentiates TPUs from traditional chip architectures, particularly in the context of matrix operations which are central to neural network processing.

Furthermore, key aspects of TPU functionality, such as compilation techniques and the integration with supporting frameworks like TensorFlow, PyTorch, and JAX, are examined. This analysis underpins the understanding of how TPUs optimize the execution of deep learning models, thus providing a clear insight into their operational efficiency on a programmatic level. The poster also delves into a comprehensive comparative analysis, evaluating the performance of Cloud and Edge TPUs against other established chip architectures like CPUs and GPUs. This comparison is crucial in demonstrating the substantial performance improvements TPUs offer in both cloud and edge computing scenarios.

Additionally, the poster underscores the imperative need for further research in optimization techniques for efficient deployment of AI architectures on the Edge TPU and benchmarking standards for a more robust comparative analysis in edge computing scenarios. The primary motivation behind this push for research is that efficient AI acceleration, facilitated by TPUs, can lead to substantial savings in terms of time, money, and environmental resources.

Keywords: TPU · HPC · Edge Computing · AI Accelerator · Hardware

K. Daimi and A. Al Sadoon (Eds.): ACR 2024, LNNS 956, p. 559, 2024.
https://doi.org/10.1007/978-3-031-56950-0_47

The Controversies and Challenges of Developing Beneficial Artificial Intelligence

Louis Golding(✉) and Robert Polding

Department of Data and Business Analytics, School of Science and Technology, IE University, Madrid, Spain
lgolding.ieu2021@student.ie.edu, robert.polding@ie.edu

Abstract. Artificial Intelligence (AI) technology is constantly advancing. Intelligent hardware and software that reason like human beings is beginning to affect many critical areas of human life. However, there are many challenges accompanying these innovations. The challenges that need to be vitally considered to get broader advantages of AI are technical and ethical.

Learning, adoption, and retention are essential in the technical challenges that we face. To learn humans' goals, AI must not merely reason about what we do, but also about why we do it. Humans carry out this task without realizing how complicated it is for computing systems to do. It is thus hard for AI systems to strictly digest our motives, but it could be conceivably argued that if intelligent systems are provided with huge amounts of data, they would possibly be able to come up with reasonable conclusions. With regards to adoption, even if AI systems can absorb our goals, there would be no assurance they can inevitably adopt them. To discuss retention, let's assume an AI system that can learn and adopt our goals is constructed. Can these systems maintain these goals regardless of the endless enhancements these systems endure? When AI systems continue to be more intelligent, it is likely their potential to fulfill our goals will increase. However, their comprehension of the nature of these goals may progress ahead of our knowledge.

Ethical challenges deal with expressing morals that AI systems should meet. In this case, it is hard to envision the types of morals that need to be encoded in AI systems, the people who will identify them, their accomplishments on an international scale, and employing consistent laws and morals in different countries and cultures. As a result, there is a great demand for sensible solutions to these requirements. For AI to be beneficial, these solutions should be sought promptly.

Keywords: Artificial Intelligence · Learning · Adoption · Retention · Ethical Challenges

K. Daimi and A. Al Sadoon (Eds.): ACR 2024, LNNS 956, p. 560, 2024.
https://doi.org/10.1007/978-3-031-56950-0_48

Author Index

K. Daimi and A. Al Sadoon (Eds.): ACR 2024, LNNS 956, pp. 561–563, 2024.
https://doi.org/10.1007/978-3-031-56950-0

Printed in the United States
by Baker & Taylor Publisher Services